REA's Test Prep Books Ar

(a sample of the <u>hundreds of letters</u> REA receives each year)

" The best thing about [REA's *The Best Test Preparation for the USMLE Step 3*] is that it's updated and the information is accurate. The explanations contain information which obeys the recent guidelines for Hypertension and Diabetes. The questions are very similar to the actual questions on the exam. I would rate it an 11 out of 10. "

Medical Student, Chicago, IL

" My students report your chapters of review as the most valuable single resource they used for review and preparation. "

Teacher, American Fork, UT

" Your book was such a better value and was so much more complete than anything your competition has produced — and I have them all! "

Teacher, Virginia Beach, VA

" Compared to the other books that my fellow students had, your book was the most useful in helping me get a great score. "

Student, North Hollywood, CA

" Your book was responsible for my success on the exam, which helped me get into the college of my choice... I will look for REA the next time I need help. "

Student, Chesterfield, MO

" Just a short note to say thanks for the great support your book gave me in helping me pass the test... I'm on my way to a B.S. degree because of you! "

Student, Orlando, FL

(more on next page)

(continued from front page)

" I just wanted to thank you for helping me get a great score
on the AP U.S. History... Thank you for making great test preps! "
Student, Los Angeles, CA

" Your Fundamentals of Engineering Exam book was the absolute best
preparation I could have had for the exam, and it is one of the major
reasons I did so well and passed the FE on my first try. "
Student, Sweetwater, TN

" I used your book to prepare for the test and found that the advice and the
sample tests were highly relevant... Without using any other material, I earned
very high scores and will be going to the graduate school of my choice. "
Student, New Orleans, LA

" What I found in your book was a wealth of information sufficient to shore up
my basic skills in math and verbal... The section on analytical ability was
excellent. The practice tests were challenging and the answer explanations
most helpful. It certainly is the Best Test Prep for the GRE! "
Student, Pullman, WA

" I really appreciate the help from your excellent book. Please keep
up with your great work."
Student, Albuquerque, NM

" I used your *CLEP Introductory Sociology* book and rank it 99% — thank you! "
Student, Jerusalem, Israel

" The painstakingly detailed answers in the sample tests are the most helpful
part of this book. That's one of the great things about REA books. "
Student, Valley Stream, NY

The Best Test Preparation for the

USMLE STEP 3

United States Medical Licensing Examination

Rose S. Fife, MD
Professor of Medicine, Biochemistry,
and Molecular Biology
Indiana University School of Medicine
Indianapolis, IN

John Min, MD
Faculty
Washington University
School of Medicine
St. Louis, MO

Vijay Shah, MD
Postdoctoral Fellow
Section of Digestive Diseases
Yale University School of Medicine
New Haven, CT

Douglas Monasebian, MD, DMD
Private Practice
Plastic & Reconstructive Surgery
New York, NY

Vartan Tarakchyan, MD
Resident Physician
Harbor-UCLA Medical Center
Torrance, CA

Gopi Rana-Mukkavilli, MD, FACP
Department of Medicine
New York University
New York, NY

T. M. Worner, MD
Clinical Associate Professor of
Public Health
Cornell University
New York, NY

And the Staff of Research & Education Association
Dr. M. Fogiel, Director

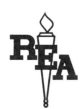 **Research & Education Association**
61 Ethel Road West
Piscataway, NJ 08854

The Best Test Preparation for the
UNITED STATES MEDICAL LICENSING
EXAMINATION (USMLE) STEP 3

Year 2001 Printing

Printed in the United States of America

Library of Congress Control Number 00-132033

International Standard Book Number 0-87891-076-X

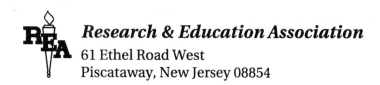 **Research & Education Association**
61 Ethel Road West
Piscataway, New Jersey 08854

TABLE OF CONTENTS

About Research & Education Association

Research & Education Association (REA) is an organization of educators, scientists, and engineers specializing in various academic fields. Founded in 1959 with the purpose of disseminating the most recently developed scientific information to groups in industry, government, and universities, REA has since become a successful and highly respected publisher of study aids, test preps, handbooks, and reference works.

Created to extensively prepare students and professionals with the information they need, REA's Test Preparation series includes study guides for the Tests of General Educational Development (GED), the Scholastic Assessment Tests (SAT I and SAT II), the Advanced Placement Exams (AP), the Test of English as a Foreign Language (TOEFL), as well as the Graduate Record Examinations (GRE), the Graduate Management Admission Test (GMAT), the Law School Admission Test (LSAT), and the Medical College Admission Test (MCAT).

Whereas most Test Preparation books present practice tests that bear little resemblance to the actual exams, REA's series presents tests that accurately depict the official exams in both degree of difficulty and types of questions. REA's practice tests are always based on the most recently administered exams and include every type of question that can be expected on the actual exams.

REA's publications and educational materials are highly regarded and continually receive an unprecedented amount of praise from professionals, instructors, librarians, parents, and students. Our authors are as diverse as the subjects represented in the books we publish. They are well-known in their respective fields and serve on the faculties of prestigious high schools, colleges, and universities throughout the United States and Canada.

Acknowledgments

In addition to our authors, we would like to thank the following: Dr. Max Fogiel, President, for his overall guidance, which brought this publication to its completion; Nicole Mimnaugh, New Book Development Manager, for directing the editorial staff throughout each phase of the project; Larry B. Kling, Quality Control Manager of Books in Print, for supervising revisions; Gary J. Albert, Project Editor, for coordinating the development of the book and revisions; Dr. Floyd Donahue, Dr. Jeffrey Smith, Dr. Cindy Taylor, Carol Carter, Ellen Gong, Malcolm Macdonald, Kathleen Roberts, Jeanette Segal, Lansing Wagner, and Dominique Won for their editorial contributions to the book; Kristin Massaro, Project Manager, and Jennifer Payulert and Jason Twomey, Editorial Assistants, for their editorial contributions to the revised edition; Jeanne Gruver for keying in the manuscripts; and Marty Perzan for typesetting the book.

INDEPENDENT STUDY SCHEDULE

Day	Time	Activity
Day 1	2 hours	Read the Coaching Review for the USMLE Step 3 to familiarize yourself with the format of the examination and the types of questions you will encounter on it.
Day 2	5 hours	Take Practice Test 1 to determine your strengths and weaknesses. Check your answers against the answer keys given after the practice test. Carefully study the detailed explanations for the questions you answered incorrectly. Make sure you understand why you got each question wrong.
Day 3	4 hours	Review the topics of questions you answered incorrectly in Practice Test 1. Use textbooks, lecture notes, or any reference material available to you to review these topics. Be sure to take notes during your review.
Day 4	5 hours	Take Practice Test 2. Check your answers against the answer keys given after the practice test. Carefully study the detailed explanations for the questions you answered incorrectly. Make sure you understand why you got each question wrong.
Day 5	4 hours	Review the topics of questions you answered incorrectly in Practice Test 2. Use textbooks, lecture notes, or any reference material available to you to review these topics. Be sure to take notes during your review.
Day 6	5 hours	Take Practice Test 3. Check your answers against the answer keys given after the practice test. Carefully study the detailed explanations for the questions you answered incorrectly. Make sure you understand why you got each question wrong.
Day 7	4 hours	Review the topics of questions you answered incorrectly in Practice Test 3. Use textbooks, lecture notes, or any reference material available to you to review these topics. Be sure to take notes during your review.
Day 8	2 hours	Study your notes from the review sessions. Read the Coaching Review for the USMLE Step 3 again. Study the topics covered in questions you answered incorrectly on all three practice tests.

USMLE STEP 3

Coaching Review for
the USMLE Step 3

COACHING REVIEW FOR THE USMLE STEP 3

INTRODUCTION TO THE UNITED STATES MEDICAL LICENSING EXAMINATION

The United States Medical Licensing Examination (USMLE) is the single, three-step, examination for medical licensure in the United States. The USMLE provides a fair way to evaluate all applicants for medical licensure. The USMLE has replaced the Federation Licensing Examination (FLEX) and the NBME Parts I, II, and III.

In 1999, all steps of the USMLE were switched from a paper-and-pencil administration to computer-based. Once the computer-based administration for a step has been implemented, the paper-and-pencil examination for that step will no longer be scheduled.

The practice exams included in this book contain more questions than the computer-based USMLE Step 3 in order to provide a score that is roughly comparable to the actual computer-based examination. The practice exams in this book may vary in format from the computer-based examination, but the same knowledge is tested. Because of the complex, interactive nature of the Computer-based Case Simulation (CCS) questions (which will be explained in greater detail later), the practice exams in this book contain only multiple-choice questions. It would be impossible to provide Computer-based Case Simulation questions in book form. We would like to stress, however, that the practice tests contained in this book will provide comparable scores to those one would receive taking the actual USMLE Step 3 computer-based examination.

Contact the USMLE Secretariat to obtain material that will introduce and explain all elements of the USMLE Step 3 computer-based examination. You can also contact that office to order booklets, sample tests, or the *USMLE Bulletin of Information* mentioned later in this section. Write, call, or point your browser as follows:

USMLE Secretariat
3750 Market Street
Philadelphia, PA 19104–3190
Telephone: (215) 590–9600
Website: http://www.usmle.org

INTRODUCTION TO THE PURPOSE OF THE USMLE STEP 3

The purpose of the USMLE Step 3 is to determine whether a physician has the knowledge and comprehension of clinical medicine to enable him/her to practice unsupervised medicine. Emphasis is placed on the management of patients in an outpatient setting, but also includes inpatient and emergency environments. Questions are written in such a way as to create a situation resembling one that might be encountered in clinical practice.

Who Takes the USMLE Step 3 and What is it Used for?

Step 3 is taken by eligible physicians and it is used to assess whether the examinee has the knowledge base and understanding of clinical medicine to practice unsupervised medicine. To be eligible to take Step 3, an examinee must: meet the requirements determined by the local licensing authority (see the next paragraph); have obtained the M.D. degree (or its equivalent) or the D.O. degree; passed Steps 1 and 2; and obtain ECFMG certification or successfully complete a "Fifth Pathway" program if he/she is a foreign medical school graduate.

The USMLE program suggests that all licensing authorities (usually state medical boards) establish an eligibility requirement for Step 3. This requirement may be the completion, or near completion, of at least one postgraduate training year in a program or graduate medical education accredited by the Accreditation Council for Graduate Medical Education, or the American Osteopathic Association. Please see the *USMLE Bulletin of Information* for further details.

Who Administers the Test?

Step 3 is administered by individual medical licensing authorities in the United States and its territories. The local licensing authority should be contacted for eligibility guidelines, deadlines, fees, etc. Please see the *USMLE Bulletin of Information* for further details.

When Should the USMLE Step 3 be Taken?

The USMLE Step 3 is usually taken after graduation from medical, osteopathic, or an equivalent school and while one is in a residency program, usually during the internship (or first) year, or as determined by the individual medical licensing authority.

When and Where is the USMLE Step 3 Given?

Step 3 is given by the local medical licensing authority, and this authority should be contacted to ascertain time, location, deadline, and fee for the test.

Is There a Registration Fee?

There is a registration fee for Step 3, and the local licensing authority should be contacted regarding the cost.

FORMAT OF THE USMLE STEP 3

Are There any Time Limits for the Examination?

Unlike Steps 1 and 2, which are one-day exams, Step 3 is a two-day examination. The exam consists of multiple-choice questions and Computer-based Case Simulations (CCS). The first day-and-a-half consists solely of multiple-choice questions. The last half day is made up of the CCS questions.

What are the Multiple-Choice Questions?

The multiple-choice questions on the USMLE Step 3 are presented in "blocks" of about 30 to 60 minutes. During the time given to complete the questions in each block, test-takers may answer the test questions in any order, review their responses, and change answers. Once you exit a block, or when time expires, further review of test questions or changing answers within that block is not possible. The specific types of multiple-choice questions are discussed in the next section.

What are the Computer-based Case Simulations (CCS)?

The Computer-based Case Simulations (CCS) are unique and complex test questions designed to allow the test-taker to provide care for a simulated patient. The CCS questions are NOT presented in multiple-choice format. Instead, the test-taker must balance the clinical information presented in a question with the severity of the clinical problem in deciding which treatment to start and when to start it—all the while monitoring the patient's response. The testing computer records each action made by the test-taker to care for the patient and scores overall performance. The CCS questions are designed to permit evaluation of the test-taker's clinical decision-making skills in a more realistic and integrated manner than is possible with multiple-choice questions.

In the CCS questions, the test-taker may request information from the patient's history and physical examination; order laboratory studies, procedures, or consultants; and begin medication and/or other therapy. It is possible to enter thousands of commands or orders, which the test-taker types on an "order sheet" that is processed and verified by the "clerk." When the test-taker has determined that there is nothing further to be done for a patient, the test-taker decides when to re-evaluate the patient by advancing time. As time advances, the patient's condition is changed by evaluating the underlying problem and the test-taker's intervention. Also, results of tests are reported and outcomes of interventions must be monitored. As the test-taker, you can suspend the movement of time as you determine your next steps. While you cannot reverse time, you can change your orders to reflect changes to your treatment plan. The patient's chart contains, in addition to the order sheet, the reports returned from your orders. By choosing the proper chart tabs, you can review vital signs, progress notes, nurses' notes, and test results. You may see and move patients from the office, home, emergency department, intensive care unit, and ward.

As part of the scoring process, your treatment strategy will be compared with those of practicing physicians and content experts. Strategies closer to the ideal will produce a higher score. Thoroughness, efficiency, avoidance of risk, and timeliness should be appropriate to the clinical situation. Potentially dangerous and unnecessary actions will lower your score.

As stated previously, we urge you to contact the USMLE Secretariat to obtain more information on the CCS questions and how best to prepare for them.

How is the Examination Organized?

The USMLE Step 3 consists of two major question formats: multiple-choice questions and Computer-based Case Simulations (CCS). Because of the complex, interactive nature of the CCS questions, it is not possible to present strategies or examples for these questions in book form. Instead, we will focus on only the multiple-choice questions in this section. To learn more about the CCS questions, contact the USMLE Secretariat.

There are several types of multiple-choice questions on the USMLE Step 3. These include the following:

If the overall test is examined from the system perspective, it would be divided as follows:

- 8–12% of the questions are devoted to Obtaining History and Performing Physical Examination

- 8–12% of the questions are devoted to Using Laboratory and Diagnostic Studies

- 8–12% of the questions are devoted to Formulating Most Likely Diagnosis

- 8–12% of the questions are devoted to Evaluating Severity of Patient's Problems

- 8–12% of the questions are devoted to Applying Scientific Concepts and Mechanisms of Disease

- 45–55% of the questions are devoted to Managing the Patient covering the following categories:

  —Health Maintenance

  —Clinical Intervention

  —Clinical Therapeutics

  —Legal and Ethical Issues

From the Clinical Encounter Frame perspective, the examination is divided approximately as follows:

- 20–30% of the questions are devoted to Initial Workups

- 55–65% of the questions are devoted to Continued Care

- 10–20% of the questions are devoted to Emergency Care

The following clinical settings are included in Step 3:

- Unscheduled Patients/Clinic

- Scheduled Appointments/Office

- Hospital Rounds

- Emergency Department

- Other Encounters

The *USMLE Bulletin of Information* and the USMLE Step 3 application material will provide a more detailed outline of what topics are covered on the exam.

DESCRIPTION OF TYPES OF MULTIPLE-CHOICE QUESTIONS FOUND ON THE USMLE STEP 3

Explanation of the Question Types

The USMLE Step 3 consists of several types of multiple-choice questions. These include the following:

- Positively-Phrased One-Best-Answer questions—these are standard multiple-choice questions;

- Negatively-Phrased One-Best-Answer questions—these are similar to the One-Best-Answer type, but they are phrased in the negative using words such as NOT, LEAST, or EXCEPT;

- Matching Sets—these consist of a set of words or phrases that are interrelated in some fashion and that must be matched with one of a series of descriptors, each of which can be used once, more than once, or not at all;

- Multiple-Item Sets—these consist of a clinical scenario which is introduced by a paragraph or two and followed by several (usually four) related questions;

- Case Clusters—these consist of a clinical vignette that is introduced by a paragraph or two and followed by several (usually eight) questions related to the setting. These questions should be answered in order, since preceding answers can influence subsequent answers, and time may have passed between questions.

Specific Directions for Each Question Type

- For the Positively-Phrased One-Best-Answer format, an unfinished statement is made or a question is posed. Four or five possible answers are given, and only one can be selected.

- For the Negatively-Phrased One-Best-Answer format, a negatively-phrased statement or question is given, and only one of the four or five possible answers can be chosen.

- For the Matching Sets, an answer in the right column might be correct for a phrase in the left column. Each answer may be used once, more than once, or not at all, but only one answer can be selected for each problem.

- For the Multiple-Item Sets, several multiple-choice questions follow a clinical synopsis. Each question has only one correct or best answer. These may be of the One-Best-Answer or the Negatively-Phrased One-Best-Answer format.

- For the Case Clusters, multiple-choice questions (usually about eight) follow a clinical vignette. Again, each question has only one correct answer and may be either Positively- or Negatively-Phrased One-Best-Answer questions. These questions should be answered in order, since time may pass between questions, and additional information may be provided.

Suggested Strategies for Each Question Type

Specific strategies to assist in approaching each type of question are given below. However, the most important strategy of all, which applies equally to all of the different types of questions, is to read the question/statement carefully. If a case or cluster is involved, read the entire introductory statement before attempting to answer the questions. Careful attention to detail cannot be overemphasized here. It is critical to understand what is being asked before an answer is given.

One-Best-Answer Questions

First, read the question/statement closely and make sure that you understand it. Once you recognize the salient points of the case or cluster, if that is what the question is contained in, eliminate those answers that you are sure are incorrect.

You may be left with only one answer or with more than one. Choose the answer you think is correct and be sure to enter it into the correct spot on the answer form. If you are not sure which of the remaining answers is correct, make an "educated" guess, since you will not be penalized for wrong answers and you will be rewarded for correct ones.

Negatively-Phrased One-Best-Answer Questions

This represents a variation of the One-Best-Answer questions. In negatively-phrased questions, the question is stated in the negative and you must choose the one correct answer. In most cases, these questions can be recognized by one of the following capitalized words: EXCEPT, NOT, or LEAST. Again, read the question carefully, particularly since you need to recognize that it is of the negative variety. Then go through the same process of elimination as you did for the One-Best-Answer questions, always keeping in mind that you are answering a negatively-phrased question or statement. An important concept to remember when working on negatively-phrased questions is that the correct choice is often the *incorrect* function, activity, phenomenon, etc.

Matching Sets

Read all of the numbered items in the left-hand column closely: these are the "questions." Then read all of the lettered items in the right-hand column: these are the "answers." The numbered items are related to each other. Go through the answers and select the best match for each numbered item. Remember that a given answer may be used once, more than once, or not at all, so consider each question separately. It is sometimes helpful if you can decide on a correct answer to a numbered item and then look for it or a related word or phrase in the answer column on the right.

Multiple-Item Sets

Read the case vignette carefully, even more than once if necessary. Then approach the questions, basing your answers on the vignette. The questions are all related to the synopsis. Pay close attention to whether the question is a Positively- or Negatively-Phrased One-Best-Answer type of question. Use the same approach you would in choosing an answer in any other similar One-

Best-Answer type of question, i.e., eliminate the answers that you can and select the best answer among those remaining.

Case Clusters

Again, read the case synopsis carefully. The questions are based on the vignette, but time may elapse between each question and new information may be provided, so be sure to answer the questions in order. Be sure you notice whether the questions are of the Positively- or Negatively-Phrased One-Best-Answer formats. Use the same approach that you would for other similar One-Best-Answer questions.

EXAMPLE OF EACH QUESTION TYPE AND APPROACHES TO IDENTIFYING THE CORRECT ANSWER

Example of a Positively-Phrased One-Best-Answer Question

Choose the correct answer.

1. A 45-year-old man with a history of hypertension and cigarette smoking presents to the emergency room with acute onset of chest pain. His electrocardiogram shows T-wave inversion. You suspect that he has

    (A) esophagitis.

    (B) myocardial ischemia.

    (C) old myocardial infarction.

    (D) costochondritis.

    (E) aortic aneurysm.

The correct answer choice is (B)

Strategy: Read the question carefully. Understand what the patient's presentation represents and consider the possible diagnoses. T-wave inversion is not a component of esophagitis or costochondritis or aortic aneurysm. That leaves two possible answers. Myocardial infarction is characterized by the presence of q waves, while ischemia (B) is associated with T-wave inversion.

Example of a Negatively-Phrased One-Best-Answer Question

Choose the correct answer.

2. A 36-year-old man presents to your office with an acutely swollen, painful, and red knee. He has a fever of 102° F. He has been in good health but had some dental work a few weeks ago. All of the following are possible explanations for his arthritis EXCEPT

    (A) gout.

    (B) septic arthritis.

    (C) pseudogout.

    (D) osteoarthritis.

    (E) rheumatoid arthritis.

The correct answer choice is (D)

Strategy: First, notice that the question is *negatively-phrased*. Therefore, all but one of the answers is actually *correct*. Gout and pseudogout can both cause an acute arthritis associated with a fever, as can septic arthritis. The patient's history of a recent dental procedure should raise the suspicion of septic arthritis here. While a monoarticular arthritis in an adult male is unusual as the initial presentation of rheumatoid arthritis, it is not impossible. Osteoarthritis (D), by definition, does not cause acute inflammatory arthritis with fever unless an infection is superimposed on the underlying condition.

Example of Matching-Set Questions

For each numbered item in the left column, choose the one best lettered item from the right column. Each answer may be used once, more than once, or not at all.

3. Digitalis toxicity	(A) Peaked T waves
4. Hypercalemia	(B) U waves
5. Hyperkalemia	(C) Prolonged Q-T
6. Hypocalcemia	(D) Downward sloping ST
7. Quinidine toxicity	(E) Shortened Q-T
	(F) Torsades de Pointes

The correct answer choices are 3. (D); 4. (E); 5. (A); 6. (C); and 7. (F)

Strategy: Each numbered item has one best correct answer, although each answer may be used once, more than once, or not at all. Read all of the numbered items and think of words or phrases that describe or are related to each item. Note that all of these items relate to different types of cardiac toxicity. Now look through the lettered answers and find the one that best matches each numbered item. In this case, no answer is used more than once, and (B) is not used at all.

Example of Multiple-Item-Set Questions

Questions 8 through 11 refer to the following:

A 43-year-old woman presents to the emergency room with severe abdominal pain, nausea, and emesis. She admits to binge-drinking but has not ingested any alcohol for about two days because of her pain. She denies having a history of delirium tremens but does admit to shakiness sometimes when she stops drinking.

8. On physical examination, her abdomen is painful but not rigid. You can hear some rushes of bowel sounds. She has no ascites. You do all of the following EXCEPT

    (A) draw an amylase.

    (B) order an abdominal radiograph.

    (C) order an abdominal MRI.

    (D) call for a surgical consult.

    (E) start an intravenous line.

The correct answer choice is (C)

Strategy: This is a Negatively-Phrased One-Best-Answer question. A serum amylase level is useful in evaluating acute abdominal pain, as is a radiograph of the abdomen. A surgical consult is usually necessary for pain such as this. Since you do not know the condition of the patient's bowel, it is best to make her NPO and hydrate her via the IV route. An abdominal MRI (C) would not be called for at this point in the evaluation.

9. The amylase is elevated, as is the patient's white blood cell count. Her differential shows a left shift. The abdominal film shows some air-filled loops of small bowel but no air-fluid levels. The surgical consultant is likely to do all of the following EXCEPT

    (A) operate.

    (B) tell you to admit the patient to the medical service.

    (C) tell you to keep her NPO.

    (D) recommend antibiotics.

    (E) recommend follow-up amylase levels and blood counts.

The correct answer choice is (A)

Strategy: This is another Negatively-Phrased One-Best-Answer question. The surgeon will probably want the patient admitted, not fed, hydrated, given antibiotics, and subjected to the follow-up lab tests. This patient does not appear to have a condition requiring immediate surgical intervention (A).

10. The likeliest diagnosis in this patient at this time is

    (A) diverticulosis.

    (B) pancreatitis.

    (C) colon cancer.

    (D) cholecystitis.

    (E) hepatitis.

The correct answer choice is (B)

Strategy: This is a Positively-Phrased One-Best-Answer question. Of all of these conditions, only pancreatitis (B) is associated with all of the findings and symptoms that this patient manifests.

11. You admit the patient to the hospital and keep her NPO and on intravenous fluids. The next day she is confused and does not know where she is or how she got there. She is likely to be suffering from

    (A) dementia.

    (B) acute viral encephalitis.

    (C) a cerebrovascular event.

    (D) a subdural hematoma.

    (E) impending delirium tremens.

The correct answer choice is (E)

Strategy: This is a Positively-Phrased One-Best-Answer question. The patient is fairly young and probably does not have dementia or multiple strokes. She has no findings to suggest viral encephalitis or a subdural hematoma. Since she has now spent three days without alcohol, impending delirium tremens (E) is a likely etiology for her confusion.

Summary strategy: Read the initial vignette carefully. Answer the questions in order based on the vignette and on any additional information provided with each question. Make sure you notice whether a question is a Positively- or Negatively-Phrased One-Best-Answer type.

Example of Case-Cluster Questions

Questions 12 though 17 refer to the following:

A 33-year-old man is admitted to your service because of acute pneumonia. He is extremely ill with tachypnea, fever, and tachycardia. He is straining to get enough air when he breathes and has retractions. You notice a few spots of reddish raised skin lesions on his trunk and legs. He is new to your city and you have no old records on him.

12. The first thing you do is

    (A) draw blood cultures.

    (B) perform a history and physical exam.

    (C) draw a CBC.

    (D) draw an arterial blood gas.

    (E) wait until a relative or friend arrives.

The correct answer choice is (B)

Strategy: The very first thing that you should do with any patient is at least a cursory history (if he/she is responsive) and a physical exam (B).

13. The patient is somewhat confused and you are not sure he understands what you want to do. You draw a blood gas and find that his PO_2 is 55 on room air. His tachypnea has increased to 40 respirations per minute. You think he should be intubated but you do not think he is capable of understanding the explanation you try to give him. You should

    (A) wait until someone shows up who can give permission.

    (B) try to get a court order.

    (C) intubate him.

    (D) try to get him to tell you if he wants to be resuscitated.

    (E) give him an anti-psychotic agent.

The correct answer choice is (C)

Strategy: The patient is acutely ill, and you do not know what his underlying illness is. You cannot wait for a relative who may or may not arrive or for a court order. The patient cannot tell you what he wants you to do. You do not want to give him drugs that may further alter his mental status. You can only do what you judge to be the best medical intervention in this patient at this time, which is intubation (C).

14. The white count comes back from the laboratory at 1,000, and his platelet count is 55,000. His chest radiograph shows diffuse bilateral infiltrates. Your physical exam has demonstrated some genital warts. His tongue is coated with a white material. The lesions on his legs and trunk are likely to be

    (A) bacterial infection.

    (B) squamous carcinoma.

    (C) cherry angiomata.

    (D) Kaposi's sarcoma.

    (E) livedo reticularis.

The correct answer choice is (D)

Strategy: The questions are leading you toward a specific diagnosis. Given the overall picture, you should be suspecting the underlying diagnosis. This combination of infections and skin lesions would not be likely to result from a bacterial infection or squamous cancer. Cherry angiomata and livedo reticularis are specific skin lesion not associated with this patient's other problems. Kaposi's sarcoma (D) is likely to be associated with his other findings.

15. The likeliest underlying disease that would explain all of this patient's symptoms and physical findings is

    (A) bacterial sepsis.

    (B) histoplasmosis.

    (C) HIV/AIDS.

    (D) tuberculosis.

    (E) metastatic lung cancer.

The correct answer choice is (C)

Strategy: This constellation of symptoms and findings and laboratory results is not typical for bacterial sepsis, histoplasmosis, tuberculosis, or metastatic lung cancer, but is very characteristic of HIV/AIDS (C).

16. You stabilize the patient and get his fever and respirations under control. A young man arrives who tells you he is the patient's significant other and that the patient has been diagnosed in San Diego and does not want to be intubated or have any other form of resuscitation. You explain the situation to him and he understands. He presents you with his power of attorney and the patient's living will. You should do all of the following EXCEPT

    (A)   put the living will in the chart.

    (B)   write a DNR order in the chart.

    (C)   explain the patient's condition to his friend.

    (D)   explain his condition to your staff.

    (E)   refuse to honor his wishes.

The correct answer choice is (E)

Strategy: This is a Negatively-Phrased One-Best-Answer question. All but one answer (E) are correct. You should honor the patient's wishes and let his significant other and the staff know his status.

17. The patient's pneumonia resolves over a few days with antibiotics and fluid and he is able to be weaned from the ventilator. He apologizes to you for not having his papers with him so that you would not have had to intubate him, but he does not resent the process. He tells you he was diagnosed with AIDS about 4 years ago and has been having some trouble lately with his memory, which is why he had not remembered to carry his living will. The likeliest cause of his memory loss is

    (A)   AIDS dementia.

    (B)   cerebral lymphoma.

    (C)   Western equine encephalitis.

    (D)   Alzheimer's disease.

    (E)   multi-infarct dementia.

The correct answer choice is (A)

Strategy: Both AIDS dementia and cerebral lymphoma are associated with HIV/AIDS, while the

other conditions are not. Lymphoma, though, would not be as likely to cause memory loss as would AIDS dementia (A).

Summary strategy: As in the case of the multiple-item set, first read the introductory vignette. Read each question carefully and try to answer them in order. Even if you cannot answer each question, make sure you read it for all the information it may provide before you try to answer a subsequent question. These questions are of the Positively- or Negatively-Phrased One-Best-Answer sort.

SCORING THE USMLE STEP 3

The scoring of the USMLE Step 3 varies from one licensing authority to the next. For information on score reporting, examinees should contact the FSMB (Federation of State Medical Boards) or the medical licensing authority in the jurisdiction where they registered for Step 3. However, test-takers should be aware that there is a **Minimum Passing Score**. After you sit for a Step, the number of items you answered correctly (raw score) is converted to two equivalent scores, one on a three-digit scale and one on a two-digit scale, for the purpose of score reporting and for making pass/fail decisions. The mean score for those reported on a three-digit scale is 200 (177 is usually the passing score for Step 3). A two-digit score of 82 is always equivalent to the three-digit score of 200. The two-digit score is derived in such a way that a score of 75 always corresponds to the minimum passing score. Individual licensing authorities have the option of shifting the minimum passing score or scoring each examination on a pass/fail basis. In any case, however, to attain a passing score you must answer approximately 55%–65% of the questions correctly.

The practice tests contained in this book are longer than the actual USMLE Step 3 computer-based test. This has been done to allow scores on the practice tests to be comparable to those scores that would be received on the computer-based test.

To determine whether you have achieved a passing score on a practice test, divide the number of questions you answered correctly by 720. This will give you the percentage of questions you answered correctly. If this percentage is 55 percent or higher (approximately 396 questions correct), then you have achieved a passing grade for that practice test.

USMLE STEP 3

Practice Test 1

NOTE:
The following practice test contains more questions than the actual USMLE Step 3 computer-based examination. This is necessary to provide a score that is roughly comparable to the computer-based exam which contains Computer-based Case Simulations (CCS) questions. Due to the interactive nature of CCS questions, it would be impossible to present them in book form. Although the format is different, this test will give you an accurate idea of your strengths and weaknesses, and provide guidance for further study.

USMLE STEP 3 PRACTICE TEST 1

Day One – Morning Session

(Answer sheets appear in the back of this book.)

TIME: 3 Hours
180 Questions

DIRECTIONS: Each of the following numbered items or incomplete sentences is followed by an answer or a completion of the statement. Choose the **ONE** choice that **BEST** answers the question or completes the sentence.

Questions 1-4 refer to the following:

Match the following scleral conditions with the appropriate diagnosis.

(A) Yellow sclera

(B) Brown sclera

(C) Red sclera

(D) Blue sclera

(E) Scleral protrusion

1. Icterus

2. Osteogenesis imperfecta

3. Melanin deposition

4. Staphyloma

Questions 5-12 refer to the following:

A 58-year-old man presents to your emergency room with acute onset of shortness of breath, chest pain, nausea, vomiting of undigested food, and diaphoresis. Focused history reveals that these symptoms began about 40 minutes previously and that he has never had these symptoms before. His past medical history includes hypertension and non-insulin-dependent diabetes mellitus, for which he is taking a calcium channel blocker and an oral hypoglycemic.

5. Of the following illnesses on the differential diagnosis, it would be appropriate to attempt to rule all of them out immediately EXCEPT

(A) acute myocardial infarction.

(B) acute pulmonary embolism.

(C) acute bacterial pneumonia.

(D) acute aortic dissection.

(E) acute pericardial tamponade.

6. All of the following findings on physical examination would be consistent with an acute myocardial infarction EXCEPT

(A) inspiratory rales on auscultation of the lungs.

(B) elevated jugular venous distension.

(C) hypotension.

(D) pulses paradoxis.

(E) chest radiograph that is normal.

7. On physical examination, you find a well-developed white man in severe distress. His blood pressure is 180/75, his heart rate is 48, his respiratory rate is 35, and he is afebrile. Focused physical examination reveals significantly elevated jugular venous distention to 12 centimeters, lungs that are clear, and an abdominal exam that is benign. Cardiac exam reveals a normal S1 and S2 with no murmurs or S3 or rubs. Extremities reveal equal pulses bilaterally. Rectal exam is guaiac-negative. All of the following tests would be appropriate to order immediately EXCEPT

    (A) electrocardiogram.

    (B) chest radiograph.

    (C) arterial blood gas.

    (D) initial blood tests including cardiac enzymes.

    (E) ventilation perfusion scan.

8. Initial testing reveals that his chest radiograph has no infiltrates or effusions and the cardiac silhouette is within normal limits. Electrocardiogram reveals sinus bradycardia with 3 mm ST elevation in leads II, III, avL, and 2 mm ST depression in leads VI and V2. No other abnormalities are noted. The other tests that you have ordered are in the lab. The diagnosis of an acute myocardial infarction is made. All of the following would be appropriate to consider for initial treatment in this patient EXCEPT

    (A) immediate treatment with aspirin.

    (B) immediate treatment with intravenous heparin.

    (C) immediate treatment with thrombolytic therapy.

    (D) immediate treatment with intravenous lidocaine.

    (E) immediate triage to the cardiac catheterization suite.

9. The findings on electrocardiogram most likely represent an acute infarction in

    (A) the inferior wall.

    (B) the lateral wall.

    (C) the anterior wall.

    (D) the septal wall.

    (E) each area of the heart.

The patient is taken to the cardiac catheterization suite where it is found that he has an acute occlusion of his proximal right coronary artery, which is successfully opened by percutaneous transluminal coronary angioplasty. His other coronary arteries appear normal. He returns to you with a blood pressure of 120/75, heart rate of 80, and respirations of 16. He denies any discomfort and is on a nitroglycerin drip. During his hospitalization, his subsequent labs show that he had a peak creatinine phosphokinase-MB of 48.

10. All of the following would be appropriate for risk stratification before discharge EXCEPT

    (A) two-dimensional echocardiogram.

    (B) fasting lipid profile.

    (C) hemoglobin A1C.

    (D) maximal exercise treadmill test.

    (E) discussion of diet and smoking cessation.

11. Of the following, the preferred medication to be used in this patient would be a(n)

    (A) beta-blocker.

    (B) calcium channel blocker.

    (C) ACE inhibitor.

    (D) diuretic.

    (E) direct vasodilator.

12. If the patient's hospital course after his cardiac catheterization remains uncomplicated, the appropriate time to discharge him to home with close follow-up would be

    (A) 1 day.

    (B) 3 days.

    (C) 7 days.

    (D) 14 days.

    (E) 21 days.

13. A 44-year-old smoker comes to you complaining of a painful, productive cough. Examination reveals a temperature of 101.2°F and rales on auscultation of the lungs. The most likely diagnosis is

    (A) asthma.

    (B) lung carcinoma.

    (C) bronchitis.

    (D) viral upper respiratory tract infection.

    (E) pneumothorax.

14. A 50-year-old man presents with two days of headaches. He notes them to be lancinating and occurring behind his right eye. He notes associated ipsilateral lacrimation and nasal congestion. They occur a few times a day and last about an hour each. He denies any recent head trauma, but does note that he's been under more pressure recently than usual. The most likely diagnosis of this headache is

    (A) tension headache.

    (B) migraine headache.

    (C) subdural hematoma.

    (D) cluster headache.

    (E) subarachnoid hematoma.

15. A 32-year-old male is concerned over his tongue that has a small, white, hairy patch. You, as a clinician, should be concerned for

    (A) carcinoma.

    (B) herpes.

    (C) HIV.

    (D) streptococcus.

    (E) trauma.

16. A physician is submitting bills to Medicare for procedures on his patients that he has not performed. This is considered

    (A) an honest mistake.

    (B) fraud.

    (C) trivial.

    (D) acceptable medical practice.

    (E) clever.

17. A 10-year-old male immigrant is brought to the emergency room by "friends." The history of his illness is difficult to obtain due to a language barrier. He complains of shock-like sensations on forward flexion. His calf and thigh muscles fatigue easily. He has no fever and his appetite is good. He was treated with unknown medications for a "long time" in his own country. Physical examination reveals a temperature of 98°F, pulse of 74, respiration of 16, and blood pressure of 100/70. He has rigid gibbus, no scoliosis, and lungs WNL. Neuro exam reveals paraparesis. An MRI is shown in the figure. You immediately

    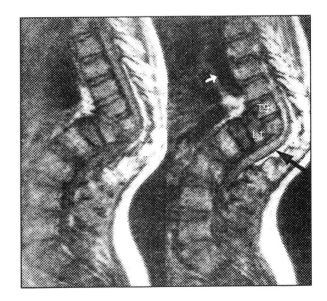

    (A) perform a lumbar puncture.

    (B) obtain an orthopedic consultation.

    (C) begin IV vancomycin, 30 mg/kg Q 4H.

    (D) arrange for immediate radiotherapy.

    (E) obtain a bone scan.

18. A 48-year-old man is hospitalized for acute renal failure. His serum potassium level is 6.0 mg/dl. All of the following are EKG findings associated with hyperkalemia EXCEPT

(A) peaked T-waves.

(B) PR interval lengthening.

(C) prominent U-waves.

(D) QRS widening.

(E) P-wave flattening.

19. A 67-year-old female presents for a periodic health examination. She has no complaints. All of the following measurements should be performed as part of her routine check-up EXCEPT

(A) serum cholesterol.

(B) plasma glucose.

(C) blood pressure.

(D) body weight.

(E) body height.

20. An 80-year-old male, who recently relocated, arrives for a check-up. Examination is significant for a nontender, midabdominal mass, which is confirmed by the abdominal computed tomography scan, shown in the figure. You recommend

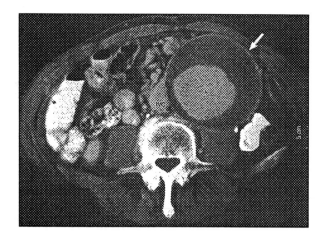

(A) reevaluation in one year.

(B) consultation with an oncologist.

(C) vascular surgery consultation.

(D) immediate CAT of the brain.

(E) carotid Doppler studies.

21. A 35-year-old female from Brazil presents to her physician with complaints of palpitations, shortness of breath, and orthopenia for several weeks. She also has symptoms of bloating, heartburn, and dysphagia. There is no associated fever or chills. Her chest X-ray reveals an enlarged heart. What is the diagnostic test of choice to make the diagnosis?

(A) Echocardiogram

(B) Barium swallow

(C) Serological testing

(D) Peripheral smear examination

(E) Electrocardiogram

For Questions 22-25, identify the most likely causative organism.

(A) *Streptococcus pneumoniae*

(B) *Streptococcus pyogenes*

(C) *Haemophilus influenzae*

(D) *Staphylococcus aureus*

(E) *Klebsiella pneumoniae*

22. A 30-year-old man presents with fevers to 103°F and a sore throat for three days. He denies any difficulty swallowing or breathing. He has had no significant past medical illnesses and is not on any medications. On physical examination, he has a temperature of 102.7°F, a blood pressure of 130/70, a heart rate of 70, and a respiratory rate of 20. His lungs are clear and his heart exam is without murmurs or gallops. His abdominal exam is benign and his extremities are without edema. His oropharynx is notable for erythema with tonsillar exudates. He also has bilateral painful cervical lymphadenopathy.

23. A 52-year-old presents with fevers to 103°F, and shortness of breath. He noted, about two weeks previously, that he had the "flu," and that he was feeling better until two days previously, when he began to feel more ill with high fevers and cough productive of sputum. He denies taking any medications and denies any sick contacts. On physical examination, he has a temperature of 103°F, a

heart rate of 100, a blood pressure of 120/70, and a respiratory rate of 22. His lungs reveal consolidation in the left lower lobe, and his cardiac exam is with a regular rate and rhythm without S3 or murmurs. His abdominal exam is benign and he has no peripheral edema.

24. A 30-year-old woman underwent an open cholecystectomy three days previously and has done well until today. She notes fevers to 102°F, and pain over the incision site. On examination, you note an erythematous and swollen area around the incision site with a small amount of purulent discharge.

25. An 18-year-old man with a history of intravenous drug abuse presents with fevers to 100°F. He denies any symptoms of shortness of breath, cough, nausea, vomiting, chest pain, dysuria, abdominal pain, diarrhea, or constipation. He denies any significant past medical illnesses and is not taking any medications. His blood pressure is 110/70, heart rate is 110, respiratory rate is 20, and temperature is 101°F. His lungs are clear and his cardiac exam reveals a normal S1 and S2 with a III/VI systolic blowing murmur. His abdominal exam is without abnormalities and his extremities are without abnormalities. On chest radiograph, he has numerous small lesions consistent with septic emboli.

26. While examining a woman's abdomen you detect a peritoneal friction rub. This may represent all of the following EXCEPT

   (A) splenic infarction.
   (B) carcinoma of the liver.
   (C) syphilitic hepatitis.
   (D) ileus.
   (E) liver abscess.

Questions 27-34 refer to the following:

A 38-year-old man with a history of cirrhosis presents with four episodes of hematemesis. His past medical history is significant for cirrhosis secondary to alcoholism.

27. Of the following, the most common cause of upper gastrointestinal bleeding in this patient would be

   (A) esophageal varices.
   (B) gastric varices.
   (C) Mallory-Weiss tear.
   (D) peptic ulcer disease.
   (E) esophageal cancer.

28. His vital signs reveal that he is tachycardiac to 120, and has a blood pressure of 100/60 which decreases to 85/40 upon standing. An approximate estimation of blood lost is

   (A) 0-15%.
   (B) 15-25%.
   (C) 25-35%.
   (D) 35-45%.
   (E) greater than 45% of blood volume.

29. Appropriate initial maneuvers to stabilize the patient would be

   (A) initiation of beta-agonist, such as dobutamine.
   (B) initiation of a selective pressor, such as norepinephrine.
   (C) initiation of a pressor and an inotrope, such as dopamine.
   (D) fluid resuscitation.
   (E) None of the above.

30. Besides the above, other appropriate initial measures would include all of the following EXCEPT

   (A) insertion of two large-bore intravenous needles.
   (B) type and cross.
   (C) complete blood count.
   (D) coagulation studies.
   (E) placement of a pulmonary artery catheter.

31. The appropriate initial interventions are done and the patient is stabilized with a heart rate of 100 and a blood pressure of 120/70. NG lavage reveals bright red blood with clots. Of the following diagnostic tests, the most appropriate immediate intervention is

    (A) CT scan of the abdomen.

    (B) tagged red cell scan.

    (C) esophagogastroduodenoscopy.

    (D) colonoscopy.

    (E) barium swallow.

32. While awaiting the diagnostic test, the patient becomes hypotensive again and begins to vomit several hundred cc's of bright red blood. He is intubated for airway protection. All of the following are appropriate temporizing measures EXCEPT

    (A) intravenous vasopressin.

    (B) intravenous octreotide.

    (C) insertion of a Sengstaken-Blakemore tube.

    (D) rapid infusion of blood.

    (E) All of the above.

33 Esophagogastroduodenoscopy reveals bleeding esophageal varices. Of the following, which one is true regarding treatment?

    (A) Sclerotherapy remains the most effective treatment.

    (B) Band ligation has been shown to be more effective in treatment of variceal bleed.

    (C) Ligation and sclerotherapy have the same efficacy.

    (D) Neither are effective in the treatment of esophageal varices.

    (E) Sclerotherapy is effective for bleeding gastric varices.

34. Of the following medications, the one that has been shown to decrease recurrent bleeding is

    (A) cimetidine.

    (B) Carafate.

    (C) omeprazole.

    (D) propranolol.

    (E) antibiotics.

35. A 19-year-old male is seen at your office for urethral mucoid discharge. The discharge followed symptoms of urgency and frequency lasting three days. Physical examination is otherwise normal. Regarding this patient's condition, which one of the following statements is NOT true?

    (A) *Chlamydia trachomatis* can be a cause.

    (B) *Ureaplasma urealyticum* can be a cause.

    (C) *Neisseria gonorrhea* can be a cause.

    (D) This condition may be asymptomatic in men.

    (E) This condition may be asymptomatic in women.

36. A 29-year-old woman who is 19 weeks pregnant presents to the emergency room complaining of abdominal pain, nausea, and vomiting. After a complete physical examination, the presumptive diagnosis of appendicitis is made, and an emergency appendectomy is scheduled. In respect to nonobstetric surgery in this pregnant patient, which one of the following statements is correct?

    (A) The incidence of surgery for nonobstetric procedures is about four percent.

    (B) Appendectomy is the second most common operative procedure during pregnancy.

    (C) Ketamine is a relatively safe anesthetic agent for both the mother and the fetus and, therefore, can be used in premedicating pregnant women.

    (D) If general anesthesia is to be employed, generous administration of fluids would minimize the side effects that are associated with this procedure.

(E) If regional anesthesia is to be employed, hypotension in a pregnant patient can be avoided with fluid preloading.

37. The mother of a playful five-year-old girl brings her daughter to you complaining that she has had a scaling patch on her scalp for two weeks. After close examination, you suspect that the child has tinea capitis. The most appropriate treatment for tinea capitis is

    (A) an antifungal ointment.

    (B) a topical antibacterial ointment.

    (C) a combination topical antifungal with a steroid ointment.

    (D) oral griseofulvin.

    (E) amoxicillin.

38. You have admitted a 17-year-old male with enlarged epitrochlear nodes. These may come from all of the following areas EXCEPT

    (A) the little finger.

    (B) the ring finger.

    (C) the ulnar aspect of the arm.

    (D) the radial aspect of the arm.

    (E) the ulnar half of the long finger.

39. A 33-year-old female comes to the emergency room complaining of passing black tarry stools for several days. She has no abdominal pain but has had some dyspepsia. She was recently seen for a sprained ankle sustained while playing tennis. You are most interested in her ingestion of

    (A) acetaminophen.

    (B) nonsteroidal anti-inflammatory agents.

    (C) penicillin.

    (D) sulfa.

    (E) birth control pills.

40. A 36-year-old male who is known to have HIV/AIDS comes to the emergency department because of a recent onset of a rash. He denies any recent exposures. You ask about all of the medications he takes and suspect which one of the following of causing his rash?

    (A) Pentamidine

    (B) Zidovudine

    (C) Trimethoprim-sulfamethoxazole

    (D) Clarithromycin

    (E) Didanosine

41. A 21-year-old male with asthma comes to the emergency room because of nausea, vomiting, and a sense of dizziness. After asking about his medications, you order

    (A) a theophylline level.

    (B) a chest radiograph.

    (C) a urinalysis.

    (D) a stool culture.

    (E) blood cultures.

42. A 64-year-old male with congestive heart failure comes to the emergency room because of nausea, vomiting, and some visual changes affecting his perception of colors. He is slightly confused. His wife tells you that he was recently started on a "water pill" in addition to his "heart medicines." His serum potassium is 2.8 mEq/dl. You suspect

    (A) viral gastroenteritis.

    (B) cardiac decompensation.

    (C) schizophrenia.

    (D) dementia.

    (E) digoxin toxicity.

43. A 45-year-old woman comes in because of a sore throat. She teaches second grade. She has a history of sore throats as a child but has not had one for years. Her tonsils are covered with exudates and she has cervical lymphadenitis. After obtaining cultures, you treat her with

    (A) Xylocaine mouth wash.

(B) guaifenesin.

(C) penicillin.

(D) isoniazid.

(E) acyclovir.

44. A 78-year-old man with severe osteoarthritis is brought in because of confusion. His liver function tests are elevated. He takes no prescription drugs but does take over-the-counter medications for his joint pain. His family thinks he has increased his ingestion of pills lately because of more pain. He has no evidence of bleeding. While awaiting the arrival of a family member with the bottle of medicine that the patient has taken, you suspect it will be

(A) aspirin.

(B) vitamin E.

(C) diphenhydramine.

(D) acetaminophen.

(E) iron.

45. A two-year-old male was admitted for the evaluation of recurrent syncopal episodes which have occurred over the past few months. Based on the electrocardiogram, shown in the figure, you tell the concerned parents that

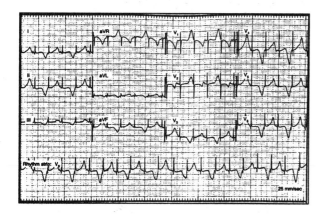

(A) this condition most often occurs sporadically.

(B) the risk of sudden death is increased.

(C) syncopal episodes are unrelated to underlying cardiac disease.

(D) family therapy is advised.

(E) neurologic consultation is recommended.

46. An 18-year-old male presents with gynecomastia; small, firm testicles; azoospermia; and a eunuchoidal habitus. He was found to have low testosterone levels, elevated gonadotropin levels, and impairment of spermatogenesis. What is the most likely diagnosis?

(A) Kartagener's syndrome

(B) Klinefelter's syndrome

(C) Noonan's syndrome

(D) Mumps orchitis

(E) Congenital adrenal hyperplasia

47. A 32-year-old male presents to the doctor's office with complaints of persistent low back pain for the last six months, which is worse in the morning and gradually improves after activity. The physical examination is normal except for decreased flexion of the lumbar spine. The HLA-B27 test is positive. Which one of the following tests will also assist us in arriving at the correct diagnosis and subsequent management?

(A) Plain X-rays of the sacroiliac joint

(B) Serum rheumatoid

(C) Arthrocentesis of the first metatarsophalangeal joint

(D) Spinal films

(E) Straight-leg testing

For Questions 48-51, match the pulmonary function flow volume curves, shown in the figure, with the clinical diagnosis.

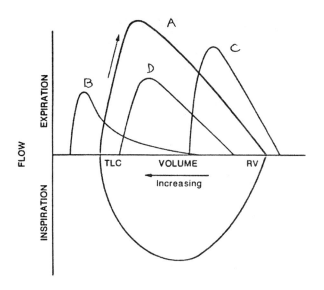

Panel A

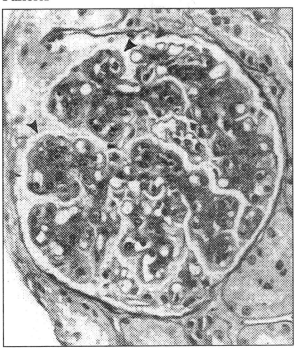

(A)   Curve A

(B)   Curve B

(C)   Curve C

(D)   Curve D

48.   Normal

49.   Asthma

50.   Sarcoidosis

51.   Diaphragmatic paralysis

52.   A renal biopsy, shown in the figures to the right and on the next page, was done on an 8-year-old girl to evaluate persistent proteinuria and microscopic hematuria. Your diagnosis is

    (A)   nodular glomerulosclerosis.

    (B)   membranoproliferative glomerulonephritis.

    (C)   focal segmental glomerulosclerosis.

    (D)   IgA nephropathy.

    (E)   minimal change disease.

Panel B

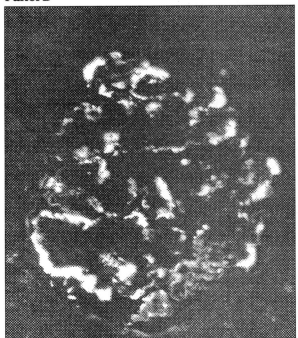

Panel C

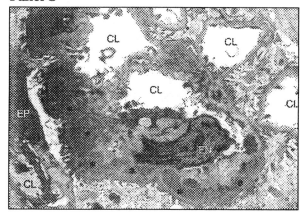

Questions 53-57 are together.

53. You evaluate a 50-year-old male with dysplasia of the cavernous sheaths and contracture of the investing fascia of the corpora. This disease is known as

    (A) priapism.

    (B) Peyronie's disease.

    (C) inguinal hernia.

    (D) varicocele.

    (E) torsion.

54. The penis will usually

    (A) deviate to the involved side.

    (B) deviate to the uninvolved side.

    (C) remain erect and straight at all times.

    (D) remain flaccid at all times.

    (E) be uninvolved.

55. Erection

    (A) is impossible.

    (B) is painful.

    (C) is painless.

    (D) is painful only during intercourse.

    (E) is painful only during ejaculation.

56. You offer treatment to this patient which may include all of the following EXCEPT

    (A) surgical removal of the involved plaque.

    (B) steroid injections.

    (C) ultrasonic treatment.

    (D) oral steroids.

    (E) radiation.

57. You wish to convert a tension pneumothorax to a routine pneumothorax. You can do this by

    (A) placing a chest tube.

    (B) placing a 13-gauge needle in the chest over absent breath sounds

    (C) performing a tracheostomy.

    (D) intubating the patient.

    (E) positive pressure ventilation.

58. Following a fatal automobile accident, the family of a 75-year-old male requests an autopsy. The man, who was a passenger in the car, was noted to have increasing memory impairment over the past several months. A section of the frontal cerebral cortex is shown in the figure. Based on the pathologic findings, you discuss all of the following with the family EXCEPT

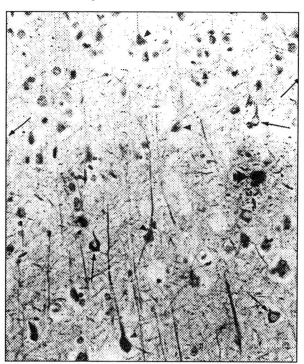

(A) in 20-25% of cases, there is another affected relative.

(B) similar neuropathic changes develop in persons with Down's syndrome.

(C) ApoE4 homozygotes are at increased risk compared to E2 or E3 homozygotes.

(D) some of these pathologic changes have been observed in dementia pugilistica.

(E) this is a rare, reportable case.

Questions 59-62 refer to the following:

A 15-year-old white teenager is seen in the clinic because of symptoms of malaise, anorexia, jaundice, and unsteady gait. There is no history of prior drug use or past medical history. There is no history of exposure to shellfish. There is a family history of liver disease. The lab data reveals elevation of serum aminotransferases. On examination, the liver is enlarged and there is evidence of a mild tremor. Also on examination, the limbus of the cornea has a brownish-green discoloration.

59. All of the following can be used to diagnose this disease EXCEPT

(A) serum ceruloplasmin level.

(B) quantitative liver biopsy.

(C) quantitative urine analysis.

(D) slit-lamp examination.

(E) hepatitis profile.

60. All of the following are complications of this disease EXCEPT

(A) hemolytic anemia.

(B) hepatic encephalopathy.

(C) dystonic postures.

(D) disseminated intravascular coagulation (DIC).

(E) severe arthropathy.

61. The excess accumulation of the metabolite causing this disorder begins in

(A) adulthood.

(B) infancy.

(C) teen years.

(D) a fetus.

(E) toddlerhood.

62. Which one of the following is the treatment of choice for this disease?

(A) D-penicillamine

(B) Prednisone

(C) Zinc

(D) No treatment available.

(E) Dimercaprol

63. Your son, employed as a technician at the university hospital, shows you a scanning electron microscopic section of a peripheral blood specimen from a person with anemia.

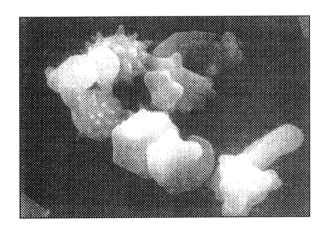

You tell him that the most likely underlying medical problem in this person is

(A) chronic renal failure.

(B) cirrhosis of the liver.

(C) pancreatitis.

(D) idiopathic cardiomyopathy.

(E) pulmonary tuberculosis.

64. A 32-year-old woman presents to your office with feelings of generalized fatigue for about three months. She also has noted decreased appetite, cold intolerance, and some thinning of her hair. The most appropriate screening test in this woman would be a

   (A) serum TSH.

   (B) cosyntropin suppression test.

   (C) T4.

   (D) 24-hour calorie count.

   (E) None of the above.

65. A patient you have seen occasionally for hypertension comes in because she wants you to write a letter to her insurance company documenting medical necessity for reduction mammoplasty. She wants you to say she has back problems due to her large breasts and that she has a chronic recalcitrant inframammary rash. You examine her and find no evidence of any medical necessity for the procedure. You

   (A) agree to write the letter anyway.

   (B) call the insurance company to tell them she wants to commit fraud.

   (C) tell her you will write the letter only if she pays you extra.

   (D) tell her you cannot write the letter because it is not true.

   (E) refer her to a colleague who will write such a letter.

66. Which one of the following statements about the "impaired physician" is NOT true?

   (A) Impairment may result from physical or emotional disability which is likely to lead to inability to function effectively and safely.

   (B) The most common causes of physician impairment are advancing age or premature senility, alcohol abuse, and drug abuse.

   (C) The "impaired physician" does not care much about the accepted standards of patient care.

   (D) Increasing impairment may lead to professional incompetence.

   (E) Forgetfulness, confusion, or loss of dexterity are components of the impairment.

Questions 67-74 refer to the following:

A 73-year-old man with metastatic prostate cancer who has failed orchiectomy and chemotherapy comes in with his wife. He is having a lot of leg and back pain and is using a walker.

67. You tell him that you want to obtain radiographs of his femur and spine. He tells you that he and his wife have agreed to his having a living will with advanced directives stating that no resuscitation should be attempted if he arrests. The wife has power of attorney should the patient become incompetent. The wife questions the need for the radiographs. You tell her

   (A) you are doing them to be complete.

   (B) if he has metastatic lesions you would recommend radiotherapy.

   (C) it would be malpractice not to get radiographs.

   (D) you do not agree with his living will.

   (E) they should not question the physician's decisions.

68. The wife asks why he should have radiotherapy since he has a living will. You tell her

   (A) she should go to the waiting room and not question you.

   (B) you know what is best.

   (C) you do not agree with the living will.

   (D) radiotherapy could relieve a lot of his pain.

   (E) the insurance company has approved radiotherapy.

69. This therapy would be consistent with the concept of improving

    (A) the patient's appearance.

    (B) the hospital's revenue.

    (C) the patient's quality of life.

    (D) the patient's prognosis.

    (E) your malpractice company's guidelines.

70. The patient does, indeed, have metastatic lesions in the painful bones. He undergoes a course of radiation therapy and feels much better. He is able to walk for a while without any assistive devices. However, he gradually deteriorates, losing weight, becoming weaker, and occasionally getting confused. The wife calls you and says she cannot take care of him at home by herself any more. You recommend all of the following EXCEPT

    (A) admission to the ICU.

    (B) admission to a hospice.

    (C) home nursing care.

    (D) admission to a nursing home.

    (E) a home health aide.

71. The patient is admitted to a nursing home. When you visit him, you find him somnolent and difficult to arouse. The wife has already told you she wants nothing done except supportive care. You should

    (A) do a lumbar puncture.

    (B) transfer him to the emergency room.

    (C) tell the nurses to be prepared to conduct a full code.

    (D) call the wife and suggest intravenous fluids.

    (E) start a central line.

72. The patient's wife says she does not want IV fluids administered. You do not agree and

    (A) give him IV fluids.

    (B) call the nursing home attorney.

    (C) transfer him to the hospital.

    (D) refuse to care for him.

    (E) explain to her what you think should be done.

73. The wife still does not agree with you. You

    (A) start an IV line and give him fluids.

    (B) honor her wishes.

    (C) transfer care to another physician.

    (D) tell her she does not know what she is doing.

    (E) try to have the patient made a ward of the state.

74. The next day, while you are visiting the patient, he has a full cardiopulmonary arrest. You

    (A) call a full resuscitation.

    (B) call an ambulance to transfer him to the ICU.

    (C) note the time of death and call the wife.

    (D) begin an IV line.

    (E) intubate him.

Questions 75-77 refer to the following:

A 29-year-old HIV-positive female postal worker presents to the free-standing health center complaining of painful urination, malaise, anorexia, and tender lymph glands in the groin area over the course of two weeks. She is sexually active. On examination, she has a fever and bilateral tender inguinal adenopathy. There are painful, weeping, vesicles on the vulva, vagina, and cervix of this patient.

75. To make the correct diagnosis, what would one visualize on the cytology of the cells scraped from the oozing lesion?

    (A) Branching hyphae

    (B) Dysplastic squamous cells

    (C) Intranuclear inclusion bodies and multinucleated giant cells

(D) Gram-negative diplococci embedded in neutrophils

(E) Gram-positive, filamentous branching rods that have a beaded appearance

76. Six weeks later, this patient is brought into the emergency room by the ambulance because she is unconscious, febrile, and found to have new onset seizures. Her family states that she has been having headaches for the last week and bizarre behavior. Which one of the following tests would make the definitive diagnosis in this case?

(A) Lumbar puncture

(B) CT of the brain

(C) Electroencephalogram (EEG)

(D) Ophthalmoscopic examination

(E) Brain biopsy

77. What is the treatment of choice for this disorder?

(A) Acyclovir

(B) Amphotericin

(C) Doxycycline

(D) Steroids

(E) Ganciclovir

For Questions 78-81, match the appropriate cardiomyopathy with the appropriate clinical case.

(A) Dilated cardiomyopathy

(B) Hypertrophic cardiomyopathy

(C) Restrictive cardiomyopathy

(D) None of the above.

78. A 76-year-old man with three-vessel coronary artery disease with symptoms of angina and leg swelling.

79. A 35-year-old female with shortness of breath. Cardiac examination reveals a systolic heart murmur which increases with Valsalva.

80. A 46-year-old female with history of breast cancer who develops shortness of breath and pedal edema after completion of chemotherapy.

81. A 26-year-old female, one month postpartum, with shortness of breath and echocardiogram showing decreased wall motion and mural thrombus.

82. One of your colleagues is staunchly opposed to abortion. A young woman who is one month pregnant and is scheduled to have an abortion next week comes to the emergency department because she is having abdominal pain. Your colleague refuses to take care of her. All of the following statements are true EXCEPT

(A) he does not have to perform an abortion if he objects to it.

(B) he does not have to take care of this patient's abdominal pain.

(C) you can take care of this patient.

(D) he does not have to recommend an abortion to a patient.

(E) he should not work in an emergency room.

Questions 83-89 refer to the following:

The university has recently opened a clinic for diagnosis and treatment of children with short stature. You are evaluating a six-year-old male with the growth curve shown in the figure on the following page. The child was adopted at birth. There have been no systemic illnesses. Examination reveals normal skeletal proportions and a pudgy, youthful appearance.

83. Chemistry panel, CBC, and skull films are reported as normal. You now order a(n)

(A) renal sonogram.

(B) thyroid profile.

(C) urinary sodium, phosphate, and creatinine.

(D) barium enema.

(E) parathyroid hormone.

Boys From 2 to 18 Years
STATURE FOR AGE

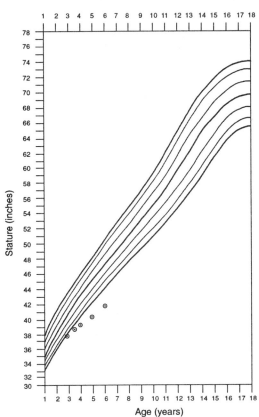

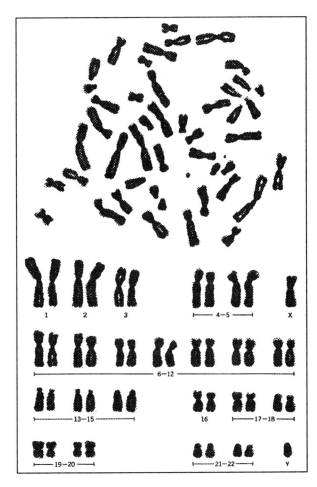

84. Following the report of normal thyroid function, you ordered a chromosomal analysis, which is shown in the figure in the next column. You indicate to the mother that

   (A) gonadal dysgenesis is the most likely etiology of his short stature.

   (B) there is no evidence of a chromosomal abnormality.

   (C) the child has Laron dwarfism.

   (D) the child has the Prader-Willi syndrome.

   (E) the child is short due to genetic predisposition.

85. The report of the X rays of the left wrist and hand indicate that the skeletal age, compared with the chronological age, is greater than 2.5 standard deviations. You discuss all of the following with the parents EXCEPT

   (A) one of every 20 normal children may have skeletal age retarded by two standard deviations.

   (B) one of every 20 normal children may have skeletal age advanced by two standard deviations.

   (C) the hand and wrist are useful sites for measuring bone age throughout childhood.

(D) boys are more advanced than girls in skeletal development at all ages.

(E) bone age, determined by X-rays, is one of the best indices of general growth.

86. You now order which one of the following tests?

(A) Bone biopsy

(B) L-dopa stimulation test

(C) Baseline growth hormone level

(D) Insulin level

(E) Glucagon level

87. You confirm your findings with a clonidine stimulation test. Peak growth hormone level is 8.9 ng/mL. You now

(A) perform a CAT scan of the pituitary.

(B) perform a CAT scan of the hypothalamus.

(C) begin treatment with growth hormone, 0.1 U/kg.

(D) begin treatment with prednisone, 7.5 mg/day.

(E) begin treatment with ergocalciferol, 1,250 IU/day.

88. The child responded to your therapy. Seven years later, the mother reports that the child has become a behavioral problem. In addition, his scholastic performance has deteriorated. On examination, you note myoclonus, tremor, and cerebellar ataxia. You now

(A) refer the child to a psychiatrist.

(B) decrease the medication dosage by half.

(C) admit the child to the hospital.

(D) order a urine toxicology.

(E) begin propranolol, 20 mg/day.

89. Several months later, the child dies. An autopsy, which was limited to the brain, shows depletion of cortical neurons, marked reactive astrocrytosis, intracellular vacuolar changes, and plaques. There is an absence of inflammatory changes. Immunochemical stains are positive for protease-resistant protein. You discuss all of the following disease issues with his family EXCEPT

(A) its incidence peaks in the second decade.

(B) it usually occurs sporadically.

(C) it has been transmitted by corneal transplantation.

(D) in children, it has been transmitted by contaminated cadaveric hormone preparations.

(E) it has developed in women treated with pituitary gonadotropin for infertility.

90. Regarding immunizations in HIV-positive individuals, which one of the following vaccinations is NOT recommended by the U.S. Preventive Services Task Force on Periodic Health Examination?

(A) IPV

(B) Measles

(C) Mumps

(D) Rubella

(E) Hepatitis B

For Questions 91-94, select the most likely pathogen in these patients with diarrhea.

(A) Cryptosporidium

(B) Shigella

(C) *Giardia lamblia*

(D) *Clostridium difficile*

(E) Rotavirus

91. A 24-year-old female with a urinary tract infection

92. A 50-year-old female returning from a hiking trip in the Rocky Mountains

93. A 30-year-old intravenous drug user with thrombocytopenia

94. A 50-year-old banker with dysentery

95. You are attending a course on alternative health care. The current session is focusing on acupuncture. The opacities evident on the chest X-ray, shown in the figure below, represent fragments of acupuncture needles. Regarding this type of therapy, you are taught all of the following EXCEPT

    (A) the needles are aligned along vertical meridians of the torso.

    (B) the needles were intentionally broken by the acupuncturist.

    (C) the patient believes that the needles absorb energy from his surroundings.

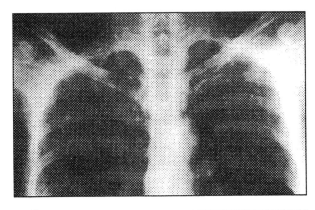

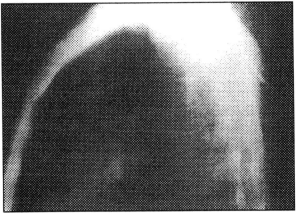

    (D) the fragments will be removed after 10 years.

    (E) by balancing the yin and yang forces, these needles improve the patient's health.

96. A 12-year-old boy is brought to the walk-in clinic in which you work. He was playing baseball and fell while running from first base to second. He hyperextended his wrist to break his fall. You order a radiograph because you suspect

    (A) Legg-Calve-Perthes disease.

    (B) a Colles' fracture.

    (C) a march fracture.

    (D) osteochondritis dissecans.

    (E) avascular necrosis.

97. A 25-year-old female is brought to the emergency room by friends. She is comatose. Her friends say they had been at a party where there were drugs and alcohol, but they do not know what the patient ingested. Her pupils are contracted. You decide to treat with

    (A) naloxone.

    (B) methadone.

    (C) gastric lavage.

    (D) ipecac.

    (E) a chelating agent.

98. A 34-year-old man comes into your walk-in clinic complaining of episodic headaches and nosebleeds. His blood pressure is 180/130. You call his family physician who says that the patient is usually normotensive but does have episodic elevations, which the physician thinks are due to stress. The patient is flushed and sweaty. You treat his blood pressure acutely and recommend evaluation for

(A) Cushing's syndrome.

(B) renal artery stenosis.

(C) polycystic kidney disease.

(D) pheochromocytoma.

(E) carcinoid syndrome.

99. A 52-year-old woman has been placed on sulfasalazine for her ulcerative colitis. She is relatively asymptomatic and has a routine colonoscopy performed and, as per the usual protocol, is monitored by ear oximetry. She is found to have a significant hypoxia. The gastroenterologist stops the procedure and questions the patient regarding her breathing. She is surprised he has stopped and states that she feels fine. The likeliest cause of this hypoxia is

(A) a pulmonary embolus.

(B) pneumonia.

(C) carboxymethemoglobinemia.

(D) thalassemia.

(E) COPD.

100. A 44-year-old woman who runs for exercise and used to play basketball in high school comes to your walk-in clinic because she has noticed that her right knee has been giving out lately and she has almost fallen several times. You examine the knee and palpate a small effusion. She has some ligamentous laxity. You refer her to an orthopedist with a working diagnosis of

(A) osteoarthritis.

(B) osteochondromatosis.

(C) osteosarcoma.

(D) anterior cruciate ligament insufficiency.

(E) popliteal cyst.

101. A 49-year-old woman comes to your walk-in clinic because of pain in her right wrist. She has noticed this for a month or two but it is getting worse. No other joints bother her and she feels relatively well, though perhaps a little more tired than usual. You question her about her activities and she tells you she is an avid gardener and has a large assortment of roses. Her wrist is warm, swollen, and

slightly tender. Which one of the following conditions is the likeliest diagnosis?

(A) Rheumatoid arthritis

(B) Sporotrichosis

(C) Candidiasis

(D) Tuberculosis

(E) Lyme disease

102. A baby is born with complete heart block. He is otherwise healthy. As the obstetrician, you have noted that the mother has had a mild facial rash throughout her pregnancy and some aching in her joints which she has attributed to pregnancy. The most likely explanation for these events is

(A) tetralogy of Fallot.

(B) transposition of the great vessels.

(C) myocarditis in the newborn.

(D) rubella.

(E) maternal lupus.

103. A 15-year-old male with sickle cell anemia comes to the emergency room because of progressively worsening right hip pain. It has gotten to the point that he cannot bear weight on his right leg. He has had no fevers or chills and has been feeling fairly well otherwise. Your working diagnosis is

(A) avascular necrosis of the femur.

(B) rheumatoid arthritis.

(C) osteoarthritis.

(D) factitious pain.

(E) reflex sympathetic dystrophy.

104. You examine a patient with a painful rectum in the emergency room and perform an examination revealing a diffuse rectal ulcer. This most likely represents

(A) bacillary dysentery.

(B) tuberculosis.

(C) irradiation.

(D) trauma.

(E) lymphogranuloma venereum.

105. A previously healthy, athletic male was brought in by ambulance because of fever, pain, and erythema in the left forearm, decreased strength in the left forearm, and diminished pulses in that extremity. He also had a decreased sensation and swelling in that arm. Blood cultures grew *Strep. pyogenes*. What would be the immediate intervention needed in this case?

    (A) Surgical fasciotomy

    (B) Clindamycin

    (C) Hyperbaric oxygen chamber

    (D) CT of the head

    (E) Thrombolytic agents

106. Which one of the following is NOT true of cyanosis?

    (A) Its degree is modified by the quality of cutaneous pigment and the thickness of the skin.

    (B) Clinical detection correlates well with oximetric values.

    (C) If anemia is severe, marked arterial desaturation does not produce it.

    (D) Local passive congestion may produce it.

    (E) Carboxyhemoglobin produces a cherry-colored flush, rather than cyanosis.

107. A 35-year-old man comes to your clinic complaining of urethral discharge. You treat him empirically, thinking that gonococcal infection is the likeliest diagnosis. The culture subsequently returns positive for *Neisseria gonorrhea*. You must

    (A) call all of the patient's sexual contacts.

    (B) call his wife.

(C) tell all of your colleagues.

(D) notify the Board of Health.

(E) call the patient's employer.

108. A 23-year-old woman presents to the emergency room with abdominal pain. You want to test for cervical and vaginal infection because you suspect PID. All of the following tests can be done with a pelvic and cervical exam EXCEPT

    (A) gonococcal culture.

    (B) KOH prep.

    (C) Gram stain.

    (D) *Chlamydia* culture.

    (E) peritonitis.

109. As part of a CME program, you are evaluating the slide shown in the figure. Which one of the following diagnoses is LEAST likely?

    (A) Status post total gastrectomy

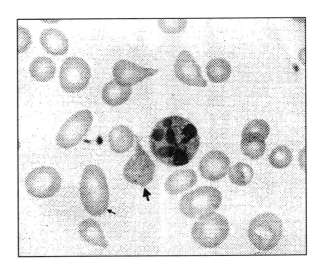

    (B) Tropical sprue

    (C) True vegetarianism

    (D) Heinz body anemia

    (E) Pernicious anemia

110. The case fatality rate for disease X is 15% within four years of the initial diagnosis. The probability that three randomly selected patients with this disease will die within the same time period is

(A) 0.3375.

(B) 0.03375.

(C) 0.00375.

(D) 0.000375.

(E) 0.0000375.

111. You have just seen a 23-year-old woman who is 16 weeks pregnant for a prenatal visit. You should schedule the next visit in

(A) one week.

(B) two weeks.

(C) one month.

(D) two months.

(E) three months.

Questions 112 and 113 refer to the following:

A patient presents to your office for a routine physical, and upon auscultation of the heart you hear a midsystolic click.

112. The patient most likely has

(A) tricuspid stenosis.

(B) tricuspid regurgitation.

(C) mitral valve prolapse.

(D) aortic stenosis.

(E) aortic regurgitation.

113. The patient above is also found to have a right upper quadrant mass in the abdomen. This may represent all of the following EXCEPT

(A) pulsatile liver.

(B) enlarged gallbladder.

(C) ptotic right kidney.

(D) enlarged right kidney.

(E) transverse colon carcinoma.

Questions 114-117 refer to the following:

A 19-year-old woman presents to your office after having been seen in the emergency room four days ago for a painful lump on her buttocks. She's been changing the dressings twice a day and has noted continued drainage. She denies any fevers, chills, or nausea, but does complain of continued pain in the area of the cyst. On physical examination, you note a two centimeter openly draining lump on the superior area between her gluteal folds. The drainage is serosanguinous in character, and the area is very painful to palpation.

114. The most likely diagnosis is

(A) pilonidal cyst.

(B) genital wart.

(C) Bartholin's cyst.

(D) squamous cell cancer.

(E) None of the above.

115. Appropriate initial treatment in the office would be

(A) repack the draining lump to keep it open and redress the wound.

(B) do not repack the draining lump and allow it to close and redress the wound.

(C) under local anesthesia, probe with a scalpel to attempt to open the wound further.

(D) immediate admission for surgical incision and drainage.

(E) None of the above.

116. She asks you how long it will take to heal. You tell her that likely it will

(A) take several months to heal and that if it doesn't, surgical therapy may be indicated.

(B) heal in a few weeks if she continues to apply clean dressing changes to it.

(C) heal in a few more days.

(D) never heal.

(E) None of the above.

117. Appropriate decisions regarding treatment would be

(A) to begin antibiotics and refer her to a surgeon to assist in her care.

(B) to not begin antibiotics and refer her to a surgeon to assist in her care.

(C) to begin antibiotics and not refer her to a surgeon.

(D) to not begin antibiotics and not refer her to a surgeon.

(E) admit her to the hospital to a surgical service.

118. During hospital rounds, you see one of your partner's patients with thrombotic thrombocytopenic purpura (TTP). The patient has numerous abnormal signs and symptoms. Which one of the following is NOT generally seen in patients with TTP?

(A) Fever

(B) Elevated creatinine

(C) Schistocytes on blood smear

(D) Reduced platelet count

(E) Positive Coombs' test

Questions 119 and 120 refer to the following:

A 79-year-old woman comes to your clinic with a throbbing temporal headache.

119. Your first course of action is to

(A) advise her to avoid bright light and loud noises.

(B) prescribe analgesics.

(C) perform a temporal artery biopsy.

(D) start steroids.

(E) schedule a head CAT scan.

120. You would be concerned for what disease in the above situation?

(A) migraine headache.

(B) cluster headache.

(C) temporal arteritis.

(D) a brain tumor.

(E) subdural hematoma.

121. In the management of persons with diabetes mellitus, which of the following is NOT true concerning the clinical usefulness of a hemoglobin A1C level?

(A) The percent of glycated hemoglobin gives an estimate of diabetic control for the preceding 6-12 week period.

(B) The "normal range" must be established for each laboratory.

(C) Levels exceeding 12% are associated with poor diabetic control.

(D) It provides the same information as a glycated albumin level.

(E) Conditions which increase red cell turnover spuriously lower glycohemoglobin.

122. A 36-year-old man comes to the emergency room because of a high fever, cough, and weight loss. He looks cachectic. He confesses to you that he is bisexual. However, he refuses to let you obtain an HIV test. You should

(A) refuse to take care of him.

(B) draw it anyway.

(C) try to diagnose the cause of his acute symptoms and treat them symptomatically.

(D) call the Board of Health.

(E) call the patient's family.

Questions 123-126 refer to the following:

You are asked to determine which of two tests, leukocyte esterase or urinary nitrates, would be the best screening test to use in your clinic for the rapid diagnosis of urinary tract infections (UTI). Upon reviewing the records of patients treated for UTI in the clinic over the last three years, you find the following: 811 patients were evaluated for UTI. 503 patients were diagnosed with UTI based on positive urine culture. All of these patients underwent leukocyte esterase and urinary nitrate testing of the urine. Of the 393 patients with a negative leukocyte esterase, 240 also had a negative urine culture, while of the 284 patients with a negative nitrate assay, 206 also had a negative urine culture.

123. Which of the two tests has the greater sensitivity?

    (A)   Leukocyte esterase

    (B)   Urinary nitrate

    (C)   Same sensitivity

    (D)   The value cannot be determined without knowing the prevalence of the condition in the population.

124. What is the approximate false-positive rate of the leukocyte esterase test?

    (A)   10%

    (B)   20%

    (C)   30%

    (D)   40%

    (E)   50%

125. What is the approximate false-negative rate of the nitrate test?

    (A)   5%

    (B)   10%

    (C)   15%

    (D)   20%

    (E)   25%

126. Which one of the following statements is true?

    (A)   Leukocyte esterase is the better of the two tests.

    (B)   The urinary nitrate test is more specific.

    (C)   The urinary nitrate test is less sensitive.

    (D)   Both tests have a poor reproducibility.

    (E)   None of the above.

127. A 23-year-old woman presents to the emergency room with left knee pain and erythema. She has been previously healthy and takes no medications. Aspirate reveals yellow fluid that has a cell count of 50,000 and no crystals. The most likely etiology for this is

    (A)   septic joint.

    (B)   trauma.

    (C)   normal.

    (D)   gout.

    (E)   inflammatory disease, such as systemic lupus erythematosus.

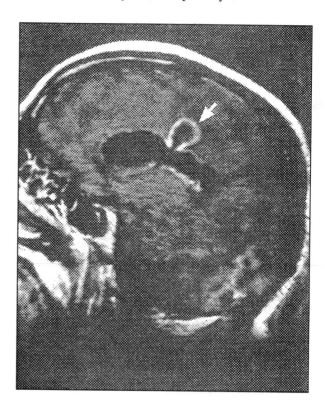

128. A 48-year-old male presents with a one-week history of headache, disorientation, and ataxia. He was in good health until three months ago when he developed a dental abscess, which improved with antibiotics. He is a nonsmoker and a social alcohol user. Physical examination reveals a temperature of 99°F, pulse of 80, respiration of 18, and blood pressure 140/90. He is lethargic, with no evidence of trauma. HEENT is WNL, with no nuchal rigidity and right hemiparesis. As part of the initial work-up, you order a gadolinium-enhanced MRI, shown in the figure on the previous page. Your diagnosis is

   (A) subdural empyema.

   (B) epidural abscess.

   (C) cerebral abscess.

   (D) subdural hematoma.

   (E) venous sinus thrombosis.

129. A 33-year-old hemophiliac male comes in with head trauma sustained in a motor vehicle accident in which he was not wearing a helmet. You have taken care of him before and warned him of the risks of riding a motorcycle with and especially without a helmet. You now

   (A) refuse to take care of him.

   (B) call the neurosurgeon to assess him and treat as needed.

   (C) admit him to the ICU.

   (D) admit him to the psychiatric service.

   (E) commit him.

130. Which one of the following is NOT a standard intra-operative anesthesia monitor?

   (A) Capnograph

   (B) Pulse oximeter

   (C) Electroencephalogram

   (D) Non-invasive blood pressure

   (E) Temperature probe

131. A 38-year-old woman presents to your office for the first time and tells you that she has a history of glucose-6-phosphate dehydroge-

nase deficiency. She asks you which medications she should avoid. You tell her she should avoid all of the following medications EXCEPT

   (A) nitrofurantoin.

   (B) dapsone.

   (C) aspirin.

   (D) sulfamethoxazole.

   (E) She should avoid all of the above.

Questions 132-135 refer to the following:

You are asked to see a 34-year-old male with a prolonged, persistent, penile erection caused without sexual desire.

132. This condition is known as

   (A) Peyronie's disease.

   (B) penile hyperplasia.

   (C) cavernositis.

   (D) priapism.

   (E) epispadias.

133. Local mechanical causes for this condition include all of the following EXCEPT

   (A) thrombosis.

   (B) hemorrhage.

   (C) neoplasm.

   (D) inflammation.

   (E) urinary retention.

134. The condition may be associated with

   (A) leukemia.

   (B) diabetes.

   (C) hypertension.

   (D) benign prostatic hypertrophy.

   (E) lupus.

135. The condition resulting when the orifice of the prepuce is so small that the foreskin cannot be retracted from the glans is known as

   (A) phimosis.

   (B) paraphimosis.

(C) hypospadias.

(D) epispadias.

(E) balanitis.

136. An unknown young male is brought to the emergency room after being hit at 30 mph by a motor vehicle. He has bilateral open lower extremity fractures, is bleeding from a large scalp laceration, and is disoriented and combative. Initial measures include all of the following EXCEPT

(A) large bore intravenous access.

(B) arterial blood gas.

(C) digital rectal exam.

(D) peritoneal lavage.

(E) endotracheal intubation.

137 Which one of the following is NOT true of radiation injury?

(A) Single-strand breaks and base alterations result from low linear energy transfer radiation.

(B) Large doses of radiation may produce direct cell death due to membrane or cytoplasmic structural damage.

(C) Free radicals generated by ionizing radiation are primarily responsible for DNA and chromosomal alterations.

(D) Chromosomal breaks, with rearrangements associated with loss of chromosomal mass, may cause cell death at the first postradiation mitotic divisions.

(E) Repair of radiation-induced DNA and chromosomal damage is directly related to the rate at which the radiation is absorbed.

Questions 138-145 refer to the following:

A 23-year-old woman, with a history of gonorrhea five years previously, presents to your emergency room with two days of suprapubic pain that has been gradually worsening, now to the point of severe abdominal discomfort. Her last bowel movement was yesterday and she denies any emesis, although she has had some nausea. Her past medical history has been essentially unremarkable except for the gonorrhea five years previously. She has never been pregnant. She denies any surgical history of medications. She is currently sexually active, and her last menstrual period was seven weeks prior to admission. On physical examination, the patient is an ill-appearing female in distress, but lying still. She is tachycardiac to 120 and has a blood pressure of 90/60. She is afebrile and she has a respiratory rate of 30. Her lungs are clear and her cardiac exam is without murmurs or gallops. Her abdominal exam reveals no bowel sounds and diffuse guarding. She has significant rebound tenderness on examination.

138. Appropriate initial testing should include all of the following EXCEPT

(A) urine hCG.

(B) complete blood count.

(C) type and cross.

(D) pelvic examination.

(E) right upper quadrant ultrasound.

139. Her abdominal examination is concerning for

(A) acute peritonitis.

(B) ischemic bowel disease.

(C) small bowel obstruction.

(D) biliary colic.

(E) nephrolithiasis.

140. Testing is done and lab tests reveal a positive urine hCG and a normal right upper quadrant ultrasound. The complete blood count reveals a white blood count of 20,000 and a

hematocrit of 23%. The pelvic examination reveals cervical motion tenderness and focal tenderness over the right adnexa; no masses are noted. The most appropriate test to confirm the diagnosis is

(A) abdominal CT.

(B) transvaginal ultrasound.

(C) laparoscopy.

(D) culdocentesis.

(E) laparotomy.

141. Appropriate testing confirms the diagnosis of ruptured ectopic pregnancy. Appropriate treatment is

(A) immediate laparotomy.

(B) medical treatment.

(C) close observation with intravenous fluids.

(D) intravenous antibiotics.

(E) None of the above.

142. If the patient above had NOT had a ruptured ectopic pregnancy, a possible medication that could induce evacuation of the ectopic pregnancy is

(A) prolactin.

(B) vasopressin.

(C) beta-blockers.

(D) methotrexate.

(E) corticosteroids.

143. Which one of the following statements is true regarding treatment with RhoGAM?

(A) All patients with an ectopic pregnancy should receive RhoGAM.

(B) Only patients who are treated with laparotomy should receive RhoGAM.

(C) Only patient who are treated with medications should receive RhoGAM.

(D) All Rh-negative women with an ectopic pregnancy should receive RhoGAM.

(E) All Rh-positive women with an ectopic pregnancy should receive RhoGAM.

144. Risk factors for ectopic pregnancy include all of the following EXCEPT

(A) history of pelvic inflammatory disease.

(B) history of intrauterine device for contraception.

(C) prolonged infertility.

(D) more than one therapeutic abortion.

(E) previous history of ectopic pregnancy.

145. The patient asks you what her chances are of having another ectopic pregnancy. You tell her that

(A) it is not known what the reoccurrence rate is because the incidence of ectopic pregnancies is so low.

(B) history of an ectopic pregnancy does not increase the chance of having another ectopic pregnancy.

(C) history of an ectopic pregnancy increases the chance of having another ectopic pregnancy by five percent.

(D) history of an ectopic pregnancy increases the chance of having another ectopic pregnancy by 25%.

(E) history of an ectopic pregnancy makes it nearly impossible to have a subsequent normal pregnancy.

146. A 29-year-old woman stumbles into the emergency room where you work as a resident on-duty. Her pulse is 90 beats/min, her

blood pressure is 160, and she is diaphoretic. She is tremulous and is having difficulties relating a history. She believes your chair is a ghost in the room. In response to your questioning on her drinking habits, she admits to being a social drinker for over ten years. She also complains of sleeplessness in the past three days. The most appropriate follow-up treatment of this patient would be which one of the following?

- (A) Referral to a psychiatrist

- (B) Referral to a social worker

- (C) Obtaining a complete history and physical examination with emphasis on liver, GI, and neurologic functioning

- (D) Imipramine PO

147. An elderly, confused man has been brought to the emergency room by someone who has left without speaking to the staff. The patient is disheveled, smells of alcohol, and has a flat-footed gait. He can give you no useful medical history but says he has met you recently at Joe's, a bar down the street. Your working diagnosis is

- (A) Alzheimer's disease.

- (B) Wernicke-Korsakoff syndrome.

- (C) meningitis.

- (D) brain tumor.

- (E) schizophrenia.

148. A 46-year-old female comes to the emergency room complaining of right upper quadrant discomfort for the past several weeks, associated with mild nausea and worse at night. Physical examination reveals mild right upper quadrant tenderness. You order an ultrasound exam, which reveals gallstones. Which one of the following is the most likely composition of this patient's gallstones?

- (A) Pigment

- (B) Cholesterol

- (C) Calcium

- (D) Phospholipid

- (E) None of the above.

149. A 16-year-old woman presents to your office with bilateral eye irritation. She's noted that for three days, she's had red eyes that are watery and pruritic. On physical examination, you note a mild conjunctivitis with watery discharge. Of the following possible findings on physical examination, which one would classically be consistent with viral conjunctivitis?

- (A) Preauricular adenopathy

- (B) Anterior cervical adenopathy

- (C) Absence of an upper respiratory infection

- (D) Erythema in the posterior pharynx

- (E) Otorrhea

150. Which one of the following is NOT true of chromosomal abnormalities?

- (A) Chromosome deletion results in an abnormal number of chromosomes.

- (B) In uniparenteral disomy, both chromosomes, either totally or partially, are inherited from a single parent.

- (C) Prader-Willi syndrome is an example of genomic imprinting.

- (D) A Barr body results from lyonization.

- (E) Some rare X-linked dominant disorders occur only in heterozygous females.

151. A 67-year-old male, previously adequately treated for pulmonary tuberculosis, was admitted for evaluation of persistent hemoptysis, associated with cough, dyspnea, and fatigue. He denied fever or recent weight loss.

Lobectomy was performed, based on the results of computed tomographic studies of the chest, shown in Panel A. Your pre-operative diagnosis, confirmed by the methenamine-stained tissue section, shown in Panel B, was

    (A)   recurrent pulmonary tuberculosis.

    (B)   multidrug resistant pulmonary tuberculosis.

Panel A

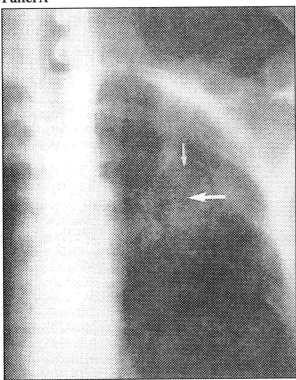

Panel B

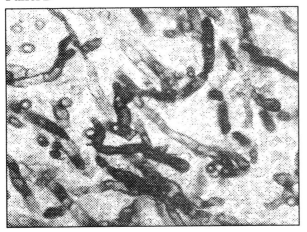

    (C)   pulmonary aspergilloma.

    (D)   mycetoma.

    (E)   pulmonary candidiasis.

152. In most states, in order to be committed to a psychiatric ward, it is necessary

    (A)   to go to court to prove the patient is insane.

    (B)   get a psychiatrist to sign a paper.

    (C)   get a minimum of two other physicians, one of whom is a psychiatrist, besides the attending to agree that the patient is mentally ill.

    (D)   to call the police.

    (E)   to give the patient a trial of a psychotropic agent.

Questions 153-160 refer to the following:

A 40-year-old woman presents to the emergency room with a painful right calf for three days. She denies any medical illnesses and is taking only oral contraceptives. She denies alcohol usage or illicit drugs, but smokes one pack each day. She denies any shortness of breath, chest pain, nausea, vomiting, fevers, or chills.

153. All of the following are risk factors for deep venous thrombosis EXCEPT

    (A)   oral contraceptives.

    (B)   ovarian cancer.

    (C)   immobility.

    (D)   recent trauma.

    (E)   All of the above are potential risk factors.

154. All of the following are risk factors for hypercoagulability EXCEPT

    (A)   protein C deficiency.

    (B)   protein S deficiency.

    (C)   anti-thrombin III deficiency.

    (D)   lupus anti-coagulant deficiency.

(E) elevated anti-phospholipid levels.

155. On physical examination, you note that her right calf is swollen compared to the left side. She also has calf tenderness to palpation on the right side. Pain in the calf with flexion of the ankle is called

(A) Courvoisier's sign.

(B) Murphy's sign.

(C) Tinel's sign.

(D) Homan's sign.

(E) None of the above.

156. Which one of the following is correct regarding the accuracy of the clinical test above?

(A) It's generally about 50% sensitive and 50% specific.

(B) It's very specific but not very sensitive.

(C) It's very sensitive but not very specific.

(D) It's very sensitive and very specific.

(E) None of the above are true.

157. Of the following, the gold standard test to diagnose a deep venous thrombosis is

(A) venogram.

(B) lymphangiogram.

(C) duplex scanning.

(D) ultrasound Doppler.

(E) physical examination.

158. With appropriate testing, the diagnosis of a deep venous thrombosis is made. Which one of the following statements is correct regarding anticoagulation?

(A) Anticoagulation therapy should be continued indefinitely.

(B) Anticoagulation therapy should be continued for six months.

(C) Anticoagulation therapy should

be continued for six weeks.

(D) Anticoagulation therapy should be continued during the hospital course.

(E) Anticoagulation therapy should be continued only if the patient has symptoms of a pulmonary embolism.

159. If, on hospital day two, while on anticoagulation, the patient has a large lower gastrointestinal bleed, what would be the next appropriate intervention?

(A) Stop anticoagulation and discharge to home.

(B) Stop anticoagulation and place an inferior vena cava filter.

(C) Stop anticoagulation and place an inferior vena cava filter only if the patient has symptoms of a pulmonary embolism.

(D) Continue anticoagulation and place an inferior vena cava filter.

(E) Continue anticoagulation and discharge to home.

160. The patient is treated appropriately for her deep venous thrombosis. What can you tell her regarding the possibilities of reoccurrence of deep venous thrombi?

(A) Because she has already been treated, she will not likely get another deep venous thrombosis.

(B) Her chances of getting a deep venous thrombosis are the same as the general population.

(C) Her chances of getting a deep venous thrombosis are approximately 30% greater because of her history of deep venous thrombi.

(D) Her chances of getting a deep venous thrombosis are approximately 75% greater because of her history of deep venous thrombi.

(E) None of the above are true.

161. A 52-year-old white male presents to the emergency room with symptoms of progressive unilateral ptosis and diplopia at the end of the day for the last few months. He also states that after walking for a few blocks, his legs become weaker and weaker. There is no atrophy in any of the limbs. All of the following can be used in the initial work-up of this patient EXCEPT

   (A) serum anticholinesterase receptor antibody.

   (B) electromyography.

   (C) edrophonium chloride testing.

   (D) CT of the anterior mediastinum.

   (E) oral pyridostigmine testing.

162. A 60-year-old man who is post-myocardial infarction day number three is noted to have a wide complex tachycardia on the monitor. Upon reaching his bed, he is not responsive and he does not have a pulse. Chest compressions are begun and the airway is secured. The most appropriate initial intervention is

   (A) intravenous adenosine.

   (B) intravenous lidocaine.

   (C) intravenous amiodarone.

   (D) intravenous adenosine.

   (E) electrical cardioversion.

163. You see a patient in the emergency room and perform a Gram stain. All of the following are Gram-positive rods EXCEPT

   (A) *Corynebacterium.*

   (B) *Bacillus.*

   (C) *Listeria.*

   (D) *Clostridium.*

   (E) *Neisseria.*

For Questions 164-167 you want to perform a pulmonary function test on your 65-year-old male patient with COPD. Match the descriptions with the following terms.

   (A) Tidal volume

   (B) Total lung capacity

   (C) Residual volume

   (D) Vital capacity

   (E) Forced vital capacity

164. The volume of air remaining in the lungs at the end of a maximal exhalation

165. The volume of air in the lungs after maximal inspiration

166. The volume of air moved during normal, quiet respiration

167. Maximum volume of air that can be forcibly exhaled after a full inspiration

168. A 40-year-old man comes to your office asking for help in quitting smoking. He has smoked for 20 years and is smoking two packs per day. The most correct statement regarding smoking cessation is

   (A) the success of smoking cessation depends only on nicotine replacement.

   (B) the success of smoking cessation depends on behavior modification with reinforcement.

   (C) if a patient can't quit the first time, he'll never quit.

   (D) nicotine patches with behavior modification have a 90% success rate in smoking cessation.

   (E) None of the above.

169. All of the following can cause secondary amenorrhea EXCEPT

   (A) pregnancy.

   (B) prolonged, intense exercise.

   (C) hypothyroidism.

   (D) hyperprolactinemia.

(E) diabetes insipidus.

170. A 21-year-old man was involved in a motor vehicle accident. He was not wearing his seat belt. On physical exam, he had ecchymosis of the left external ear, blue-gray discoloration behind the mastoid process (Battle's sign), and bilateral peri-orbital ecchymosis (raccoon eyes). He also had unilateral hearing loss and anosmia. What type of injury did he suffer from?

(A) Frontal sinus fracture

(B) Nasal fracture

(C) Orbital floor (blow-out) fracture

(D) Basilar skull fracture

(E) Transverse fracture

171. You are called about a patient with a potassium of 6.5 mmol/L. All of the following will raise a serum potassium EXCEPT

(A) diuretics.

(B) Addison's disease.

(C) hemolysis of specimen.

(D) acidosis.

(E) renal failure.

172. A 63-year-old male requests an appointment today for evaluation of increasingly severe back pain. He was compliant with the medical regimen you recently prescribed for treatment of his urinary tract infection. His fever has decreased. Examination shows tenderness to percussion over the thoracic spine, with spasm of the paraspinal muscles. X-rays suggest irregular erosions of the end plates at T8 and T9. To further evaluate this lesion, an unenhanced computed axial tomographic scan of the spine, shown in the figure, was performed. You now begin treatment for

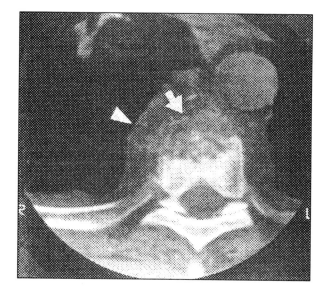

(A) Gaucher's disease.

(B) pathologic fracture secondary to multiple myeloma.

(C) osteoporotic fracture.

(D) metastatic prostate cancer.

(E) vertebral osteomyelitis.

173. Which one of the following is a midline cervical cyst?

(A) Hygroma

(B) Branchial cyst

(C) Thyroglossal cyst

(D) Zenker's diverticulum

(E) Laryngocele

174. A 42-year-old male presents with arthralgias, lower extremity rash, and abdominal pain associated with bloody diarrhea that is worse after eating meals. On examination, he has palpable purpura on both lower extremities and buttocks, and his stool guaiac test is positive. Urine analysis reveals both proteinuria and hematuria. Biopsy of the kidneys and immunoflourescent staining revealed IgA deposits in the glomeruli. What is the correct diagnosis?

(A) Henoch-Schonlein purpura

(B) Essential mixed cryoglobinemia

(C) Thrombotic thrombocytopenic purpura

(D)   Waldenstrom's hyperglobuli-
      nemic purpura

(E)   Systemic lupus erythematosus

175. Treatment of acute pancreatitis in a patient
      that is euglycemic and hypocalcemic may
      include all of the following EXCEPT

      (A)   volume replacement.

      (B)   narcotics.

      (C)   nasogastric suction.

      (D)   insulin.

      (E)   calcium.

176. In the following figures, you are reviewing a
      small bowel biopsy with the hospital pa-
      thologist. You report that the patient is a 42-
      year-old male with a 25-pound weight loss
      over the past two to three months. He has as-
      sociated diarrhea, steatorrhea, abdominal
      pain, and arthralgias. Your diagnosis is

Panel A

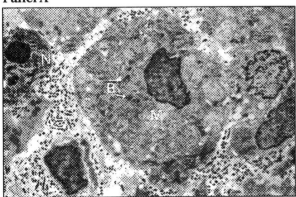

Panel B

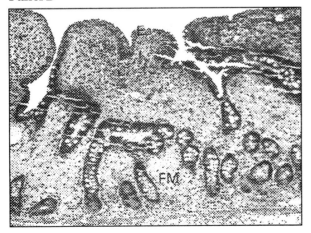

Panel C

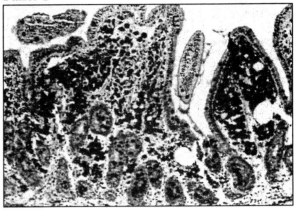

      (A)   intestinal lymphoma.

      (B)   amyloidosis.

      (C)   Whipple's disease.

      (D)   regional enteritis.

      (E)   eosinophilic enteritis.

177. A 25-year-old female presents to your office
      with profuse menstrual bleeding. This con-
      dition is known as

      (A)   menarche.

      (B)   menorrhagia.

      (C)   metrorrhagia.

      (D)   amenorrhea.

      (E)   dysmenorrhea.

178. Which one of the following is NOT true of
      the anion gap?

      (A)   It is calculated by subtracting the
            sum of the serum chloride and
            bicarbonate from the serum
            sodium.

      (B)   It may be decreased in multiple
            myeloma.

      (C)   It is increased in renal failure due
            to retention of sulfates and
            phosphates.

      (D)   Albumin and other proteins
            usually account for half of it.

      (E)   It is usually more than 25 mEq/L.

179. Your diabetic patient is scheduled for surgery and has been NPO. She normally receives 20 units of insulin in the morning. The morning of surgery she should receive

    (A)   no insulin.

    (B)   5 units.

    (C)   10 units.

    (D)   20 units.

    (E)   40 units.

180. You have seen a patient several times in the ER because of depression. His employer calls you a few weeks later and asks you what you have treated him for. You

    (A)   tell the employer.

    (B)   inform the employer that you cannot discuss the patient with him without the patient's permission via a signed release of information.

    (C)   tell the employer you must call the patient first.

    (D)   tell the employer you have never seen the patient.

    (E)   tell the employer he is immoral for calling you.

USMLE STEP 3 PRACTICE TEST 1

Day One – Afternoon Session

(Answer sheets appear in the back of this book.)

TIME: 3 Hours
180 Questions

DIRECTIONS: Each of the following numbered items or incomplete sentences is followed by an answer or a completion of the statement. Choose the **ONE** choice that **BEST** answers the question or completes the sentence.

Questions 1-4 refer to the following:

A 30-year-old woman presents to the emergency room with three weeks of galactorrhea. She is otherwise healthy and is not taking any medications. On physical examination, she has a slight decrease in vision in her temporal fields bilaterally. Otherwise, physical examination is without abnormalities. Her urine hCG is negative.

1. The most likely pathologic etiology of the patient's symptoms is

   (A) prolactin-secreting microadenoma.

   (B) surreptitious medications.

   (C) pregnancy.

   (D) macroadenoma.

   (E) breast cancer.

2. Initial appropriate treatment would be

   (A) surgery.

   (B) chemotherapy.

   (C) bromocriptine.

   (D) prochlorperazine.

   (E) radiation therapy.

3. Of the following statements regarding appropriate treatment, which one is correct?

   (A) Treatment should be continued indefinitely.

   (B) Treatment should be continued until prolactin levels return to normal.

   (C) Treatment should be continued until there is no further galactorrhea.

   (D) Treatment should be continued for six weeks.

   (E) None of the above.

4. Which one of the following statements is true regarding the association of prolactin-secreting macroadenomas in women?

   (A) They will induce infertility.

   (B) They will make a woman more fertile.

   (C) They can enlarge during pregnancy.

(D) They can shrink during pregnancy.

(E) Surgical resection is not necessary in women who will become pregnant.

Questions 5-8 refer to the following:

A 45-year-old black female presents to the clinic with complaints of difficulty getting up from a chair, climbing stairs, and combing her hair. She has been slowly getting weaker, with morning stiffness and fatigue. The patient has a normal neurological examination with decreased deep-tendon reflexes secondary to motor weakness. The ESR is 27 mm/hR.

5. All of the following are criteria used to define this disorder EXCEPT

(A) electromyographic changes consistent with inflammatory myopathy.

(B) symmetric weakness of limb girdle muscles and anterior neck flexors.

(C) elevation of creatinine phosphokinase levels.

(D) elevation of titers of anticentromere antibody.

(E) muscle biopsy evidence of an inflammatory exudate.

6. Two weeks later, this patient developed periorbital edema, raised and scaly patches over the knuckles, and a violaceous rash over the upper eyelids. Which one of the following is associated with this disorder?

(A) Breast and lung cancers

(B) Intracranial hemorrhages

(C) Type II diabetes mellitus

(D) Pneumonia

(E) Leukemia

7. All of the following are treatment options for this syndrome EXCEPT

(A) steroids.

(B) physical therapy.

(C) immunosuppressive agents.

(D) antacids.

(E) D-penicillamine.

8. All of the following statements regarding overall prognosis of this disease are correct EXCEPT

(A) patients with associated pulmonary, cardiac, and gastrointestinal involvement have a poor prognosis.

(B) children have the best prognosis.

(C) patients with inclusion body myositis usually improve.

(D) patients with Jo-l antibodies do not respond well to therapy.

(E) the overall five-year survival rate is approximately 80%.

9. A 25-year-old male was brought to the emergency room by paramedics because of smoke inhalation. He is unconscious and his lips and nail beds are cherry-red. His carboxyhemoglobin level is sixty percent. Later on, lung auscultation revealed ronchi, and this patient was diagnosed with respiratory failure. What would be the most immediate intervention?

(A) Hyperbaric oxygen therapy

(B) One hundred percent oxygenation via a non-rebreather venti-mask

(C) Indirect laryngoscopy

(D) Intubation and ventilation with one hundred percent oxygen

(E) Diuretic therapy

10. Concerning BCG vaccine, all of the following statements are false EXCEPT

(A) BCG vaccine is not FDA approved and, therefore, it is not used in the United States.

(B) it may be considered for infants and children with positive PPD if they have had continuous exposure to persons with active TB and cannot tolerate INH therapy.

(C) BCG vaccine is contraindicated in persons with symptomatic HIV infection.

(D) if combined with BCG vaccine, INH loses its hepatotoxicity.

(E) All of the above statements are false.

11. A glomus tumor is

(A) found within the neck.

(B) found beneath the nail.

(C) black or dark brown.

(D) non-tender.

(E) highly malignant.

Questions 12 and 13 refer to the following:

Your 72-year-old male patient with chronic obstructive pulmonary disease (COPD) comes to your office for a routine office visit. He notes an increased production of mucus and worse cough. You decide to order a chest X-ray.

12. All of the following are radiographic findings commonly associated with COPD EXCEPT

(A) diaphragmatic depression.

(B) diaphragmatic testing.

(C) increased AP diameter.

(D) large bullae.

(E) pleural-based densities.

13. All of the following are disorders that may lead to radiographic findings associated with obstructive lung disease EXCEPT

(A) cystic fibrosis.

(B) alpha 1 antitrypsin deficiency.

(C) second-hand smoke exposure.

(D) asthma.

(E) Goodpasture's syndrome.

14. A healthy 38-year-old woman presents to your office for a routine check-up. She denies any complaints and is not on any medications. Her physical examination is unremarkable. Screening laboratory tests reveal a slightly elevated hypercalcemia at 10.8 mg/dl. The most likely diagnosis causing her hypercalcemia is

(A) sarcoidosis.

(B) hypercalcemia of malignancy.

(C) primary hyperparathyroidism.

(D) iatrogenic.

(E) None of the above.

Questions 15-18 refer to the following:

An attractive 24-year-old woman has come to the emergency room several times during your shift complaining of bronchitis. Each time you (a male) find very minimal, if any, abnormal physical findings.

15. On this visit, she has no abnormalities and is asking you if you are married or "seeing someone." You should

(A) ask her out.

(B) tell her you are single even though you are married.

(C) gently tell her this is irrelevant to her care.

(D) tell her you are married but separated.

(E) tell her you are divorced.

16. She tells you she does not really care about your marital status, but a friend of hers is having a party Saturday night and she wants you to go with her. You tell her

(A) you are busy.

(B) it would be inappropriate for you to date a patient.

(C) you would love to.

(D)   you would rather go to dinner with her.

(E)   your wife will not let you.

17.   She is disappointed. On her next visit to the emergency room, again during your shift, she complains of a vaginal discharge. You should

(A)   do a pelvic exam.

(B)   tell her you know nothing is wrong with her.

(C)   ask her to leave you alone.

(D)   ask one of your colleagues to see her instead of you.

(E)   ask the nurses to tell her you are not in the ER.

18.   If the patient came in with an acute pelvic problem and you were the only physician in the ER at the time, you should

(A)   do a pelvic exam.

(B)   refuse to treat her.

(C)   do a pelvic exam only in the presence of a nurse.

(D)   send her to another hospital.

(E)   admit her.

Questions 19-26 refer to the following:

A 25-year-old man comes to your clinic for the first time complaining of cough, weight loss, and fatigue. He has not felt well for several months. He denies any unusual exposures.

19.   All of the following diagnoses are likely in this patient EXCEPT

(A)   tuberculosis.

(B)   AIDS.

(C)   histoplasmosis.

(D)   osteogenesis imperfecta.

(E)   coxsackievirus.

20.   Which one of the following conditions, if diagnosed in this patient, would have to be reported to the State Board of Health?

(A)   Lung cancer

(B)   Histoplasmosis

(C)   Tuberculosis

(D)   Sarcoidosis

(E)   Systemic lupus erythematosus

21.   You need the patient's signed informed consent for which one of the following procedures?

(A)   Sputum culture

(B)   Urethral culture

(C)   Throat culture

(D)   HIV test

(E)   ASO titer

22.   The patient's chest radiograph shows a hazy infiltrate in the left upper lobe and a few calcified hilar nodes. The patient has some mild hemoptysis. The next test(s) you order should be

(A)   blood cultures.

(B)   sputum culture.

(C)   urinalysis.

(D)   Lyme titer.

(E)   ASO titer.

23.   You describe a PPD test to the patient and he denies having ever had one. You place

(A)   a PPD test and control antigen skin tests.

(B)   a PPD.

(C)   a concentrated PPD.

(D)   histoplasmin skin test.

(E)   *Candida* antigen.

24.   The patient's PPD is positive. You should

(A)   begin appropriate antibiotic treatment.

(B) withhold treatment until cultures are back.

(C) call in his family and treat them.

(D) call in his family and test them.

(E) watch him for worsening of his condition.

25. You also must

(A) inform all of the patient's contacts.

(B) inform the Health Department.

(C) call the police.

(D) quarantine the patient on a special isolation ward.

(E) send the patient to a sanatorium.

26. It is very important to

(A) warn the patient to stay away from everyone for three weeks.

(B) warn the patient to stay in his home for a month.

(C) explain the disease, the need for and duration of treatment, and complications that can result from noncompliance.

(D) give a face mask to all of the patient's contacts.

(E) notify the patient's next-of-kin.

Questions 27-30 refer to the following:

A 38-year-old woman presents to your office for the first time with the concern that she may have diabetes mellitus. She tells you that over that past four months, she's noted polyuria and polydipsia. She denies any other medical problems and is not taking any medications. She notes that she has a strong family history of adult-onset diabetes mellitus. Physical examination reveals a blood pressure of 150/95, heart rate of 70, temperature of 98.5°F, and a respiratory rate of 14 in a slightly obese female. Physical examination otherwise is unremarkable.

27. The simplest way to diagnose diabetes mellitus in this patient would be to

(A) find that a random plasma glucose level is greater than 160 mg/dl.

(B) find that a fasting plasma glucose level is greater than 100.

(C) find that urinalysis reveals glucose.

(D) find that urinalysis reveals protein.

(E) find that a hemoglobin A1C is greater than 10%.

28. By laboratory examination, you diagnose diabetes mellitus. Other pertinent laboratory findings reveal that the serum creatinine is 2.7, serum potassium is 4.0, and the urinalysis reveals trace protein. Of the following, initial treatment would appropriately be

(A) dietary therapy.

(B) oral sulfonylureas.

(C) oral metformin.

(D) insulin therapy.

(E) insulin pump.

29. Of the following statements regarding metformin for type II diabetes mellitus, which one is true?

(A) Metformin can be used, but not with an oral sulfonylurea.

(B) Metformin can be used, but not if the patient has G6PD deficiency.

(C) Metformin can be used, but not if the patient has chronic renal insufficiency.

(D) Metformin can be used, but not if the patient is obese.

(E) Metformin is safe for any patient with type II diabetes mellitus.

30. Appropriate screening and preventive care for patients with type II diabetes mellitus include all of the following EXCEPT

    (A) bi-yearly exercise treadmill tests.

    (B) yearly urinalysis testing for microscopic proteinuria.

    (C) yearly ophthalmology follow-up.

    (D) immunization with pneumococcal vaccine.

    (E) close attention to the feet for ulcers and sores.

31. A 19-year-old primigravida presents at 12 weeks of gestation for a well-care examination. Obstetrical screening of this pregnant woman at this time should include all of the following EXCEPT

    (A) complete blood count.

    (B) blood group.

    (C) Rh factor.

    (D) alpha-fetoprotein.

    (E) HBV.

Questions 32–39 refer to the following:

You are notified that a 29-year-old woman is experiencing severe hemorrhage immediately after delivery of a baby. Medical records of the patient show that a C-section was performed and the surgery was uneventful. A regional, T4 level of anesthesia was obtained via the epidural catheter.

32. Considering the case cited, what are some of the conditions that should be included in your differential diagnosis?

    (A) Retained products of conception and placenta accreta

    (B) Inverted uterus and coagulopathy

    (C) Uterine atony and cervical lacerations

    (D) Preeclampsia and vaginal laceration

    (E) All of the above should be included in the differential diagnosis of this patient's condition.

33. Which one of the following is NOT a risk factor for uterine atony?

    (A) Multiple births

    (B) Multiple gestation

    (C) Multiparity

    (D) Prolonged labor

    (E) Oligohydramnios

34. You quickly diagnose uterine atony and start the treatment. Your management includes massaging the uterus through the abdominal wall and vagina, IV oxytocin, IM ergot derivatives, and prostaglandin F2-alpha directly into the uterus to increase myometrial tone and the force of contractions. Although bleeding is somewhat reduced in intensity, it has not stopped. If your suspicion of retained placenta is confirmed, which one of the following actions should you consider as your next step in the management of this patient?

    (A) Increasing the force of massage will help the retained placental tissues to separate.

    (B) Continuing infusion of IV oxytocin

    (C) Continuing infusion of IV ergot derivatives

    (D) Manually removing the placenta

    (E) None of the above.

35. Your clinical suspicion of retained placenta is not confirmed on ultrasonography. Consulting your colleagues brings you to the original diagnosis of uterine atony. All of the following procedures can be choices in managing uncontrolled uterine atony EXCEPT

    (A) manual removal of the placenta.

    (B) hypogastric artery ligation.

    (C) hysterectomy.

    (D) pelvic artery embolization.

    (E) (A) and (C).

36. Techniques that are available to the mother for pain relief during labor include

    (A) systemic narcotics.

    (B) inhalation analgesia.

    (C) epidural anesthesia.

    (D) hypnosis.

    (E) All of the above.

37. Considering the anesthesia that has been used to achieve surgical analgesia during the caesarean section, which one of the following statements is correct?

    (A) Epidural anesthesia is rarely used for anesthesia during a C-section.

    (B) Conduction anesthesia permits the mother to remain awake during delivery.

    (C) There are many contraindications to regional anesthesia.

    (D) Spinal anesthesia is technically more difficult to perform than epidural anesthesia.

    (E) Epidural anesthesia is technically easier to perform than spinal anesthesia.

38. The patient's bleeding is now controlled; however, she complains of severe headache. Concerning the headache in this patient, which one of the following statements is INCORRECT?

    (A) It results from decreased amount of fluid available to cushion the brain secondary to persistent leakage of CSF.

    (B) Headache follows 15-20 minutes after discontinuing the anesthesia.

    (C) The headache is classically located over the occipital or frontal regions.

    (D) The headache improves in the supine position and exacerbates in the erect position.

    (E) Noninvasive therapy includes mild analgesics, hydration, and caffeine.

39. Regarding advantages and disadvantages of general anesthesia over regional anesthesia for a caesarean section, which one of the following statements is NOT true?

    (A) The preoperative preparatory time is shorter in general anesthesia.

    (B) Coagulopathy that is common in regional anesthesia is rare in general anesthesia.

    (C) Maternal aspiration and neonatal depression are the disadvantages of the general anesthesia.

    (D) General anesthesia may delay maternal bonding.

    (E) (A) and (D).

Questions 40-43 refer to the following:

You are conducting a clinical trial for a pharmaceutical company for which you receive a grant of $5,000 per patient who completes the protocol. The protocol takes four months. During it, at least one-third of the patients receive a placebo medicine. Per study protocol, you cannot give them anything except propoxyphene for the pain they may experience during the study. If a patient cannot tolerate the pain, he or she must drop out of the study so a definitive treatment can be administered.

40. Mrs. Jones is a 55-year-old woman whom you have been seeing as a patient for many years. She has stayed with the protocol for two months, but is now very uncomfortable. She wants you to give her something for her pain. You tell her

    (A) if she does not finish the study you will not treat her any more.

    (B) she may leave the study and you will give her appropriate medicine for her pain.

(C) she can take some codeine occasionally as long as she does not tell anyone.

(D) she cannot leave the study and must bear the discomfort.

(E) you will pay her extra if she stays on the study for the entire four months.

41. You meet one of your colleagues at a meeting and you learn that he is also conducting the same study in his patients. You tell him about your frustrations with the study because of patients like Mrs. Jones. He tells you he routinely gives these patients codeine if they are having pain and just does not record it in his chart or tell the pharmaceutical company. You

(A) decide to do the same thing.

(B) tell him he is dishonest.

(C) explain to him that this is not proper management and he should not do it.

(D) send your potential "drop-outs" to him.

(E) tell everyone you know how dishonest he is.

42. You had originally told the pharmaceutical company you would be able to get ten patients into the study. The study is about to end, and you have only recruited seven. You

(A) make up three other patients so you can get the maximum money.

(B) make up one more patient.

(C) use a patient who dropped out of the study.

(D) tell the company you could only find seven patients.

(E) tell the company your recruiting nurse was sick and you need more time.

43. One of your patients has had an episode of chest pain during the study. This is considered

(A) an adverse event and should be reported to the Institutional Review Board and the company.

(B) an incidental occurrence.

(C) an adverse event that does not need to be reported.

(D) insignificant.

(E) something that you do not document in the chart.

44. A 53-year-old woman with a bleeding peptic ulcer has been admitted to your service. Her hemoglobin is 6, down from a documented baseline of 12. She is known to be a Jehovah's Witness. You want to transfuse her because you think this is a life-threatening situation. You

(A) transfuse her despite her requests to the contrary.

(B) call the Ethics Committee for a consult.

(C) discuss the situation with her and then honor her decision.

(D) try to get a court injunction to transfuse her.

(E) try to get her declared mentally incompetent so you can transfuse her.

45. Swelling and tenderness behind the tissues of the ear is diagnostic of

(A) sinusitis.

(B) otitis externa.

(C) mastoiditis.

(D) folliculitis.

(E) basilar skull fracture.

46. A 72-year-old male with a urinary tract infection was admitted to your service four nights ago. He was treated with antibiotics and defervesced. Tonight, the nurse calls you to

tell you the patient has a fever of 38°C, feels uncomfortable, but has no other physical findings. You decide to

    (A)   stop the antibiotics because he is probably having a drug reaction.

    (B)   change the antibiotics empirically.

    (C)   draw blood cultures and send off another urine sample for culture.

    (D)   do nothing because it is probably just residual to his infection.

    (E)   get an emergency infectious diseases consultation.

47.   A 34-year-old man was admitted to you in the afternoon because of significant hypertension and tachycardia. He denied any relevant medical history. You have given him antihypertensive agents and his blood pressure has become normal but he is still tachycardiac. You are called to see him at 8 p.m. because he is agitated. He does not remember you and he is yelling at the nurses. His pulse is now 140 and his blood pressure is elevated again to 170/110. You suspect that the patient

    (A)   has presenile dementia.

    (B)   is withdrawing from alcohol.

    (C)   has schizophrenia.

    (D)   has meningitis.

    (E)   has thyrotoxicosis.

48.   A 53-year-old male is transferred to your service from the CCU after suffering an anterolateral myocardial infarction. He is doing well until a routine electrocardiogram demonstrates atrial fibrillation, which he has never had before. An echocardiogram suggests a mural thrombus. You decide to

    (A)   give him Tapazole.

    (B)   give him radioactive iodine.

    (C)   cardiovert him.

    (D)   begin anticoagulation.

    (E)   give him lidocaine.

49.   A 23-year-old sexually active female is admitted to your service with a painful swollen left knee. The knee discomfort started 24 hours earlier. She has a fever and a leukocytosis with a left shift. The most likely cause of her symptoms is

    (A)   gout.

    (B)   pseudogout.

    (C)   Reiter's syndrome.

    (D)   lupus.

    (E)   gonococcal arthritis.

50.   A 16-year-old with chronic asthma has been admitted to your service because of a severe asthma attack. He had been away from home in basketball camp for the last two weeks. His serum theophylline level is below therapeutic on admission. You stabilize him, getting his symptoms under control, and then

    (A)   you increase his theophylline dose.

    (B)   you suggest desensitization shots for allergies.

    (C)   you tell him not to exercise again.

    (D)   you ask him how frequently he has been taking theophylline while at camp.

    (E)   you order home oxygen for him.

51.   A 33-year-old woman presents with three weeks of galactorrhea and three months without menses. She denies any abdominal pain and denies sexual activity. She takes numerous medications for several different illnesses. Physical examination reveals galactorrhea and no abnormalities on pelvic examination. Of the following medications, the one most likely to cause her symptoms would be

    (A)   risperidone.

    (B)   insulin.

    (C)   alprazolam.

    (D)   nifedipine.

    (E)   None of the above.

Questions 52-54 refer to the following:

A 46-year-old truck driver is brought by ambulance to the emergency room because his wife complained that the patient was confused and subsequently called 911 for an ambulance. This patient had no prior past medical history and no known allergies or known drug abuse. In the emergency room, his serum calcium level was 15.4 mg/dl.

52. All of the following are clinical findings seen in hypercalcemia EXCEPT

   (A) polyuria.

   (B) fatigue.

   (C) diarrhea.

   (D) nausea.

   (E) lethargy.

53. Upon admission to the medical ward, further work-up revealed an elevated parathyroid hormone level. What would be the appropriate management of choice?

   (A) Biphosphonates

   (B) Calcitonin

   (C) Indomethacin

   (D) Surgical resection of the involved parathyroid tissue

   (E) Low-dose prednisone

54. This patent's condition deteriorates rapidly and he falls into a stupor. His serum calcium level is repeated and found to be 16.2 mg/dl. What would be the immediate management of choice?

   (A) Perform an electrocardiogram

   (B) Intravenous insulin

   (C) Intravenous normal saline and subsequent furosemide

   (D) Hemodialysis

   (E) Mithramycin

Question 55 refers to the following:

A 70-year-old female smoker requests evaluation for an aching pain of the lower ex-

tremities, which is relieved by elevation and aggravated by dependency. Examination of the digits shows clubbing. There is tenderness to pressure applied over the affected area of the legs.

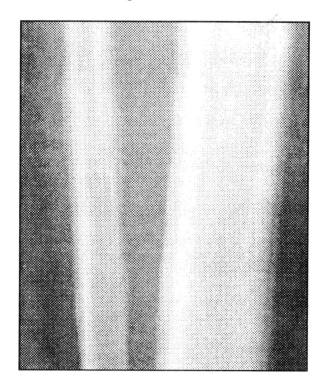

55. An X-ray of the tibia and fibula is shown in the figure above. You diagnose

   (A) osteomyelitis.

   (B) metastatic carcinoma.

   (C) osteomalacia.

   (D) hypertrophic osteoarthropathy.

   (E) Paget's disease.

56. Tuberculin skin testing of asymptomatic individuals is recommended for all EXCEPT

   (A) people newly arrived from third-world countries.

   (B) all family members of a symptomatic patient.

   (C) all individuals prior to their employment at health care facilities.

   (D) individuals prior to commencing their volunteer work at schools.

(E) individuals with a history of compromised immune system.

57. A 32-year-old gravida 1, para 0 black female comes to your office for a routine check-up at 25 weeks gestation. Her blood pressure is 180/110, and she has 3+ proteinuria on dipstick. You admit her to the hospital with a diagnosis of preeclampsia and for aggressive monitoring of maternal and fetal status. Which one of the following antihypertensive drugs is contraindicated in this patient?

(A) Hydralazine

(B) Labetalol

(C) Captopril

(D) Nifedipine

58. A 14-year-old boy is brought in by ambulance after being struck by a hit-and-run driver. He has multiple fractures and a concussion. You should

(A) call the police.

(B) refuse to treat him until his parents are found.

(C) try to find the driver.

(D) call the priest.

(E) look for witnesses.

Questions 59-62 refer to the following:

You refer your 18-year-old male patient to a urologist for evaluation of a possible hydrocele.

59. The most likely description of a hydrocele is

(A) tender testicular swelling.

(B) non-tender testicular swelling.

(C) tender penile swelling.

(D) non-tender penile swelling.

(E) None of the above.

60. Evaluation for the above would include all of the following EXCEPT

(A) inspection.

(B) palpation.

(C) transillumination.

(D) pinching.

(E) auscultation.

61. All of the following may be confused with hydrocele EXCEPT

(A) hematocele.

(B) chylocele.

(C) gumma.

(D) tuberculosis.

(E) orchitis.

62. Usually the epididymis is

(A) in front of the testis.

(B) behind the testis.

(C) on top of the testis.

(D) below the testis.

(E) None of the above.

Questions 63-66 refer to the following:

A 54-year-old white male with a long history of alcoholism presents with severe abdominal pain associated with nausea and vomiting. There was no history of trauma. On examination, he has abdominal distension with fever and mild ascites. Lab data reveals a serum amylase level of 400 U/L and lipase level of 250 U/L. His glucose level was 100 mg/dl, hematocrit was 43%, and he showed no evidence of jaundice.

63. The most likely diagnosis is

(A) pancreatic carcinoma.

(B) chronic pancreatitis.

(C) cholecystitis.

(D) acute pancreatitis.

(E) bowel perforation.

64. The most useful test to make the correct diagnosis would be

(A) laparoscopy.

(B) CT scan of the abdomen.

(C) ultrasound of the abdomen.

(D) X-rays of the abdomen.

(E) clinical examination.

65. What could be the most likely cause for this disorder?

(A) Biliary sludge

(B) Medications

(C) Alcoholism

(D) Gallstones

(E) Infection

66. How would the physician manage this patient?

(A) Intravenous antibiotics

(B) Oxygenation

(C) Morphine for pain

(D) Peritoneal lavage

(E) Nasogastric tube placement and hydration

67. A 58-year-old male smoker presents to the clinic suddenly with complaints of blood-tinged productive sputum on coughing and weight loss. He was found to have a temperature of 100.0°F and significant weight loss. There is no family history of cancer. What would be the next step in establishing the diagnosis?

(A) PPD skin test

(B) Culture of the sputum for acid-fast bacteria

(C) Chest X-ray

(D) Bronchoscopy

(E) Starting therapy for bronchitis and waiting to see if the patient's symptoms are alleviated

68. A 38-year-old black man with a history of sickle cell disease is hospitalized for sickle cell crisis. On hospital day number three, he becomes very short of breath and has a low-grade temperature of 101°F. He denies cough or sputum. Chest radiograph reveals bilat-

eral interstitial pulmonary infiltrates, and room air arterial blood gas reveals a pH of 7.48, a pCO_2 of 20, and a pO_2 of 58. The most likely diagnosis is

(A) pulmonary embolism.

(B) congestive heart failure.

(C) acute chest syndrome.

(D) bacterial pneumonia.

(E) fungal pneumonia.

Questions 69-75 refer to the following:

A 36-year-old woman with a history of diabetes presents to the hospital with fever and a decreasing level of consciousness for two days. She is difficult to arouse when you see her. Her family tells you that she was well until two days previously when she began to note fevers, and her family began to note that she became more and more somnolent. She has a history of diabetes mellitus, for which she is taking insulin. The family denies that she uses any illicit drugs, tobacco products, or ethanol. On physical examination, the patient is an obese female who is responsive only to deep sternal rub. She has a temperature of 103°F, heart rate of 110, blood pressure of 140/70, and a respiratory rate of 28. Pupils are equal and reactive to light, and the patient has a doll's eye reflex. Lungs are clear and cardiovascular exam is without murmurs or gallops. Abdominal exam reveals normoactive bowel sounds and no distension.

69. Appropriate initial interventions may include

(A) lumbar puncture.

(B) head computed tomography scan.

(C) blood cultures.

(D) urine cultures.

(E) All of the above.

70. Appropriate diagnostic interventions are done. Laboratory results show a white blood count of 24,000, a hematocrit of 39%, and a platelet count of 330,000. Her serum chem-

istries are all within normal limits except for a glucose level of 204. Lumbar puncture reveals 1,200 total cells, 1,100 of them nucleated (90% segmented neutrophils), and Gram stain with Gram-positive cocci in chains. Head CT shows no abnormalities. Chest radiograph shows a left lower lobe consolidated infiltrate. Urine and blood cultures are pending. Sputum shows numerous segmented neutrophils and Gram-positive cocci in chains. Of the following statements regarding the patient's cerebrospinal fluid, which one is correct?

(A) The studies are consistent with a bacterial meningitis, most likely *Streptococcus* pneumoniae.

(B) The studies are consistent with a bacterial meningitis, most likely *Neisseria meningitis.*

(C) The studies are consistent with a bacterial meningitis, most likely *Staphylococcus aureus.*

(D) The studies are consistent with an aseptic meningitis, most likely tuberculous meningitis.

(E) The studies are consistent with an aseptic meningitis, most likely viral meningitis.

71. Of the following statements regarding the association between the pneumonia and meningitis, which one is most likely correct?

(A) The patient most likely had a primary bacterial meningitis which then caused an aspiration pneumonia.

(B) The patient most likely had a primary bacterial meningitis which then spread by bacteremia to cause a focal pneumonia.

(C) The patient most likely had a primary bacterial pneumonia which then spread by bacteremia to cause meningitis.

(D) The patient most likely had a primary pulmonary tuberculosis which then spread by bacteremia to cause the meningitis.

(E) The two findings are independent of each other.

72. The most appropriate initial antibiotic regimen is

(A) intravenous vancomycin.

(B) intravenous ceftriaxone (third-generation cephalosporin).

(C) intravenous ampicillin.

(D) intravenous aminoglycosides.

(E) intravenous vancomycin and ceftriaxone.

73. 24 hours after beginning antibiotics, the patient begins to seize. She is intubated for airway protection and continues to seize. The most appropriate next intervention would be

(A) intravenous benzodiazepines.

(B) intravenous paralytics.

(C) intravenous phenytoin.

(D) intravenous pentobarbital.

(E) intravenous calcium.

74. The seizures stop after treatment. However, in spite of appropriate treatment, she continues to seize intermittently and continues to have high fevers to 105°F in spite of antipyretics and cooling blankets. You note that her CPK begins to rise steadily to 80,000 IU/L. Also, her serum creatinine rises and her urine output decreases. The most likely complication occurring now is

(A) dehydration causing pre-renal azotemia.

(B) renal artery stenosis causing pre-renal azotemia.

(C) rhabdomyolysis causing intrinsic acute renal failure.

(D) antibiotic-induced acute renal failure.

(E) post-renal obstruction.

75. Appropriate treatment for this includes all of the following EXCEPT

(A) aggressive hydration.

(B) intravenous infusion of sodium bicarbonate.

(C) intravenous mannitol.

(D) control of seizures.

(E) intravenous calcium.

Questions 76-79 refer to the following:

An 80-year-old man comes to your office with symptoms of exertional chest pain and shortness of breath. Physical examination reveals a midsystolic murmur. Chest X-ray and EKG suggest left ventricular hypertrophy. Echocardiogram reveals an elevated flow gradient across the aortic valve.

76. The most common cause of this disorder is

(A) rheumatic heart disease.

(B) arteriosclerotic degeneration.

(C) congenital bicuspid aortic valve.

(D) ankylosing spondylitis.

(E) syphilis.

77. The most useful method to assess the severity of this condition would be

(A) endomyocardial biopsy.

(B) thallium stress test.

(C) left-heart catheterization.

(D) Swan-Ganz catheterization.

(E) coronary arteriography.

78. All of the following are potential therapeutic options EXCEPT

(A) prosthetic valve replacement.

(B) porcine valve replacement.

(C) valvuloplasty.

(D) beta-blocker therapy.

79. Sublingual nitroglycerin therapy is not commonly used for the treatment of chest pain in patients with severe aortic stenosis because

(A) tachyphylaxis develops with use of this agent.

(B) the systemic vasodilatory effects associated with these agents will increase cardiac afterload.

(C) nitrate therapy is only effective in patients with coronary artery occlusion.

(D) it only aids the reduction in cardiac preload.

(E) oral nitrate therapy has a greater bioavailability.

Questions 80-83 refer to the following:

You are called by the nurse to evaluate a patient who is receiving a transfusion of packed RBCs. She is concerned that the patient is having a transfusion reaction.

80. All of the following are indications of a transfusion reaction EXCEPT

(A) back pain.

(B) fever.

(C) vomiting.

(D) hypotension.

(E) hemolysis.

81. Management of a hemolytic transfusion reaction include all of the following EXCEPT

(A) vigorous IV hydration.

(B) return blood to blood bank with new sample of patient's blood.

(C) monitor renal function.

(D) administration of O-negative blood.

(E) management of hyperkalemia.

82. All of the following blood-group antigens may trigger a hemolytic reaction EXCEPT

    (A) ABO.

    (B) Kell.

    (C) Duffy.

    (D) Lewis.

    (E) Rhesus.

83. Which one of the following statements is true regarding delayed hemolytic transfusion reactions?

    (A) Occurs more commonly in patients who have never been transfused previously

    (B) Occurs five to ten days after the transfusion

    (C) Alloantibody screen remains negative even at the time of the reaction

    (D) Is often associated with the transmission of hepatitis C

    (E) The diagnosis can be made by an elevated arterial blood ammonia level

84. A five-year-old white girl presents to the ER with a one-week history of arthritis, severe crampy abdominal pain, bloody diarrhea, hematuria, and a purpuric rash on the dorsal aspect of both feet. She has a normal platelet count. What is the most common cause of morbidity and mortality in this normally self-limiting disorder?

    (A) Ischemic heart disease

    (B) DIC

    (C) Septic arthritis

    (D) Renal failure

85. You have admitted a non-insulin-dependent diabetic patient to the ward because of an infection. The most appropriate diet is

    (A) 2 grams of sodium.

    (B) 4 grams of sodium.

    (C) low cholesterol.

    (D) 1,800 calorie ADA.

    (E) 2,400 calorie ADA.

86. The signs of gonadal dysgenesis, or Turner's syndrome, include all of the following EXCEPT

    (A) tall stature.

    (B) webbed neck.

    (C) shieldlike chest.

    (D) delayed growth of pubic hair.

    (E) extremity lymphedema.

87. An asymptomatic pregnant woman is routinely screened for which one of the following combinations of disease entities?

    (A) Syphilis/gonorrhea/CMV/HSV-2

    (B) Syphylis/parvovirus/CMV/HSV-2

    (C) Syphilis/gonorrhea/HBV/rubella

    (D) Gonorrhea/toxoplasmosis/HBV/rubella

    (E) Gonorrhea/parvovirus/HBV/HSV-2

Questions 88-91 refer to the following:

A 48-year-old man whom you follow in clinic for mild hypertension presents to the emergency department with a complaint of a three-week history of increasingly frequent episodes of left shoulder pain, neck pain, occasional left upper arm numbness, and shortness of breath. He did not pay much attention to these episodes at first, but recently he has been having as many as three a day. They now seem to be precipitated by walking quickly, climbing a flight of stairs, and getting upset. Sometimes they awaken him during the night. His physical examination is essentially normal, except for a blood pressure of 150/96 and a pulse of 110. His blood count is normal except for a white count of 12,000 with a slight left shift. His electrolytes are normal. His urinalysis is negative. A chest radiography is unremarkable. An electrocardiogram shows sinus tachycardia with nonspecific ST-T wave changes. The patient has an episode of shortness of breath and neck pain while lying flat on the gurney while you are writing up your findings.

88. Which of the following would you do first?

    (A) Give him intravenous morphine sulfate.

    (B) Administer sublingual nitroglycerine.

    (C) Draw a CPK.

    (D) Repeat the electrocardiogram.

    (E) STAT page a cardiologist.

89. The patient responds to your treatment. You would then do all of the following EXCEPT

    (A) obtain intravenous access.

    (B) repeat an electrocardiogram.

    (C) draw a CPK.

    (D) administer oxygen.

    (E) administer sedatives.

90. The new electrocardiogram shows minimal ST elevations in leads 2, 3, and AVF that were not evident in the original tracing. You suspect that

    (A) the patient has inferior ischemia.

    (B) the patient has had an inferior infarction.

    (C) the patient has anterolateral ischemia.

    (D) the patient had an infarction long ago.

    (E) the patient has hypertension.

91. The patient's wife arrives in the emergency department, having been called at home by the nurse. You tell her

    (A) her husband is in critical condition.

    (B) you are going to admit her husband for observation for a possible myocardial infarction.

    (C) she can take her husband home.

    (D) you are going to obtain an emergency cardiac catheterization and need her permission.

    (E) you are going to call the cardiac surgeons to evaluate him for possible bypass.

92. Which of the following beta-blocking agents would be most suitable to administer to an asthmatic patient?

    (A) Labetalol

    (B) Propranolol

    (C) Atenolol

    (D) Metoprolol

    (E) Timolol

For Questions 93–96, which of the following data would be most helpful?

    (A) Sensitivity

    (B) Specificity

    (C) Positive-predictive value

    (D) Negative-predictive value

    (E) Incidence of the disease in the specific population

93. A 43-year-old man with multiple risk factors for HIV tests positive for HIV. He wants to know the chance that he truly has the disease.

94. You have been doing research on a diagnostic test for disease X. A marketing company asks you what percentage of patients who have the disease will test positive for the disease by your diagnostic test.

95. A patient of yours calls to tell you that her son has just been tested positive for *Helicobacter pylori* infection with serum IgG levels. You know that the sensitivity and specificity of this are not optimal. In order to give her an accurate estimate of the chances that her son is infected, what do you need to know?

96. A 30-year-old woman without significant past medical problems presents to your office with intermittent episodes of chest pain. She denies family history of heart disease or any history of smoking. You order a stress test, which comes back as negative for ischemia.

97. A 22-year-old male presents to the emergency room with a broken jaw. The single best film to appreciate this fracture is the

    (A) Water's view.

    (B) lateral skull.

    (C) anterior skull.

    (D) panorex view.

    (E) submentovertex view.

98. A 35-year-old white female with breast cancer presents to her oncologist's office for a routine follow-up appointment. She had received chemotherapy 10 days ago and her total white blood cell count is 214. On examination she has a temperature of 100.5°F. All of the following should be performed in this neutropenic cancer patient EXCEPT

    (A) full set of blood cultures.

    (B) granulocyte colony stimulating factor injections.

    (C) respiratory isolation.

    (D) intravenous antibiotics.

    (E) reverse isolation precautions.

99. A 45-year-old male comes to see you off-schedule. You have only seen him a few times, usually for bronchitis or minor trauma. He has been having episodes of severe headaches, strange olfactory sensations, and thinks he needs new glasses. You are concerned that he may have

    (A) transient ischemic attacks.

    (B) a brain tumor.

    (C) hypertension.

    (D) subacute bacterial endocarditis.

    (E) meningitis.

100. The laboratory calls you to report a serum potassium of 8.2 mEq/L. Since the blood test was obtained on a healthy male as part of an annual executive physical, you consider the possibility of pseudohyperkalemia. Possibilities include all of the following EXCEPT

    (A) thrombocytosis.

    (B) leukocytosis.

    (C) obtaining the specimen through too small a needle.

    (D) acidosis.

    (E) prolonged, excessively tight tourniquet, with repeated fist-clenching.

101. A 54-year-old man with mild chronic obstructive pulmonary disease returned from a business convention and developed a fever and cough. He was treated for pneumonia by his family physician with amoxicillin/clavulanic acid (Augmentin$^{(r)}$) but failed to improve. The antimicrobial most likely to be helpful in this situation is

    (A) trimethoprim/sulfamethoxazole.

    (B) erythromycin.

    (C) tobramycin.

    (D) amantadine.

    (E) aztreonam.

102. A 62-year-old man suffered a heart attack. One month later he underwent an exercise stress test. All of the following are goals of post-myocardial infarction exercise treadmill stress testing EXCEPT

    (A) to determine the extent of the left main coronary artery disease.

    (B) to evaluate the hemodynamic response to exercise.

    (C) to monitor the effect of medications.

(D) to rule out exercise-induced ventricular arrhythmias.

(E) to determine prognosis.

103. A four-year-old boy presents with inability to bear weight on his right lower extremity. He has moderate pain at the extremes of internal and external rotation of the right hip. He is afebrile, with a normal white blood cell count (WBC) and an erythrocyte sedimentation rate (ESR) of 10. X-rays are normal and ultrasound of the hip shows a small effusion.

The most likely diagnosis is

(A) normal hip.

(B) transient synovitis of the hip.

(C) septic arthritis of the hip.

(D) Perthes' disease of the hip.

(E) developmental dysplasia of the hip (DDH).

Questions 104-111 refer to the following:

A 63-year-old man who had an inferior myocardial infarction about a month ago comes to your office for an unscheduled visit. He had an uncomplicated course after his MI and underwent an uneventful angioplasty. He had been doing well and was attending his cardiac rehabilitation sessions, but recently noted the onset of a burning pain in his left hand. The pain is diffuse and seems unrelated to activity. Your examination of the hand reveals that it is hyperesthetic and perhaps a bit puffy.

104. Your next action is to

(A) send him for an emergency radiograph.

(B) admit him to the hospital.

(C) do a complete physical examination.

(D) call an orthopedist.

(E) try to aspirate the hand for a culture.

105. On physical examination, he is normotensive and has a regular heart rate and rhythm. He has a clear chest and an unremarkable cardiovascular examination. He has no synovitis and no other tender areas except slightly decreased range of motion of the left shoulder. You order laboratory tests. All of the following tests are indicated EXCEPT

(A) CBC.

(B) differential.

(C) radiograph of the hand.

(D) antinuclear antibody.

(E) electrocardiogram.

106. The patient's electrocardiogram most likely shows

(A) Q waves in 1 and AVL.

(B) Q waves in 2, 3, and AVF.

(C) Q waves in V1-V3.

(D) 4 mm ST-T segment elevation in V1-V3.

(E) bigeminy.

107. The radiograph is normal. The white count is 8,000 with a normal differential. Upon closer examination of the affected hand you observe that it is very sweaty. You now suspect

(A) cellulitis.

(B) osteomyelitis.

(C) autonomic dysfunction.

(D) Raynaud's phenomenon.

(E) causalgia.

108. Your leading diagnosis now is

(A) shoulder-hand syndrome.

(B) Dressler's syndrome.

(C) Shy-Drager syndrome.

(D) diabetic neuropathy.

(E) multiple sclerosis.

109. You write a prescription for the patient. The treatment you choose is

    (A) Coumadin.

    (B) a benzodiazepine.

    (C) prednisone.

    (D) acetaminophen.

    (E) penicillin.

110. You schedule the patient for a course of

    (A) penicillin shots.

    (B) desensitization shots.

    (C) more cardiac rehabilitation.

    (D) physical therapy.

    (E) radiation therapy.

111. If this patient had not come in for another few months, you would have expected to find all of the following EXCEPT

    (A) an abnormal radiograph.

    (B) an abnormal bone scan.

    (C) ST elevation on electrocardio-gram.

    (D) a flexion contracture of the hand.

    (E) adhesive capsulitis of the shoulder.

112. A 33-year-old Chinese patient calls you wanting to be skin tested for tuberculosis because she may have been exposed. She immigrated to the United States when she was 10 years old and has no other medical illnesses. You tell her that skin testing, for her, is

    (A) not appropriate because of her age.

    (B) not appropriate because of her likely treatment with the BCG vaccine.

    (C) not appropriate because of the low pretest clinical probability.

    (D) appropriate and should be done now.

    (E) appropriate and should be done now and repeated in six months.

113. A 40-year-old woman, who has previously refused surgery for hyperparathyroidism, complains of severe colicky flank pain, fever of 102°F, and hematuria. Physical examination reveals a temperature of 103°F, pulse of 90, blood pressure of 140/90, and respiration of 18. She is moderately distressed, with CVA tenderness bilaterally. An abdominal film, obtained as part of the evaluation, is shown in the figure below. Your diagnosis is

    (A) renal cell carcinoma.

    (B) medullary sponge kidney.

    (C) nephrocalcinosis.

    (D) vitamin D intoxication.

    (E) gouty nephropathy.

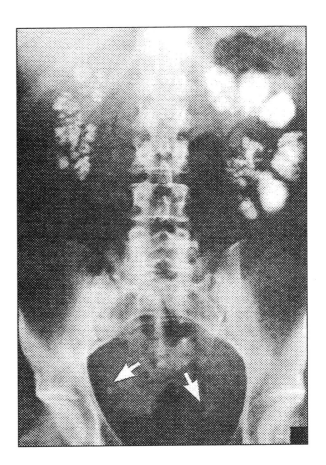

For Questions 114-117, match the most appropriate intervention with the symptoms presented.

(A) Admission for observation

(B) Admission to the intensive care unit

(C) Formal work-up in the emergency room

(D) Discharge with treatment and follow-up with primary physician in a few days

(E) Discharge without treatment and follow-up with primary physician as needed

114. A 19-year-old woman presents with periumbilical discomfort for two days. She has also noted nausea and vomiting, and has had anorexia. She denies any change in bowel habits. On physical examination, she has a temperature of 100.5°F, and vitals otherwise are within normal limits. Her abdominal examination reveals that she has periumbilical tenderness with rebound tenderness. Rectal examination reveals guaiac-negative stool and periumbilical pain during the rectal examination.

115. A 58-year-old man presents with chest pain. He tells you that until two days previously he had no symptoms; however, two days previously, he noted moderate substernal chest discomfort with minimal exercise. His past medical history includes diabetes mellitus treated with diet and hypertension. His physical examination reveals no abnormalities and his electrocardiogram is normal.

116. A 38-year-old woman presents with two days of cough productive of rusty brown sputum. She has noted fevers to 101.9°F and chills. She denies any other medical problems or shortness of breath. Her physical examination reveals bronchial breath sounds in the right inferior aspect of the lung.

117. A 59-year-old man presents with five days of nausea, vomiting, and abdominal pain. He had previously been drinking large amounts of alcohol but stopped when he continued to vomit. Physical examination reveals a blood pressure of 90/58, heart rate of 110, and respirations of 22. Abdominal exam reveals tenderness to palpation over the left upper quadrant with normal bowel sounds. Laboratory results reveal a white blood count of 18,000, a hematocrit of 42%, and a platelet count of 330,000. Serum sodium is 140, potassium is 3.0, chloride is 108, bicarbonate is 24, glucose is 308, SGOT is 380, LDH is 470, amylase is 48, and lipase is 508.

Questions 118-121 refer to the following:

An 18-year-old male presents to the dermatologist on a referral from his primary doctor regarding a "lesion" on his arm that has been present for several days. Your job is to describe the possible lesion by matching the diagnosis with the description.

(A) Macule

(B) Nodule

(C) Wheal

(D) Pustule

(E) Vesicle

118. A lesion caused by edema of the skin

119. A lesion caused by the accumulation of fluid between the upper layers of the skin, producing an elevation covered by a thin epithelium

120. A solid and elevated lesion with extension deep into the dermis

121. A localized change in skin color

For Questions 122-126, you are asked to work in a radiology clinic and to specify the best radiographic test to help determine a diagnosis. Using the following tests, choose the one that will most help a clinician determine the correct diagnosis.

(A) CAT scan

(B) MRI

(C) Ultrasound

(D) Angiogram

(E) Plain film

122. A 67-year-old male about to undergo revascularization of his lower extremity

123. A 44-year-old male with a herniated cervical disc

124. A 33-year-old male with a questionable kidney cyst

125. A 24-year-old male with a fractured femur

126. A 35-year-old male with an orbital fracture with questionable eye involvement

127. All of the following statements about suicide and adolescents are true EXCEPT

    (A) many automobile accidents involving adolescent drivers may be a suicidal attempt.

    (B) all adolescents showing signs of depression should be evaluated for possible suicidal thoughts.

    (C) scratching veins may be an example of a suicidal gesture rather than an attempt.

    (D) routine screening for suicidal intent is recommended.

    (E) depressed adolescents with suicidal thoughts should be asked if they use alcohol and other drugs.

128. Which one of the following is a true statement about treatment of cancer pain?

    (A) Identifying the cause of the pain is not included in palliative care.

    (B) Fear and anxiety modify pain threshold without affecting its management.

    (C) The confusion and drowsiness of a narcotic analgesic can be treated by switching to another narcotic analgesic.

    (D) Intractable, chemotherapy-induced nausea and vomiting can be managed by a serotonin antagonist.

    (E) IV administration of narcotics is the route of choice for patients in severe discomfort and with inability to take medication by mouth.

129. If a physician is HIV-positive, he must

    (A) tell all his co-workers.

    (B) tell his patients.

    (C) practice universal precautions.

    (D) quit his job.

    (E) never deal with patients.

130. An employer calls asking for information regarding a patient's psychiatric history. You

    (A) tell him what you know.

    (B) tell him you must charge him for the information.

    (C) tell him to call the patient's psychiatrist.

    (D) tell him you do not talk to employers.

    (E) tell him you cannot discuss the patient with him without the patient's written permission.

131. A 32-year-old woman returns for the results of her Pap smear. You note the result to be atypical squamous cells of undetermined significance or ASCUS. You advise your patient that

    (A) she might have cervical cancer and will need colposcopic evaluation as soon as possible.

    (B) this is a benign finding and no further follow-up is necessary.

    (C) she has cervical cancer and will need a hysterectomy.

    (D) this is a lab error and a repeat Pap smear needs to be done.

    (E) a Pap smear should be obtained every six months for two years. Annual Pap smears may be instituted after three consecutive negative smears.

Questions 132-135 refer to the following:

132. An eight-year-old boy is brought to the hospital because of a raccoon bite. You suspect rabies. All of the following symptoms may be present EXCEPT

    (A)   radiating dystonia.

    (B)   malaise.

    (C)   increased appetite.

    (D)   nausea.

    (E)   restlessness.

133. When performing your neurologic examination, deep tendon reflexes are

    (A)   absent.

    (B)   hypoactive.

    (C)   normal.

    (D)   hyperactive.

    (E)   initially absent and then hypoactive.

134. You perform an examination of the lungs, and most likely will find the pattern of breathing to be

    (A)   shallow and regular.

    (B)   shallow and irregular.

    (C)   deep and regular.

    (D)   deep and irregular.

    (E)   normal.

135. All of the following can make the diagnosis of rabies EXCEPT

    (A)   observation of the animal.

    (B)   microscopic examination of the brain of the animal.

    (C)   microscopic examination of the spinal cord of the animal.

    (D)   microscopic examination of the tongue of the animal.

    (E)   analysis of the saliva of the animal.

136. A 14-month-old male is brought in by his parents for evaluation. The child fell while attempting to walk across the living room. He is in severe pain. They observed swelling and discoloration of the right knee. There have been no prior medical problems with this child, but another son had a bleeding problem following a circumcision. Physical examination reveals acutely distressed crying child with hemarthrosis of the right knee. Laboratory tests show PT of 12 seconds and PTT of 160 seconds. The test most likely to confirm your diagnosis is

    (A)   bleeding time.

    (B)   Factor VIII assay.

    (C)   platelet count.

    (D)   Factor V assay.

    (E)   Factor X assay.

Questions 137-140 refer to the following:

A 45-year-old woman comes to the emergency room with bloody diarrhea and you suspect ulcerative colitis.

137. To confirm your diagnosis, you may perform a

    (A)   rectal examination.

    (B)   ultrasound.

    (C)   colonoscopy.

    (D)   flat plate of the abdomen.

    (E)   deep palpation of the lower abdomen.

138. You are concerned with this patient because of a severe presentation. The causes of death from ulcerative colitis include all of the following EXCEPT

    (A)   perforation.

    (B)   sepsis.

    (C)   hemorrhage.

    (D)   toxemia.

    (E)   electrolyte imbalance.

139. Treatment of ulcerative colitis may include all of the following EXCEPT

    (A) surgery.

    (B) intravenous fluids.

    (C) nasogastric tube.

    (D) low-fat diet.

    (E) antibiotics.

140. An elective prophylactic colectomy may be needed because of the high risk of

    (A) colonic bleeding.

    (B) perforation.

    (C) infection.

    (D) cancer.

    (E) adhesions.

Questions 141 and 142 refer to the following:

A 61-year-old woman comes to the office complaining of unilateral ear pain. On physical examination, you note that vesicles are present in the affected external ear.

141. Which one of the following is the pathogen responsible for this syndrome?

    (A) *Rhabdovirus*

    (B) Herpes zoster virus

    (C) *Coronavirus*

    (D) Influenza virus

    (E) Hepatitis C virus

142. Which one of the following cranial nerves is affected in this patient?

    (A) Trigeminal nerve

    (B) Vagus nerve

    (C) Accessory nerve

    (D) Facial nerve

    (E) Vestibulocochlear nerve

For Questions 143-146, match the most likely diagnosis with each numbered question.

    (A) Zollinger-Ellison syndrome

    (B) Pheochromocytoma

    (C) Chronic active gastritis

    (D) Medullary thyroid carcinoma

    (E) Hyperparathyroidism

143. A 57-year-old female presents with severe right flank pain and dysuria. She also has signs of osteopenia on radiographs.

144. A 42-year-old debilitated female presents with weight loss, malaise, and an elevated serum calcitonin level.

145. A 36-year-old construction worker presents with intractable diarrhea and abdominal pain. He visits another gastroenterologist for a second opinion. The previous physician was prescribing cimetidine, which was not alleviating his symptoms. His serum gastrin level was 1,000 ng/L.

146. A 52-year-old executive presents to the corporation's employee health clinic with symptoms of epigastric pain and dyspepsia. An upper endoscopy and subsequent cultures revealed a spiral shaped, Gram-negative bacterium.

147. A 10-year-old Chinese boy is brought to your clinic by his baby-sitter. The boy has punctured his foot on a nail while playing in a nearby construction facility. He is a recent immigrant and does not speak English. His parents are not going to be available until next month. The baby-sitter does not know anything about the child's immunization history. Which one of the following actions should you consider for the prevention of tetanus in this child?

    (A) A single dose of tetanus toxoid should be administered regardless of prior immunizations.

    (B) A single dose of tetanus immunoglobulin should be administered regardless of prior immunizations.

(C) You should immediately find an infectionist and ask for professional assistance.

(D) You should consider both tetanus toxoid and immunoglobulin.

(E) Initiate a search of a close relative who would know the immunization history of this child.

148. Which of the following statements regarding maternal prenatal surveillance is true?

(A) Blood pressure should be measured at every visit.

(B) Amount of change in blood pressure should be measured at every visit.

(C) Weight and amount of change should be measured starting in the second trimester. @ Qvist

(D) (A) and (B).

(E) All of the above.

Questions 149-152 refer to the following:

Panel A

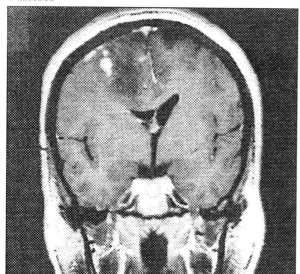

Panel B

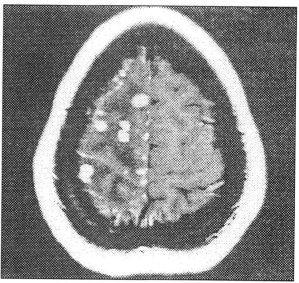

The gadolinium-enhanced T1 weighted MRI, shown in the figure, was performed to evaluate a new onset seizure in a 26-year-old female with AIDS. One year previously she had received a single intramuscular dose of penicillin. Serum RPR was 1:32. Serum treponemal IgG antibody was positive. Cerebrospinal fluid VDRL was negative.

149. Your diagnosis is

(A) primary syphilis.

(B) secondary syphilis.

(C) late benign syphilis.

(D) meningovascular syphilis.

(E) tabes dorsalis.

150. The differential diagnosis of chronic granulomatous conditions of the central nervous system includes all of the following EXCEPT

(A) tuberculosis.

(B) sarcoidosis.

(C) leprosy.

(D) blastomycosis.

(E) herpes.

151. The prozone phenomena explains

    (A) nonreactive or weakly reactive VDRL in secondary syphilis.

    (B) false-positive VDRL in malaria.

    (C) congenital false-positive VDRL.

    (D) positive VDRL in primary syphilis.

    (E) false-positive VDRL in persons older than 75 years.

152. Chronic false-positive tests for syphilis may occur in all of the following EXCEPT

    (A) intravenous drug abusers.

    (B) persons over age 70.

    (C) systemic lupus erythematosus.

    (D) mycoplasma pneumonia.

    (E) leprosy.

153. A 45-year-old female with rheumatoid arthritis complains of paresthesias of both hands, associated with pain in the forearm. Tingling, which is especially pronounced at night, is relieved by "shaking the hand." Physical examination reveals decreased abduction and opposition of the thumb, positive Tinel's sign, and positive Phalen's maneuver. Nerve conduction studies are shown in the figure below. You diagnose

    (A) fibromyalgia.

    (B) psychogenic rheumatism.

    (C) neuropathic joint disease.

Motor Nerve Conduction	Distance cm	Latency ms	CV m/s	Amplitude mV	Intensity mA
R nerve medianus					
Wrist---APB	4.0	6.8		5.70	63.00
Elbow---wrist	22.0	11.5	46.8	5.60	53.00
R nerve ulnaris					
Wrist---ADQ	6.0	2.6		11.10	71.00
Bl elbow--wrist	20.0	6.0	58.8	10.60	89.00
Ab elbow--bl elbow	7.0	7.3	53.8	10.30	89.00
Erb's pt--ab elbow	0.0	0.0	0.0	0.00	0.00

Standard F-wave analysis	M-response Amplitude µV	M-response Latency ms	Min-F-Ml ms
R nerve medianus	5,800	6.7	25.6
R nerve ulnaris	10,700	2.3	24.4

Sensory Nerve Conduction	Distance cm	Latency ms	CV m/s	Amplitude µV	Intensity mA
R nerve ulnaris					
Digit V----wrist	10.0	2.3	43.4	15.60	16.00
R nerve medianus					
Digit II---palm	12.0	4.4	27.2	6.90	5.40
L nerve medianus					
Digit II---palm	12.5	3.1	40.3	17.70	4.20

(D)   carpal tunnel syndrome.

(E)   reflex sympathetic dystrophy.

154.   A 76-year-old carpenter presents to the emergency room complaining of severe left knee pain associated with fever. This pain has been present for four days and has become worse over time. The patient denies trauma or any other past medical history. On exam, he has a temperature of 101.8°F, a tender, erythematous swollen left knee without crepitus, and no radiation of the pain. Aspiration of the affected knee joint reveals synovial fluid, which shows weakly positive, birefringent crystals in rhomboid shapes under the polarizing microscope. What is the diagnosis and treatment?

   (A)   Acute gouty arthritis treated with colchicine

   (B)   Septic arthritis treated with antibiotics

   (C)   Osteoarthritis treated with nonsteroidal anti-inflammatory drugs

   (D)   Rheumatoid arthritis treated with injecting steroids into the joint space

   (E)   Calcium pyrophosphate dihydrate disease treated with oral prednisone and indomethacin

155.   Which one of the following statements should NOT be included in your recommendations for the patient with suspected essential hypertension on the first visit?

   (A)   Daily food should include no more than 300 mg of cholesterol, no more than 30% of calories from fat, and no more than 10% of calories from saturated fat.

   (B)   Daily activities should include a walking program.

   (C)   Insist on trying nonpharmacologic maneuvers first, even if the patient says he is not going to comply with your advice.

(D)   Any of the above.

(E)   None of the above.

156.   A 23-year-old man with a history of sickle cell disease presents with sickle cell crisis. He tells you that he had feelings of myalgias, generalized malaise, and dry cough for two days previously. His laboratory tests reveal that his hematocrit is down from his baseline of 28% to 21% and his reticulocyte count is 0.3%, down from his normal of 2.0%. The most likely infection which precipitated this sickle cell crisis is

   (A)   parvovirus B10.

   (B)   human papillomavirus.

   (C)   hepatitis A virus.

   (D)   coxsackievirus.

   (E)   human immunodeficiency virus.

157.   A previously healthy 30-year-old woman presents to the emergency room with one day of fever, neck stiffness, and myalgias. She denies any other medical problems or medications. On physical examination, she has a temperature of 100°F, a heart rate of 87, a blood pressure of 110/70, and a respiratory rate of 14. Her neck is slightly stiff to movement. Her lungs are clear and her cardiac exam is without murmurs. Her abdominal exam is benign. Her neurological exam reveals a patient who is alert and oriented to time, place, and person. She has no focal deficits. You perform a lumbar puncture, which reveals normal glucose and slightly elevated total protein. The cell count comes back with 18 total cell: 15 nucleated cells, 98% of them being lymphocytes. No xanthochromia is noted. The most likely diagnosis is

   (A)   pneumococcal meningitis.

   (B)   meningococcal meningitis.

   (C)   viral meningitis.

   (D)   subarachnoid hemorrhage.

   (E)   None of the above.

158. A 44-year-old male is brought to the emergency room with absent breath sounds on the right and a deviated trachea. The oxygen saturation is 84% on 100% O_2 by face mask. The next step is

    (A) placement of a chest tube.

    (B) needle thoracostomy.

    (C) tracheotomy.

    (D) chest X-ray.

    (E) intubation.

159. A 60-year-old man is admitted for four large episodes of bright red blood per rectum. This has never happened previously, and he denies any history of medical illnesses. His vital signs are stable and his abdominal exam reveals normoactive bowels. His abdomen is not tender or distended. The most likely etiology of his hemorrhage is

    (A) diverticulosis.

    (B) peptic ulcer disease.

    (C) colon cancer.

    (D) hemorrhoids.

    (E) aorto-enteric fistula.

For Questions 160-163, match the management of choice with each numbered case question.

    (A) Paracentesis

    (B) Nasogastric tube insertion

    (C) Endoscopic retrograde cholangiopancreatography

    (D) Liver transplantation

    (E) Flexible sigmoidoscopy

160. A 52-year-old female has symptoms of pruritus, jaundice, right upper quadrant fullness, malaise, anorexia, and fatigue. She presents to the clinic and has findings of hepatosplenomegaly, portal hypertension, xanthomatous lesions around the eyelids, and an elevated alkaline phosphatase level.

161. A 34-year-old alcoholic male presents to the emergency room with symptoms of severe abdominal pain, nausea, vomiting, and fever. He is subsequently admitted to the intensive care unit because of severe hypotension and volume depletion. His lipase level is 200 mg/dl.

162. A 53-year-old physician presents to his primary care doctor for a routine yearly physical examination.

163. A 49-year-old Hispanic florist is admitted to the University Hospital for a work-up of elevated liver function enzymes. On examination she is found to have ascites, jaundice, weight loss, telangiectases of exposed areas on the skin, palmer erythema, and hepatosplenomegaly. Her serum hepatitis B surface antigen is positive. Her serum hepatitis B antibody is negative. On the tenth hospital day, she complains of worsening abdominal pain and fever. Later on that day, she has an upper GI bleed.

164. Your friend, who is doing a third-year clerkship in radiology, calls you to see this "fascinoma," shown in the figures. You indicate that the lesion

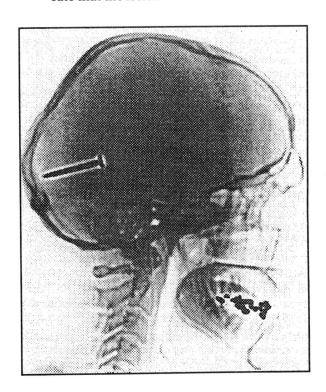

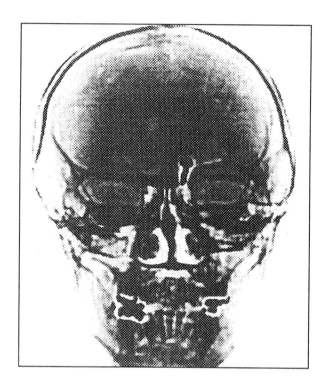

(A) is an artifact.

(B) is incompatible with life.

(C) is intracranial.

(D) is extracranial.

(E) is best evaluated by an MRI of the brain.

For Questions 165-168 match the case description with the most likely diagnosis

(A) Allergic rhinitis

(B) Sinusitis

(C) Migraine headache

(D) Pneumonia

(E) Acute bronchitis

165. A 57-year-old man with a productive cough and known COPD

166. A 33-year-old woman who has right hemifacial congestion, photophobia, and a severe right-sided headache

167. A 37-year-old alcoholic male with a productive cough

168. A 22-year-old woman with bifrontal headaches and purulent postnasal drainage

169. You are consulting at an institution for the mentally retarded. The nurse reports that several of the children recently have had trouble sleeping. Some of them have perianal excoriations. Anal examination of one of the children is shown in the figure. You diagnose

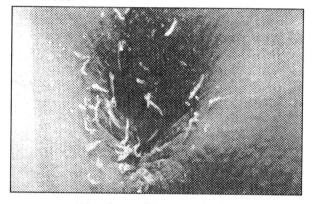

(A) *Enterobius vermicularis.*

(B) *Trichuris trichiura.*

(C) *Strongyloides stercoralis.*

(D) *Ascaris lumbricoides.*

(E) *Necator americanus.*

170. A 57-year-old woman whom you have been following for mild hypertension comes in to see you with her daughter, who has a grocery bag full of herbal remedies that she wants to give her mother. You look through them and ascertain that there is nothing particularly toxic among them. You

(A) tell the daughter that the herbal treatments are ridiculous.

(B) tell the patient you cannot follow her if her family wants to interfere.

(C) tell the patient and her daughter that she can probably try a small amount of a few of these treatments in succession but that you do not think they are likely to help.

(D) tell them she can take as much as she likes of all of them.

(E) tell the daughter not to bother her mother with such things.

171. A 53-year-old woman comes to see you two weeks before her scheduled visit because she has been having nightsweats and has been very irritable. She smokes and has noticed a slight increase in her chronic cough. She is worried that she has cancer. Your examination is completely normal, showing the patient has a clear chest. Her lab tests and chest radiograph are unremarkable. You question her about

(A) her family history.

(B) how many cigarettes she is smoking.

(C) the date of her last menstrual period.

(D) her recent travels.

(E) gardening.

172. A 23-year-old woman in her 30th week of pregnancy comes in off-schedule because of increased thirst and nocturia. You order

(A) a brain MRI.

(B) a glucose tolerance test.

(C) an electroencephalogram.

(D) a barium swallow.

(E) a urine culture.

173. Which one of the following is NOT considered a significant risk factor for the development of transitional cell carcinoma of the urinary bladder?

(A) Cigarette smoking

(B) Phenacetin administration

(C) Cyclophosphamide administration

(D) Alcohol abuse

(E) Infection by *schistosoma spp.*

174. Which one of the following patients is NOT likely to develop thrush?

(A) A 43-year-old man with HIV/AIDS and *pneumocystis carinii* pneumonia.

(B) A 65-year-old woman with diabetes mellitus and a blood glucose of 300.

(C) A 37-year-old female who has received a bone marrow transplant for acute leukemia 2 weeks earlier.

(D) A 55-year-old man who completed a course of chemotherapy for small cell carcinoma of the lung three weeks earlier.

(E) A seven-year-old with otitis media.

175. A 58-year-old female was brought in by her family because of depression, memory loss, and abnormal gait. On exam, she was disoriented, with impaired position sense and paresthesias. Lab data shows she has megaloblastic anemia with hypersegmented neutrophils. Her cobalamin level (B12) was low—100 pg/mg. This patient was taking no medication and has no prior surgery. All of the following can be seen in vitamin B12 deficiency EXCEPT

(A) elevated methylmalonic acid levels.

(B) decreased homocysteine levels.

(C) elevated anti-parietal cell antibody levels.

(D) elevated mean corpuscular volume.

(E) normal serum cobalamin levels.

176. A patient is brought to the trauma unit following a high-speed motor vehicle accident in which the patient sustained blunt abdominal trauma. There were no other areas of injury. The patient is hemodynamically unstable despite attempted resuscitation with plenty of fluids and packed red blood cells. Coagulation factors and fibrin split

products are normal. X-rays show a displaced pelvic fracture. Exploratory laparotomy is negative and the patient continues to be unstable despite external fixation of the pelvic fracture. The next step in management would be

(A) transfusion of fresh frozen plasma (FFP).

(B) removal of the external fixator.

(C) open reduction of the pelvic fracture.

(D) arterial embolization.

(E) observation.

177. A 35-year-old male sees you in the walk-in clinic. He has thrush and has lost about 30 pounds in the last six months. He is feeling tired. He adamantly denies any history of homosexual activity or intravenous drug abuse. However, he does boast of his multitude of female sexual partners. Your working diagnosis is

(A) HIV/AIDS in a heterosexual man with multiple different partners.

(B) leukemia.

(C) lymphoma.

(D) gastric cancer.

(E) histoplasmosis.

178. A 23-year-old graduate student comes to the walk-in clinic because of several episodes of severe right-sided headache in the last few months. She has no aura but does feel slightly nauseated with the pain. She has never had such headaches before. She has no visual impairment. You order

(A) imitrex for migraines.

(B) a lumbar puncture kit.

(C) brain MRI.

(D) electroencephalogram.

(E) a sedative.

179. A 38-year-old mildly obese female presents to the clinic for her quarterly evaluation for hypercholesterolemia. She now has new complaints of fatigue, constipation, cold intolerance, and menorrhagia. On examination, the relaxation phase of the deep-tendon reflexes are prolonged and she exhibits periorbital puffiness. Which one of the following tests should be completed in the initial work-up of this patient?

(A) Technetium-99m pertechnetate thyroid scanning

(B) Thyroid stimulating hormone (TSH)

(C) Serum calcitonin

(D) Ultrasound of the thyroid gland

(E) Thyroid-releasing hormone stimulation test

180. A five-year-old male presents to your office with high fevers lasting for six days, cervical adenopathy, bilateral conjunctivitis, a "strawberry tongue," dry chapped lips, a truncal exanthem, and descuamation of his fingertips and toes. With these signs and symptoms, a diagnosis of Kawasaki syndrome is made. What would you NOT do for this patient?

(A) Administer IV gammaglobulin

(B) Administer aspirin

(C) Obtain an echocardiogram

(D) Administer corticosteroids

USMLE STEP 3
PRACTICE TEST 1

Day Two – Morning Session

(Answer sheets appear in the back of this book.)

TIME: 3 Hours
180 Questions

DIRECTIONS: Each of the following numbered items or incomplete sentences is followed by an answer or a completion of the statement. Choose the **ONE** choice that **BEST** answers the question or completes the sentence.

For Questions 1-4, match each of the following poisonings with its management.

   (A)   Assessment and support of ABCs

   (B)   Antidote administration

   (C)   Obtaining history

   (D)   Naloxone

   (E)   Induction of emesis with syrup of ipecac

1.   A 22-year-old man is brought to the ER by his friends. He is unconscious. Drug overdose is suspected.

2.   A five-year-old girl is seen in the ER. Her mother tells you that the daughter was found unconscious beside her bed with a half-empty bottle of Tylenol. The patient has been assessed in a local family care clinic, decontaminated, and is sent to you with a detailed note stating that the patient has been stabilized.

3.   A two-year-old boy is evaluated for ingestion of his grandmother's pills that she takes for insomnia. The drug appears to be flurazepam. The boy is assessed for vital signs and decontaminated with gastric lavage and syrup of ipecac. You have to prevent systemic intoxication of the already digested portion of the drug.

4.   Aspirin overdose is suspected in a 73-year-old comatose patient who has been on prophylactic aspirin therapy for recurrent, unstable angina pectoris.

Questions 5-8 refer to the following:

You are asked to see a 12-year-old boy in the emergency room who sustained a laceration on his right forearm the day before from a broken piece of glass. Examination now reveals a 3-centimeter laceration over the distal ulna with a visible cut nerve and tendon.

5.   The tendon exposed is most likely

   (A)   palmaris longus.

   (B)   flexor carpi ulnaris.

   (C)   flexor carpi radialis.

   (D)   pronator teres.

   (E)   flexor indicis propius.

6. The patient complains of numbness of his fingers. You would expect numbness of the

    (A) index and long fingers.

    (B) long and ring finger.

    (C) ring and little finger.

    (D) little finger only.

    (E) None of the above.

7. The patient is asked to flex his wrist. You notice

    (A) normal flexion.

    (B) radial deviation.

    (C) ulnar deviation.

    (D) no flexion at all.

    (E) limited straight flexion.

8. The canal most closely associated with the injury is

    (A) cubital.

    (B) carpel.

    (C) Guyon's.

    (D) Allen.

    (E) brachial.

For Questions 9-12, select the antiarrhythmic agent that would be an appropriate first-line medication.

    (A) Lidocaine

    (B) Quinidine

    (C) Amiodarone

    (D) Adenosine

    (E) Disopyramide

9. A 60-year-old man, post-MI day two, is noted to have sustained ventricular tachycardia on the monitor. During this time, he denies any chest pain, shortness of breath, nausea, or light-headedness, and his blood pressure is 140/70.

10. A 50-year-old woman with a history of hypertension is noted to have a new onset of atrial fibrillation. She denies any other medical problems and is taking no other medications. She asks what kind of medication she can take to try to stay in a normal heart rhythm.

11. A 70-year-old man with a history of coronary artery disease, hypertension, and diabetes mellitus presents with chest pain. While in the hospital, he has an episode of ventricular tachycardia which progresses to ventricular fibrillation. Fortunately, appropriate cardiopulmonary resuscitation brings him back to sinus rhythm within two minutes.

12. A 30-year-old woman without significant past medical history presents with feelings of palpitations. She denies any associated chest pain or shortness of breath. Her blood pressure is 140/70, heart rate is 150, respiratory rate is 22, and temperature is 98.7°F. She is noted to have a narrow complex tachycardia at 150, although it is difficult to assess the underlying rhythm.

For Questions 13-16, select the test that is most useful in arriving at a diagnosis for each patient.

    (A) Serum alcohol level

    (B) Chest radiograph

    (C) Lumbar puncture

    (D) CPK

    (E) Rheumatoid factor

13. An agitated, confused, combative 34-year-old man who was brought in by a friend who then left

14. A febrile, crying eight-month-old boy with no focal findings

15. A 58-year-old male with fever, chills, and productive cough

16. A 69-year-old man with proximal muscle weakness and pigmented lesions on his knuckles

17. A 59-year-old female patient is seen for assessment of a chronic cough which has become bothersome lately. The cough is accompanied by mucoid sputum. She has

been smoking two packs of cigarettes/day for 16 years. On physical examination her blood pressure is 150/90 mm Hg and pulse is 88 and regular. She weighs 240 lb. You notice that she wheezes while she talks. Chest X-ray reveals significant bronchial wall thickening. Regarding this patient's condition, which one of the following pulmonary test abnormalities is NOT expected to be present?

(A) Decreased residual volume

(B) Decreased FEV

(C) Decreased ratio of FEV1/FVC

(D) Decreased FEV 25-75

(E) Normal or increased functional residual capacity

18. A patient reports black tarry stools to you, and a guaiac test is negative. This may result from

(A) epistaxis.

(B) gastric ulcer.

(C) esophageal varix.

(D) black cherries.

(E) hemoptysis.

Questions 19-22 refer to the following:

A 39-year-old man presents with fever of unknown origin. He has a history of diabetes mellitus that has been treated with oral hypoglycemics. He denies any history of intravenous drug use. On physical examination, he is a slightly obese male in no acute distress. His temperature is 101.8°F, heart rate is 80, blood pressure is 140/70, and respiratory rate is 14. Lungs are clear, and cardiac exam reveals a II/VI systolic murmur. Abdominal exam is benign. Blood cultures are drawn and come back in three days, diagnosing the patient with bacterial endocarditis.

19. Of the following, which one is not commonly seen with subacute bacterial endocarditis?

(A) Painful nodules on the palms

(B) Ungual splinter hemorrhages

(C) Splenomegaly

(D) Spider angiomatous

(E) Hematuria

20. Of the following, which is the most common organism to cause subacute bacterial endocarditis?

(A) *Streptococcus spp.*

(B) *Staph spp.*

(C) *Haemophilus spp.*

(D) *Eikenella spp.*

(E) Fungal organisms.

21. Subacute bacterial endocarditis most commonly affects

(A) the tricuspid valve.

(B) the pulmonic valve.

(C) the mitral valve.

(D) the aortic valve.

(E) more than one valve.

22. A history of intravenous drug abuse would predispose the patient particularly to

(A) *Streptococcus spp.*

(B) *Staph spp.*

(C) *Haemophilus spp.*

(D) *Eikenella spp.*

(E) Fungal organisms.

Questions 23-30 refer to the following:

A 40-year-old man presents to the emergency room, brought in by his family, for being somewhat lethargic over the last three days. Per his family, over the last three weeks he's had less energy, and over the last three days, he's been sleeping much more and has been more lethargic. Over the last two weeks, he's had several episodes per day of vomiting of maroon-colored emesis and has also had some episodes of black-colored stools. Per the family, he fell down about three weeks ago during an alcohol binge and hit his head. He has no other medical illnesses and has never had any surgeries. He drinks quite heavily, often drinking one or two "fifths" each day, and smokes two packs of cigarettes each day. He takes no medications and does not take any illicit drugs.

23. The most likely cause of the patient's symptoms is

    (A) sepsis.

    (B) inflammatory bowel disease.

    (C) gastrointestinal bleed secondary to alcoholism.

    (D) subdural hematoma.

    (E) acute myocardial infarction.

24. On physical examination, the patient is a disheveled middle-aged male who is difficult to arouse. His blood pressure is 90/60, heart rate is 110, respiratory rate is 20, and temperature is 98°F. His lungs are clear and his cardiac exam reveals a tachycardiac rate without murmurs or gallops. His abdomen has normoactive bowel sounds, and there is no distension or pain to palpation. Rectal examination reveals guaiac-positive black stool. Extremities reveal no edema. Appropriate initial interventions include all of the following EXCEPT

    (A) type and cross.

    (B) insertion of two large-bore intravenous needles.

    (C) electrocardiogram.

    (D) complete blood count.

    (E) All of the above are appropriate.

25. Nasogastric lavage reveals bright red blood which clears after 3 liters of saline. Head CT reveals no bleed. Electrocardiogram reveals sinus tachycardia without evidence of ischemia or infarction. Chest radiograph reveals no infiltrates or effusions. Blood studies are pending. His blood pressure continues to drop to 70/50. The most appropriate immediate intervention is

    (A) initiation of dopamine.

    (B) initiation of norepinephrine.

    (C) initiation of wide open crystalloids.

    (D) initiation of antibiotics.

    (E) pericardiocentesis.

26. The blood bank calls to tell you that he has some antibodies which will make it difficult to cross him for blood and it may take a little bit longer. Instead of blood transfusions, you can try

    (A) intravenous hetastarch.

    (B) intravenous sterile water.

    (C) intravenous lactated Ringer's solution.

    (D) intravenous normal saline.

    (E) intravenous half-normal saline.

27. Of the following, which one is the most appropriate intervention?

    (A) Immediate computed tomography of the abdomen

    (B) Immediate upper endoscopy

    (C) Immediate barium swallow

    (D) Immediate laparotomy

    (E) Immediate tagged red blood cell scan

28. The appropriate testing is done and it shows a bleeding gastric ulcer which is sclerosed. However, in spite of this, the patient continues to be hypotensive. The most appropriate next therapy is

    (A) insertion of a triple lumen catheter for resuscitation.

    (B) insertion of a cordis for resuscitation.

    (C) insertion of another peripheral line for resuscitation.

    (D) initiation of Neo-Synephrine.

    (E) initiation of dobutamine.

29. Of the following, which statement is correct regarding intubation?

    (A) This patient does not need to be intubated, as he has no pulmonary problems.

    (B) This patient does not need to be intubated now, but may need it if he goes into heart failure from all of the intravenous fluids.

    (C) This patient needs to be intubated now for ventilation.

    (D) This patient needs to be intubated now for oxygenation.

    (E) This patient needs to be intubated now for airway protection.

30. Of the following diseases, which is the only one that can be ruled out with a normal erythrocyte sedimentation rate?

    (A) Osteomyelitis

    (B) Subacute bacterial endocarditis

    (C) Temporal arteritis

    (D) Lupus nephritis

    (E) Hepatitis

31. A 27-year-old HIV-positive Hispanic male patient presents to the virology clinic with symptoms of dysphagia and odynophagia over the course of several weeks. On exam, he is mildly emaciated with oral thrush and a low-grade fever. His CD4 count is 204. He has had no previous opportunistic infections. What is the next step in management of this patient?

    (A) Acyclovir

    (B) Fluconazole

    (C) Upper endoscopy with biopsy

    (D) Barium swallow

    (E) Ganciclovir

32. A nurse confides in you that she is HIV-positive. You

    (A) tell her supervisor.

    (B) relieve her of her duties.

    (C) remind her of the need for everyone to use universal precautions.

    (D) refuse to let her deal with your patients.

    (E) tell every patient who sees her.

33. A 24-year-old male presents with symptoms of facial flushing which spreads to the trunk and upper extremities. These episodes are accompanied by diarrhea and wheezing. On exam, the patient had erythematous facial flushing which eventually turned purplish. The liver was also enlarged. The blood pressure was low during this episode. Excretion of 5-hydroxyindoleacetic acid in the urine was elevated. What is the most likely diagnosis?

    (A) Pheochromocytoma

    (B) Carcinoid syndrome

    (C) Mastocytosis

    (D) Thyrotoxicosis

    (E) Urticaria

34. You are performing a high-school physical on a 17-year-old male and notice lateral deviation of the great toe. Your diagnosis is

    (A) hammer toe.

    (B) hallux rigidus.

    (C) hallux valgus.

    (D) hallux varus.

    (E) gout.

35. A 38-year-old female is referred to a psychiatrist. When she arrives at the physician's office, she is dressed with spiked clothing and is tattooed on both arms with piercings in several places including her nose, tongue, and nipples. She claims that beside her 36-year-old sister, she does not have anyone she can trust or refer to as a close friend. She admits to a heartfelt belief in the use of tarot cards to predict her future, and demonstrates an extreme suspicion of the psychiatrist's intentions. Which one of the following disorders does the woman most likely suffer from?

    (A) Paranoid

(B) Schizoid

(C) Schizotypal

(D) Histrionic

(E) Antisocial

36. A 24-year-old woman comes to the clinic because of her increasing anxiety over the consequences of recent unprotected sex with three different men. After obtaining history and completing the physical examination, you decide to do counseling regarding PID and associated risk factors. Which of the following is NOT a true statement regarding the epidemiology of PID?

(A) Oral contraceptives have proven to protect against gonococcal PID.

(B) Barrier contraceptive methods are protective against gonorrheal but not chlamydial forms of PID.

(C) Risk factors for acute PID include IUD and symptoms of urethritis in a male partner.

(D) Concomitant infection with *Chlamydia trachomatis* is present in approximately 45% of patients with gonorrhea.

(E) Many *N. gonorrhea* strains have become resistant to penicillin and tetracycline.

Questions 37-40 refer to the following:

A three-month-old baby has been left in a bassinet in the hospital lobby without any information. He is admitted to your service and called Baby Doe. He is cyanotic and clearly needs a cardiac catheterization and probably will need open heart surgery. He has some bruises on his extremities and an abnormal angulation of his forearm. Radiography shows a displaced fracture of the radius, with minimal callus formation.

37. The baby's vital signs are deteriorating. You call the pediatric cardiologist and

(A) agree that you need to get a court order before any procedure can be performed.

(B) schedule emergency catheterization with an operating team on standby.

(C) call the police to put out an all-points bulletin for next-of-kin.

(D) start calling hospitals in town to find out if anyone knows who the child is.

(E) interrogate the personnel on duty in the hospital lobby.

38. You will eventually need to

(A) institute legal proceedings to make the child a ward of the court.

(B) send the police out looking for relatives.

(C) send the child to a hospice.

(D) call Aid for Dependent Families.

(E) run an ad in the paper.

39. You should contact the appropriate authorities to

(A) do a house-to-house search of the parents' neighborhood.

(B) arrest the parents.

(C) find any close relatives.

(D) commit the parents.

(E) find foster parents.

40. If the parents or relatives who left the child in the hospital did show up, they would be suspected of

(A) homicide.

(B) burglary.

(C) infanticide.

(D) child abuse.

(E) intoxication.

Question 41 and 42 refer to the following:

An 18-year-old high school student presents to your office with a complaint of painful swallowing, decreased oral intake, and chills and fevers for the past two days.

41. Your physical examination should include all of the following EXCEPT

    (A) the neck.

    (B) the oropharynx.

    (C) the cranial nerves.

    (D) the lungs.

    (E) the abdomen.

42. Screening laboratory tests would include which of the following?

    (A) A CBC

    (B) A rapid streptococcal test

    (C) Liver function tests

    (D) A chest X-ray

    (E) An electrocardiogram

Questions 43-50 refer to the following:

A 40-year-old woman presents to your office with three months of intermittent aching in her hands. She notes that these symptoms are worse in the morning and improve during the day. She denies any other significant past medical problems. She takes several aspirin each day for these symptoms. She denies any fevers, chills, nausea, or vomiting. There has been a family history of arthritis in her family.

43. By history, the most likely diagnosis is

    (A) pseudogout.

    (B) gout.

    (C) rheumatoid arthritis.

    (D) osteoarthritis.

    (E) septic arthritis.

44. Concerns regarding possible extra-articular manifestations include all of the following EXCEPT

    (A) gastritis.

    (B) pulmonary fibrosis.

    (C) vasculitis.

    (D) serositis.

    (E) rheumatoid nodules.

45. On physical examination, you note some mild swelling and mild erythema of the proximal interphalangeal joints in both of her hands. The remainder of her physical examination is without abnormalities. Her rheumatoid factor returns strongly positive. The diagnosis of rheumatoid arthritis is made. Due to the patient's ingestion of aspirin, appropriate initial blood tests include all of the following EXCEPT

    (A) hematocrit.

    (B) serum creatinine.

    (C) prothrombin time.

    (D) serum transaminase levels.

    (E) serum amylase.

46. Besides nonsteroidal anti-inflammatory drugs, another appropriate medication for relief of symptoms is

    (A) glucocorticoids.

    (B) methotrexate.

    (C) acetaminophen.

    (D) cyclophosphamide.

    (E) plasmapheresis.

47. Appropriate treatment is done and the patient notes symptomatic relief for her flare. However, although her symptoms are improved, you note continued active synovitis. Considerations to adjunctive medications include all of the following EXCEPT

    (A) methotrexate.

    (B) gold.

(C) penicillamine.

(D) bleomycin.

(E) hydroxychloroquine.

48. Several weeks later, she presents to your office with a complaint of her right knee being very painful. You note it to be warm and erythematous and painful to palpation. The rest of her joints seem to be doing relatively well. The most likely explanation for this is

(A) septic joint.

(B) gout.

(C) pseudogout.

(D) exacerbation of the disease.

(E) progression of the disease.

49. You begin the administration of methotrexate. You need to explain to the patient the possibilities of side effects that commonly include all of the following EXCEPT

(A) nausea and vomiting.

(B) bone marrow toxicity.

(C) hepatitis.

(D) renal toxicity.

(E) hypersensitivity pneumonitis.

50. Appropriate treatment is done and you slow down the progression of the disease. However, in spite of optimal treatment, the disease continues and, several years later, her left hip has gradually worsened to the point that she has much difficulty walking. The appropriate treatment would be

(A) total hip replacement.

(B) administration of intra-articular corticosteroid injections.

(C) administration of chronic systemic corticosteroids.

(D) administration of sulfasalazine.

(E) None of the above.

51. A 46-year-old male presents to your office for a periodic health examination. You should perform measurements of all of the following EXCEPT

(A) visual acuity.

(B) total serum cholesterol.

(C) blood pressure.

(D) height.

(E) weight.

52. Which one of the following is seen with hypercalcemia?

(A) Perioral paresthesias

(B) Lethargy

(C) Irritability

(D) Prolonged QT interval on EKG

(E) Anorexia

Questions 53-56 refer to the following:

An 80-year-old man comes to your office with symptoms of exertional chest pain and shortness of breath. Physical examination reveals a midsystolic murmur. Chest X-ray and EKG suggest left ventricular hypertrophy. Echocardiogram reveals an elevated flow gradient across the aortic valve.

53. The most common cause of this disorder is

(A) rheumatic heart disease.

(B) arteriosclerotic degeneration.

(C) congenital bicuspid aortic valve.

(D) ankylosing spondylitis.

(E) syphilis.

54. The most useful method to assess the severity of this condition would be

(A) endomyocardial biopsy.

(B) thallium stress test.

(C) left-heart catheterization.

(D) Swan-Ganz catheterization.

(E) coronary arteriography.

55. All of the following are potential therapeutic options EXCEPT

    (A) prosthetic valve replacement.

    (B) porcine valve replacement

    (C) valvuloplasty.

    (D) beta-blocker therapy.

56. Sublingual nitroglycerin therapy is not commonly used for the treatment of chest pain in patients with severe aortic stenosis because

    (A) tachyphylaxis develops with use of this agent.

    (B) the systemic vasodilatory effects associated with these agents will increase cardiac afterload.

    (C) nitrate therapy is only effective in patients with coronary artery occlusion.

    (D) it only aids the reduction in cardiac preload.

    (E) oral nitrate therapy has a greater bioavailability.

57. A 39-year-old homosexual AIDS patient presents to the virology clinic at the university hospital complaining of painful, plaque-like purplish lesions of the chest and lower extremities. These lesions are nodular and tender on palpation. The CD4 count is 100. On further questioning, this patient also has symptoms of dyspnea on exertion and abdominal pain. He has had no previous opportunistic infections in the past. What should be the initial work-up in this patient?

    (A) Skin biopsy

    (B) CT of the chest and abdomen

    (C) Bone marrow aspiration and biopsy

    (D) Lumbar puncture

    (E) Bronchoscopy

58. A 45-year-old female presents with gross hematuria for the first time. Her past medical history is significant for hypertension and renal colic secondary to nephrolithiasis. Her father had similar symptoms. On further testing, ultrasound revealed large kidneys bilaterally with a ruptured cyst within the left kidney. What is the patient at risk for?

    (A) Nephritis

    (B) Hepatomas

    (C) Proximal renal tubular acidosis (type II)

    (D) Intracranial rupture secondary to subarachnoid hemorrhage

    (E) Transitional-cell carcinoma of the bladder

59. A 21-year-old man presents to the emergency room after stepping on a rusty nail. His last tetanus booster was seven years ago, and previously, he was up to date on his immunizations. Which one of the following is appropriate for immunization against tetanus?

    (A) He doesn't need another tetanus booster for the rest of his life.

    (B) He needs only tetanus immune globulin.

    (C) He needs only tetanus toxoid.

    (D) He needs both tetanus immune globulin and tetanus toxoid.

    (E) He needs tetanus toxoid now and six months later.

60. A 30-year-old woman presents to your office after noticing a breast lump on self-examination. Of the following possible findings on physical examination, the one most likely associated with a benign lesion is

    (A) one that is associated with a new asymmetry in the breast shape.

    (B) one that is associated with microcalcifications on the mammogram.

    (C) one that is associated with changes in size with the menstrual period.

    (D) one that is associated with a bloody nipple discharge.

(E) one that is associated with a peau d'orange appearance.

61. A patient is dying from metastatic lung cancer and has painful metastases in his bones. He is clearly suffering when you make morning rounds. You should

(A) give him an overdose of a narcotic.

(B) discuss an overdose with him.

(C) give him sufficient analgesia to make him comfortable.

(D) discuss an overdose with his family.

(E) tell him to be tough.

62. A patient is scheduled for surgery. She is taking aspirin for knee pain. Your recommendation is

(A) continue the aspirin as needed for pain.

(B) stop the aspirin right away.

(C) stop the aspirin only two weeks before surgery.

(D) stop the aspirin the night before surgery.

(E) increase the use of the aspirin.

Questions 63 and 64 refer to the following:

A 67-year-old, 175-pound male is undergoing radical prostatectomy. Intraoperative blood loss has been 1,900 cc. The patient has received back two units of packed red cells and 500 cc of cell-saver blood.

63. How much additional crystalloid should the patient receive to compensate only for his blood loss?

(A) 300 cc

(B) 400 cc

(C) 700 cc

(D) 1,200 cc

(E) 3,300 cc

64. What is the approximate normal blood volume of this man?

(A) 3,500 cc

(B) 4,200 cc

(C) 5,600 cc

(D) 6,300 cc

(E) 7,000 cc

For Questions 65-68, select the most likely diagnosis.

(A) Gout

(B) Osteoarthritis

(C) Rheumatoid arthritis

(D) Pseudogout

(E) Infective arthritis

65. A 47-year-old woman comes to the clinic complaining of low-grade fevers and joint pains involving both knees. Physical examination reveals bilateral synovitis of the metacarpophalangeal and proximal interphalangeal joints, in additional to bilateral ballottable patellae.

66. A 56-year-old female comes to the emergency room complaining of severe pain in the left wrist. White blood cell count is 16.4. Joint aspiration reveals needle-shaped crystals which appear negatively birefringent under a polarized light microscope.

67. A 50-year-old female complains of bilateral pain in the fingers. Physical examination reveals nodes in the proximal and distal interphalangeal joints. X-ray of the hands shows a loss of joint space narrowing.

68. A 55-year-old alcoholic man complains of severe pain in the right big toe. Joint aspiration reveals rhomboid crystals which are positively birefringent.

69. During a routine visit to the geriatric clinic, an 87-year-old white female presents with symptoms of right temporal headache associated with a low-grade fever and malaise. Her ESR is 100 mm/hr. What would be the immediate management in this case?

(A) Temporal artery biopsy

(B) Nonsteroidal anti-inflammatory drugs

(C) Antibiotics

(D) Steroids

(E) CT of the brain

70. A 40-year-old man has been depressed for several months. You decide to start him on an antidepressant. Which one of the following medications is considered a first-line treatment for depression?

(A) A benzodiazepine

(B) A monoamine oxidase inhibitor—MAOI

(C) A selective serotonin reuptake inhibitor—SSRI

(D) A tricyclic antidepressant—TCA

(E) A phenothiazine

71. A 69-year-old Hispanic male who has been hospitalized with a gastric ulcer presents suddenly with severe, right-sided thoracic pain radiating across the back and associated with fever. On examination, the T12 dermatomal skin lesion shows vesicular lesions, which are tender and pruritic in nature. The nurse calls the medical resident to evaluate this patient's complaints. What would be the next step in making the diagnosis?

(A) Biopsy of the skin lesion

(B) Topical corticosteroids

(C) Empiric treatment with acyclovir

(D) Tzanck prep

(E) Electrocardiogram

72. A 45-year-old man comes to the clinic for a routine employment check-up. He was found to have a reactive (10 mm) PPD skin test. He is otherwise asymptomatic. His chest X-ray is normal. His physical exam was normal. What would be the next step in management of this patient?

(A) Isoniazid and B12 prophylaxis

(B) Sputum for acid-fast bacilli smears and cultures

(C) CT scan of the chest

(D) Repeat the chest X-ray in one year if symptoms occur

(E) Repeat the PPD skin test in six months

Questions 73-76 refer to the following:

A 53-year-old man with chronic low back pain comes in complaining of radiation of his pain to his left leg. He says he is in great pain and is hardly able to walk, though you have seen him come in from the parking lot without limping or any other sign of discomfort. His physical exam is benign with only minimal lumbosacral tenderness and no objective evidence of radiation.

73. The patient has been taking an anti-inflammatory agent and eight propoxyphenes a day. You had only prescribed six propoxyphenes daily as a maximum dose for him. He is out of propoxyphene and is demanding more pain medicine. You

(A) tell him he is faking his pain.

(B) give him as many propoxyphenes as he wants.

(C) give him multiple refills.

(D) give him codeine instead.

(E) tell him too many propoxyphenes are not good for him and can be habit-forming, and only give him enough to last a month at a dose of six per day, with no refills.

74. The patient becomes irate and threatens to go to another doctor. You

(A) tell him he is a drug addict.

(B) try to explain again why you are doing this.

(C) accuse him of selling propoxyphene.

(D) call a psychiatrist.

(E) call the police.

75. The patient remains irate and accuses you of not taking proper care of him. You

    (A) give him the names of four other physicians he can see.

    (B) call a psychiatrist.

    (C) try to get him committed.

    (D) call your lawyer.

    (E) call his insurance company.

76. Two weeks later a pharmacy calls you to confirm a prescription with your name on it for this patient for 200 pills of codeine with six refills, dated the day after his last visit to you. You

    (A) tell the pharmacist to fill it.

    (B) tell the pharmacist you did not write it and it should not be filled.

    (C) call a psychiatrist.

    (D) tell the pharmacist the patient is a drug dealer.

    (E) tell the pharmacist to call the police.

77. Potassium levels are the highest in which one of the following bodily fluids?

    (A) Diarrhea

    (B) Sweat

    (C) Pancreatic juice

    (D) Gastric juice

    (E) Bile

78. A three-year-old child is brought to the emergency room by his parents because of a febrile seizure which occurred for the first time. This child's temperature was 104°F and there was no evidence of neurologic pathology on exam. The seizure was generalized and lasted for five minutes. There was no history of previous neurologic insult or CNS abnormalities. What would be the American Academy of Pediatrics recommendations in this particular case?

    (A) CT of the head

    (B) Lumbar puncture

    (C) Immediate hospitalization

    (D) Electroencephalogram (EEG)

    (E) Antipyretics

79. While shopping at a grocery store, you see an elderly man clutch his chest and pass out. Upon arrival, you find him to be pulseless and apneic. Appropriate initial intervention is

    (A) active EMS.

    (B) begin mouth-to-mouth resuscitation.

    (C) begin chest compressions.

    (D) administer a precordial thump.

    (E) check the airway for foreign objects.

Questions 80 and 81 refer to the following:

You are conducting a clinical trial of a new antihypertensive agent. One of your new patients appears to qualify.

80. You should

    (A) start the medicine if you think it is necessary.

    (B) obtain informed consent from the patient.

    (C) not offer him the medicine because he is your patient.

    (D) tell him you will not take care of him if he does not participate in the study.

    (E) call the company and ask if you can recruit your own patient.

81. To conduct a clinical trial, you must

    (A) have a good idea.

    (B) get financial support.

    (C) get the approval of an Institutional Review Board for the Protection of Human Subjects.

    (D) agree to financial terms with your boss.

    (E) have your own nurse.

82. During your hospital rounds, you see a 50-year-old female patient of yours who has been in the hospital for the past three days with a bleeding duodenal ulcer. Her bleeding has been stable and you planned to discharge her today; however, you note that she has developed a fever of 102°F. Which one of the following is the LEAST likely source of fever in this patient?

    (A) Thrombophlebitis secondary to intravenous catheter

    (B) Aspiration pneumonia secondary to recent endoscopy

    (C) Urinary tract infection secondary to indwelling Foley catheter

    (D) Drug fever secondary to medications

    (E) Infected pressure sore secondary to bed rest

Questions 83 and 84 refer to the following:

A 34-year-old male is involved in a motorcycle accident and you suspect an abdominal injury. You have decided to perform a peritoneal lavage.

83. Which one of the following findings is suggestive of intra-abdominal trauma?

    (A) Hematocrit <1%

    (B) RBC <50,000 cells/cc

    (C) Amylase <50 units

    (D) WBC >500 cells/cc

    (E) Absence of bile

84. All of the following are complications of peritoneal lavage EXCEPT

    (A) infection.

    (B) perforation.

    (C) bleeding.

    (D) death.

    (E) pneumothorax.

Questions 85 and 86 refer to the following:

A 45-year-old woman with high cholesterol presents to your office with generalized skin deposits.

85. These are known as

    (A) juvenile xanthoma.

    (B) xeroderma pigmentosa.

    (C) xanthoma disseminatum.

    (D) xanthelasma.

    (E) hyperkeratosis.

86. These skin deposits may occur on all of the areas listed below EXCEPT

    (A) the oral mucosa.

    (B) the face.

    (C) the trunk.

    (D) the axillae.

    (E) the flexor surfaces of the limbs.

87. A nonresponsive middle-aged man presents to your emergency room. Nothing more is known about him. He has spontaneous respirations and his blood pressure is 130/70. All of the following are appropriate initial interventions EXCEPT

    (A) naloxone.

    (B) dextrose.

    (C) thiamine.

    (D) insert an intravenous line.

    (E) insulin.

88. A 32-year-old female has missed her menstrual period for three consecutive cycles. Her serum pregnancy test was negative. She is otherwise in good health and has no other complaints. What would be the next step in managing this patient?

    (A) Endometrial biopsy

    (B) Colposcopy

    (C) Oral medroxyprogesterone

(D)   Oral estrogen

(E)   Obtaining serum prolactin

For Questions 89-92, match the biopsy with the diagnosis.

Several of your patients were admitted for evaluation of possible underlying liver disease. Four of them underwent liver biopsy. Match the biopsies, shown in the figures, with the clinical diagnosis.

(A)

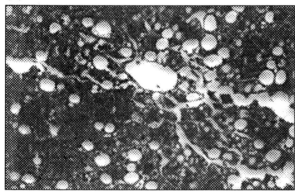

(B)

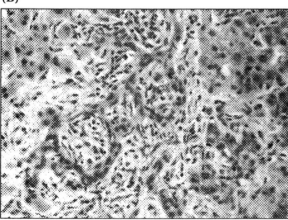

(C)

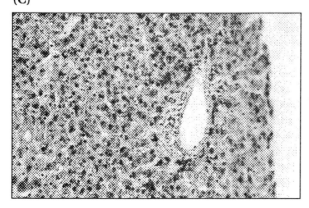

(D)

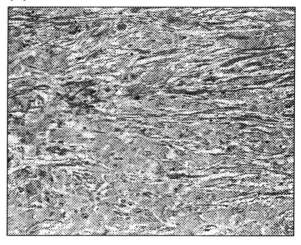

89.   Alcoholic steatosis

90.   Primary biliary cirrhosis

91.   Normal liver

92.   Hepatocellular carcinoma

Questions 93 and 94 refer to the following:

A 34-year old male has a third-degree burn over 50% of each arm.

93.   His percentage of body burn is closest to

(A)   2%.

(B)   10%.

(C)   20%.

(D)   30%.

(E)   50%.

94.   You are informed that this burn patient weighs 70 kg. His fluid requirement for the first 24 hours of admission is closest to

(A)   1,400 cc.

(B)   2,800 cc.

(C)   4,200 cc.

(D)   5,600 cc.

(E)   7,000 cc.

95. A 32-year-old female has been evaluated by you for the recent onset of throbbing headaches. A physician in the local emergency room contacts you today, reporting that she was brought in by the Emergency Medical Service for evaluation following a seizure. A cerebral angiogram, shown in the figure, was performed following the report of an abnormal magnetic resonance imaging study, also shown here. Treatment options include all of the following EXCEPT

Panel A

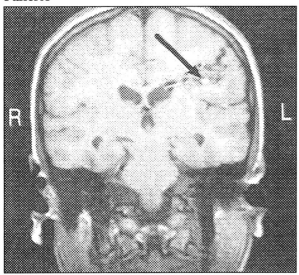

Panel B

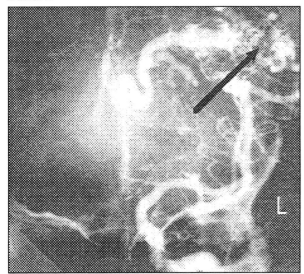

(A) surgical resection.

(B) arterial embolization.

(C) gamma-ray-induced thrombosis.

(D) proton-beam-induced thrombosis.

(E) chemotherapy with BCNU.

Questions 96-103 refer to the following:

A 22-year-old male is brought to the emergency room after being involved in a motor vehicle accident as an unrestrained driver. He had lost consciousness at the scene. His vital signs are 80/40 blood pressure, 120 pulse, 20 bagged respirations/minute, and a temperature of 36.7°C. He has no relatives to give you a history. You arrive as part of the trauma team and are assigned to do the initial survey.

96. Your head and neck exam should include all of the following EXCEPT

(A) inspection and palpation for lacerations and fractures.

(B) inspection of the pupils.

(C) inspection for otorrhea and rhinorrhea.

(D) mobility of the neck.

(E) position of the trachea.

97. Upon listening to the heart and lungs, you hear a rapid heart rate, no breath sounds on the right, and a deviated trachea is noted. You suspect

(A) esophageal intubation.

(B) right main stem intubation.

(C) tension pneumothorax.

(D) hemothorax.

(E) atelectasis.

98. The next step that should be performed is

(A) confirmation with a chest X-ray.

(B) repositioning of the endotracheal tube.

(C) needle thoracostomy.

(D) chest tube.

(E) positive pressure.

(D) 8.

(E) 10.

99. You now move on to examine the abdomen and notice faint ecchymosis around the umbilicus. This is known as

(A) Grey-Turner's sign.

(B) Cullen's sign.

(C) Murphy's sign.

(D) McBurney's sign.

(E) Cushing's sign.

100. The patient cannot give you information, so plain radiographs are ordered to give you more information. The X-ray giving you the least information would be

(A) skull film.

(B) mandible film.

(C) lateral C-spine.

(D) chest X-ray.

(E) pelvis film.

101. You are palpating the pulses of the lower extremities. The right dorsalis pedis and posterior tibial are normal, the left dorsalis pedis and posterior tibial are absent. Which one of the following would also be present?

(A) Warm left toes with normal capillary refill

(B) Fractured left femur

(C) Fractured right femur

(D) Left popliteal pulse

(E) Absent left brachial pulse

102. The patient opens his eyes to pain and has no motor response and no verbal response. His Glasgow coma scale score is

(A) 3.

(B) 4.

(C) 6.

103. Computerized tomography of the brain reveals midbrain compression. The respiratory pattern characterized by this is

(A) normal.

(B) hyperventilation.

(C) deep sighs and yawns.

(D) hypoventilation.

(E) Cheyne-Stokes.

Questions 104 and 105 refer to the following:

A patient you have not treated before presents to your clinic with visual complaints and you perform an examination of visual fields. You detect left homonymous hemianopsia.

104. The lesion is at the

(A) left optic tract.

(B) right optic tract.

(C) left optic nerve.

(D) right optic nerve.

(E) optic chiasm.

105. The father of the above patient drove the patient to your office and you note that he has drooping of his upper eyelids. This disease is known as

(A) ectropion.

(B) entropion.

(C) ptosis.

(D) enophthalmos.

(E) exophthalmos.

Questions 106-113 refer to the following:

Your practice is located in rural Montana. Your nurse interrupts your staff advisory meeting with the following information. A 50-year-old male with hyperlipidemia and hypertension, who is scheduled to see you in

15 minutes, just arrived at your office with complaints of severe indigestion. There is associated nausea, anxiety, weakness, and diaphoresis. While parking his car this morning, he had an altercation with a delivery man, who wanted the same parking spot. Vital signs are blood pressure 150/100, pulse of 100, respiration of 16, and temperature of 98.6°.

106. You advise her to

  (A) administer Mylanta, 30cc po STAT.

  (B) calm him down and indicate that you will see him at the appointed time.

  (C) obtain a STAT electrocardiogram.

  (D) administer diazepam, 10 mg intravenously STAT.

  (E) verify that his insurance coverage is still in effect.

107. You have obtained a more detailed history and completed your examination. Blood has been sent for analysis. Chest X-ray is unremarkable. The electrocardiogram is shown in the figure below. You now

  (A) administer streptokinase, 1.5 million units over 60 minutes.

  (B) administer aspirin, 500 mg po.

  (C) administer atenolol, 100 mg intravenously.

  (D) arrange for an immediate upper gastrointestinal endoscopy.

  (E) arrange for a ventilation perfusion lung scan.

108. The patient responded to your treatment. He returns several months later for a reevaluation. He is asymptomatic. Physical examination is significant for a blood pressure of 140/95. Laboratory results are CBC: WNL; chemistry panel: chol 400 mg/dL, otherwise WNL; and HDL chol: 45 ng/dL, LDL chol: 145 ng/dL. You discuss with him all of the following NCEP guidelines EXCEPT

  (A) for persons with coronary artery disease, the target LDL cholesterol is 100 mg/dL or lower.

  (B) in persons without coronary artery disease, the desirable cholesterol level is less than 200 mg/dL.

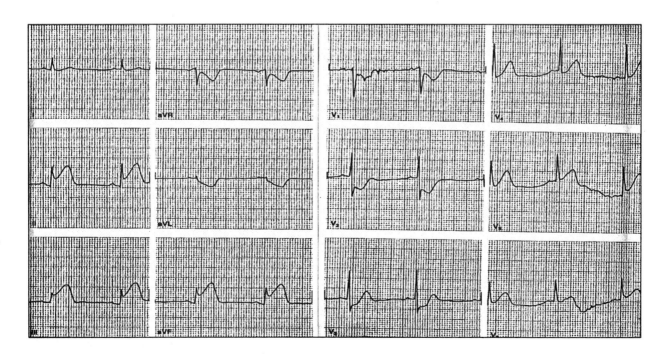

(C) an HDL cholesterol greater than 60 mg/dL is a negative risk factor for coronary artery disease.

(D) an HDL cholesterol less than 35 mg/dL is a risk factor for coronary artery disease.

(E) total cholesterol should always be measured in the fasting state.

109. Two years later while attending his son's graduation from medical school, he devel-

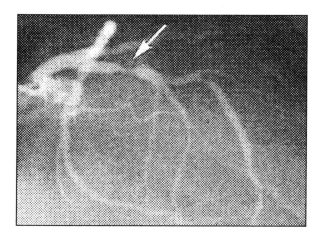

ops crushing substernal chest pain. Following admission to the intensive care unit, a coronary angiogram, shown in the figure, is performed. You diagnose

(A) coronary artery stenosis.

(B) aneurysm of the coronary artery.

(C) normal study.

(D) polyarteritis nodosa.

(E) stent occlusion.

110. Which one of the following is NOT true regarding the use of cardiac troponin I and T levels in coronary syndromes?

(A) Monoclonal antibodies against cardiac troponin T and I have very little cross-reactivity with corresponding skeletal muscle isoforms.

(B) A quantitative relationship between long-term clinical outcome and cardiac troponin T

levels has been reported in persons with unstable angina.

(C) Together with troponin C, these proteins regulate the calcium-dependent interactions between myosin and actin.

(D) Levels of these proteins are sensitive and specific markers of myocardial cell injury.

(E) Measurement of these proteins is the most cost-effective way to monitor persons with acute cardiac events.

111. Three years later he returns with complaints of increasing cramping, numbness, and fatigue of his calves. He is unable to perform his normal activities. The symptoms are more severe in the right as compared to the left leg. Rest pain is now present. Physical examination reveals absent pulses below the femoral on the right, decreased DP and PT pulses on the left; thickened nail beds and dry, cool, smooth, shiny skin with decreased hair bilaterally as well as trace edema bilaterally. An arteriogram, performed as part of his diagnostic evaluation, is shown in the figure. You suggest all of the possible options EXCEPT

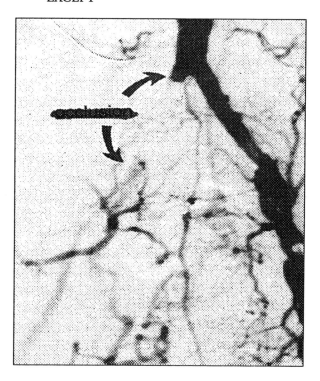

(A)   pentoxifylline, 100 mg orally TID.

(B)   percutaneous transluminal angioplasty.

(C)   rotational atherectomy.

(D)   intravascular stent.

(E)   aortofemoral bypass.

112. The patient responds to your treatment. Two years later, he presents to the emergency room with complaints of the sudden onset of left-sided weakness. Physical examination reveals blood pressure of 150/100, pulse of 60, respiration of 20, temperature of 98.6°F, left hemiplegia and hemianesthesia, and left hyperreflexia left positive Babinski. Laboratory tests are CBC: WNL, chemistry panel: glucose 140 mg/dL, chol 300 mg/dL; and PT WNL, PTT WNL. Noncontrast computed tomographic scans (obtained 2-1/2 hours following symptom onset) are shown in the figures. The section in panel B was taken slightly cephalad to that in panel A. You diagnose

Panel A

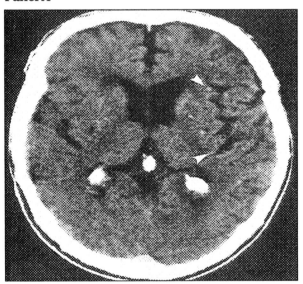

Panel B

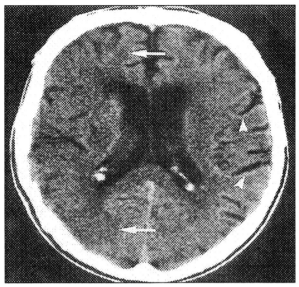

(A)   right middle cerebral artery infarction.

(B)   lateral medullary syndrome.

(C)   basilar artery occlusion.

(D)   posterior cerebral artery occlusion.

(E)   transient ischemic attack.

113. His condition continues to deteriorate. Two days later, a repeat computerized tomographic scan is performed to evaluate a progressive decline in his level of consciousness. The figures shown here are at comparable levels to those obtained at admission (Question 112). These studies demonstrate all of the following EXCEPT

Panel A

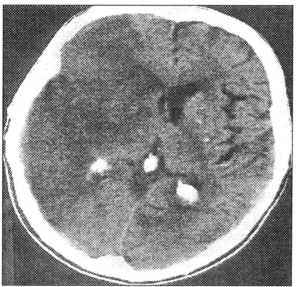

Panel B

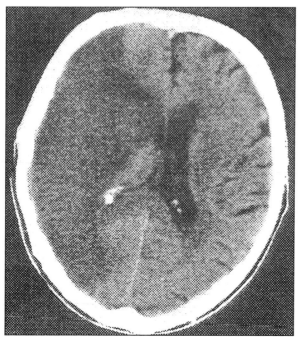

(A) a left-to-right midline shift.

(B) a right-to-left midline shift.

(C) severe hypodensity in the distribution of the right middle cerebral artery.

(D) a mass effect on the ventricular system.

(E) right cerebral infarction.

114. You are looking for some bandages in a supply closet and discover one of the interns assigned to the ER slumped on the floor with a tourniquet on his arm, a bottle of morphine, and a used syringe on the floor next to him. You call for help and awaken him with naloxone. When he has recovered, you

(A) get everyone to promise that they will not report him.

(B) fire him.

(C) call the police.

(D) commit him.

(E) discuss his problem with him and admit him to a drug recovery unit.

115. Your 68-year-old healthy female patient comes to you for routine follow-up care. She is concerned about the development of osteoporosis. Which one of the following statements is NOT true regarding osteoporosis?

(A) Asymptomatic osteoporosis is uncommon.

(B) Osteoporosis is the most common underlying disorder in fracture.

(C) Back pain is the most common complaint in patients with osteoporosis.

(D) Blood levels of calcium, phosphate, and alkaline phosphate are normal in osteoporosis.

(E) Long-term heparin use predisposes towards the development of osteoporosis.

116. A 60-year-old woman is hospitalized for urosepsis. Due to her age and other comorbidities, intravenous access is difficult, and you are asked to place central access. During an attempt at central access to the right internal jugular artery, she begins to complain of chest pain and shortness of breath and becomes tachycardiac. Of the following possible complications, which one of the following is most likely to be causing the above symptoms?

    (A)   Hemorrhage

    (B)   Tension pneumothorax

    (C)   Plyocardial rupture

    (D)   Infection

    (E)   None of the above.

117. A 45-year-old poorly controlled insulin-dependent diabetic female complains of low-grade fever, dull sinus pains and nasal congestion that has progressed over the past few days to facial and periorbital swelling. Physical examination reveals an inflamed, friable nasal mucosa with the appearance of dried blood on the turbinates, periorbital edema, and mild proptosis. A computed axial tomographic scan of the head, done as part of your initial workup, is shown in the figure below. You now

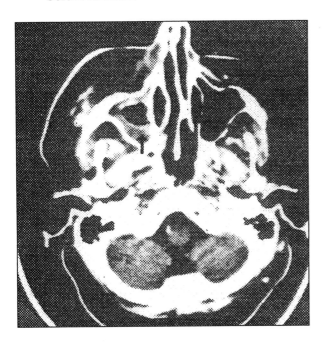

(A)   admit her to the hospital.

(B)   begin therapy with 12 million units penicillin IV daily.

(C)   begin antihistamines and broad spectrum antibiotics.

(D)   schedule a biopsy for the following morning.

(E)   begin acyclovir, 800 mg po X5 daily.

118. A patient in a clinical trial you are conducting has a minor adverse reaction to the drug late in the course of the study. You do not feel the reaction is serious or will affect the patient adversely. If you notify the company, they will probably tell you to withdraw the patient and will not pay you the remaining fee for the patient's enrollment. You should

    (A)   not tell the company.

    (B)   explain to the patient that he has nothing to worry about if you do not tell anyone.

    (C)   discuss the issue with your colleagues.

    (D)   call a lawyer.

    (E)   report the adverse reaction.

119. The bleeding of dysentery is due to

    (A)   ulcerative erosions into arterial feed vessels.

    (B)   colonic mucosal invasion of the pathogen.

    (C)   a systemic coagulopathy.

    (D)   thrombosis of submucosal capillaries.

    (E)   bowel necrosis.

For Questions 120-123, match each of the following organizations with its correct description.

    (A)   Centers for Disease Control

    (B)   Environmental Protection Agency (EPA)

    (C)   American Cancer Society

(D)   Food and Drug Administration (FDA)

(E)   Professional Review Organizations (PROs)

120. Investigates epidemic diseases

121. Sets guidelines for hazardous waste control

122. Is supported by voluntary donations

123. Sets standards for the quality of care provided to Medicaid and Medicare patients

124. A 65-year-old asymptomatic male, with a 30-year history of smoking two packs of cigarettes a day, presents to your office. According to the U.S. Preventive Services Task Force on the Periodic Health Examination, you should perform

(A)   sputum cytology for lung carcinoma.

(B)   chest X-ray for lung carcinoma.

(C)   tonometry for glaucoma.

(D)   endoscopic examination to detect laryngeal cancer.

(E)   None of the above.

125. An 18-year-old female comes to your office with frontal and maxillary sinus tenderness. The next step is to

(A)   prescribe antibiotics.

(B)   order sinus plain films.

(C)   order sinus CAT scans.

(D)   aspirate the sinuses in question.

(E)   schedule the patient for surgery for sinus exenteration.

126. A 56-year-old female patient comes to the emergency room complaining of low back pain. Physical exam reveals spinal and paraspinal tenderness at the L4 vertebrae. X-rays reveal a lytic lesion at this site, suggesting metastatic cancer. The most likely primary site of cancer is

(A)   ovary.

(B)   uterus.

(C)   breast.

(D)   colon.

(E)   stomach.

127. A 26-year-old woman presents to your office, having tested positive for HIV. She brings copies of the results to you, and it shows that she had a positive ELISA and a negative Western blot. She has no significant medical illnesses. She is sexually active and uses condoms "most of the time," although she denies any sexual contact in the last nine months. She denies any history of intravenous drug use. The most appropriate statement regarding the results of her test is

(A)   she has AIDS.

(B)   she is infected with the human immunodeficiency virus.

(C)   she may or may not be infected; you don't know.

(D)   she is not infected, but should change her lifestyle habits.

(E)   she is not infected and may continue her present lifestyle.

128. A 29-year-old woman presents to your clinic with a burning tongue. The most likely cause is

(A)   oral cancer.

(B)   tobacco smoking.

(C)   odontalgia.

(D)   myxedema.

(E)   thyrotoxicosis.

129. A 40-year-old female patient comes to your office requesting screening for hemochromatosis due to a family history of the disease. You order screening blood tests for hemochromatosis including HLA typing. Which one of the following bloodtest results are consistent with the diagnosis of hemochromatosis?

(A) Decreased percent transferrin saturation

(B) Increased plasma iron

(C) Increased iron binding capacity

(D) Decreased serum ferritin

(E) None of the above.

130. A 28-year-old patient complains of diffuse back pain. In addition, he claims that he has headaches, his stomach aches, and he has had several episodes of diarrhea. He claims that he has vomited several times in the past four weeks. History further reveals that the man is impotent, and wonders whether the impotency is related to the pain on urination that he experiences. No organic cause can be identified. Which one of the following disorders does the patient most likely suffer from?

(A) Somatization disorder

(B) Undifferentiated somatoform disorder

(C) Conversion disorder

(D) Pain disorder

(E) Hypochondriasis

131. A 42-year-old woman presents to your office with recurrent abdominal pain. She states that periodically, several times a year, she notes severe pain in her right upper quadrant. She describes it as crampy in character and worsened with food when it occurs. She denies having any fevers or chills associated with the symptoms. An appropriate initial diagnostic test would be

(A) serum levels of amylase and lipase.

(B) esophagoduodenoscopy.

(C) serum levels of IgG for *Helicobacter pylori*.

(D) right upper quadrant ultrasound.

(E) CT of the abdomen.

Questions 132-134 refer to the following:

A 32-year-old babysitter presents to the clinic with an unscheduled appointment be-cause she has symptoms of palpitations, weight loss, heat intolerance, and increased anxiety and restlessness. She has had these symptoms for over two weeks, and they have been getting progressively worse. On exam, she has warm and smooth skin, mild systolic hypertension, tremors, and hyperactive deep tendon reflexes.

132. All of the following tests are appropriate in order to confirm the presence of thyrotoxicosis EXCEPT

(A) serum thyroglobulin concentrations.

(B) a thyroid radionucleotide scan.

(C) thyroid-stimulating hormone assay.

(D) antithyroid microsomal antibody.

(E) free thyroxine level.

133. All of the following abnormalities are seen in the lab data in Grave's disease EXCEPT

(A) elevated antithyroglobulin antibody.

(B) modest anemia.

(C) sinus tachycardia on the EKG.

(D) increased bone density on CT scan.

(E) increased uptake on thyroid scan.

134. What is the current recommended treatment of choice for Grave's disease?

(A) L-thyroxine

(B) Prednisone

(C) Radioactive iodine thyroid ablation

(D) Nonsteroidal anti-inflammatory agents

(E) Tapazole

135. An eight-year-old boy gets bitten on his arm by the family dog, whose rabies status is known. The wound is sutured closed and

you then ask the boy to return to the clinic for follow-up in

(A) 1 day.

(B) 5 days.

(C) 7-10 days.

(D) 10-14 days.

(E) 14-21 days.

Questions 136 and 137 refer to the following:

A mother brings in her one-year-old child with "pink eye" and a purulent ocular discharge. There is no visual problem.

136. The most likely diagnosis is

(A) viral conjunctivitis.

(B) bacterial conjunctivitis.

(C) upper respiratory infection.

(D) blepharitis.

(E) None of the above.

137. If you were to treat the above patient, the mother should be treated

(A) all of the time.

(B) some of the time.

(C) only if she is symptomatic.

(D) never.

(E) only until the child improves.

138. A 78-year-old female presents with inability to control her urine flow. She was diagnosed with mixed incontinence by her physician. All of the following can assist her in regaining control of her bladder EXCEPT

(A) alpha-adrenergic blockers.

(B) biofeedback therapy.

(C) anticholinergic therapy.

(D) bladder training.

(E) toilet assistance.

139. A 25-year-old female comes to your office with complaints of a foul-smelling vaginal discharge. A KOH wet mount gives off a fishy odor, and "clue cells" are observed on microscopic exam. The most likely etiology of her discharge is infection with

(A) *Trichomonas.*

(B) *Gardnerella.*

(C) human papilloma virus.

(D) *Candida albicans.*

(E) *Chlamydia.*

Questions 140-147 refer to the following:

You are called by the frantic mother of a 30-year-old depressed female, who was scheduled to see you today. Following an altercation, the young woman locked herself in the bathroom, where she ingested "a bottle of Tylenol."

140. You advise the mother to

(A) call the emergency medical service.

(B) immediately administer two tablespoonfuls of sodium bicarbonate (baking soda) in orange juice.

(C) immediately administer activated charcoal, 10 grams.

(D) immediately administer syrup of ipecac, 10 ml.

(E) begin forced diuresis with Gatorade.

141. The patient initially refused transport to the emergency room. She arrives eight hours later. She is vomiting and diaphoretic. Physical examination, except for depression, is unremarkable. You now order all of the following EXCEPT

(A) liver function tests.

(B) prothrombin time.

(C)   urine drug toxicology.

(D)   urine acetaminophen level.

(E)   serum BUN.

142.   The laboratory reports the plasma acetaminophen level as 800 micrograms/mL. Based on the nomogram, shown in the figure, you now administer

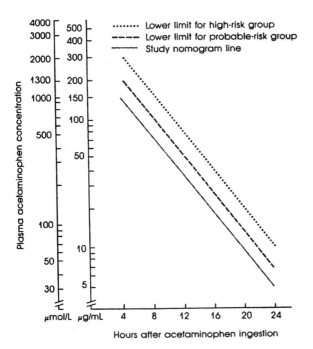

(A)   activated charcoal, 50 grams orally.

(B)   acetylcysteine, 140 mg/kg orally.

(C)   phytonadione, 10 mg IM.

(D)   dimercaprol, 5.0 mg/kg IM (L).

(E)   deferoxamine mesylate, 1 gram IM.

143.   You explain to the family that this treatment is thought to work by

(A)   acting as a sulfhydryl donor.

(B)   inhibiting synthesis of glutathione.

(C)   depleting hepatic stores of glutathione.

(D)   promoting the conversion of glyoxalase to glycine.

(E)   reactivating cholinesterase.

144.   Four hours after admission (12 hours after ingestion) the woman complains of right upper quadrant abdominal pain, nausea, and diarrhea. Physical examination reveals a blood pressure of 100/70, pulse of 100, respiration of 18, temperature of 99°F, and right upper quadrant tenderness to palpation. Admission CBC and chemistry panel were within normal limits. You now order

(A)   abdominal sonogram.

(B)   liver spleen scan.

(C)   repeat chemistry profile and PT.

(D)   upper gastrointestinal X ray.

(E)   stool culture.

145.   Three hours later, the laboratory reports that the prothrombin time and liver transaminases are within normal limits. As you discuss the results with the woman, she reports that her symptoms have resolved. She further admits that her behavior, which precipitated this admission, was impulsive. She denies current symptoms of depression. You now

(A)   discharge her to the care of her psychiatrist.

(B)   discuss the need to repeat liver transaminases and prothrombin time in 24 hours.

(C)   tell the family that you think there is a laboratory error.

(D)   ask the laboratory to repeat the transaminases after diluting the specimen.

(E)   discharge the patient, with a follow-up appointment in one month.

146.   The woman's condition has progressively deteriorated over the past five days. Physical examination is positive for clouding of con-

sciousness, asterixis, fetor hepaticas, purpura, and jaundice. Abnormal laboratory tests include

Alanine aminotransferase: 4,000 U/L
Aspartate aminotransferase: 4,500 U/L
Glucose: 60 mg/dL
Prothrombin time: 24 seconds

You advise the family that

(A) if the woman survives the acute episode, nursing home care will be necessary to manage chronic encephalopathy.

(B) survivors of acute toxicity rarely have residual liver damage.

(C) most survivors of acute toxicity have compensated cirrhosis.

(D) it is very unlikely that this clinical picture is due to acute drug toxicity.

(E) with this clinical picture, there have been no survivors.

147. All of the following laboratory test abnormalities may be present with chronic, as opposed to acute, acetaminophen toxicity EXCEPT

(A) sterile pyuria.

(B) "ring sign" on an intravenous pyelogram.

(C) proteinuria greater than 10 grams/day.

(D) serum creatinine greater than 3 mg/dL.

(E) positive urine cytology.

148. You are called to review a CXR after Swan-Ganz catheter placement. The proper location for the tip of a Swan-Ganz catheter is

(A) 5 cm distal to the pulmonic valve.

(B) the junction of the right atrium and superior vena cava.

(C) 4 cm distal to the aortic valve.

(D) the right subclavian vein.

(E) 4 cm distal to the tricuspid valve.

149. A 47-year-old man is brought to the emergency room with delirium. Laboratory exam reveals the following: NA: 142, K: 5.0, Cl: 109, HCO_3: 9. All of the following conditions are consistent with this type of anion-gap disturbance EXCEPT

(A) Type IV renal tubular acidosis.

(B) renal failure.

(C) diabetic ketoacidosis.

(D) sepsis.

(E) ethylene glycol ingestion.

Questions 150-157 refer to the following:

A 23-year-old woman presents to your office with one day of urinary frequency, hematuria, and dysuria. She denies flank pain, fevers, or chills. Physical examination reveals mild tenderness over the suprapubic area with palpation.

150. Besides a simple cystitis, the disease that is most associated with the above symptoms is

(A) acute glomerulonephritis.

(B) acute renal failure.

(C) acute nephrolithiasis.

(D) acute renal artery thrombosis.

(E) renal cell carcinoma.

151. A urinalysis reveals positive leukocyte esterase, nitrite, blood, and no other abnormalities. Of the following statements regarding urinalysis, the LEAST accurate one is

(A) a urinalysis must be submitted within six hours or it's not valid.

(B) leukocyte esterase is a by-product of white blood cells which are found in a urinary tract infection.

(C) nitrite is a by-product of bacteria.

(D) a urine culture does not need to be sent off.

(E) trace of blood is commonly seen in acute cystitis.

152. Of the following possibilities for treatment, the most appropriate initial therapy would be to

(A) treat for three days with oral Trimethoprim/sulfamethox-azole.

(B) admit for intravenous ceftazi-dime.

(C) treat with one intramuscular shot of ceftriazone.

(D) treat with two doses of oral vancomycin.

(E) treat with 10 days of cephalexin.

153. In two days, the patient returns to your office and tells you that she continues to have urinary frequency, dysuria, and hematuria. In addition, she now complains of severe suprapubic crampy pain. On physical examination, she has moderate pain to tenderness over her suprapubic area without rebound. Pelvic examination reveals a small amount of vaginal discharge and a normal appearing cervix. You prepare a sample of the vaginal discharge to observe under the microscope. Of the following findings on physical examination, the one that would make you LEAST concerned that the patient is having pelvic inflammatory disease is

(A) a friable cervical mucosa.

(B) adnexal tenderness.

(C) the presence of genital warts.

(D) cervical motion tenderness.

(E) None of the above.

154. Of the following findings on microscopic examination of the vaginal discharge, the one most likely to suggest bacterial vaginosis is

(A) the presence of pear-shaped flagellated organisms.

(B) the presence of epithelial cells dotted with dark spots and with blurry margins.

(C) the presence of hyphae.

(D) the presence of white blood cells.

(E) the presence of red blood cells.

155. The vaginal discharge appears normal under microscopic examination. The patient continues to deny fevers or chills. The most likely cause of the patient's symptoms are

(A) vaginal candidiasis.

(B) trichomoniasis.

(C) bladder spasm.

(D) renal colic.

(E) None of the above.

156. The most appropriate medication for the treatment of the patient's symptoms is

(A) prazosin.

(B) phenazopyridine.

(C) alprazolam.

(D) metronidazole.

(E) morphine.

157. The patient takes your prescription and notes significant improvement after one day. The most appropriate follow-up after resolution of the symptoms is

(A) a repeat urine culture.

(B) urodynamic testing.

(C) cystoscopy.

(D) laparoscopy.

(E) discussion of bladder suspension.

158. All of the following are true of vertigo EXCEPT

(A) reading exacerbates motion sickness by miscuing the visual system.

(B) height vertigo results from a mismatch of normal body sway and the lack of its visual detection.

(C) benign positional vertigo is the most common form of physiologic vertigo.

(D) benign positional vertigo results from free-floating calcium carbonate crystals that inadvertently enter the long arm of the posterior semicircular canal.

(E) seasickness results from maladaptation of the vestibular system when it is subjected to unfamiliar head movements.

Questions 159-166 refer to the following:

A 30-year-old female, diagnosed with systemic lupus erythematosus (SLE) in another city, has relocated to your city. She has chosen you as her "gatekeeper" from the information provided by her HMO. She walks into your office today requesting a refill of her medications. She has obtained a copy of her prior laboratory tests and wants to discuss them with you.

159. You first discuss antinuclear antibodies, indicating all of the following EXCEPT

(A) if they are negative, there is less than a one percent chance of developing SLE.

(B) less than ten percent of SLE patients are positive if the substrate contains human nuclei HEP-2.

(C) the frequency of positivity increases with age.

(D) they may be positive in low titer in normal persons.

(E) they develop in 50-75% of persons taking procainamide.

160. She has many questions regarding other autoantibodies in SLE. You discuss all of the following EXCEPT

(A) antibodies to double-stranded DNA are relatively specific for SLE.

(B) antibodies to Sm are relatively specific for SLE.

(C) high serum levels of anti-dsDNA antibodies usually correlate with renal disease activity.

(D) anti-Ro (SSA) is common in ANA negative SLE.

(E) antibodies to single-stranded DNA are more specific for SLE than antibodies to double-stranded DNA.

161. In SLE, which one of the following is NOT true regarding complement?

(A) Low levels of complement usually reflect renal disease activity.

(B) Total functional hemolytic complement (CH50) levels are the most sensitive measure of complement activation.

(C) Total functional hemolytic complement (CH50) levels are most subject to laboratory error.

(D) Very low levels of CH50 with normal levels of C3 suggest an inherited deficiency of a complement component.

(E) C1 INH is commonly deficient in SLE.

162. You indicate that all of the following are included in the American Rheumatism Association hematologic criteria for classification of SLE EXCEPT

(A) hemolytic anemia with reticulocytosis.

(B) leukopenia less than 4,000/mm^3 total on at least two occasions.

(C) lymphopenia less than 1,500/mm^3 on at least two occasions.

(D) thrombocytopenia, less than 100,000/mm^3 in the absence of offending drugs.

(E) aplastic anemia.

163. Which one of the following is true of the lupus anticoagulant?

    (A) It is recognized by prolongation of the prothrombin time.

    (B) It is recognized by prolongation of the partial thromboplastin time.

    (C) It corrects with the addition of normal plasma.

    (D) It is more sensitive than the Russell viper venom time.

    (E) It is more sensitive than the rabbit brain neutral phospholipid test.

164. She has been treated with several drugs in the past and wonders how you distinguish the drug-induced form of lupus from SLE. After discussing the distinguishing clinical features, you also discuss the distinguishing laboratory features. You indicate, that in comparison with SLE, drug-induced lupus is characterized by all of the following EXCEPT

    (A) antibodies to double-stranded DNA are rare.

    (B) hypocomplementemia is rare.

    (C) ANA positively is rare.

    (D) anti-histone antibodies are very common.

    (E) HLA-DR4+ persons are at increased risk.

165. She is considering pregnancy and wants to be informed of the potential risks both during the pregnancy and to her baby. You discuss all of the following EXCEPT

    (A) antiphospholipid antibodies predispose to recurrent midtrimester fetal loss.

    (B) an elevated creatinine has no effect on fetal outcome.

    (C) transmission of maternal anti-Ro antibodies across the placenta may cause neonatal lupus.

    (D) transient neonatal thrombocytopenia may result from maternal antiplatelet antibodies.

    (E) congenital heart block is associated with anti-Ro antibodies.

166. She returns six months later with deterioration of renal function. You indicate that renal biopsy is helpful in distinguishing between the various types of nephritis, assessing fibrosis/sclerosis, and excluding other forms of renal disease. Possible pathologic lesions in SLE include all of the following EXCEPT

    (A) Berger's nephritis.

    (B) mesangial nephritis.

    (C) diffuse proliferative glomerulonephritis.

    (D) membranous glomerulonephritis.

    (E) focal proliferative nephritis.

Question 167-170 refer to the following:

A 67-year-old man comes to your office complaining of difficulty in swallowing.

167. Which one of the following is LEAST helpful in determining the etiology of his symptoms?

    (A) Symptoms related to solids versus liquids

    (B) Duration of symptoms

    (C) History of peptic ulcers

    (D) Associated heartburn

    (E) Weight loss

168. A barium swallow is obtained, which reveals a dilated esophagus and a narrowing at the gastroesophageal junction. Which one of the following diagnoses is most likely based on this finding?

    (A) Esophageal cancer

    (B) Schatzki's ring

    (C) Diffuse esophageal spasm

(D) Peptic stricture

(E) Achalasia

169. The best test to confirm this diagnosis is

(A) esophageal manometry.

(B) 24-hour pH probe.

(C) therapeutic trial with a proton pump inhibitor.

(D) upper endoscopy with full-thickness esophageal biopsy.

(E) pneumatic balloon dilation of the gastroesophageal junction.

170. If this patient was found to have dysphagia secondary to an esophageal cancer at the gastroesophageal junction, the most likely histopathology of the tumor would be

(A) squamous cell carcinoma.

(B) smooth muscle sarcoma.

(C) adenocarcinoma.

(D) carcinoma-in-situ.

(E) Barrett's mucosa.

Questions 171-173 refer to the following:

A 59-year-old arthritic golfer, with a recent history of a knee arthroscopy, presents to the emergency room with severe left knee pain and fever. On examination, his knee is tender, swollen, and a fluctuance is present. He has decreased active range of motion.

171. The next best test is

(A) a CBC, Chem 7, ABG, and MAI serologies.

(B) joint aspiration of synovial fluid.

(C) X-rays of the knee.

(D) MRI of the knee.

(E) blood cultures.

172. During your diagnostic evaluation, an X-ray and MRI of the knee are performed that reveal soft tissue swelling; no destructive changes are seen. The most appropriate treatment is

(A) systemic antibiotics.

(B) bed rest.

(C) frequent joint aspirations.

(D) Both (A) and (C).

(E) Both (B) and (C).

173. The patient's most likely predisposing factor is his history of

(A) perennial golfing.

(B) diabetes mellitus.

(C) arthritis.

(D) endocarditis.

(E) recent joint surgery.

174. Your 44-year-old patient, who is an asthmatic under good control, presents to your office wheezing and extremely short of breath. Your first action should be

(A) have him register and wait his turn.

(B) obtain an arterial blood gas and wait for the result before initiating therapy.

(C) obtain a chest X-ray.

(D) intubate for impending respiratory distress.

(E) administer a nebulizer treatment and reassess the patient after the result.

175. You are called to the floor to evaluate a 67-year-old male who is in respiratory distress three days post small bowel resection for tumor. Oxygen saturation by pulse oximeter is reading 89%. What will be the patient's approximate PaO_2 by arterial blood gas analysis?

(A) 300 mm Hg

(B) 26 mm Hg

(C) 57 mm Hg

(D) 125 mm Hg

(E) 80 mm Hg

Questions 176 and 177 refer to the following:

A 38-year-old female with rheumatoid arthritis comes to the office complaining of cough and shortness of breath.

176. All of the following are pulmonary complications of rheumatoid arthritis EXCEPT

    (A) small cell carcinoma.

    (B) pulmonary nodules.

    (C) obliterative bronchiolitis.

    (D) pleural effusion.

    (E) fibrosing alveolitis.

177. In addition to pulmonary disease, other extra-articular features of rheumatoid arthritis include all of the following EXCEPT

    (A) vasculitis.

    (B) episcleritis.

    (C) splenomegaly.

    (D) pericarditis.

    (E) urethral discharge.

Questions 178 and 179 refer to the following:

A 30-year-old woman has had an increasing pain in her neck for two months with no resolve. Recently she has noticed pain in her upper arm.

178. Your next step would be

    (A) examination of the neck and neurologic systems.

    (B) cervical spine X-rays.

    (C) CT of the neck.

    (D) MRI of the neck.

    (E) myelogram of the neck.

179. You diagnose a herniated disc of the cervical region. All of the following would be appropriate treatment modalities EXCEPT

    (A) traction.

    (B) surgery.

    (C) nonsteroidal anti-inflammatory drugs.

    (D) muscle relaxants.

    (E) neck exercises.

180. Which one of the following conditions is the LEAST likely cause of prolonged fevers of undetermined origin?

    (A) Diverticulitis

    (B) Hodgkin's disease

    (C) Bacterial meningitis

    (D) Factitious fever

    (E) Temporal arteritis

USMLE STEP 3 PRACTICE TEST 1

Day Two – Afternoon Session

(Answer sheets appear in the back of this book.)

TIME: 3 Hours
180 Questions

DIRECTIONS: Each of the following numbered items or incomplete sentences is followed by an answer or a completion of the statement. Choose the **ONE** choice that **BEST** answers the question or completes the sentence.

Questions 1-9 refer to the following:

Your 50-year-old patient with a family history of melanoma comes to your office with a skin lesion on the neck. You biopsy the lesion and make a diagnosis of basal cell carcinoma.

1. Which one of the following statements is true regarding basal cell carcinoma (BCC)?

    (A) Tumors are locally invasive and metastatic.

    (B) Tumors are rapid growing.

    (C) Hemorrhage from the lesion is common.

    (D) Pearly margin, telangiectatic vessels, and central ulceration are classic findings.

    (E) None of the above.

2. Physical examination is significant for 2+pitting edema of both lower extremities. You suspect that the patient may have a renal abnormality and order a 24-hour urine for protein, which returns with a value of 4.7 grams in 24 hours. Which of the following conditions would be LEAST likely to be a cause of this patient's symptoms?

    (A) Right-heart failure

    (B) Obstruction of the inferior vena cava

    (C) Constrictive pericarditis

    (D) Deep venous thrombosis

    (E) Liver failure

3. All of the following renal conditions may cause proteinuria in this range EXCEPT

    (A) diabetes mellitus.

    (B) amyloidosis.

    (C) minimal change disease.

    (D) poststreptococcal glomerulopathy.

    (E) focal and segmental glomerulosclerosis.

4. Which one of the following blood tests is LEAST likely to be normal in this patient?

    (A) C3, C4 levels

    (B) Cholesterol

(C) Creatinine

(D) Potassium

(E) Blood urea nitrogen

5. You proceed with renal biopsy, which reveals basement glomerular basement membrane thickening and IgG and C3 deposits in a uniform, finely granular pattern, outlining the capillary loops, consistent with membranous glomerulopathy. Which lesion is associated with all of the above conditions EXCEPT

(A) lung carcinoma.

(B) systemic lupus erythematosus.

(C) multiple myeloma.

(D) chronic hepatitis B infection.

(E) gold therapy.

6. All of the following are pathophysiologic processes involved in this condition EXCEPT

(A) activation of renin-angiotensin syndrome.

(B) renal sodium retention.

(C) increased tubular secretion of albumin.

(D) fluid migration into the interstitium.

(E) increased hepatic lipoprotein synthesis.

7. Your patient wishes to know the prognosis of his disease. You should tell him which one of the following?

(A) Almost half the patients with his condition will progress to end-stage renal disease in 10 years.

(B) Most patients with his condition will have a remission with steroid therapy.

(C) Therapy is not necessary as the condition is usually self-limited.

(D) There is no increase in the risk of bacterial infections.

(E) None of the above.

8. You continue to follow the patient at your office. The patient returns to your office complaining of hematuria. Blood tests reveal a sudden deterioration in renal function from a creatinine of 1.4 from the results of three weeks prior to a creatinine of 3.2. Which one of the following is an appropriate course of action?

(A) Repeat renal biopsy to evaluate disease progression

(B) Ultrasound/Doppler study of renal veins

(C) Initiation of therapy with intravenous Cytoxan

(D) Listing for renal transplantation

(E) None of the above.

9. Which one of the following serum levels is LEAST likely to be elevated in patients with a deterioration in renal function?

(A) Potassium

(B) Phosphorus

(C) Magnesium

(D) Uric acid

(E) None of the above.

For Questions 10-13, match the vitamin deficiency with each numbered case question.

(A) Thiamine

(B) Vitamin A

(C) Ascorbic acid

(D) Folate

(E) Vitamin K

10. A 56-year-old alcoholic male presents to the emergency room with symptoms of shortness of breath, anorexia, vomiting, an ataxic gait, and ophthalmoplegia. On examination, he had signs of congestive heart failure.

11. A 96-year-old female is a resident of a nursing home. She is seen routinely by a staff physician and found to have lethargy, malaise, perifollicular hemorrhages, and swollen, bleeding gums. She is pale and her teeth are loose.

12. A 45-year-old male is taken to jail because he continues to drive even after having his driver's license revoked due to multiple traffic accidents at night. On a routine ophthalmologic examination, he was found to have a small perforation of the cornea.

13. A newborn baby girl is given intravenous antibiotics for group B streptococci infection. She develops bleeding from her umbilical cord site and epistaxis.

14. A 71-year-old male presents with cardiogenic shock and acute pulmonary edema. Nine years earlier he had both his mitral and aortic valves replaced with Bjork-Shiley prostheses. A frame from the cinefluoroscopy study, shown in the figure, demonstrates all of the following EXCEPT

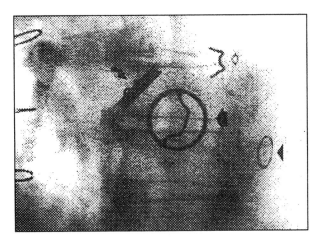

    (A) intact aortic valve prosthesis.

    (B) intact mitral valve prosthesis.

    (C) severed minor strut.

    (D) free-floating disk.

    (E) defective valve prosthesis.

Questions 15-18 refer to the following:

A previously healthy 24-year-old man presents to the emergency room with one month of gradually increasing shortness of breath to the point now that he has shortness of breath at rest. He also has noted a cough that is occasionally productive of yellow sputum. He denies any previous significant medical problems. He denies smoking and drinks alcohol only socially. He is currently sexually active and has been with a number of partners over the past several years. He has been treated for gonorrhea and syphilis. He is unsure about his HIV status. On physical examination, he has a heart rate of 120, a blood pressure of 120/70, a respiratory rate of 30, and a temperature of 100.7°F. His lungs reveal dry crackles on inspiration throughout and no wheezes. Cardiac exam reveals no rubs, gallops, or murmurs. Abdominal exam is benign. Chest radiograph reveals bilateral interstitial infiltrates consistent with pneumocystis carinii pneumonia.

15. The appropriate diagnostic test to confirm the diagnosis is

    (A) sputum sent for direct fluorescent antibody.

    (B) sputum sent for culture.

    (C) sputum sent for Gram stain.

    (D) serum antibody for pneumocystis carinii.

    (E) urinary antigen for pneumocystis carinii.

16. The treatment of choice is

    (A) atovaquone for 21 days.

    (B) dapsone for 21 days.

    (C) Clindamycin for 21 days.

    (D) aerosolized pentamidine for 21 days.

    (E) trimethoprim/sulfamethoxazole for 21 days.

17. The indication for adding systemic glucocorticoid therapy is

    (A) CD4 count less than 500.

    (B) CD4 count less than 250.

    (C) negative HIV ELISA test.

    (D) respiratory rate greater than 30.

    (E) room air PaO_2 <75 mm Hg.

18. Once the patient is treated for this acute illness, appropriate treatment for prophylaxis is

    (A) dapsone.

    (B) pentamidine.

    (C) trimethoprim/sulfamethoxazole.

    (D) inhaled corticosteroids.

    (E) None of the above; the patient should only be treated for prophylaxis if his CD4 count is less than 200.

19. Patients with a penicillin allergy should avoid

    (A) cephalosporins.

    (B) vancomycin.

    (C) gentamicin.

    (D) erythromycin.

    (E) clindamycin.

20. You instruct your 44-year-old paraplegic in the care of pressure sores and inform him he must shift his weight every

    (A) 2 hours.

    (B) 4 hours.

    (C) 8 hours.

    (D) 12 hours.

    (E) 24 hours.

Question 21-27 refer to the following:

A 43-year-old male with bullous emphysema was admitted with increasing shortness of breath, chest pain, cough productive of yellow-greenish sputum, fever, and malaise. Physical examination reveals an acutely ill-appearing male in respiratory distress, with decreased breath sounds throughout, and rales present at the right lower base.

21. The admission chest X-ray, shown in the figure below, demonstrates

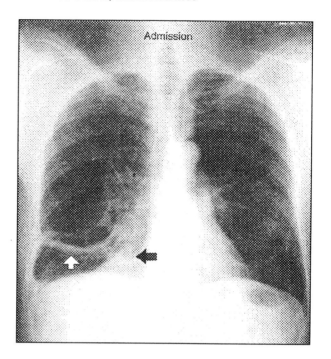

    (A) right lower lobe pneumonia only.

    (B) large bulla only in the right lung field.

    (C) right lower lobe pneumonia and a large bulla in the right lung field.

    (D) dextrocardia.

    (E) rib fracture with a small pneumothorax.

22. Treatment is instituted. The chest radiograph, shown below, obtained on the third admission day, now shows

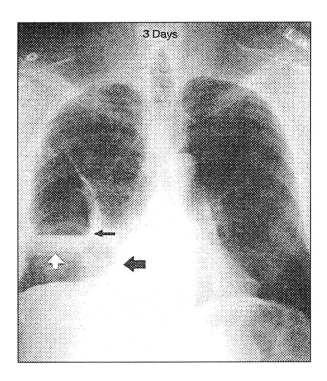

(A) expanding pneumothorax.

(B) air fluid level within the bulla.

(C) left subdiaphragmatic effusion.

(D) malposition of the endotracheal tube.

(E) left tension pneumothorax.

23. He responds to your treatment and is discharged from the hospital. Two months later, he returns for a follow-up evaluation. He offers no complaints. He has discontinued smoking. He has gained 10 pounds since discharge. He is compliant with your prescribed medical regimen. After reviewing the X-ray, shown in the figure below, you indicate

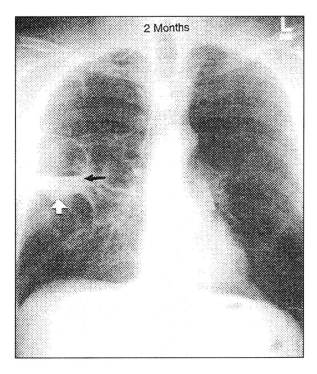

(A) the right lower lobe infiltrate has resolved.

(B) family members and close contacts should be tested for tuberculosis.

(C) immediate surgical consultation is necessary.

(D) bronchoscopic biopsy/aspiration is indicated immediately.

(E) a pneumothorax is present at the left lower base.

24. He returns for a follow-up examination two months later. He has still discontinued smoking. He felt well enough to return to his job as an account executive. He has gained another 10 pounds. He offers no complaints. Repeat chest X-ray is shown in the figure below. You now diagnose

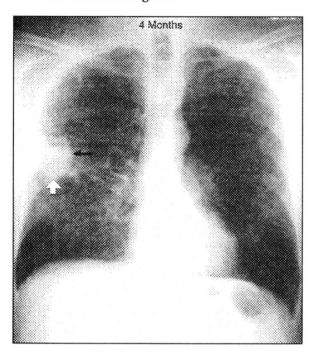

(A) squamous cell carcinoma.

(B) resolving parapneumonic effusion.

(C) malignant mesothelioma.

(D) pulmonary infarction.

(E) hamartoma.

25. In persons with cor pulmonale and clinical signs of right-heart failure, which one of the following is an indication for continuous supplemental oxygen therapy?

(A) PaO$_2$ less than 80 mm Hg

(B) PaO$_2$ less than 70 mm Hg

(C) PaO$_2$ less than 55 mm Hg

(D) PaCO$_2$ greater than 60 mm Hg

(E) PaCO$_2$ greater than 75 mm Hg

26. He returns two years later with complaints of an acute upper respiratory infection. His sputum is greenish in color and has increased in volume and viscosity. He has not stopped smoking and otherwise feels well. Physical examination reveals a temperature of 99.8°F, pulse of 90 and regular, blood pressure 110/70, respiratory of 20, nasal congestion, mild pharyngeal erythema, scattered rhonchi and wheezing in the lungs bilaterally, and decreased breath sounds throughout. The chest X-ray is shown in the figure below. You now recommend

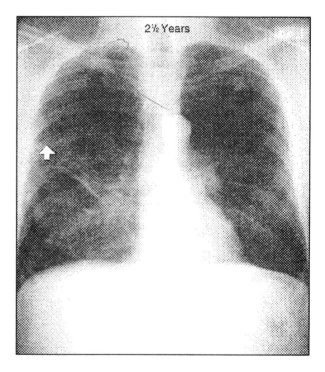

(A) admission to the hospital.

(B) a one-week course of broad spectrum antibiotics.

(C) an immediate ventilation-perfusion lung scan.

(D) a pulmonary arteriogram.

(E) intravenous corticosteroids.

27. Which one of the following tests would be most helpful in evaluating emphysema occurring in several family members, all of whom are nonsmokers?

(A) Serum IgA

(B) C'1 esterase

(C) Serum alpha$_1$antitrypsin

(D) Serum ceruloplasmin

(E) Serum angiotensin converting enzyme

28. A woman who says she represents an insurance company that is considering issuing a life insurance policy to your patient calls you asking for information on his health. You must

(A) give her the information she wants.

(B) refer her to the medical records department.

(C) refuse to talk to her.

(D) tell her you can only discuss the patient with her after he has given you a release of information permitting you specifically to talk to her.

(E) tell her you do not talk to insurance companies.

Questions 29-36 refer to the following:

A 32-year-old woman without significant past medical illnesses presents with a breast lump found on physical examination. She is very worried about this, as her mother and older sister have both been diagnosed with breast cancer. She denies any other medical illnesses and is not taking any medications. She denies smoking, alcohol use, or illicit drug use.

29. Of the following, the most common breast lesion is

(A) fibrocystic disease.

(B) fibroadenoma.

(C) intraductal papilloma.

(D) inflammatory cancer.

(E) medullary carcinoma.

30. The patient asks you about the risk factors of breast cancer. You tell her that all of the following have been shown to be associated with an increased risk in breast cancer EXCEPT

(A) female gender.

(B) age.

(C) positive family history.

(D) nulliparity.

(E) history of fibrocystic disease.

31. Which one of the following can be ruled out on the basis of the patient's age alone?

(A) Fibrocystic disease

(B) Fibroadenoma

(C) Inflammatory cancer

(D) Medullary carcinoma

(E) None of the above.

32. On physical examination, you note no asymmetry in breast shape. She has no notable adenopathy. There is no peau d'orange appearance to either breast. Her left breast has a 1 centimeter firm nodule at 3:00, about 4 centimeters from the nipple. It is freely movable and smooth. She has no nipple discharge. With this information, which one of the following can be ruled out?

(A) Fibrocystic disease

(B) Fibroadenoma

(C) Inflammatory cancer

(D) Medullary carcinoma

(E) None of the above.

33. You attempt to aspirate the mass and no fluid is obtained. Of the following, which one is true regarding mammograms in this case?

(A) A mammogram that is not consistent with cancer can rule out cancer.

(B) A mammogram that is notable for microcalcifications is cancer.

(C) A mammogram is a poor screening tool for elderly patients.

(D) A mammogram has good sensitivity in younger patients.

(E) A mammogram can only increase or decrease the suspicion of cancer.

34. A mammogram is obtained and reveals no change in breast architecture or microcalcifications. The next most appropriate intervention is

   (A) biopsy.

   (B) fine needle aspiration.

   (C) close observation.

   (D) repeat mammogram in six months.

   (E) reassurance.

35. Which one of the following statements regarding the incidence of breast cancer is correct?

   (A) About 9% of all women will be diagnosed with breast cancer.

   (B) About 20% of all women will be diagnosed with breast cancer.

   (C) About 35% of all women will be diagnosed with breast cancer.

   (D) About 10% of all patients with breast cancer are men.

   (E) None of the above are true.

36. Which one of the following statements is true regarding the use of anti-estrogen agents?

   (A) They should be used in premenopausal patients with positive axillary nodes.

   (B) They should be used in all premenopausal patients.

   (C) They should be used in postmenopausal patients with positive axillary nodes receptors.

   (D) They should be used in postmenopausal patients with positive axillary nodes and negative receptors.

(E) They should be used in all postmenopausal patients.

Questions 37–43 refer to the following:

A 34-year-old male comes to your office after being hit in the face with a rock. On examination, he is swollen over his left face and eye. The left eyeball cannot look up and the face is numb. There is also a severe malocclusion.

37. You order plain films and a CAT scan of the facial skeleton and expect to find a

   (A) nasal and zygoma fracture.

   (B) orbit and nasal fracture.

   (C) orbit and mandible fracture.

   (D) maxillary and mandible fracture.

   (E) frontal bone fracture.

38. The inability of the left eye to look up is known as

   (A) entrapment.

   (B) ectropion.

   (C) entropion.

   (D) ptosis.

   (E) None of the above.

39. The muscle involved in this phenomenon is the

   (A) inferior rectus.

   (B) inferior oblique.

   (C) superior rectus.

   (D) superior oblique.

   (E) medial rectus.

40. Appropriate management includes all of the following EXCEPT

   (A) observation.

   (B) exploration.

   (C) repair.

   (D) antibiotics.

   (E) elevation of head of bed.

41. Long-term-problems may include all of the following EXCEPT

    (A) infection.

    (B) diplopia.

    (C) malocclusion.

    (D) paresthesias.

    (E) bleeding.

42. Postoperative care should include

    (A) discharge home after surgery.

    (B) regular diet.

    (C) full activity.

    (D) observation in hospital postoperatively.

    (E) postoperative anticoagulation.

43. Bone healing can be expected to occur in

    (A) one week.

    (B) three weeks.

    (C) six weeks.

    (D) three months.

    (E) six months.

44. A 50-year-old previously healthy man presents to your office with cough productive of sputum for two days. He denies any chest pain, fevers, chills, shortness of breath, weight loss, night sweats, or orthopnea. He states that his sputum has been yellow-green in color. He has no other medical problems and is not taking any medications. He has smoked one pack of cigarettes per day for 25 years. Physical examination reveals that he is afebrile, and that his respiratory rate is 14. Lungs are clear without any dullness to percussion. An in-office chest X-ray reveals no infiltrates or effusions. The most appropriate intervention would be to

    (A) admit for IV antibiotics.

    (B) place a purified protein derivative (PPD) and begin isoniazid therapy.

    (C) initiate outpatient treatment with trimethoprim/sulfamethoxazole.

    (D) initiate outpatient treatment with doxycycline.

    (E) order a chest CT to rule out cancer.

45. A 32-year-old woman comes to your clinic complaining of right lower quadrant pain. On examination, she has guarding and rigidity in that region. You send her to see the surgeon in the emergency room because your leading diagnosis is

    (A) an ectopic pregnancy.

    (B) pelvic inflammatory disease.

    (C) acute appendicitis.

    (D) acute pancreatitis.

    (E) ruptured diverticulum.

46. The laboratory calls you with the following test results

    CBC: WBC: 22,000/mm^3 (84% neutrophils and bands)

    Hgb:12.0 g/dL

    Platelets: 175,000/mm^3

    Chemistry panel:

    Na: 131 mEq/L

    K: 5.1 mEq/L

    Cl: 95 mEq/L

    HCO$_3$: 10 mEq/L

    Gluc: 675 mg/dL

    BUN: 30 mg/dL

    Cr: 0.9 mg/dL

    Arterial blood gas:

    pH: 7.20

pO$_2$: 100 mm Hg

pCO$_2$: 28 mm Hg

Based on this information, you begin treatment for

(A) lactic acidosis.

(B) hyponatremia.

(C) hyperkalemia.

(D) diabetic ketoacidosis.

(E) renal tubular acidosis.

Questions 47 and 48 refer to the following:

An 18-month-old toddler is brought in for a routine checkup. You note that her skin is very pale and that she is above the 95% for weight. The results of her blood work show that she is anemic.

47. The most common cause of anemia in infants and children in the United States is

(A) lead poisoning.

(B) iron deficiency.

(C) folate deficiency.

(D) hemolytic uremic syndrome.

(E) thalassemia.

48. This patient's venous lead level is found to be 15 micrograms/dl. What recommendations for treatment will you give?

(A) None. This is an acceptable lead level for a child of this age.

(B) Hospitalization and parenteral chelation therapy with BAL (British antilewisite) and calcium disodium edetate.

(C) Oral chelation therapy with DMSA.

(D) Only environmental interventions and care-giver education about how to avoid lead exposure are necessary at this time.

(E) Oral chelation therapy with D-penicillamine.

49. A six-year-old girl is brought to the ER by her mother. The mother says that the child fell off a sofa and broke her left leg. Physician examination shows a swollen, bruised left leg. You also notice old bruises and old abrasions in various stages of healing. The child is otherwise normal. You decide to hospitalize the child. The mother insists on taking her daughter home. You should ensure that

(A) you have the mother's written authorization to hospitalize her child.

(B) you have written authorization from both parents allowing you to hospitalize the child.

(C) the child is in a safe environment, and keep the patient in a hospital against the mother's will.

(D) your decision is legal and request an immediate court hearing.

(E) your decision is ethical and request intervention of the hospital's ethics committee.

50. A 65-year-old woman with chronic hypertension that has been well-controlled with one agent for a long time now presents for her routine visit with a blood pressure of 170/120. The best course of action is to

(A) order an intravenous pyelogram.

(B) schedule a kidney biopsy.

(C) change her antihypertensive regimen.

(D) order a renal angiogram.

(E) refer her to an endocrinologist.

51. A 45-year-old woman comes for her annual examination and you notice a 1-cm mass in her right breast. She says she has had it for at least nine months and it has not changed. You

(A) schedule a mammogram.

(B) reassure her.

(C) order a fine needle biopsy.

(D) order breast ultrasound.

(E) tell her to come back in three months for another exam.

52. A 63-year-old man who comes in for an annual check-up has no complaints. He stopped smoking cigarettes a year ago and now smokes a pipe. His chest radiograph shows a new solitary lesion in the right upper lobe. Your working diagnosis is

(A) aspergilloma.

(B) pneumonia.

(C) tuberculosis.

(D) lung cancer.

(E) metastatic cancer.

53. A 27-year-old female with a history of recurrent streptococcal infections in her childhood comes in with a sore throat. You recommend

(A) an oral antiseptic.

(B) prophylactic antibiotics at bedtime.

(C) vaccination.

(D) that no intervention is needed since she has probably outgrown streptococcal infections.

(E) a streptococcal throat culture.

54. A 34-year-old man with chronic seasonal allergic rhinitis comes to see you because the antihistamines you have prescribed are not helping much. You order serologic tests for antibodies to various antigens with the intention of

(A) changing antihistamines.

(B) beginning allergy desensitization shots.

(C) scheduling nasoseptal surgery.

(D) treating with antibiotics.

(E) reassuring him that there is nothing to worry about.

55. The wife of a previously healthy 45-year-old man accompanies him to his routine appointment for the first time. She is concerned because he is having blackout spells and has had several automobile accidents. An important question to ask is

(A) family history of strokes.

(B) family history of hypercholesterolemia.

(C) whether the patient has had a lipid profile.

(D) how much alcohol the patient drinks.

(E) whether the patient has a psychiatric history.

56. A 54-year-old woman whom you see occasionally tells you she had the first seizure of her life two weeks earlier. Her husband observed it and told her she was "shaking." She did have urinary incontinence. A likely diagnosis is

(A) a recent stroke.

(B) a brain tumor.

(C) meningitis.

(D) simple epilepsy.

(E) amyotrophic lateral sclerosis.

57. A 55-year-old woman who has complained of vague joint pains for a long time comes in with itchy eyes and some difficulty swallowing because of dry mouth. You suspect

(A) fibromyalgia.

(B) hysteria.

(C) Sjögren's syndrome.

(D) lupus.

(E) allergic conjunctivitis.

58. Which one of the following statements about the association between barrier methods of contraception and cervical cancer is true?

(A) There is fair evidence to suggest that barrier methods of contraception significantly reduce the incidence of cervical cancer.

(B) There is no ample evidence at this time to suggest any association.

(C) There is some evidence to suggest a direct association between barrier methods of contraception and the development of cervical neoplasia.

(D) There is some evidence to suggest an indirect association.

(E) None of the above statements reflects the true association.

59. Which one of the following agents cannot be used to achieve skeletal muscle relaxation during surgery?

(A) Vecuronium

(B) Midazolam

(C) Lidocaine

(D) Bupivacaine

(E) Desflurane

60. The most common cause of community-acquired bacteria pneumonia is

(A) pneumococcal.

(B) staphylococcal.

(C) streptococcal.

(D) klebsiella.

(E) herpetic.

61. The mental foramen is located

(A) over the maxillary central incisors.

(B) by the maxillary molars.

(C) by the mandibular incisors.

(D) by the mandibular premolars.

(E) by the mandibular molars.

62. The nerve transversing the mental foramen will give sensation to

(A) the upper lip.

(B) the cheek.

(C) the lower lip and chin.

(D) the posterior mandible.

(E) the neck.

63. Which one of the following statements about polyvalent pneumococcal vaccine is true?

(A) It covers 50% of bacteremic diseases reported annually in the U.S.

(B) It covers all cases of bacteremic diseases reported annually in the U.S.

(C) Current research data promise higher effectiveness for children.

(D) The vaccine is widely recommended for the elderly.

(E) The vaccine has recently been losing its effectiveness.

64. All of the following cancers are common in farmers and other people who are exposed to pesticides EXCEPT

(A) malignant melanoma.

(B) cancer of the prostate.

(C) Hodgkin's disease.

(D) pancreatic cancer.

(E) cancer of the lip.

65. As a family physician, you see a six-year-old girl on well-child examination. Provided that the child has received timely immunizations, which one of the following vaccinations would be most appropriate at this time?

(A) DTP booster

(B) Hib

(C) MMR

(D) Hepatitis B vaccine

(E) OPV vaccine

66. A five-year-old boy is brought to your office for a routine physical examination. You should screen for

    (A) high serum cholesterol.

    (B) growth retardation.

    (C) mental retardation.

    (D) learning disabilities.

    (E) misalignment of pupils.

67. A 42-year-old man with a long history of chronic alcohol use presents with symptoms of upper GI bleeding. On exam, he has orthostatic hypotension, melena, testicular atrophy, spider angiomas, jaundice, ascites, splenomegaly, asterixis, and confusion secondary to hepatic encephalopathy. He was diagnosed with end-stage liver cirrhosis (Childs Class D) and portal hypertension. Lab data revealed an elevated creatinine level. All of the following could have precipitated the decompensation of his liver cirrhosis EXCEPT

    (A) viral hepatitis.

    (B) Nyquil and acetaminophen ingestion.

    (C) bacterial peritonitis.

    (D) beta-blockers.

    (E) diuretics.

68. Splenomegaly may result from all of the following EXCEPT

    (A) lymphoma.

    (B) Gaucher's disease.

    (C) myeloid metaplasia.

    (D) hereditary spherocytosis.

    (E) Fanconi's syndrome.

69. Complications of Paget's disease include all of the following EXCEPT

    (A) high output failure.

    (B) pathologic fractures.

    (C) urolithiasis.

    (D) hearing loss.

    (E) hypercalcemia.

70. A 12-year-old girl is brought to the ER after her father found her jerking spasmodically. History reveals that the "spastic" episode, as the father termed it, consisted of jerking of both arms and both legs. The girl is bleeding from the mouth after biting her tongue. Which one of the following represents the most likely diagnosis?

    (A) Partial simple seizure

    (B) Partial complex seizure

    (C) Generalized absence seizure

    (D) Generalized tonic-clonic seizure

    (E) Alcohol withdrawal seizure

Questions 71-74 refer to the following:

A 55-year-old comes to the walk-in clinic because of acute severe abdominal pain. He has never had anything like this. He does have a history of gout. He has been working extra hours lately and has been drinking a lot of coffee to stay awake. He describes his pain as "worse than" stabbing. It is the worst pain he has ever had.

71. You order all of the following tests EXCEPT

    (A) urinalysis.

    (B) electrolytes.

    (C) hemoglobin electrophoresis.

    (D) abdominal radiograph.

    (E) CBC.

72. A useful piece of family history that the patient remembers is

    (A) his father had cancer.

    (B) his brother has gout.

    (C) his mother had diabetes.

    (D) his father had kidney stones.

    (E) his son has asthma.

73. The urinalysis shows hematuria, but the abdominal radiograph is negative. Your leading diagnosis is

(A)   pyelonephritis.

(B)   nephrolithiasis.

(C)   perforated viscus.

(D)   urethritis.

(E)   discitis.

74.   All of the following modalities are indicated in the management of this patient EXCEPT

(A)   hydration.

(B)   analgesics.

(C)   saving all urine.

(D)   rest.

(E)   allopurinol.

75.   A 50-year-old man comes to your office with a history of proximal muscle stiffness for the past several weeks, visual disturbances, and unilateral throbbing headaches. You obtain an ESR, which is 120. Which one of the following statements is true regarding this patient and his diagnosis?

(A)   The patient should be started on high-dose corticosteroids as soon as possible.

(B)   The patient should be scheduled for an elective diagnostic biopsy.

(C)   This condition usually affects younger patients.

(D)   Additional symptoms may include delirium and psychosis.

(E)   None of the above.

76.   A 60-year-old man presents with left flank pain for three days. He denies any fevers, chills, hematuria, or dysuria. His past medical history includes hypertension, diabetes mellitus, and hypercholesterolemia. His physical examination reveals mild tenderness to palpation on the left costovertebral angle. Initial laboratory results that are abnormal are a serum creatinine of 4.6, BUN of 67, potassium of 4.8, and LDH of 807. His baseline creatinine was 2.4. Of the following, the test that would most likely make the diagnosis would be

(A)   a 24-hour urinary protein excretion.

(B)   a 24-hour urinary collection for creatinine clearance.

(C)   a renal ultrasound with Doppler.

(D)   a urinalysis with urine culture.

(E)   urine electrolytes.

Questions 77-80 refer to the following:

A 33-year-old bisexual man is HIV-positive. He is married and says he has not told his wife about his positivity.

77.   You ask him

(A)   if he feels guilty.

(B)   if he uses a condom with his wife.

(C)   how he feels about this.

(D)   who he thinks infected him.

(E)   if he has told his coworkers.

78.   You tell him he should

(A)   use condoms.

(B)   see a psychiatrist.

(C)   take more vitamins.

(D)   do nothing.

(E)   take out more life insurance.

79.   The patient refuses to use condoms or tell his wife. You should

(A)   call a psychiatrist.

(B)   try to get the patient committed.

(C)   inform the patient's wife.

(D)   call the patient's employer.

(E)   call his minister.

80.   This situation invokes the physician's obligation of

(A)   legal necessity.

(B)   duty to warn.

(C)   patient-physician trust.

(D) need to report to the Board of Health.

(E) *primum non nocere.*

Questions 81 and 82 refer to the following:

81. You are debating whether to intubate a patient for respiratory failure. All of the following are signs of respiratory failure EXCEPT

    (A) tachypnea > 35 breaths per minute.

    (B) pH < 7.25.

    (C) vital capacity < 15 ml/kg.

    (D) $PaO_2 < 70$ mm Hg on 50% O_2.

    (E) $PaCO_2 = 40$ mm Hg.

82. After intubation, all of the following should be performed EXCEPT

    (A) chest X-ray.

    (B) auscultation of bilateral breath sounds.

    (C) arterial blood gas.

    (D) chest tube.

    (E) securing of the tube.

83. A 52-year-old white male presents to the emergency room with symptoms of progressive unilateral ptosis and diplopia at the end of the day for the last few months. He also states that after walking for a few blocks, his legs become weaker and weaker. There is no atrophy in any of the limbs. All of the following can be used in the initial work-up of this patient EXCEPT

    (A) serum anticholinesterase receptor antibody.

    (B) electromyography.

    (C) edrophonium chloride testing.

    (D) CT of the anterior mediastinum.

    (E) oral pyridostigmine testing.

84. One of your colleagues has been covering your service for you for a few days. When you return, you find that he has missed a significant drop in hemoglobin in a patient with a history of peptic ulcer disease. You

    (A) berate him in the middle of his morning rounds with his team.

    (B) write to the chief of your service telling him your colleague is dangerous.

    (C) talk to your colleague in private.

    (D) discuss the problem with your colleague in the patient's room with the patient present.

    (E) do nothing, but decide not to let your colleague cover your service again.

85. Although a preventable disease, it is estimated that, worldwide, 800,000 neonates die annually from tetanus. All of the following are true concerning infection with tetanus EXCEPT

    (A) in developing countries, tetanus may be acquired following application of animal dung to the umbilical stump.

    (B) in the United States, most cases of tetanus occur in inadequately immunized persons.

    (C) the change in the oxidation-reduction potential at the site of injury is conducive to reversion of spores into a vegetative form which produces tetanospasmin.

    (D) at the presynaptic terminals, the toxin produced by *Clostridium tetani* blocks release of excitatory neurotransmitters.

    (E) "cephalic tetanus," characterized by cranial nerve dysfunction, results from a head injury or an ear infection.

86. A 16-year-old woman presents with bloody and purulent vaginal discharge. She denied having been sexually active. You should do all of the following EXCEPT

    (A) obtain a Pap smear.

    (B) evaluate for gonorrhea.

    (C) evaluate for HIV infection.

(D) test for urine hCG levels.

(E) screen for breast cancer.

For each of the patients in Questions 87-90, select the most appropriate initial antibiotic choice.

(A) A third-generation cephalosporin

(B) An extended penicillin

(C) An aminoglycoside

(D) Vancomycin

(E) Sulfamethoxazole

87. A 38-year-old previously healthy female who is post-op day five from a cholecystectomy; her surgical wound reveals purulent drainage.

88. A 70-year-old man with chronic obstructive pulmonary disease is hospitalized for pneumonia.

89. A 76-year-old woman with pancreatic cancer presents with right upper quadrant pain, jaundice, and fevers to 104.5°F.

90. A 35-year-old woman with cirrhosis who presents with esophageal variceal bleeding is incidentally noted to have a urinary tract infection.

91. A 38-year-old female complains of severe lower back pain and bilateral anterior rib pain. X-rays of the lumbar spine showed compression fracture and evidence of osteopenia. The serum calcium level was 13.7 mg/dl. All of the following can cause osteopenia and hypercalcemia EXCEPT

(A) thyrotoxicosis.

(B) multiple myeloma.

(C) hyperparathyroidism.

(D) chronic renal failure.

(E) metastatic breast cancer.

92. A 66-year-old male presents to the emergency room with acute bone pain. The most likely diagnosis is

(A) staphylococcal infection.

(B) osteosarcoma.

(C) tendon rupture.

(D) Paget's disease of bone.

(E) hyperparathyroidism.

93. An immigrant from Santo Domingo comes to the urgent-care center with symptoms of severe myalgias, diarrhea, and fever. On further testing, he was found to have a marked eosinophilia and his creatinine phosphokinase level was elevated. He does not remember any new changes in his dietary habits. What is the treatment of choice in this patient?

(A) Discontinue L-tryptophan

(B) Thrombolytic therapy

(C) Vigorous intravenous hydration

(D) Thiabendazole

(E) Steroids

Questions 94-97 refer to the following:

A 78-year-old man who has had a massive cerebrospinal accident has been comatose for two weeks and is intubated. He had not written a living will or directed his family as to his wishes prior to his illness.

94. The anesthesiologist recommends a tracheostomy because of impending tracheomalacia with continued intubation. You

(A) turn off the respirator.

(B) extubate the patient.

(C) agree to the tracheostomy.

(D) order an EEG.

(E) do nothing.

95. Electroencephalographic studies show no organized higher cortical activity. You

    (A) discuss the patient's terminal condition with the family and recommend turning off the respirator.

    (B) turn off the respirator without talking to the family.

    (C) schedule the tracheostomy.

    (D) remove all intravenous lines.

    (E) do nothing.

96. The patient's wife, who is totally competent, agrees with your assessment and tells you to turn off the respirator. The patient's sister says she thinks it is wrong. You tell the family

    (A) you will turn off the respirator.

    (B) to let you decide.

    (C) to decide among them and tell you their decision.

    (D) you will call in the Ethics Committee to make an independent judgment and present their results to the family.

    (E) to do nothing.

97. Everyone agrees with turning off the respirator. The patient does not initiate spontaneous respirations when the machine is off. You

    (A) call a code.

    (B) do an emergency tracheostomy.

    (C) pronounce him dead.

    (D) reintubate him.

    (E) give him cardiostimulants.

98. A 43-year-old female presents with an acute onset of malaise, fever, chills, and neck pain. On exam, she was tachycardic and febrile with an enlarged, tender thyroid gland. Biopsy revealed follicular cell destruction and infiltration with lymphocytes, multinucleated giant cells, and polymorphonuclear leukocytes. Lab data showed an elevated white blood cell count, elevated ESR, and a low radioactive iodine uptake. This patient had a recent viral respiratory tract infection. There is no family history of thyroid disorders. What is the most likely diagnosis?

    (A) Hashimoto's thyroiditis

    (B) Graves' disease

    (C) Subacute granulomatous thyroiditis

    (D) Subacute lymphocytic thyroiditis

    (E) Medullary cell carcinoma of the thyroid gland

99. A 23-year-old woman presents to your office with two days of feeling ill. She tells you that she has had low-grade fevers and feelings of malaise. She also has noted a sore throat, dry cough, and myalgias. She denies any rigors, sputum, or chest pain. She has no other medical problems. On physical examination, you find that her heart rate is 80, blood pressure is 120/75, respiratory rate is 12, and temperature is 99.3°F. Her lungs are clear, and her oropharynx is slightly erythematous without exudates. The most appropriate treatment would be to

    (A) reassure her and tell her to take acetaminophen as needed and drink plenty of liquids.

    (B) begin a short course of antibiotic therapy for pneumonia.

    (C) begin a short course of antibiotic therapy for Strep throat.

    (D) order a monospot test.

    (E) order a chest radiograph.

Questions 100-103 refer to the following:

A 30-year-old man with a history of seizures presents after having had a seizure at home. His family denies that he hit his head. In addition to a history of seizures, he also has had a history of non-insulin-dependent diabetes mellitus. He is currently taking phenytoin and an oral hypoglycemic for his diabetes mellitus. On presentation, he is postictal, but his vital signs are stable and he is afebrile. His lungs are clear and his cardiac exam is without S3 or murmurs. His abdominal exam is benign and his extremities have no edema.

100. If the patient begins to seize again, what is an appropriate immediate medication to stop the seizures?

   (A) Diazepam

   (B) Phenobarbital

   (C) Phenytoin

   (D) Pentobarbital

   (E) Vecuronium

101. All of the following are common causes of a decrease in the seizure threshold EXCEPT

   (A) hyponatremia.

   (B) hypoglycemia.

   (C) hypercalcemia.

   (D) hyperosmolar non-ketotic state.

   (E) sub-therapeutic medication levels.

102. If the serum levels of his phenytoin reveal that he hasn't been taking his medication, and you decide to load him intravenously, what side effect do you need to be careful about acutely?

   (A) Hypotension

   (B) Ventricular arrhythmias

   (C) Airway closure

   (D) Intracranial bleeding

   (E) Anaphylaxis

103. With recurrent seizures, all of the following are common complications and should be watched for EXCEPT

   (A) aspiration.

   (B) rhabdomyolysis.

   (C) myoglobinuria.

   (D) ventricular arrhythmias.

   (E) hyperthermia.

104. On a weekend call, a patient calls to complain of severe abdominal pain. She tells you that she is seeing your partner and has been treated for this abdominal pain in the past with oral meperidine, but that she has run out of the medication. You tell her that

   (A) you will be happy to prescribe her another refill.

   (B) you will only prescribe her enough to last through the weekend.

   (C) you don't feel comfortable treating this severe abdominal pain over the telephone and that she should go to the nearest emergency room if her pain is severe.

   (D) she should call her physician after the weekend.

   (E) None of the above.

105. A 16-year-old teenager came to the walk-in clinic without an appointment because he was bitten by a dog on the dorsum of his left hand. On examination, the laceration was deep and the lesion was painful. Lab data revealed a white blood cell count of 19,000 and an ESR of 78 mm/hr. All the joints had full range of motion. All of the following should be done in the continued care of this patient EXCEPT

   (A) tetanus prophylaxis.

   (B) rabies prophylaxis.

   (C) beta-lactam/beta lactamase antibiotics.

   (D) suturing the laceration.

   (E) irrigation of the wound.

106. A 58-year-old white male presents to the emergency room with complaints of severe substernal chest pain radiating to the left shoulder which awoke him in the middle of the night. This pain is associated with diaphoresis, shortness of breath at rest, and anxiety. There is no prior past medical history except for hypercholesterolemia. The electrocardiogram shows 3 mm ST-T wave elevations in the anteriolateral leads. The

creatinephosphokinase level was elevated to over 1,000 mg/dl. The pulse is 42 and the blood pressure is 70/50 mm/hg. What would be the initial step in managing this patient?

(A) Aspirin

(B) Intravenous nitroglycerin

(C) Beta-blockers

(D) Lasix

(E) Synchronized defibrillation with 100 joules

107. Which of the following statements concerning screening procedures during pregnancy is in accord with the Canadian Task Force recommendations?

(A) All pregnant women should be screened for HIV infection at least once.

(B) Only pregnant women with a prior history of preeclampsia or eclampsia should receive systolic and diastolic pressure measurements.

(C) Rh (D) immune globulin is given to all Rh-positive pregnant women.

(D) Every pregnant woman should receive one prenatal ultrasound in the second trimester.

(E) Amniocentesis should only be offered to women with diagnosed fetal distress.

108. A 38-year-old man comes in with severe lower right quadrant pain for the last two days, associated with nausea, vomiting, and a low-grade fever. On physical examination, he has pain to palpation with guarding in his lower abdomen. His peripheral white count is 15,000 with a left shift. What do you do next?

(A) Order an abdominal radiograph.

(B) Perform a paracentesis.

(C) Start antibiotics.

(D) Call a STAT surgical consult.

(E) Pass a nasogastric tube.

109. A 45-year-old disheveled male presents to the emergency department complaining of shaking chills and some shortness of breath. He smells of ethanol. A chest radiograph shows a right lower lobe infiltrate. Your working diagnosis is

(A) delirium tremens.

(B) pneumonia.

(C) asthma.

(D) atelectasis.

(E) bronchitis.

110. A 67-year-old man comes in with abdominal pain. He has not had a bowel movement in almost a week. Upon careful questioning, he admits that he has had less of an appetite recently and has lost weight. Abdominal radiograph is consistent with an ileus. Your working diagnosis is

(A) Hirschsprung's disease.

(B) toxic megacolon.

(C) ulcerative colitis.

(D) intestinal obstruction due to colon cancer.

(E) Crohn's disease.

111. A 38-year-old woman presents because of severe abdominal pain, nausea, and vomiting. Her symptoms began a few days earlier. She admits to drinking "a few" beers a day. Her abdomen is very tender to palpation. All of the following laboratory tests should be ordered now EXCEPT

(A) amylase.

(B) CBC.

(C) abdominal CT.

(D) lipase.

(E) urinalysis.

112. A 25-year-old woman comes in because of acute shortness of breath. She has a history of nasal polyps and has been taking an over-the-counter agent for menstrual cramps. She has wheezes on auscultation. You diagnose asthma which you think is due to

(A)   use of a nonsteroidal agent in a patient with nasal polyps.

(B)   seasonal allergies.

(C)   anxiety.

(D)   cold intolerance.

(E)   hormone imbalance.

113. A 52-year-old diabetic man comes in because he has noticed that his ankle is "crooked." He is unaware of any trauma and has no pain in the area. His ankle is grossly deformed and unstable. You order a radiograph which shows multiple fractures and dislocations, as well as loss of joint space and demineralization. You are amazed that the patient has no symptoms. The likeliest diagnosis is

(A)   metastatic cancer.

(B)   tuberculosis.

(C)   rheumatoid arthritis.

(D)   Charcot arthropathy.

(E)   multiple myeloma.

114. A 43-year-old woman presents to your office for a routine office checkup. She has been doing well and has no complaints. She is taking no medications. Her vital signs reveal that she is normotensive and afebrile. Her lungs are clear, and her cardiac exam reveals no murmurs or gallops. No masses or dimpling are noted on her breast exam. Abdominal exam is benign, as is her pelvic exam. Routine laboratory testing reveals serum chemistries all within normal limits except for a calcium level of 12.0 mg/dl. The most likely etiology for hypercalcemia in this patient is

(A)   metastatic breast cancer.

(B)   renal failure.

(C)   primary hyperparathyroidism.

(D)   myeloma.

(E)   sarcoidosis.

115. A 50-year-old man presents to your office with symptoms of daytime somnolence. He denies any medications and admits to only occa-

sional alcohol ingestion. His wife tells you that he snores loudly. Physical examination reveals an obese white male in no distress. His vital signs are stable, and he is afebrile. His lungs reveal decreased breath sounds throughout. His cardiac examination reveals no murmurs or gallops. You tell him that the most likely etiology of his symptoms is

(A)   primary pulmonary hypertension.

(B)   obstructive sleep apnea syndrome.

(C)   bacterial pneumonia.

(D)   uremia.

(E)   multi-infarct dementia.

Questions 116-119 refer to the following:

An 83-year-old woman is undergoing total knee replacement. She has a history of anaphylaxis to penicillin.

116. Which one of the following antibiotics would be most appropriate for perioperative prophylaxis?

(A)   Gentamicin

(B)   Imipenem

(C)   Cefotetan

(D)   Vancomycin

(E)   Cefazolin

117. Prior to surgery, preparations are made for intravenous access and fluid administration. Flow through a 10 cm 10-gauge trauma intravenous line is how much greater than flow through a 20-gauge 5 cm intravenous line?

(A)   2X

(B)   4X

(C)   8X

(D)   16X

(E)   32X

118. What platelet count is generally regarded as minimally adequate for providing surgical hemostasis?

(A) 25,000

(B) 50,000

(C) 75,000

(D) 100,000

(E) 10,000

119. Surgical stimulation results in the release of all of the following EXCEPT

(A) norepinephrine.

(B) cortisol.

(C) aldosterone.

(D) insulin.

(E) antidiuretic hormone.

120. A 33-year-old patient with known ovarian cancer presents to your office for a scheduled appointment. Her cancer was diagnosed a year ago, and since that time she is receiving radio- and chemotherapy. With respect to the prognosis of this cancer patient, which one of the following statements is true?

(A) Chemotherapy has resulted in significant reduction of cancer mortality.

(B) Radiotherapy has resulted in significant reduction of cancer mortality.

(C) In order to achieve any significant reduction in cancer death rates, the use of both chemotherapy and radiotherapy must be combined.

(D) The overall results of chemotherapy and radiotherapy are ambiguous; further investigations may be needed to come up with conclusive data.

(E) Combining chemotherapy with radiotherapy has resulted in decreased numbers of cancer deaths over the past two decades in the United States.

121. Which one the following statements is NOT true of refractive errors?

(A) In myopia, the image of a distant object focuses in front of the retina.

(B) In hyperopia, the image of a distant object focuses behind the retina.

(C) The accommodative loss resulting in an inability to focus on near objects is known as presbyopia.

(D) In young persons, accommodation compensates for minor degrees of hyperopia.

(E) In anisometropia, the image of a near object focuses in front of the retina.

For Questions 122-125, match the procedure with its associated complication.

(A) Total peripheral nutrition

(B) Bronchopulmonary dysplasia

(C) PEEP

(D) Mechanical ventilation

(E) CPR

122. Muscle weakness

123. Decrease in cardiac output

124. Metabolic hypercarbia

125. Congestive heart failure

Questions 126-129 refer to the following:

A 25-year-old patient presents with blood in his urine.

126. This is termed

(A) hemoptysis.

(B) hematuria.

(C) hematemesis.

(D) epistaxis.

(E) hemothorax.

127. Your work up for this would initially include all of the following EXCEPT

(A)	detailed history and physical.

(B)	bleeding studies.

(C)	urinalysis.

(D)	cystoscopy or IVP.

(E)	MRI of the kidneys.

128.	The etiology of this disease includes all of the following EXCEPT

(A)	trauma.

(B)	coagulopathy.

(C)	tumor.

(D)	kidney stones.

(E)	diabetes mellitus.

129.	After an extensive work-up, the diagnosis is urethritis. The appropriate antibiotic is

(A)	cleocin.

(B)	vancomycin.

(C)	Flagyl.

(D)	tetracycline.

(E)	doxycycline.

130.	A 35-year-old man with known HIV infection presents with severely decreased vision in his left eye. You send him to the ophthalmologist because of the likelihood of

(A)	glaucoma.

(B)	chlamydial infection.

(C)	CMV retinitis.

(D)	staphylococcal infection.

(E)	retro-orbital tumor.

131.	A 24-year-old male with sickle cell anemia comes to the clinic with acute shortness of breath. Your immediate management of him should include all of the following EXCEPT

(A)	oxygen.

(B)	allopurinol.

(C)	analgesia.

(D)	hydration.

(E)	blood gases.

For Questions 132-135, match the recommended treatment of choice with each numbered question.

(A)	Vancomycin

(B)	Trimethoprim-sulfamethoxazole

(C)	Erythromycin

(D)	Ceftazadime

(E)	Nafcillin

132.	A 22-year-old college student presents to the emergency room with fever, non-productive cough, bullous myringitis, and patchy infiltrates on chest X-ray. Her serum cold-agglutinin titers were positive.

133.	A 67-year-old female, who has been hospitalized in the intensive care unit for sepsis, presents with fever, chills, productive cough, and malaise.

134.	A 19-year-old AIDS patient presents to the emergency room with a dry, non-productive cough, fever, and substernal pleuritic chest pain associated with shortness of breath, hypoxia, and an elevated LDH. Chest X-ray reveals bilateral diffuse interstitial infiltrates.

135.	A 78-year-old nursing home resident, with a long-standing sacral decubitus, presents with fever, chills, low-back pain, and an ESR over 100 mm/hr. The bone scan was positive for osteomyelitis. The bone biopsy revealed an organism that was resistant to penicillin.

136.	Which one of the following is NOT true of malignant hyperthermia?

(A)	Sudden massive muscle contractions lead to a rapid rise in body temperature.

(B)	A linkage to mutations of the skeletal muscle ryanodine receptor has been observed in some cases.

(C)	Muscle biopsies from susceptible individuals may contract when exposed to caffeine.

(D)	Screening with CPK is the best way to identify susceptible individuals.

(E) Triggering anesthetics release calcium from the membrane of the muscle cell's sarcoplasmic reticulum.

Questions 137 and 138 refer to the following:

A 44-year-old executive presents to your office stating that he is under a lot of stress. He also has a lot of pain in his jaw and jaw joint.

137. You suspect

   (A) myocardial infarction.

   (B) temporomandibular joint disease.

   (C) peptic ulcer.

   (D) osteoarthritis.

   (E) rheumatoid arthritis.

138. For the patient above, you would prescribe all of the following EXCEPT

   (A) soft diet.

   (B) analgesics.

   (C) rest.

   (D) MRI.

   (E) follow-up appointment in two weeks.

Questions 139 and 140 refer to the following:

A 61-year-old woman comes to the office complaining of unilateral ear pain. On physical examination, you note that vesicles are present in the affected external ear.

139. Which one of the following is the pathogen responsible for this syndrome?

   (A) Rhabdovirus

   (B) Herpes zoster virus

   (C) Coronavirus

   (D) Influenza virus

   (E) Hepatitis C virus

140. Which one of the following cranial nerves is affected in this patient?

   (A) Trigeminal nerve

   (B) Vagus nerve

   (C) Accessory nerve

   (D) Facial nerve

   (E) Vestibulocochlear nerve

141. Which of the following has NOT been implicated as a clinical complication of sleep apnea?

   (A) Left-heart failure

   (B) Pulmonary hypertension

   (C) Behavioral disorders

   (D) Systemic hypotension

   (E) Nocturnal death

142. A hemophiliac patient comes in with a massive bleed after minor trauma. He has received many transfusions in the past and gets another six now. You suggest he should get an HIV test. He tells you he wants to think about it. You

   (A) draw it without telling him.

   (B) do as he asks.

   (C) call his parents.

   (D) call a psychiatrist.

   (E) refuse to treat him.

For Questions 143-146, choose the best lettered answer for each numbered question.

   (A) Give medically necessary transfusion

   (B) Perform necessary emergency procedures

   (C) Do not give transfusion

   (D) Obtain consent from parents

143. Adult Jehovah's Witness refusing blood transfusion for himself

144. Adult Jehovah's Witness refusing blood transfusion for his minor child

145. A 10-year-old runaway who is comatose and needs emergency surgery

146. A 12-year-old girl who meets criteria for an experimental drug

Questions 147-154 refer to the following:

A 35-year-old man is brought to your office because of progressively worsening heart failure. He has a hypertrophic cardiomyopathy with an ejection fraction of 25%. His creatinine is 2.5 and his BUN is 36. He has 2+ peripheral edema.

147. Since his renal function is worsening and diuretics and cardiotropic agents are not helping him, you recommend

    (A) long-term renal dialysis.

    (B) renal transplant.

    (C) cardiac catheterization.

    (D) renal biopsy.

    (E) heart transplant.

148. The family is surprised by this suggestion, but you explain why you think it is necessary. They ask about the steps involved in obtaining a heart and you tell them

    (A) he will have to wait until one of his immediate family dies.

    (B) he will need to go through a pre-transplant evaluation and then will be placed on an organ waiting list.

    (C) he should have a new heart in a few weeks.

    (D) he will have a normal lifespan if he gets a well-matched heart.

    (E) you have contacts who can get him a heart sooner than usual.

149. All of the following are important in evaluating someone for appropriateness for this transplant EXCEPT

    (A) wealth.

    (B) compliance with medical regimen.

    (C) alcoholism within the last six months.

    (D) support network.

    (E) psychiatric evaluation.

150. The patient admits to drinking an occasional beer lately because he has been "nervous." He denies ever drinking more than one beer a day. You tell him

    (A) he cannot get a transplant.

    (B) he must stop drinking completely for at least six months.

    (C) he must stop drinking and go through an Alcoholics Anonymous program.

    (D) he is still eligible for a transplant but should not drink any more.

    (E) you will have to talk to a psychiatrist.

151. The transplant team and the patient's insurance company inform you that he is a good candidate for a transplant. You now can tell the family

    (A) he can expect a heart within days.

    (B) the length of time until a heart becomes available is unpredictable.

    (C) he needs to wait for a relative to die.

    (D) if they pay the transplant team he may get a heart sooner.

    (E) he can expect a heart within weeks.

152. While waiting for a transplant, the patient develops a severe ventricular arrhythmia. You

    (A) treat his arrhythmia.

    (B) tell the family there is nothing to be done at this point.

    (C) tell them he can only be on an experimental drug.

    (D) tell them he cannot receive an experimental drug.

(E)   tell them he is no longer a transplant candidate.

153. Depending on the severity and recurrence of the arrhythmia, it is possible

(A)   that he will no longer be eligible for a transplant.

(B)   that he may be moved up higher on the transplant list.

(C)   that he will be moved further down on the list, i.e., have to wait longer for a transplant.

(D)   that no heart will be found.

(E)   that he will need a lung transplant, too.

154. The patient continues to have recurrent ventricular arrhythmias and no donor heart has been found yet. You tell the family

(A)   he may have to stay in the CCU until he can be transplanted.

(B)   he will probably never receive a transplant.

(C)   he can go home and wait for a transplant.

(D)   he should move to another city.

(E)   they should tell him he will probably die soon.

For Questions 155-158 match the following respiratory diseases with the patients in which they are most likely to occur.

(A)   Asthma

(B)   Bronchitis

(C)   Croup

(D)   Epiglottitis

(E)   COPD

155. A 75-year-old woman with a 150 pack-year history who constantly gasps for air

156. A one-year-old child with a recent upper respiratory tract infection with a current sore throat and high temperature.

157. A 35-year-old smoker who gets a productive cough two to three times a year with normal to low-grade temperatures

158. A seven-year-old boy who presents to your office urgently stating that breathing feels like "sucking air through a straw."

159. A 24-year-old male patient comes to the clinic complaining of urethral discharge. Physical examination reveals mild groin lymphadenopathy. Culture of urethral discharge reveals Gram-negative cocci. Which one of the following statements is true regarding this condition?

(A)   Single-dose therapy with intramuscular penicillin is an effective therapy.

(B)   The pathogenic organism is *Hemophilus ducreyi*.

(C)   VDRL is usually positive.

(D)   The condition is associated with specific serotypes of human papillomavirus.

(E)   Spontaneous resolution is the rule.

160. A 23-year-old woman presents to your office with a sore throat for three days. She states that she has had some difficulty swallowing and a fever to 102°F. On physical examination, she has some difficulty opening her mouth completely, and you are able to note an uvula that is slightly deviated to the right. She has left tender cervical lymphadenopathy. The most appropriate intervention would be

(A)   send the patient with an urgent referral to an otolaryngologist.

(B)   begin treatment for bacterial pharyngitis.

(C)   send off a throat culture.

(D)   send off a monospot test.

(E)   assure the patient that it is likely a viral illness and to rest and drink plenty of fluids.

Questions 161-164 refer to the following:

A 33-year-old man known to be HIV positive comes to see you for the first time. He has been in good health and continues to work full-time as an accountant. On physical examination, you note some axillary lymphadenopathy. He admits to having noticed this recently while taking a shower. His CD4 count is 750.

161. Your differential diagnosis of the lymphadenopathy includes all of the following EXCEPT

  (A) lymphoma.

  (B) reactive lymphadenopathy.

  (C) lymphadenitis.

  (D) metastatic lung cancer.

  (E) a fungal infection.

162. To make the correct diagnosis, you order

  (A) an axillary lymph node dissection.

  (B) a chest CT scan.

  (C) ultrasound of the axilla.

  (D) MRI of the axilla.

  (E) fine needle aspiration.

163. You learn that the patient does not have lymphoma. You give him a follow-up visit for two months. He comes in two weeks later complaining of a left-sided headache. A repeat CD4 count comes back at 100. You refer the patient to

  (A) a neurologist.

  (B) an ophthalmologist.

  (C) a neurosurgeon.

  (D) a psychiatrist.

  (E) an oncologist.

164. You now decide that this patient has AIDS because

  (A) he is very sick.

  (B) he has had two different problems.

  (C) he needs to see an infectious diseases specialist.

  (D) he has a low CD4 count.

  (E) he has an opportunistic infection.

165. A 52-year-old homeless male, who is a chronic smoker, presents to the clinic without an appointment. He complains of worsening dyspnea, excessive purulent, blood-streaked sputum production, and a low-grade fever. On examination, he had an increased A-P diameter and diffuse wheezing and bronchi. Chest X-ray reveals diffuse interstitial markings, and spirometry demonstrates a decline in peak expiratory flow rates. The arterial blood gas is: Ph-7.38, PC02-50 P02-60. What would be the next immediate step in management of this patient?

  (A) Ventilation-perfusion scan

  (B) Bronchoscopy

  (C) PPD panel and sputum for acid-fast bacilli cultures

  (D) Inhaled nebulizer beta-adrenergic agonists

  (E) Diuretics

Questions 166-173 refer to the following:

A 33-year-old female is brought to the clinic by a friend because she has been complaining of heartburn for several days. She is known to be mentally impaired and her parents are her legal guardians. They are out of the country at present and she is staying home alone. You examine her and find no physical abnormalities. She is unable to describe the pain well.

166. You are concerned that she may have had some bleeding. Her old hospital records indicate a baseline hemoglobin of 13. You should

  (A) do nothing because her parents are not available.

  (B) obtain a blood count.

(C) call the hospital lawyer to have the patient declared a ward of the state.

(D) arrange a hearing so guardianship can be transferred to the hospital temporarily.

(E) schedule endoscopy.

167. You find no evidence of blood loss. You

    (A) can do nothing else until her parents come back.

    (B) schedule endoscopy.

    (C) commit the patient for observation.

    (D) tell her to take antacids and return if her symptoms get worse.

    (E) hospitalize her until her parents return.

168. You are running a clinical trial involving a new H2-blocker. You

    (A) sign up the patient for the study.

    (B) give her the drug without telling her it is experimental.

    (C) cannot enter her into the study without her parents' consent.

    (D) hospitalize her to give her the new agent.

    (E) can have her friend sign the informed consent to enroll her into the trial.

169. The patient returns to the emergency room three days later by ambulance because she has been found in her bathroom in a puddle of blood. You

    (A) deny ever seeing her before.

    (B) remove your notes from the chart.

    (C) admit her to the hospital and have her endoscoped on an emergency basis.

    (D) give her the study drug.

(E) refuse to do anything further until her parents return.

170. Endoscopy reveals an actively bleeding gastric ulcer that cannot be cauterized completely. She already has required 10 units of blood transfusion. You

    (A) arrange for emergency surgery.

    (B) keep giving her blood and cauterizing the lesion.

    (C) refuse to do anything else until her parents return.

    (D) give her your study drug.

    (E) call your malpractice insurance carrier.

171. She undergoes emergency partial gastrectomy and vagotomy, requiring more blood transfusions. By the time she has stabilized, her parents have been found and have come home. They should

    (A) sue you.

    (B) report you to your insurance company.

    (C) report you to the Board of Health.

    (D) talk to your chairman.

    (E) thank you.

172. The reason you can authorize emergency surgery without the parents' consent, but cannot do a routine workup, is

    (A) without the surgery the patient was at high risk of dying.

    (B) a routine workup is unnecessary.

    (C) surgery is cheaper.

    (D) the patient can consent to a life-saving procedure.

    (E) you thought it was the right thing to do.

173. You have another clinical trial for patients who have just undergone gastrectomy. You should

(A) talk the parents into permitting the patient to participate.

(B) enroll the patient without permission because you have saved her life.

(C) give her the drug and not tell anyone.

(D) tell the parents she will die without the drug.

(E) not try to enroll her because there is no compelling reason to include a mentally impaired subject in the study.

For Questions 174-177, match the test results with their corresponding causes.

A young woman consults you for an elevated free T4 level. You ask the third-year medical student, who is doing an elective in your office, to distinguish the various causes of abnormal thyroid test results which are illustrated below.

	Free T4	T3	TSH
(A)	Normal	Increased	Decreased
(B)	Increased	Normal	Decreased
(C)	Increased	Decreased	Increased
(D)	Increased	Increased	Increased

174. Pregnancy

175. Levothyroxine

176. Radiographic contrast agents

177. Pituitary thyroid hormone resistance syndrome

For Questions 178-180, you are filling in for the neurologist in the emergency room and are asked to evaluate a chief complaint of headache. Based on the following descriptions of the headaches, identify the location.

(A) Occipital

(B) Maxilla

(C) Temple

(D) Periorbital

(E) Frontal

178. A 55-year-old male with a migraine

179. A 19-year-old college student who has been studying a lot with a complaint of headache and eyestrain

180. A 77-year-old female with a cranial arteritis

USMLE STEP 3 – PRACTICE TEST 1

Day One – Morning Session

ANSWER KEY

1. (A)	31. (C)	61. (B)	91. (D)
2. (D)	32. (E)	62. (A)	92. (C)
3. (B)	33. (C)	63. (B)	93. (A)
4. (E)	34. (D)	64. (A)	94. (B)
5. (C)	35. (C)	65. (D)	95. (D)
6. (D)	36. (E)	66. (C)	96. (B)
7. (E)	37. (D)	67. (B)	97. (A)
8. (D)	38. (D)	68. (D)	98. (D)
9. (A)	39. (B)	69. (C)	99. (C)
10. (D)	40. (C)	70. (A)	100. (D)
11. (A)	41. (A)	71. (D)	101. (B)
12. (C)	42. (E)	72. (E)	102. (E)
13. (C)	43. (C)	73. (B)	103. (A)
14. (D)	44. (D)	74. (C)	104. (E)
15. (C)	45. (B)	75. (C)	105. (A)
16. (B)	46. (B)	76. (E)	106. (B)
17. (B)	47. (A)	77. (A)	107. (D)
18. (C)	48. (A)	78. (D)	108. (E)
19. (B)	49. (B)	79. (B)	109. (D)
20. (C)	50. (C)	80. (A)	110. (C)
21. (D)	51. (D)	81. (A)	111. (C)
22. (B)	52. (B)	82. (B)	112. (C)
23. (A)	53. (B)	83. (B)	113. (E)
24. (D)	54. (A)	84. (B)	114. (A)
25. (D)	55. (B)	85. (D)	115. (C)
26. (D)	56. (E)	86. (B)	116. (A)
27. (A)	57. (B)	87. (C)	117. (A)
28. (C)	58. (E)	88. (C)	118. (E)
29. (D)	59. (E)	89. (A)	119. (D)
30. (E)	60. (D)	90. (D)	120. (C)

121. (D)	136. (D)	151. (C)	166. (A)
122. (C)	137. (E)	152. (C)	167. (E)
123. (B)	138. (E)	153. (E)	168. (B)
124. (B)	139. (A)	154. (D)	169. (E)
125. (C)	140. (B)	155. (D)	170. (D)
126. (E)	141. (A)	156. (A)	171. (A)
127. (E)	142. (D)	157. (A)	172. (E)
128. (C)	143. (D)	158. (B)	173. (C)
129. (B)	144. (D)	159. (B)	174. (A)
130. (C)	145. (D)	160. (C)	175. (D)
131. (C)	146. (C)	161. (E)	176. (C)
132. (D)	147. (B)	162. (E)	177. (B)
133. (E)	148. (B)	163. (E)	178. (E)
134. (A)	149. (A)	164. (C)	179. (C)
135. (A)	150. (A)	165. (B)	180. (B)

USMLE STEP 3 – PRACTICE TEST 1

Day One – Afternoon Session

ANSWER KEY

1. (A)	31. (D)	61. (E)	91. (B)
2. (C)	32. (E)	62. (B)	92. (D)
3. (B)	33. (E)	63. (D)	93. (C)
4. (C)	34. (D)	64. (B)	94. (A)
5. (D)	35. (A)	65. (C)	95. (E)
6. (A)	36. (E)	66. (E)	96. (C)
7. (E)	37. (B)	67. (C)	97. (D)
8. (C)	38. (B)	68. (C)	98. (C)
9. (D)	39. (B)	69. (E)	99. (B)
10. (C)	40. (B)	70. (A)	100. (D)
11. (B)	41. (C)	71. (C)	101. (B)
12. (E)	42. (D)	72. (E)	102. (A)
13. (E)	43. (A)	73. (A)	103. (B)
14. (C)	44. (C)	74. (C)	104. (C)
15. (C)	45. (C)	75. (E)	105. (D)
16. (B)	46. (C)	76. (C)	106. (B)
17. (D)	47. (B)	77. (C)	107. (C)
18. (C)	48. (D)	78. (D)	108. (A)
19. (D)	49. (E)	79. (D)	109. (C)
20. (C)	50. (D)	80. (C)	110. (D)
21. (D)	51. (A)	81. (D)	111. (C)
22. (B)	52. (C)	82. (D)	112. (B)
23. (A)	53. (D)	83. (B)	113. (C)
24. (A)	54. (C)	84. (D)	114. (A)
25. (B)	55. (D)	85. (D)	115. (A)
26. (C)	56. (E)	86. (A)	116. (D)
27. (B)	57. (C)	87. (C)	117. (A)
28. (B)	58. (A)	88. (B)	118. (C)
29. (C)	59. (B)	89. (E)	119. (E)
30. (A)	60. (E)	90. (A)	120. (B)

121.	(A)	136.	(B)	151.	(A)	166.	(C)
122.	(D)	137.	(C)	152.	(D)	167.	(D)
123.	(B)	138.	(E)	153.	(D)	168.	(B)
124.	(C)	139.	(D)	154.	(E)	169.	(A)
125.	(E)	140.	(D)	155.	(C)	170.	(C)
126.	(A)	141.	(B)	156.	(A)	171.	(C)
127.	(D)	142.	(D)	157.	(C)	172.	(B)
128.	(D)	143.	(E)	158.	(B)	173.	(D)
129.	(C)	144.	(D)	159.	(A)	174.	(E)
130.	(E)	145.	(A)	160.	(D)	175.	(B)
131.	(E)	146.	(C)	161.	(B)	176.	(D)
132.	(C)	147.	(D)	162.	(E)	177.	(A)
133.	(D)	148.	(D)	163.	(A)	178.	(C)
134.	(B)	149.	(C)	164.	(C)	179.	(B)
135.	(D)	150.	(E)	165.	(E)	180.	(D)

USMLE STEP 3 – PRACTICE TEST 1

Day Two – Morning Session

ANSWER KEY

1. (A)	31. (B)	61. (C)	91. (D)
2. (B)	32. (C)	62. (C)	92. (C)
3. (B)	33. (B)	63. (D)	93. (B)
4. (A)	34. (C)	64. (C)	94. (B)
5. (B)	35. (C)	65. (C)	95. (E)
6. (C)	36. (B)	66. (A)	96. (D)
7. (B)	37. (B)	67. (B)	97. (C)
8. (C)	38. (A)	68. (D)	98. (C)
9. (A)	39. (C)	69. (D)	99. (B)
10. (B)	40. (D)	70. (C)	100. (A)
11. (C)	41. (C)	71. (D)	101. (B)
12. (D)	42. (B)	72. (D)	102. (B)
13. (A)	43. (C)	73. (E)	103. (B)
14. (C)	44. (A)	74. (B)	104. (B)
15. (B)	45. (E)	75. (A)	105. (C)
16. (D)	46. (A)	76. (B)	106. (C)
17. (A)	47. (D)	77. (A)	107. (A)
18. (D)	48. (A)	78. (E)	108. (E)
19. (D)	49. (D)	79. (D)	109. (A)
20. (A)	50. (A)	80. (B)	110. (E)
21. (C)	51. (A)	81. (C)	111. (A)
22. (B)	52. (E)	82. (E)	112. (A)
23. (C)	53. (C)	83. (D)	113. (A)
24. (E)	54. (C)	84. (E)	114. (E)
25. (C)	55. (D)	85. (C)	115. (A)
26. (A)	56. (D)	86. (A)	116. (B)
27. (B)	57. (A)	87. (E)	117. (A)
28. (B)	58. (D)	88. (C)	118. (E)
29. (E)	59. (C)	89. (A)	119. (B)
30. (C)	60. (C)	90. (B)	120. (A)

121. (B)	136. (B)	151. (D)	166. (A)
122. (C)	137. (A)	152. (A)	167. (C)
123. (E)	138. (A)	153. (E)	168. (E)
124. (E)	139. (B)	154. (B)	169. (A)
125. (A)	140. (A)	155. (C)	170. (C)
126. (C)	141. (D)	156. (B)	171. (B)
127. (D)	142. (B)	157. (C)	172. (D)
128. (B)	143. (A)	158. (C)	173. (E)
129. (B)	144. (C)	159. (B)	174. (E)
130. (A)	145. (B)	160. (E)	175. (C)
131. (D)	146. (B)	161. (E)	176. (A)
132. (D)	147. (C)	162. (E)	177. (E)
133. (D)	148. (A)	163. (B)	178. (A)
134. (C)	149. (A)	164. (C)	179. (E)
135. (A)	150. (A)	165. (B)	180. (C)

USMLE STEP 3 – PRACTICE TEST 1

Day Two – Afternoon Session

ANSWER KEY

1. (D)	31. (E)	61. (D)	91. (D)
2. (D)	32. (E)	62. (C)	92. (C)
3. (D)	33. (E)	63. (D)	93. (D)
4. (B)	34. (A)	64. (D)	94. (D)
5. (C)	35. (A)	65. (C)	95. (A)
6. (C)	36. (C)	66. (B)	96. (D)
7. (A)	37. (C)	67. (D)	97. (C)
8. (B)	38. (A)	68. (E)	98. (C)
9. (E)	39. (A)	69. (E)	99. (A)
10. (A)	40. (A)	70. (D)	100. (A)
11. (C)	41. (E)	71. (C)	101. (C)
12. (B)	42. (D)	72. (D)	102. (A)
13. (E)	43. (C)	73. (B)	103. (D)
14. (B)	44. (C)	74. (E)	104. (C)
15. (A)	45. (C)	75. (A)	105. (D)
16. (E)	46. (D)	76. (C)	106. (A)
17. (E)	47. (B)	77. (B)	107. (D)
18. (C)	48. (D)	78. (A)	108. (D)
19. (A)	49. (C)	79. (C)	109. (B)
20. (A)	50. (C)	80. (B)	110. (D)
21. (C)	51. (A)	81. (E)	111. (C)
22. (B)	52. (D)	82. (D)	112. (A)
23. (A)	53. (E)	83. (E)	113. (D)
24. (B)	54. (B)	84. (C)	114. (C)
25. (C)	55. (D)	85. (D)	115. (B)
26. (B)	56. (B)	86. (E)	116. (D)
27. (C)	57. (C)	87. (D)	117. (C)
28. (D)	58. (D)	88. (A)	118. (B)
29. (A)	59. (B)	89. (C)	119. (D)
30. (E)	60. (A)	90. (E)	120. (E)

121. (E)	136. (D)	151. (B)	166. (B)
122. (A)	137. (B)	152. (A)	167. (D)
123. (C)	138. (D)	153. (B)	168. (C)
124. (A)	139. (B)	154. (A)	169. (C)
125. (E)	140. (D)	155. (E)	170. (A)
126. (B)	141. (D)	156. (D)	171. (E)
127. (E)	142. (B)	157. (B)	172. (A)
128. (E)	143. (C)	158. (A)	173. (E)
129. (E)	144. (A)	159. (A)	174. (A)
130. (C)	145. (B)	160. (A)	175. (B)
131. (B)	146. (D)	161. (D)	176. (C)
132. (C)	147. (E)	162. (E)	177. (D)
133. (D)	148. (B)	163. (B)	178. (D)
134. (B)	149. (A)	164. (E)	179. (A)
135. (A)	150. (D)	165. (D)	180. (C)

DETAILED EXPLANATIONS OF ANSWERS

USMLE Step 3 – Practice Test 1
Day One – Morning Session

1. **(A)** Icterus is associated with yellow sclera from jaundice.

2. **(D)** Osteogenesis imperfecta is associated with blue sclera, resulting from a thinning of the sclera that allows the choroid to show through.

3. **(B)** Melanin deposition or homogentisic acid is associated with brown sclera.

4. **(E)** Staphyloma is associated with scleral protrusion as a result of injury to the sclera or increased intraocular pressure.

5. **(C)** When someone presents and appears very ill, potentially life-threatening illnesses need to be ruled out first, such as myocardial infarction, pulmonary embolism, aortic dissection, and pericardial tamponade.

6. **(D)** Findings of congestive heart failure, such as inspiratory rales and elevated jugular venous pressure, can be found with massive myocardial damage, as can hypotension from cardiogenic shock. Chest radiograph can appear very normal with myocardial infarctions. A pulsus is found in a restrictive state, such as the restrictive pericardial effusion found in tamponade.

7. **(E)** With a pulmonary embolism, patients almost always present with tachycardia, not bradycardia. Bradycardia can occur with an inferior wall myocardial infarction and vagal stimulation.

8. **(D)** The treatment for an acute myocardial infarction is aspirin, heparin, and thrombolytics, or immediate angioplasty, whichever is available. Antiarrhythmics are not indicated unless ventricular tachycardiacs are noted.

9. **(A)** The ST elevations in II, III, and avL are classically inferior in distribution. The ST depressions in VI and V2 represent reciprocal changes of the posterior wall, which is not uncommonly also affected in inferior wall myocardial infarctions.

10. **(D)** For a patient with known coronary artery disease, it is important to try to rule out potentially treatable exacerbating diseases such as diabetes mellitus (HB A1C), hypercholesterolemia (fasting lipid profile), and other risk factors (smoking). A functional assessment of ejection fraction (echocardiogram) can also be helpful. In the near future, a sub-maximal stress test occasionally can be helpful, but not a maximal stress test so shortly after a myocardial infarction.

11. **(A)** In patients with coronary artery disease, unless there is a clear-cut reason why beta-blockers are contraindicated, beta-blocker therapy should be started.

12. **(C)** Life-threatening arrhythmias can occur commonly within 48 hours after a myocardial infarction. Once that time is over, patients should gradually begin to increase activity while being observed for problems, and can be discharged about seven days after a myocardial infarction.

13. **(C)** Bronchitis is commonly seen in smokers and increases in the winter months. There is inflammation of the bronchioles and breathing becomes difficult. Asthma (A) is a restrictive

disease and there is usually no fever. Lung carcinoma (B) presents with cough and occasional hemoptysis. Consolidation of a lung field may be detected on physical exam. A viral upper respiratory tract infection (D) will usually present with fever and cough. The cough is often not painful and the lungs may sound clear. A pneumothorax (E) will be occasionally painful, and resonance will be detected on lung examination.

14.   **(D)**   Classically, cluster headaches present in men as unilateral lancinating pain behind the eye or in the temporal region, and are occasionally associated with autonomic dysfunction, such as lacrimation or miosis.

15.   **(C)**   White hairy tongue results from opportunistic infection and in a 32-year-old male without any reason for a deficient immune system, one must be suspicious for HIV (C). Carcinoma (A) presents as an ulcerated erythoplakic or leukoplakic lesion. Herpes (B) presents as an ulcerated lesion that is initially vesicular. Streptococcus (D) on the tongue may not appear as anything unless it is overgrowing in an infection. Traumatic tongue lesions (E) appear hyperkeratotic.

16.   **(B)**   Billing for procedures not performed is fraudulent and punishable by fine or prison, or both.

17.   **(B)**   A diagnosis of tuberculosis of the spine (Pott's disease) is most consistent with the history, physical findings, and MRI examination. The midthoracic spine is usually affected, as illustrated by the involvement of T9-L1 in this case. Anterior erosion of the vertebral bodies causes collapse, resulting in a sharply angulated kyphosis without scoliosis, known as a gibbus deformity. In this case, the MRI demonstrates the collapsed vertebrae, with compression of the spinal cord. In the presence of new paraparesis, immediate orthopedic consultation should be obtained (B). Lumbar puncture would be difficult in this case, due to distortion of the bony architecture. Necessary studies, such as cultures and spinal fluid analysis, can be obtained at the time of surgery (A). Obtaining a bone scan will only delay the necessary treatment, which is decompression of the spinal cord (E). There is no indication of an acute infectious process. Both the dose and the frequency of administration of vancomycin are excessive (C). Nei-

ther the history nor the physical examination suggest that this child has a malignant process necessitating immediate radiotherapy (D).

18.   **(C)**   EKG changes associated with hyperkalemia are initially peaked T-waves (A) and a shortened QT interval. Then, the PR interval lengthens (B) and the QRS widens (D). Finally, the P-waves flatten (E), and the QRS widens further to form a sine wave.

19.   **(B)**   This patient's periodic health examination should include measurement of body mass index [(D) and (E)], serum cholesterol (A), and blood pressure (C). Screening for abnormal plasma glucose levels without pertinent history and clinical symptoms is not routinely recommended.

20.   **(C)**   The cross-section of the abdominal computed axial tomographic scan demonstrates an infrarenal abdominal aortic aneurysm, measuring 10 cm in diameter. The risk of rupture increases as the size of the aneurysm increases (C), reaching 95% in persons with aneurysms greater than 10 cm in diameter [(A) and (B)]. Pre-existing coronary artery disease, congestive heart failure, pulmonary disease, diabetes, and advanced age all contribute to increased operative risk. Diagnostic testing should be performed preoperatively to identify these risk factors [(D) and (E)].

21.   **(D)**   This patient has Chagas' disease, which is endemic to Central American countries. Infection with *Trypanosoma cruzi* is transmitted via reduviid bugs and can cause myocarditis, leading to congestive heart failure in its chronic stages. Diagnosis of acute Chagas' disease is by examination of a peripheral smear. Diagnosis of chronic Chagas' disease is by immunofluorescence testing and ELISA. Echocardiogram (A) would only tell us that the patient has cardomegaly and a low ejection fraction, but not the cause of congestive heart failure. The esophagram or barium swallow (B) would diagnose achalasia or dilated esophagus secondary to Chagas' disease. This would cause symptoms of dysphagia. Peripheral smear examination (D) is useful to diagnose acute Chagas' disease. Acute phase is generally limited to facial edema and nodule (chagoma) near the bite coupled with fever, lymphadenopathy, and

hepatosplenomegaly. Cardiac manifestations are associated with the chronic form of the disease in which few trypomastigotes are found in the blood. The electrocardiogram (E) may reveal conduction defects, but the specific diagnosis of Chagas' disease cannot be made from the electrocardiogram.

22. **(B)** The classic triad for Strep throat is fever, tonsillar exudates, and painful adenopathy.

23. **(A)** Although, classically, *Staphylococcus aureus* (D) pneumonia can follow a viral influenzae, the most common organism is *Streptococcus pneumoniae*.

24. **(D)** The most common organism causing wound infections is *Staphylococcus aureus*.

25. **(D)** This patient by history has a right-sided endocarditis, which is most commonly caused by a *Staph* species.

26. **(D)** A peritoneal friction rub does not detect an ileus. It resembles the sound of two pieces of leather rubbing together and occurs with peritoneal inflammation. It can be seen with splenic infarction (A), carcinoma of the liver (B), syphilitic hepatitis (C), and liver abscess (E).

27. **(A)** In patients with cirrhosis, the most common etiology of upper gastrointestinal bleeding is esophageal varices.

28. **(C)** Patients need to lose about 25% of their blood volume to become hypotensive. Less than 25% of total blood volume loss will only exhibit as orthostatic hypotension.

29. **(D)** In any kind of massive hemorrhage, the appropriate intervention is volume resuscitation. Pressors (C) are likely not to be helpful, as the patients are usually already maximally vasoconstricted. Volume resuscitation can be done with crystalloids, colloids, or blood products.

30. **(E)** Invasive hemodynamic monitoring may be helpful when the etiology of shock is not known. In this case, the etiology is easily determined and time should not be wasted on a needless procedure when the patient is unstable. When a patient has a significant gastrointestinal bleed, all of the other choices should be done, including two large-bore IV needle (A), type and cross (B), complete blood count (C), and coagulation studies (D).

31. **(C)** In an active upper gastrointestinal bleed, the first diagnostic test of choice is upper endoscopy to ascertain the location of the hemorrhage and to possibly treat with sclerotherapy.

32. **(E)** Vasopressin (A) and octreotide (B) can decrease portal hypertension temporarily. Blood infusion (D) will replace any lost volume. The Blakemore tube (C) can tamponade the hemorrhage in a patient with esophageal varices. However, these are all temporizing measures and should not be done in place of a definitive procedure.

33. **(C)** Band ligation and sclerotherapy have been shown to have the same efficacy in decreasing the reoccurrence of upper gastrointestinal bleeding.

34. **(D)** There has been some evidence that beta-blockers can decrease the recurrence rate of bleeding esophageal varices. There has been some evidence that calcium channel blockers and nitrates can do the same thing. The other choices have not been shown to decrease the recurrence rate of bleeding esophageal varices.

35. **(C)** *Neisseria gonorrhea* is the cause of gonococcal urethritis and is associated with purulent discharge. This patient has nongonococcal or atypical urethritis, which is commonly caused by *C. trachomatis* (A) or *U. urealyticum* (B). The infectious process may have an asymptomatic course both in men (D) and, even more commonly, in women (E).

36. **(E)** The incidence of nonobstetrical surgical procedure is between 0.3% and 2% (A). Appendectomy is the number-one cause of surgical interventions in pregnant women (B). Ketamine can increase uterine smooth muscle tone, lead to preterm labor, and, thus, should be avoided (C). Fluid preloading (E) is recommended both in general and regional anesthesia. It helps to avoid hypotension and hypoperfusion.

37. **(D)** Oral griseofulvin, given for at least six to eight weeks, is the treatment for tinea capitis.

Topical agents [(A), (B), and (C)] are ineffective. Antibiotics, such as amoxicillin (E), are not effective against fungal infections.

38. **(D)** Epitrochlear nodes are about 3 cm proximal to the medial humeral epicondyle in the groove between the biceps and triceps brachii. They drain the little finger (A), the ring finger (B), the ulnar aspect of the arm (C), and the ulnar half of the long finger (E). They do not drain the radial aspect of the arm (D).

39. **(B)** It is likely she received a nonsteroidal as part of the treatment of her ankle pain. This agent may have caused gastritis or even peptic ulcer disease.

40. **(C)** Trimethoprim-sulfa is a common cause of rash in this group of patients. The other agents are not usually associated with this allergic reaction.

41. **(A)** This patient is likely to be taking chronic theophylline, and its toxicity includes the symptoms with which he presents.

42. **(E)** This scenario is most compatible with digoxin toxicity, which can be precipitated by hypokalemia. The latter is a common side effect of diuretics.

43. **(C)** This patient has a history and physical findings consistent with streptococcal infections and is at risk for rheumatic fever. Penicillin is the drug of choice, provided there is no history of allergy.

44. **(D)** The absence of any bleeding abnormalities suggests an agent like aspirin (A), which acetylates platelets and can cause bleeding or bruising, is not the agent involved. Acetaminophen in excess doses causes liver dysfunction, especially in the elderly, and can cause confusion.

45. **(B)** The electrocardiogram shows marked prolongation of the QT interval, with T-wave alternates. Both autosomal dominant and recessive forms of the long QT syndrome have been described (A). Recurrent attacks of ventricular tachycardia are associated with cardiac arrest (C) and sudden death (B). Treatment, directed to the underlying cardiac condition, should be initiated immediately [(D) and (E)].

46. **(B)** Klinefelter's syndrome is associated with deficiency of sperm and androgen production. The classic Klinefelter's patient has a 47 XXY karyotype. Klinefelter's syndrome often results in a disproportionate increase in lower-extremity compared to upper-extremity long-bone growth. Mental retardation is common. Kartagener's syndrome (A) is caused by defects in the cilia resulting in immobile sperm. There is no defect in the karyotype and thus the patient has a normal body habitus. Noonan's syndrome (C) is an autosomal dominant disorder characterized by hyperelastic skin, short stature, webbed neck, micrognathia, low-set ears, and a high-arched palate. In males it results in small testes, reduced testosterone levels, and increased gonadotropin levels. Mumps orchitis (D) is an acquired disorder. It is associated with an isolated deficiency of sperm production. Congenital adrenal hyperplasia (E) is associated with 21-and 11-beta-hydroxylase deficiency and results in androgen excess, not deficiency.

47. **(A)** This patient has a spondyloarthropathy called ankylosing spondylitis, which is characterized by chronic low back pain for over three months, age below 40, improved lower back pain with increasing activity, and a positive HLA-B27. The diagnostic test of choice is plain X-rays of the sacroiliac joint which would reveal sacroiliitis. Serum rheumatoid factor (B) would be positive in rheumatoid arthritis, which is an inflammatory arthritis, usually in the metatarsophalangeal joint (wrist joint). Arthrocentesis of the first metatarsophalangeal joint (C) is diagnostic for gouty arthritis. This patient has no pain in that area. Plain films of the spine (D) would give information to diagnose degenerative joint disease, which is usually present in older patients and patients with osteoarthritis. The lumbar films would show sclerosis and joint space narrowing. The straight-leg testing examination (E) is nonspecific. It reveals sciatic pain or nerve entrapment which would cause the lower back pain.

48. **(A)**, 49. **(B)**, 50. **(C)**, and 51. **(D)** Static lung volumes typically distinguish between two types of lung disease—restrictive and obstructive. Obstructive lung diseases, such as asthma (B), chronic bronchitis, and emphysema, are characterized by a decrease in expiratory flow rates. The expiratory portion of the flow volume loop demonstrates decreased flow rates for any given volume. Nonuniform airway emptying is manifested by a coved

configuration of the curve. With very early disease, the only abnormality on the flow volume loop may be an abnormal configuration in the terminal portion of the forced expiratory flow-volume curve.

A restrictive pattern on pulmonary function testing may be caused by either pulmonary parenchymal or extrapulmonary disease. This pattern is characterized by a decrease in lung volumes, including both the total lung capacity and the vital capacity.

In the parenchymal variant, typified by diseases such as sarcoidosis (C), idiopathic pulmonary fibrosis, pneumoconiosis, and interstitial lung disease, the flow volume loop demonstrates the disproportionate relationship between flow rates and lung volumes. As shown in the figure, the expiratory portion of the curve appears relatively tall, indicating a preserved flow rate. However, the curve is narrowed due to decreased lung volumes.

In the extrapulmonary variant, characteristic of diseases such as diaphragmatic paralysis (D), obesity, and kyphoscoliosis, there is inspiratory muscle dysfunction. This results from either inspiratory muscle weakness or a stiff chest wall. Thus, an otherwise normal lung is unable to respond to adequate distending forces. Sometimes, the extrapulmonary variant is characterized by both inspiratory and expiratory dysfunction. When this occurs, there may also be an inability to expire to a normal residual volume. This may occur in diseases such as myasthenia gravis, muscular dystrophies, and Guillain-Barre syndrome.

52. **(B)** In membranoproliferative glomerulonephritis, the mesangial cells proliferate, either segmentally or diffusely, interposing themselves or their cytoplasm into peripheral capillary loops. There is increased synthesis of the mesangial matrix. The glomerular capillary wall is irregularly thickened (B). Nodular glomerulosclerosis (Kimmelstiel-Wilson lesion) is highly specific for diabetes mellitus. PAS-positive laminated, intercapillary nodules on a background of increased mesangial matrix characterize this lesion. Open glomerular capillary loops are present at the periphery of the nodule (A). In focal segmental glomerulosclerosis, areas of the glomerular capillary lumen are segmentally obliterated by basement membrane material, which stains positive for C3 and IgM by immunofluorescence. Adjacent glomerular lobules are normal (C). IgA nephropathy, also known as Berger's disease, reveals a spectrum of changes on renal biopsy, from normal to diffuse mesangial proliferative changes. Mesangial hypercellularity is commonly seen. The hallmark of the disease is diffuse mesangial deposition of IgA (D). In minimal change disease, also known as "nil disease" or "lipoid nephrosis," little or no change is evident in the glomerular capillaries on light microscopy. Immunofluorescence staining demonstrates absent or irregular and nonspecific deposits of immunoglobulin and complement components. Diffuse foot process effacement is evident on electron microscopy (E).

53. **(B)** Peyronie's disease is dysplasia of the cavernous sheaths and contracture of the investing fascia of the corpora. Priapism (A) is a painful, persistent penile erection. An inguinal hernia (C) is a herniation of the abdominal contents and may be direct or indirect. A varicocele (D) is a collection of large veins in the scrotum. A torsion (E) is a twisting of the cord.

54. **(A)** In Peyronie's disease, the penis deviates to the involved side because of the contracture. It does not remain straight (C) nor flaccid at all times (D).

55. **(B)** Erection with Peyronie's disease is painful, as well as persistent. It is very possible, not impossible (A). It is not painless (C), and it is usually always painful, not only during intercourse (D) or ejaculation.

56. **(E)** Treatment for Peyronie's disease includes surgery to remove the involved plaque (A), injections of steroids (B), ultrasonic treatment (C), and oral steroids (D). There is no role for radiation (E).

57. **(B)** A needle thoracostomy will convert a tension pneumothorax to a regular pneumothorax. A chest tube (A) will treat a regular pneumothorax. A tracheostomy (C) establishes an emergent airway. Intubation is also indicated in the event of an emergent airway (D). Positive pressure ventilation can actually cause or worsen a pneumothorax (E).

58. **(E)** This section from the frontal cerebral cortex is stained with the Cajal silver method to identify axons and neurofibrils. A neuritic plaque is shown here with a darkly stained core of amyloid. Also shown are neurites, which are

comprised of pathologically altered, distorted axons and dendrites. Neurofibrillary tangles are also evident. These findings are consistent with a diagnosis of Alzheimer's disease, the most common cause of dementia in the elderly (E). In 20-25% of patients with Alzheimer's disease, another affected relative can be identified by a careful history (A). ApoE4 homozygotes have an increased risk for this disease when compared to E3 or E4 homozygotes. ApoE4 heterozygotes have an intermediate risk (C). Similar neuropathologic changes have been observed in persons with Down's syndrome (B). Neurofibrillary tangles are present in the dementia that follows repeated boxing injuries.

59. **(E)** This patient has Wilson's disease, or hepatolenticular degeneration. This disease should be suspected in any young patient with liver disease and neurologic symptoms. It is an autosomal recessive disorder. The hepatic injury is gradual in onset. This patient does not have hepatitis A, B, or C. A hepatitis antibody test will not give us our diagnosis. Low serum ceruloplasmin concentrations (below 20 mg/dl) (A) are present in nearly all patients with Wilson's disease. Increased amounts of copper (greater than 250 ug/gm) are present in patients with Wilson's disease. This quantitative copper analysis can be obtained by biopsy of the liver (B). Greater than 100 ug of copper in a 24-hour urine collection (C) is diagnostic of hepatolenticular degeneration. Kayser-Fleischer rings are composed of copper-containing granules and are located in Descemet's membrane at the limbus of the cornea. This can be visible on a slit-lamp examination (D). This physical finding is virtually diagnostic of Wilson's disease.

60. **(D)** Disseminated intravascular coagulation is a complication of Gram-negative sepsis and acute myelocytic leukemia. It is not a known complication of Wilson's disease. Large amounts of copper may be released over a short period, creating the potential for acute erythrocyte injury and subsequent hemolytic anemia (A). Fulminant hepatic failure can occur eventually after most of the hepatocytes have been destroyed by the excess copper accumulation, and, thus, hepatic encephalopathy may occur (B). Neurologic signs may include dysarthria, rigidity, oscillating tremors of the upper extremities, and awkward dystonic postures (C). This is all due to excess copper accumulation in the lenticular basal ganglia part of the brain. Arthropathy (E) can result from excess copper accumulation in the joint spaces. Renal calculi and heart disease are other complications of Wilson's disease.

61. **(B)** Positive copper balance begins in infancy in Wilson's disease and continues thereafter unless appropriate therapy is given. The signs and symptoms are usually manifested during the ages of 15-20 years. The prevalence of the disease is approximately 30 per million. Once brain damage from excessive copper accumulation in the brain has occurred, children and teens may experience difficulty in school and intellectual deterioration as well as personality changes. The signs of Wilson's disease do not usually show up during early childhood, but the gradual damage to the liver, kidneys, and brain is still progressing during these years.

62. **(A)** Effective therapy depends upon establishing negative copper balance, thereby preventing deposition of more copper. Without effective lifetime therapy, Wilson's disease is inevitably fatal. D-penicillamine is the treatment of choice, given at the dosage of one gram per day in two divided doses. The response is usually slow but treatment should begin as early as possible. Some patients with fulminant hepatic failure could benefit from a liver transplant to prevent death. Prednisone (B) is given in conjunction with D-penicillamine when a patient develops toxicity from penicillamine treatment, such as rash and fever. Zinc treatment (C) is not the initial treatment and it is experimental. There is D-penicillamine chelating therapy available, so choice (D) is incorrect. Dimercaprol (E) is the treatment of choice for lead toxicity.

63. **(B)** This scanning electron micrograph demonstrates numerous acanthocytes, diagnostic of spur cell anemia. Severe hepatocellular disease, especially alcoholic cirrhosis, is associated with hemolytic anemia and bizarre-shaped red blood cells [(B), (C), (D), and (E)]. In renal failure, red blood cells with scalloped outlines ("burr cells") may be observed on the peripheral smear (A).

64. **(A)** This patient's symptoms are most consistent with hypothyroidism. Although serum TSH is usually a good screening test, for patients who have symptoms consistent with hypothyroidism,

a more definitive test, such as a serum T4, is more appropriate in assessing if someone is hypothyroid.

65. **(D)** It is not ethical to lie to an insurance company, or to anyone else, regarding a patient's condition so that the patient can get something he/she wants.

66. **(C)** Failure to function within the accepted standards of care characterizes the "incompetent physician." The "impaired physician" exhibits an inability to function safely and effectively. The "underlying pathology" is the physical or emotional disability to perform to accepted standards (A). Although increasing impairment will result in deteriorating performance, it must be distinguished from incompetence (D). Aging or premature senility is inescapable. Forgetfulness, confusion, and loss of dexterity are components of the "impairment" resulting from advancing age. Almost all physicians are social drinkers, and the distinction between social drinking and alcoholism is often subtle. The stresses of the profession may lead health care providers and physicians to drug abuse. This is more common in anesthesiologists who have easy access to narcotics. Note that unlike alcohol abuse, which is still considered a "pardonable weakness," physicians in drug abuse are subject to legal regulations.

67. **(B)** Radiation therapy to bony metastases can greatly alleviate his pain.

68. **(D)** As above, radiation therapy can reduce the pain of bony metastases.

69. **(C)** The best goal to strive for in the terminally ill is the best quality of life, i.e., the least pain and suffering, achievable.

70. **(A)** It would be inappropriate to admit to an ICU a terminally ill patient with a living will stating that no heroic measures should be performed.

71. **(D)** You are concerned that the patient may have some sensation, and you do not want him to starve.

72. **(E)** Explaining your recommendations to the family is always important.

73. **(B)** The patient has a living will and she is his guardian. Therefore, her decision in this case is the final one.

74. **(C)** The patient and his wife have set up the living will to prevent him from being subjected to resuscitation.

75. **(C)** This patient has classic signs and symptoms of herpes simplex virus. Individuals suffering from human immunodeficiency virus infection have a more progressive and virulent form of the disease. In this case, the woman has genital herpes, which can be diagnosed by a Tzanck prep and looking at the cytology under the microscope. Herpes type II virus would show up as inclusion bodies and multinucleated giant cells. The vesicular lesions are painful and can be recurrent if not treated permanently. The mode of transmission is mucocutaneous sexual contact with an infected partner. Women frequently have dysuria secondary to urethral involvement. Branching hyphae (A) are seen in candida infections, which present as "curd-like" discharge from the vagina. Dysplastic squamous cells (B) are seen in early cervical cancer. Gram-negative diplococci (D) are seen in chlamydia infections. Gram-positive filamentous beaded strands (E) are seen in actinomycoses and norcardia infections.

76. **(E)** This immunocompromised HIV patient has progressed to herpes encephalitis, which has a very high mortality. Herpes simplex encephalitis is characterized by hemorrhagic necrosis of the temporal lobe. Clinical manifestations include fever, headache, altered mental status changes, and even seizures. The gold standard for definitive diagnosis is a brain biopsy. A lumbar puncture (A) would show pleocytosis and an elevated protein level in the cerebral spinal fluid. This is nonspecific. A CT scan of the brain (B) may reveal hemorrhagic necrosis, but this, again, is not specific and not present in all cases. An EEG (C) is both nonspecific and nonsensitive in establishing the correct diagnosis of herpes encephalitis. An ophthalmologic retinal examination (D) would show signs of CMV retinitis, not herpes encephalitis. Only a brain biopsy with demonstration of inclusion bodies would establish the diagnosis.

77. **(A)** The immediate treatment of choice for both herpes encephalitis and genital herpes is acyclovir. Acyclovir is an antiviral drug, which has

proved useful in the management of mucocutaneous herpes simplex virus. Intravenous acyclovir is given for life-threatening conditions such as herpes encephalitis. Amphotericin (B) is the treatment of choice for fungal infections. Doxycycline (C) is the antibiotic of choice to treat chlamydial infections. Steroids (D) are only given if there is evidence of an elevated intracranial pressure that could cause herniation of the brain. If steroids are given in herpes encephalitis, it could make the condition worse. Ganciclovir (E) is given to treat cytomegalovirus infections such as colitis or retinitis. CMV is part of the herpes species, and it also has the capacity to remain in the latent state.

78. (D), **79. (B)**, **80. (A)**, and **81. (A)** Cardiomyopathy is by definition a disease intrinsic to the heart muscle itself. Coronary artery disease can result in systolic or diastolic dysfunction; however, it is not technically a cause of cardiomyopathy. Dilated cardiomyopathy may occur secondary to viral myocarditis, alcohol, toxins, medications such as Adriamycin, or may occur postpartum. Hypertrophic cardiomyopathy typically results in diastolic dysfunction with good preservation of systolic function. Idiopathic hypertrophic subaortic stenosis results in a murmur, which increases in intensity with maneuvers that reduce preload, such as Valsalva. Restrictive cardiomyopathy is less common than the other varieties and occurs as a result of infiltrative diseases, such as amyloidosis.

82. (B) A physician does not have the right to refuse to take care of a patient because he does not agree with the patient's opinion or decision, which is what this situation represents. This physician is not being asked to perform an abortion.

83. (B) Since clinical symptoms/signs of hypothyroidism may be minimal, it is recommended that thyroid function be assessed in all persons with short stature (B). Significant renal disease is unlikely with a normal CBC and chemistry panel [(A) and (C)]. Although inflammatory bowel disease is a cause of short stature, it is unlikely in the absence of symptoms. Chronic, inflammatory conditions are best initially evaluated with a sedimentation rate (D). Pseudohypoparathyroidism is best excluded with a serum calcium (E).

84. (B) The chromosomal picture is that of a normal male (B). Gonadal dysgenesis (Turner syndrome) should be suspected in females with short stature and other phenotypic characteristics (A). Prader-Willi results from a deletion of a chromosomal band 15qll (D). Laron dwarfism results from growth hormone resistance. It is characterized by high levels of growth hormone and low levels of IGF-I (C). Further testing must be performed before concluding that the child is genetically predisposed to short stature. Chromosomal analysis alone cannot exclude a genetic predisposition for short stature (E).

85. (D) Bone age, as determined by X-rays, is one of the best indices of general growth (E). Interpretation of skeletal age requires caution, since 1 out of every 20 children can be expected to have a skeletal age either advanced or retarded by two standard deviations from the mean for a particular chronological age [(A) and (B)]. The hand and wrist are useful sites for measuring bone age throughout childhood. The lower extremity may also be used in early infancy (C). Girls are more advanced than boys in skeletal development at all ages. This requires separate standards for determining bone age (D).

86. (B) Secretion of growth hormone is episodic. Consequently, plasma levels are variable. Therefore, random measurements of this hormone are not adequate for assessing deficiency (C). A variety of stimulatory tests for growth deficiency, such as L-dopa, are routinely performed to assess deficiency (B). In addition to L-dopa, insulin-induced hypoglycemia and glucagon may be used to stimulate growth hormone secretion [(D) and (E)]. An abnormal bone age is not an indication for a bone biopsy (A).

87. (C) Two stimulatory tests have indicated that there is deficient secretion of growth hormone, thus justifying treatment (C). There is no reason to perform further diagnostic evaluation [(A) and (B)]. Prednisone is the treatment for adrenal hypofunction (D). Ergocalciferol (vitamin D2) is used for the treatment of rickets and osteomalacia. Dosage is dependent on numerous factors, such as the presence of malabsorption or an underlying renal defect (E).

88. (C) A known complication of growth hormone therapy is Creutzfeldt-Jakob (CJ) disease. The disease often manifests as a behavioral or personality change. Later signs include dementia, myoclonus, and tremor. In children, the disease may appear more similar to kuru, with a prominence of cerebellar signs. The disease can be rapidly fatal (C). In the presence of physical findings, medical evaluation takes precedence over psychiatric referral (A). The disease is thought to result from a contamination of cadaveric preparations of growth hormone (B). Although drugs of abuse can produce a variety of neuropsychiatric symptoms/signs, the presence of myoclonus in this clinical setting suggests CJ disease (D). Beta-blockers have been used to treat essential tremor, but are not appropriate in this clinical setting (E).

89.   **(A)**   Creutzfeldt-Jakob disease is most often a sporadic disease (B). The disease incidence usually peaks in the fifth through the seventh decades (A). The disease has been transmitted by corneal transplantation (C). In children who received contaminated cadaveric growth hormone preparations, the disease has appeared between 4-21 years later (D). It has also occurred in women who received pituitary gonadotropins for the treatment of infertility (E).

90.   **(D)**   Rubella vaccine should not be given to people who lack evidence of immunity.

91. **(D)**, 92. **(C)**, 93. **(A)**, 94. **(B)** *Cryptosporidium* is an organism which can cause severe diarrhea in patients with AIDS (A). *Shigella* and *G. lamblia* are common in homosexual AIDS patients, but less likely in an individual contracting the disease through intravenous drug use. *Shigella* is an enterinvasive pathogen which causes bloody diarrhea (B). *G. lamblia* is commonly acquired by drinking water from streams (C). *C. difficile* is usually a superinfection related to antibiotic administration with subsequent changes in the colonic bacterial flora (D). Rotavirus is a common pathogen in children (E).

95.   **(D)**   The X-ray demonstrates fine metallic opacities in the soft tissues of the back, which were not evident on physical examination of this Japanese male. The gold acupuncture needles were aligned along vertical meridians of the torso by an acupuncturist and then broken off [(A) and (B)]. This man believes that the needles absorb energy from his surroundings, thereby balancing his yin and yang forces and ultimately improving his overall health [(C) and (E)]. The needle frag-

ments remain in the subcutaneous tissues permanently (D).

96.   **(B)**   Falling on a hyperextended wrist is a common way to cause a Colles' fracture in the forearm.

97.   **(A)**   The patient's pupillary contraction suggests opiate intoxication, which is best treated by administration of an opiate antagonist, such as naloxone.

98.   **(D)**   The episodicity of the hypertension and associated symptoms suggest the possibility of a pheochromocytoma.

99.   **(C)**   Occasional patients will develop usually asymptomatic carboxymethemoglobinemia when treated with sulfa drugs. The condition resolves when the drug is discontinued.

100.   **(D)**   The history of high-impact sports and the knee instability should suggest damage to the anterior cruciate ligament.

101.   **(B)**   Sporotrichosis can be transmitted to individuals via trauma from rose thorns. This would be an unusual presentation for rheumatoid arthritis (A) in an adult and for *Candida* (C) or tubercular (D) infections. The setting is not consistent with Lyme disease (E).

102.   **(E)**   Maternal SLE is a well-described cause of congenital heart block. The mother's symptoms are consistent with this diagnosis.

103.   **(A)**   Avascular necrosis occurs in patients with sickle cell anemia because of poor perfusion of the bone due to sickling in the blood vessels.

104.   **(E)**   Lymphogranuloma venereum is a venereal disease presenting as a diffuse rectal ulcer caused by *Chlamydia trachomatis*. Bacillary dysentery (A), tuberculosis (B), irradiation (C), and trauma (D) all present as discrete rectal ulcers.

105.   **(A)**   This patient has necrotizing fascitis, which is usually caused by the infectious organism *Streptococcus pyogenes*. It occurs suddenly and in young, healthy individuals. The immediate treatment is fasciotomy by the surgical team because death is otherwise imminent. The affected

arm is subsequently debrided and irrigated. Clindamycin alone (B) is an inappropriate choice. Antibiotic combinations, such as ampicillin/sublactam plus clindamycin, should be given only after surgery is performed. Hyperbaric oxygen chamber usage (C) is good for patients with anaerobic infections. This patient has infection with a Gram-positive aerobic toxin-producing bacteria. This patient has weakness and decreased sensation of the left upper extremity secondary to an infectious process and not to a stroke. Thus, a CT of the head (D) is useless and would only delay the necessary surgical intervention. Thrombolytic therapy (E) is also contraindicated because this patient does not have a thromboembolic stroke causing the weakness, but a severe infection affecting the subcutaneous tissue and muscles of the left upper limb.

106. **(B)** There is a poor correlation with clinical findings and oximetric values (B). Cyanosis indicates a bluish coloration of the skin and mucous membranes resulting from an increased amount of reduced hemoglobin. The degree of cyanosis is modified by the quality of cutaneous pigmentation, the thickness of the skin, and the status of cutaneous capillaries (A). All these factors make clinical detection difficult. The absolute rather than the relative quantity of reduced hemoglobin is important in producing cyanosis. For this reason, persons with severe anemia, even in the presence of marked arterial desaturation, do not manifest cyanosis (C). Local passive congestion, by causing an increase in the total amount of reduced hemoglobin in blood vessels due to increased oxygen extraction, also results in cyanosis (D). In carbon monoxide poisoning, carboxyhemoglobin produces a cherry-colored flush, rather than cyanosis (E).

107. **(D)** Gonorrhea is one of the diseases that must be reported to the Board of Health when the conclusive diagnosis is made.

108. **(E)** PID, or pelvic inflammatory disease, is a serious disease among women. It can lead to fertility problems or infertility. Gonococcal cultures (A), KOH prep (B), Gram stain (C) and *Chlamydia* cultures (D) can all be tested for during a pelvic-cervical exam. Peritonitis is inflammation of the peritoneum of the abdomen and is usually not tested for in this manner.

109. **(D)** The figure demonstrates characteristics of megaloblastic anemia: a multilobed (six or more lobes) polymorphonuclear cell, anisocytosis and poikilocytosis, macro-ovalocytes (large, oval erythrocytes), and basophilic stippling. Nucleated red blood cells may also appear in the periphery, especially if the hematocrit is low. Total gastrectomy, tropical sprue, true vegetarianism (strictly vegetarian diet), and pernicious anemia all predispose to vitamin B12 deficiency, one common cause of megaloblastic anemia [(A), (B), (C), and (E)]. Heinz bodies are produced by the oxidation of hemoglobin. The resulting denatured hemoglobin precipitates within the erythrocyte. Heinz bodies are not present on ordinary Wright's stained blood smears, but are evident only after staining with supravital stains, such as methyl violet (D).

110. **(C)** To calculate the probability for the combined occurrence of three independent events, the multiplication rule is used. The probability that the three events will occur simultaneously is calculated by the formula:

P(event 1, event 2, and event 3) = P(event 1) x P(event 2) x P(event 3) = 0.15 x 0.15 x 0.15 = 0.00375.

Thus, the probability that disease X will result in the fatality of all three cases within four years of their initial diagnosis is 0.00375.

111. **(C)** During a pregnancy, up to about 32 weeks of gestation of a normal progression, the mother may be seen monthly. After this, the visits are every two weeks until 36 weeks, and then weekly until delivery.

112. **(C)** A midsystolic click is often indicative of mitral valve prolapse. Tricuspid stenosis (A) produces a midprecordial diastolic murmur. Tricuspid regurgitation (B) produces a midprecordial systolic murmur. Aortic stenosis (D) produces a basal systolic murmur. Aortic regurgitation (E) produces a basal diastolic murmur.

113. **(E)** The transverse colon is found in the epigastrium. The liver (A), gallbladder (B), ptotic right kidney (C), and enlarged right kidney (D) are all found in the right upper quadrant.

114. **(A)** This cyst occurs between the gluteal folds superior to the anus. They can be very painful and swollen.

115. **(C)** Pilonidal cysts can be difficult to manage because the cyst extends beyond appreciable borders. Appropriate initial treatment is to attempt to open the often loculated cysts with surgical debridement under local anesthesia.

116. **(A)** These heal very slowly and occasionally will need surgical therapy to heal. In addition, once healed, they can return.

117. **(A)** Although antibiotics and local wound care are the mainstay treatment for pilonidal cysts, surgical intervention is sometimes necessary, and a surgeon can be helpful in determining the need for and the timing of surgery.

118. **(E)** Positive Coombs' test is not observed in TTP, as this condition is characterized by microangiopathic hemolysis, not by an autoimmune-mediated hemolysis. Fever (A) is common, though not specific. Renal failure (B) evidenced by an elevated creatinine is another feature of TTP. Schistocytes on blood smear (C) are consistent with the microangiopathic hemolysis present in TTP. Reduced platelet count (D) is a result of hemolysis.

119. **(D)** In an elderly patient with temporal headaches, you must worry about temporal arteritis which, left untreated or misdiagnosed, can lead to blindness. You must start the patient on steroids empirically. A biopsy needs to be performed (C), but not acutely because damage can occur while you are waiting for the results. Analgesics (B) can be prescribed later on. Avoiding bright light and noises (A) are for a migraine headache. A CAT scan (E) is not indicated now and would not be the first course of action here.

120. **(C)** Temporal arteritis should first come to mind based on the presentation of the patient. Migraine headaches (A) and cluster headaches (B) would present and manifest themselves differently. A brain tumor (D) may present with other neurologic sequelae. There is no history of trauma to suggest a subdural hematoma (E).

121. **(D)** Glycohemoglobin assays are considered the "gold standard" for measuring glycemic control. Glycohemoglobin results when glucose reacts nonenzymatically with the hemoglobin A molecule. Hemoglobin A1C is the major fraction resulting from this interaction. It varies in proportion to the average glucose level and the lifespan of the red blood cell, thereby providing an index of glycemic control over the prior 6-12 weeks (A). In addition to the ambient glucose level, conditions that increase the red blood cell turnover, such as pregnancy, spuriously lower glycohemoglobin (E). Due to the variety of assay methods in use, the lack of standardization procedures, and the precision of the analysis, a "normal range" must be established for each laboratory (B). In general, hemoglobin A1C exceeding 10-12 is associated with poor glycemic control (C). Although rarely used clinically, measurement of glycolated albumin, because of its short half-life, can be used to monitor glycemic control over one to two weeks (D).

122. **(C)** You cannot refuse care (A) but you also cannot obtain the test without his permission (B). In the absence of a proven reportable disease, you cannot notify the Board of Health (D), nor can you tell the family.

123. **(B)** Based on the data provided, the sensitivity of the leukocyte-esterase test is approximately 70% (350/503), while the sensitivity of the urinary nitrate test is approximately 85% (425/503) making the urinary nitrate test the more sensitive test [(A) and (C)]. The sensitivity is defined as the number of true positive tests divided by the sum of the number of true positive tests plus the number of false negative tests. The prevalence of the condition (D) is not a variable that is required to determine the sensitivity of the test.

124. **(B)** The false-positive rate is defined as the number of people with a positive test who do not have a disease divided by the total number of people who do not have the disease, which in this case is 22% (68/308). It can also be calculated as 1-specificity.

125. **(C)** The false-negative rate is determined by calculating the ratio of the number of people with negative tests divided by the total number of people with the disease. In this case, it is calculated as 78/503 = 15.5%.

126. **(E)** None of the above statements is true. Although the leukocyte esterase test has a greater specificity, it also has a lower sensitivity (A). The urinary nitrate test has the lower specificity (B) of the two tests (67% vs. 78%). The urinary nitrate test is the more sensitive (C) of the two tests (85% vs. 70%). Information is not provided to determine whether either test is reproducible (D).

127. **(E)** Septic joint (A) usually presents with more cells (>75,000) and trauma (B), and normal (C) joints have fewer cells (<25,000). In patients with gouty arthritis (D), crystals should be visible.

128. **(C)** CT and MRI are the diagnostic studies of choice for detecting brain abscess. MRI with intravenous gadolinium contrast is probably more sensitive than CT during the cerebritis phase. MRI interpretation is not affected by overlying bony structures. The ring-enhanced lesion shown here, located within the brain parenchyma, is typical of a cerebral abscess (C). A subdural empyema forms in the space between the arachnoid membrane and the dura mater. CT and MRI show an extra-axial, crescent, or elliptically shaped mass with an enhancing rim located just below the inner table of the skull, over the cerebral convexities or the interhemispheric fissures (A). Infections of the epidural space (located between the dura mater and the overlying bone) often coexist with subdural empyemas. CT or MRI demonstrates a hypodense peripherally enhancing lenticular-shaped lesion in the epidural space (B). Lateral or sagittal venous sinus thrombosis may occur as a complication of sepsis. Contrast CT may show a nonenhanced triangular area surrounded by contrast in the posterior sinus (empty "delta" sign), but the definitive diagnosis is made by angiography (E). Similarly to a subdural empyema, a subdural hematoma forms in the space between the arachnoid membrane and the dura mater. The appearance on CT and MRI depends on the acuteness of the lesion. Acutely, CT shows a clot. MRI may not demonstrate the lesion within the first several days. With time, the lesion becomes isodense with the brain and may not be visualized on CT (D).

129. **(B)** You must do what is medically proper for this patient, even if he has not followed your advice.

130. **(C)** The electroencephalogram is not a standard anesthesia monitor. It is used in special situations when monitoring brain wave activity is needed, such as with carotid artery surgery. All the other choices are standard anesthesia monitors that are used routinely for general anesthesia cases. Missing from the list are an oxygen sensor and an electrocardiogram.

131. **(C)** Medications that patients with G6PD deficiency should avoid include sulfonamides (D), dapsone (B), and methylene blue.

132. **(D)** Priapism is prolonged, persistent penile erection that occurs without sexual desire. It is usually painful. It is caused by ascending nervous impulses or local mechanical causes such as hemorrhage, neoplasm, or thrombosis. Peyronie's disease (A) is a painless and slowly developing induration of the penis with resultant deformity and occasional inability to have an erection. Penile hyperplasia (B) results from tumors of the adrenal gland, pineal gland, or hypothalamus. Cavernositis (C) is inflammation of the cavernous corpora. Epispadias (E) is a developmental abnormality in which there is a dorsal urethra.

133. **(E)** Urinary retention is not one of the local causes for priapism, whereas thrombosis (A), hemorrhage (B), neoplasm (C), and inflammation (D) all are. The condition is also associated with leukemia and sickle cell anemia. Surgical intervention may be emergently necessary.

134. **(A)** Priapism is associated with leukemia. It is not associated with diabetes (B), hypertension (C), benign prostatic hypertrophy (D), or lupus (E).

135. **(A)** Phimosis occurs when the preputial orifice is too tight to permit retraction of the foreskin over the glans penis. Paraphimosis (B) is the condition in which a prepuce with a small orifice has been retracted from the glans and the lips have impinged on the retroglandular sulcus. This will prevent return to the normal position. Hypospadias (C) is a congenital condition where the urethra opens on the undersurface of the shaft. Epispadias (D) is also a congenital condition in which the urethra opens on the dorsum of the shaft. Balanitis (E) is inflammation of the skin of the glans.

136. **(D)** Except peritoneal lavage, all the other interventions are routine in the initial management of a trauma victim. Peritoneal lavage is only

possibly indicated if dictated by a rigid or expanded abdomen, but even this is controversial. If the patient is hemodynamically unstable, he should be taken immediately for exploratory laparotomy, otherwise, current practice is to perform a head, abdominal, and pelvic CT scan.

137. **(E)** Repair of radiation-induced DNA and chromosomal damage is inversely related to the rate at which the radiation is absorbed (E). Damage to the genetic apparatus of the nucleus results from ionizing radiation. Low linear energy transfer (LET) radiation most commonly results in single-strand breaks and base alterations, while high LET radiation produces double-strand breaks (A). Free radicals generated by the ionizing radiation are primarily responsible for this DNA damage and the chromosomal alterations (C). Chromosomal breaks with rearrangements associated with loss of considerable amounts of chromosomal mass may lead to cell death at either the first or one of the first few postirradiation mitotic divisions (D). Large doses of radiation may produce direct cell death due to membrane or cytoplasmic structural damage (B).

138. **(E)** This test is only useful in distinguishing etiologies of right upper quadrant pain. Urine hCG (A) will rule out pregnancy, and a complete blood count (B) will rule out intraperitoneal bleed. Pelvic examination (D) should be done in every female patient with abdominal pain.

139. **(A)** Her symptoms of rebound and lying still all make peritonitis very concerning. This is usually due to hemorrhage or spillage of visceral contents into the peritoneum.

140. **(B)** The standard of care in a pregnant patient, if ectopic pregnancy is a concern, is transvaginal ultrasound. Culdocentesis (D) can be helpful, but is more invasive than ultrasound. Laparoscopy (C) and laparotomy (E) should only be done if ultrasound is not helpful.

141. **(A)** The ruptured ectopic pregnancy is a surgical emergency and needs to be treated as such. Medical treatment (B) should be reserved for patients who have not ruptured.

142. **(D)** In patients who have an ectopic pregnancy that has not ruptured, methotrexate can be used to induce evacuation of the ectopic pregnancy.

143. **(D)** All Rh-negative women with an ectopic pregnancy should receive RhoGAM. This should be done regardless of the treatment that the patient receives for the ectopic pregnancy.

144. **(D)** Risk factors include history of pelvic inflammatory disease (A), previous ectopic pregnancy (E), history of tubal sterilization, history of tubal reconstructive surgery, history of IUD usage (B), diethylstilbestrol exposure, and peritubular adhesions.

145. **(D)** The history of an ectopic pregnancy increases the chance of having another ectopic pregnancy by 25%.

146. **(C)** This patient is experiencing alcohol withdrawal syndrome (delirium tremens). Very often, what drinkers refer to as social drinking is chronic alcoholism. Your initial step in the management of this patient's condition is administering chlordiazepoxide PO. The next step should be obtaining a detailed history and physical checkup with particular emphasis on liver, GI, and nervous system functioning (C). Antidepressant (e.g., imipramine) administration would have been appropriate if the patient's psychosocial assessment determined underlying chronic psychopathology or social stressors (D). This patient is a candidate for a referral to Alcoholics Anonymous (AA).

147. **(B)** Wernicke-Korsakoff syndrome is associated with chronic vitamin B deficiency, most often seen in alcoholics, and causes the patient to confabulate.

148. **(B)** Seventy-five percent of gallstones in this country are derived from cholesterol. In some people, cholesterol becomes supersaturated in bile and precipitates, forming microscopic crystals and the nidus for stones. Pigment stones (A) account for 25% of stones and occur in patients with chronic hemolytic states. Calcium bilirubinate (C) is a major constituent of pigment stones. Phospholipids (D), such as lecithin, are responsible for solubilizing cholesterol in bile and do not make up gallstones.

149. **(A)** Classically, viral conjunctivitis is associated with preauricular adenopathy.

150. **(A)** Nondisjunction, the failure of two homologous chromosomes in the first division of meiosis or two sister chromatids in either mitosis or the second division of meiosis to pass opposite poles of the cell, results in abnormal chromosome numbers. Chromosome deletion is the loss of a chromosome segment following chromosome breakage (A). Uniparenteral disomy results when both chromosomes, either totally or partially, are erroneously inherited from a single parent (B). Genomic imprinting influences the developmental consequences of chromosomal abnormalities. Certain genetic loci are subject to functional modulation, which differs, depending on whether the genome passes through spermatogenesis or oogenesis. Deletion of the chromosome band 15q11 results in Prader-Willi syndrome if the affected chromosome is inherited from the father and the Angelman syndrome if the chromosome is inherited from the mother (C). Some rare X-linked dominant disorders are expressed only in the heterozygous female because the condition is lethal in the hemizygous affected male (E). Lyonization, the process of inactivation of one of the X chromosomes, produces a clumping of the chromatin at the periphery of the nucleus, known as a Barr body (D).

151. **(C)** A pulmonary aspergilloma (fungus ball) is composed of matted hyphae and debris, which occurs in a cavity, particularly of the upper lobes of the lung. Aspergillomas may complicate up to 11% of old tuberculous cavities (C). The methenamine-stained histopathologic section shown, demonstrates septate, dichotomously branching hyphae. There is no evidence of acid-fast organisms [(A) and (B)]. Mycetomas are chronic, suppurative infections of the skin, which typically follow minor trauma (D). Although candidal colonization of the tracheobronchial tree is common, particularly in immunosuppressed persons, pulmonary infection is rare. When it occurs, it typically presents as pneumonia (E).

152. **(C)** For commitment to a psychiatric unit, most states require three physicians to agree that a patient is mentally ill. One of these physicians should be a psychiatrist.

153. **(E)** Virchow's triad of risk factors for deep venous thrombosis include hypercoagulability, stasis (C) and vascular injury (D). Oral contraceptives (A) and cancer (B) are risk factors for hypercoagulability.

154. **(D)** Lupus anticoagulant deficiency is not a risk factor. Inherited blood disorders increasing the chances of deep venous thrombosis include protein C deficiency (A), protein S deficiency (B), antithrombin III deficiency (C), and the presence of lupus anticoagulant or antiphospholipid (E).

155. **(D)** Homan's sign is pain in the calf with ankle flexion. Courvoisier's sign (A) is painless jaundice noted with biliary tract cancer. Murphy's sign (B) is pain on inspiration with palpation in the right upper quadrant in acute cholecystitis. Tinel's sign (C) is numbness in the hands with flexion of the wrists in carpal tunnel syndrome.

156. **(A)** Although Homan's sign is described commonly in association with deep venous thrombosis, the sensitivity and specificity are very poor indicators of DVTs, and the diagnosis should be made with further testing.

157. **(A)** A venogram is the gold standard for the diagnosis of DVTs. Lymphangiograms (B) are good for the diagnosis of lymphangitic blockage. Duplex scanning (C) and ultrasound Doppler (D) are good noninvasive tests for diagnosing DVTs, but are not as good as venograms.

158. **(B)** Anticoagulation therapy should be continued for six months. DVTs should be treated for six months unless clear contraindications are present.

159. **(B)** Stop anticoagulation and place an inferior vena cava filter. With contraindications to anticoagulation, such as bleeding or fall risk, an inferior vena cava filter should be placed to avoid potentially fatal pulmonary emboli.

160. **(C)** Her chances of getting another DVT are approximately 30% greater because of her history of DVTs. This may be due to chronic injury that results from the DVT, but patients should realize that they are at a slightly increased risk of repeat DVT later in life.

161. **(E)** This patient has myasthenia gravis, which is an autoimmune disease associated with weakness and easy fatigability of skeletal muscles.

Many patients present with ocular motor disturbances and oropharyngeal weakness secondary to the immune-mediated disease of the acetylcholine receptor complex and autoantibodies, which bind to the receptor and reduce their number. This, in turn, decreases the effectiveness of the postsynaptic muscle membrane. Anticholinesterase drugs such as mestinon or pyridostigmine are the ones most commonly used in the treatment, and not the diagnosis, of myasthenia gravis. Anticholinesterase receptor antibodies (A) are highly specific for myasthenia gravis and they are virtually never present in healthy individuals. EMG studies are highly sensitive to diagnose myasthenia gravis. It would show increased jitter in some muscles in these patients. It would show abnormal neuromuscular transmission. Weakness caused by abnormal neuromuscular transmission characteristically improves with administration of the edrophonium chloride test (C). This is an excellent pharmacologic test to diagnose myasthenia gravis. A CT of the anterior mediastinum (D) is useful to search for a thymoma. Thymectomy has been shown to induce remission in myasthenia gravis patients.

162. **(E)** In any tachycardia that is hemodynamically significant, immediate electrical cardioversion should be done before any attempts at medical treatment are started.

163. **(E)** *Neisseria* is a Gram-negative cocci. *Corynebacterium* (A), *Bacillus* (B), *Listeria* (C), and *Clostridium* (D) are all Gram-positive rods.

164. **(C)** Residual volume is the volume of air remaining in the lungs at the end of a maximal exhalation.

165. **(B)** Total lung capacity is the volume of air in the lungs after maximal inspiration.

166. **(A)** Tidal volume is the volume of air moved during quiet, normal respiration.

167. **(E)** Forced vital capacity is the maximum volume of air that can be forcibly exhaled after a full inspiration.

168. **(B)** The success of smoking cessation is correlated not with the usage of nicotine replacement, but with counseling and behavior modification. Therefore, although nicotine patches may help, the force of the strength of smoking cessation comes from counseling.

169. **(E)** Central diabetes insipidus, a condition caused by lack of ADH, does not cause amenorrhea. Pregnancy (A) is the most common cause of secondary amenorrhea. The prevalence of secondary amenorrhea ranges from 5-60% in competitive endurance athletes (B). Both hypothyroidism (C) and hyperprolactinemia (D) have been associated with secondary amenorrhea.

170. **(D)** Basilar skull fractures are part of temporal bone fractures and can be detected by drainage of cerebral spinal fluid coming out of the nares instead of rhinorrhea. "Raccoon" eyes and "Battle's" sign are also present. Frontal sinus fractures (A) usually result from a dashboard injury from a motor vehicle accident. They are associated with severe frontal headaches and epistaxis. A CT scan is diagnostic. Nasal fractures (B) result in epistaxis, tenderness, and crepitations of nasal bones. A septal hematoma may be found. Orbital floor "blow-out" fractures (C) are very serious. They are secondary to blunt anteroposterior force directed against the eyeball. Diplopia and restricted upward gaze from ocular muscle entrapment occur. A transverse fracture (E) is a more serious injury to the temporal bone, resulting in complete sensorineural hearing loss and facial nerve injury.

171. **(A)** Diuretics will lower serum potassium (A) unless they are potassium sparing. Addison's disease (B), specimen hemolysis (C), acidosis (D), and renal failure (E) will all raise potassium and cause hyperkalemia.

172. **(E)** In vertebral osteomyelitis, the infecting organism reaches the well-perfused vertebral body via the spinal arteries. Infection rapidly spreads from the end plate into the disk space and then into the adjacent vertebral body. This unenhanced computed tomographic scan of the spine, taken at T8, demonstrates erosion of the inferior end plate of the vertebral body. A large surrounding area of paraspinal soft tissue density is also seen (E). This radiographic pattern is virtually diagnostic of bacterial infection, since neoplasms and other diseases of the spine rarely cross the disk space. However, the differential diagnosis requires exclusion of bone fractures, neoplasms, and bone infarcts [(A), (B), (C), and (D)].

173. **(C)** A thyroglossal cyst is a midline cervical cyst that arises from remnants of the thyroglossal duct. A hygroma (A) is a mass formed by many cysts of occluded lymphatic channels and is lateral. A branchial cyst (B) is also a lateral cyst that contains cholesterol and is deep to the sternocleidomastoid muscle. The Zenker's diverticulum (D) is a pharyngeal pouch occurring laterally in the neck. A laryngocele (E) is a herniation of the laryngeal diverticulum through the lateral thyrohyoid membrane that also occurs laterally.

174. **(A)** Henoch-Schonlein purpura is a vasculitis associated with IgA vascular deposition, oligoarticular synovitis, and bowel angina. Palpable purpura is the most sensitive and specific indicator of this entity. The purpura is usually self-limited and has a good prognosis. This disease is more common in adult males than females. Essential mixed cryoglobinemia (B) involves polyclonal IgM and monoclonal IgG deposits, and is associated with hepatitis B and Raynaud's phenomenon. Thrombotic thrombocytopenic purpura (C) is associated with neurologic symptoms. It is unusual to have gastrointestinal symptoms. Waldenstrom's hyperglobulinemic purpura (D) results in increased vascular fragility and bleeding. It is associated with polyclonal hyperglobulemia, not just IgA. Systemic lupus erythematosus (E) is associated with a malar rash and anti-double stranded DNA antibody. Palpable purpura is rare.

175. **(D)** Insulin is only necessary if there is excessive hyperglycemia. Volume replacement (A), narcotics (B) for pain control, and nasogastric suctioning (C) to place the pancreas at rest, are the principal treatment options for pancreatitis. In patients that develop hypocalcemia, calcium supplementation (E) is necessary.

176. **(C)** In Whipple's disease, the lamina propria is infiltrated with macrophages containing PAS-positive glycoproteins (Panel C). Panel B illustrates the clubbing of the epithelial villi and foamy macrophages. Electron microscopic studies (Panel A) show rod-shaped structures within and adjacent to the macrophages in the lamina propria, epithelial cells, and polymorphonuclear leukocytes (C). Intestinal lymphoma (A) is characterized by infiltration of the lamina propria and submucosa with malignant cells. Amyloidosis (B) is diagnosed with Congo red staining followed by examination with a polarizing microscope, looking for green birefringence. When present, noncaseating granulomas are a distinguishing feature of regional enteritis (D). Eosinophilic enteritis (E) is characterized by diffuse or patchy eosinophilic infiltration of the lamina propria and mucosa.

177. **(B)** Profuse menstrual bleeding is known as menorrhagia. Menarche (A) is the onset of menses. Metrorrhagia (C) is intermenstrual bleeding. Amenorrhea (D) is absence of menstruation. Dysmenorrhea (E) is painful menstruation.

178. **(E)** The anions required for electroneutrality are referred to as unmeasured anions, or as the serum anion gap. The serum anion gap is calculated by subtracting the sum of the serum chloride and bicarbonate concentrations from the serum sodium concentration (A). Normally, the negative charges on albumin and other proteins account for at least half of the anion gap (D). The normal anion gap is 10-12 mEq/L (E). The anion gap may be decreased in multiple myeloma due to the presence of negatively charged proteins (B). It is increased in renal failure due to the retention of sulfates and phosphates (C).

179. **(C)** When a diabetic patient is kept NPO for surgery, one traditionally gives only one-half the normal morning dose because there is less oral intake. Therefore, one-half of 20 units is 10 units. The normal dose would probably make the patient hypoglycemic. It is also good practice to check the blood glucose before and after the dose.

180. **(B)** Once again, patient-physician confidentiality is the issue here.

USMLE Step 3 – Practice Test 1
Day One – Afternoon Session

1. **(A)** The most common etiology of galactorrhea in a female is a prolactin-secreting microadenoma, as opposed to a macroadenoma (D) in a male. Breast cancer (E), if presenting with breast discharge, usually presents with a bloody discharge. Pregnancy (C) is not considered a pathologic etiology of galactorrhea and because of this is an incorrect answer.

2. **(C)** Initial treatment consists of bromocriptine; surgery can be considered if bromocriptine fails.

3. **(B)** Treatment should be continued until prolactin levels return to normal. Repeat MRI should be done to assess the size of the adenoma.

4. **(C)** Macroadenomas can enlarge during pregnancy. Therefore, a female patient who wants to become pregnant should undergo surgery to remove the macroadenoma.

5. **(D)** This patient has polymyositis, which is an inflammatory disease of skeletal muscle of unknown cause. Anti-Jo-1, Anti-PL-7, and Anti-P1-12 are autoantibodies associated with polymyositis and interstitial lung disease. Anticentromere antibody is associated with the CREST syndrome. Polymyositis is also called idiopathic inflammatory myopathy. The EMG (A) is abnormal in all patients with this disease. Changes include small-amplitude, short duration, polyphasic motor unit potentials, fibrillations, and spontaneous, bizarre, high-frequency discharges. Symmetric weakness of the limb girdle muscles (B) with arthralgias can make getting up from a chair and combing one's hair difficult. This weakness is insidious in nature. Serum levels of muscle-derived enzymes (C) are elevated, such as CPK, LDH, and SGOT. This is secondary to muscle necrosis and inflammation. A muscle biopsy (E) of involved skeletal muscle tissue would reveal inclusion body myositis, muscle fiber necrosis, phagocytosis, and muscle regeneration.

6. **(A)** This patient has developed dermatomyositis, which is associated with malignancies of the lung and breast in 20% of patients. She has developed Gottron's patches and a heliotrope rash. Any cutaneous rash associated with polymyositis is called dermatomyositis; one should look for an underlying malignancy within a year of diagnosis. Intracranial hemorrhages (B) are common in lupus patients secondary to fragile capillaries and arteries. Brain hemorrhages are not common in dermatomyositis. Insulin-dependent diabetes mellitus (C) is associated with this autoimmune disorder, not type II diabetes. Pneumonia (D) is associated with any immunocompromised state—not with dermatomyositis, which is an autoimmune disorder. Solid tumors, not hematologic tumors such as leukemias (E), are associated with dermatomyositis.

7. **(E)** D-penicillamine is used to treat primary biliary cirrhosis and not polymyositis. Daily high-dose prednisone (A) should be initiated and then a maintenance dose should be continued. Physical therapy (B) is essential with passive range of motion exercises to prevent contractures. Immunosuppressive agents (C), such as azathioprine or cyclophosphamide, are utilized in refractory cases of polymyositis. Antacids (D) or H2 blockers may be used to raise the pH of gastric fluids to prevent reflux esophagitis in patients with striated muscle esophageal dysfunction.

8. **(C)** If the biopsy of the skeletal muscle tissue shows inclusion body myositis, then the prognosis is poor and the patient usually develops progressive weakness without improvement in the outcome. Older patients, those with associated neoplasms, and patients with associated GI, pulmonary, and cardiac manifestation (A) have a poor prognosis. Children (B) and young adults have the best prognosis, although polymyositis is rare in this age group. Patients who are positive for Jo-1 antibody (D) do not generally respond well to treatment protocols. About half of the surviving patients with polymyositis essentially recover completely with treatment (E).

9. **(D)** The most immediate concern for patients suffering from smoke inhalation is to overcome loss of ventilation induced by CO, which damages lung tissue. Patients should be given 100% O_2 immediately by a tight-fitting mask or intubation. This patient may also require hyperbaric O_2 therapy (A), as indicated by a very high carboxyhemoglobin concentration. This method is considered adjunctive to respiratory support and is not the first step in therapy, but reduces mortality rates when initiated within six hours of poisoning. In a patient who is unconscious and who is in respiratory failure, 100% oxygen given by non-rebreather venti-masks (B) delivering only about 50% of the oxygen supplied, would not be effective for an unconscious person with an elevated carboxyhemoglobin level, which suggests a high concentration of CO in the blood. Indirect laryngoscopy (C) would be done to visualize thermal or toxic injury to the airway if stridor is present. Diuretic therapy (E) would be given if non-cardiogenic pulmonary edema is present after smoke inhalation. This medication would be given only after the patient has been intubated and given oxygen.

10. **(C)** According to the United States Preventive Services Task Force, BCG vaccine and symptomatic HIV infection are not compatible. BCG vaccine is not routinely used, but it can be valuable in high-risk populations living in the United States (A). Infants and children with negative PPDs and continuous exposure to TB may greatly benefit from vaccination with BCG. INH does not lose its hepatotoxicity in any drug combination and is not recommended for infected individuals over age 35.

11. **(B)** A glomus tumor is found beneath the nail. It is usually red or blue; it is painful, and it is benign. It is thought to arise from the pericyte in the vessel walls of the glomus body.

12. **(E)** Pleural-based densities are not a normal finding in patients with COPD and should raise the suspicion of asbestos-related disease or malignancy. Diaphragmatic depression (A) and increased AP diameter (C) are indications of hyperinflation. Diaphragmatic testing (B) is common and is a result of frequent infections. Large bullae (D) are common and are a result of destruction of alveolar septae.

13. **(E)** Goodpasture's syndrome is a condition associated with acute glomerulonephritis and pulmonary hemorrhage. It is not associated with obstructive lung disease. Cystic fibrosis (A) results in bronchiectasis and obstructive lung disease. Alpha 1 antitrypsin deficiency (B) and second-hand smoke exposure (C) both can result in the development of emphysema through an imbalance of proteases and protease inhibitors. Asthma (D) is another cause of obstructive airway disease and hyperinflation.

14. **(C)** In the outpatient population, the most common cause of hypercalcemia is primary hyperparathyroidism. In the inpatient population, the most common cause is hypercalcemia of malignancy.

15. **(C)** It is improper for a physician to date or discuss such personal matters with a patient.

16. **(B)** This would breach the acceptable limits of interaction between physicians and their patients.

17. **(D)** Since this patient has clearly expressed an interest in you, it would be best for everyone, including you, to have someone else examine her, probably with a chaperone present.

18. **(C)** In this situation, you would have to examine her, but you must have a chaperone present to protect yourself from potential legal actions.

19. **(D)** Osteogenesis is a hereditary condition of the bone that would not present in this fashion. The other diseases could present with these manifestations in someone of this age.

20. **(C)** All cases of *Mycobacterium tuberculosis* must be reported to State public health authorities.

21. **(D)** You cannot draw a patient's blood for HIV testing unless you have obtained signed informed consent.

22. **(B)** Sputum cultures would be most helpful. These radiographic findings suggest that the patient has a localized lung disease.

23. **(A)** A regular-strength PPD should be placed, along with control skin tests, since some patients with early tuberculosis are anergic, i.e., react to no skin tests.

24. **(A)** The patient is relatively young and has an acute disease consistent with tuberculosis. He has never had a PPD before, so he cannot be considered to have a "conversion" of his PPD test from negative to positive and thus has clearly been infected within a certain time period. A positive PPD in this setting warrants treatment.

25. **(B)** The Health Department will monitor the patient's compliance with his treatment and will track his contacts to test and treat them, as appropriate.

26. **(C)** The patient needs to understand the necessity for compliance in order to prevent the development of resistant organisms that can occur as a result of intermittent ingestion of medications.

27. **(B)** The other way to diagnose diabetes mellitus is to find that a random plasma glucose level on two different occasions is greater than 200 mg/dl.

28. **(B)** Usually, dietary therapy should be attempted first. However, it seems that the patient has already had some complications from diabetes mellitus and should be treated more aggressively. Only if oral medications fail should she be started on insulin.

29. **(C)** The side effect of metformin that causes the most concern is the lactic acidosis that can occur in patients with chronic renal insufficiency.

30. **(A)** There has been no evidence to show that routine stress testing for diabetes decreases mortality or morbidity. However, simple things that should be done with each diabetic patient are to have the patient follow up with ophthalmology yearly to assess for diabetic retinopathy, immunization with a pneumovax vaccine as she is immunocompromised, and to pay close attention to the feet, because diabetic patients commonly have peripheral neuropathy and don't always feel the ulcers. Yearly urinalysis should also be checked for microscopic proteinuria, because ACE inhibitor therapy has been shown to decrease the rate of progression of renal failure in these patients.

31. **(D)** According to the protocol of the American College of Obstetricians and Gynecologists, initial obstetrical screen should include complete blood count (A), blood group (B) and Rh antigen (C), rubella, and hepatitis B virus (E). The initial screening should be performed as early in the course of pregnancy as possible. Measurements of serum alpha-fetoprotein (D) titers are a component of an 18-week screen.

32. **(E)** The most common cause of postpartum hemorrhage is uterine atony, which occurs in two to five percent of all deliveries. Uterine atony is recognized by the presence of continued painless vaginal bleeding after delivery. Other causes include retained placental tissue, placenta accreta, cervical and vaginal lacerations, and inverted uterus. Postpartum hemorrhage may also result from conditions that are associated with coagulopathy, such as preeclampsia and amniotic fluid embolism.

33. **(E)** Any condition associated with overdistention of the uterus, such as multiple births, multiple gestation, polyhydramnios, or a large fetus, is a risk factor for uterine atony. Other risk factors include multiparity, retained placenta, prolonged general anesthesia, ruptured uterus, and perioperative treatment with beta-agonists.

34. **(D)** Retained placenta occurs in about one of 300 deliveries and is characterized by painless vaginal bleeding following delivery. Treatment requires manual removal of the placenta, which prevents uterine contractions. Dilatation and curettage [(D) and (C)] may be necessary to evacuate the uterus.

35. **(A)** Manually removing the placenta is a procedure that is performed for retained placenta. All of the other obstetrical interventions that are listed can be utilized in the management of uterine atony that is not controlled by conservative treatment. The goal is to increase myometrial tone, which would constrict bleeding vessels and stop the hemorrhage.

36. **(E)** Systemic narcotics (A) are frequently administered to attenuate labor pains. Low-dose

narcotics do not completely eliminate the pain. Meperidine is the narcotic most frequently used for labor. The purpose of inhalation analgesia (B) during labor is to achieve subanesthetic doses of agent intended to produce analgesia without depressing airway reflexes. Epidural anesthesia (C) is the most common form of regional anesthesia for the management of labor. Spinal and caudal anesthesia are used less commonly. Other options that are often used in combination with the above-mentioned forms of analgesia include hypnosis (D), psychoprophylaxis, and acupuncture. These, however, are still under investigation for improved results.

37. **(B)** Relatively few contraindications exist for regional anesthesia, including epidural anesthesia, which thus far is the most popular form. Awake-state of the mother during delivery that is assisted by regional anesthesia significantly decreases the risk of maternal aspiration associated with general anesthesia. Unlike epidural anesthesia, spinal anesthesia is technically easy to perform and provides reliable and rapid anesthesia for the procedure.

38. **(B)** Post-dural puncture headache can occur any time the dura is punctured. The headache occurs when persistent cerebrospinal fluid (CSF) leak decreases the amount of fluid available to cushion the brain. In the absence of an adequate fluid buffer, the brain shifts within the calvarium. This results in tension on pain-sensitive blood vessels and causes headache. The headache is located over the occipital or frontal regions. It is frequently accompanied by neck tension, tinnitus, diplopia, photophobia, nausea, and vomiting. The headache changes with position. It tends to improve in the lying position and get worse with the sitting or standing position. The conservative treatment plan includes mild analgesics, hydration, and caffeine.

39. **(B)** The pre-existing coagulation abnormalities are contraindications to regional anesthesia. The regional anesthesia itself is not known to produce defects in the coagulation pathway. Skin infection is another contraindication to performing regional anesthesia.

40. **(B)** If a patient is too uncomfortable, she should be dropped from the study, and her care should continue unaffected by her participation in the study. A statement to this effect is included in every informed consent signed by a study subject. The other options are unethical.

41. **(C)** You should explain to him why this is wrong. You do not need to accuse him of dishonesty.

42. **(D)** The only correct thing to do is to tell the truth.

43. **(A)** This is an adverse event and needs to be reported appropriately. All adverse events must be reported. It is not up to you to decide which is significant or not.

44. **(C)** Since this is a competent adult, she has the right to make this decision, even if you do not agree.

45. **(C)** Mastoiditis is a pyogenic infection of the mastoid process. It results from the transmission of *Streptococcus* or *Pneumococcus* through the eustacian tube or from the inner ear in cases of otitis media. Sinusitis (A) is an infection of the sinuses and will present with maxillary, frontal, or ethmoid tenderness. Otitis externa (B) is an infection of the outer ear. Folliculitis (D) is infection of a hair-bearing skin follicle, usually due to staphylococcus. Basilar skull fractures (E) are usually the result of severe trauma, accompanied by neurologic damage.

46. **(C)** The patient may have a new or resistant organism now, or he may have seeded another site with infection. You would not stop the antibiotics without other evidence of a drug reaction (A). You would not change the antibiotics without obtaining new cultures (B). You would not ignore the fever (D). There is no need for an emergency consultation (E).

47. **(B)** This is a typical picture of an individual developing delirium tremens, in which hypertension and tachycardia are often noted. Some patients develop fevers as well. His normal mental status on admission makes presenile dementia unlikely (A), and the latter is not associated with these sympathetic nervous system responses. Schizophrenia (C) also is not associated with hypertension and tachycardia. Patients with meningitis (D) or thyrotoxicosis (E) do not usually lose their memory or become combative.

48. **(D)** In a patient with a mural thrombus that could throw emboli to other sites and atrial fibrillation, which increases the risk of throwing such emboli, anticoagulation is the prudent first step in treatment. Medical management with an agent such as digitalis would probably be the next step. Some physicians might just go ahead and cardiovert him. The patient is not likely to have hyperthyroidism [(A) and (B)]. Lidocaine is not useful in atrial fibrillation (E).

49. **(E)** The patient has a syndrome consistent with septic arthritis, especially given her age and sex. The most common cause of septic arthritis in young sexually active adults is *Neisseria gonorrhoea.*

50. **(D)** It is quite likely for a teenager outside his normal environment to stop taking his medications regularly.

51. **(A)** Galactorrhea in a non-pregnant woman is due to underactivity of dopamine at the level of the hypothalamus. Risperidone and other antipsychotics act by blocking dopamine channels in the brain, and one of their side effects can be galactorrhea.

52. **(C)** Calcium levels above 11.8 mg/dl usually result in signs and symptoms attributable to hypercalcemia. These include weakness, fatigue (B), polyuria (A), anorexia, nausea (D), vomiting, depression, lethargy (E), and constipation. Diarrhea is not a symptom of hypercalcemia. Some of the signs suggestive of hypercalcemia include pancreatitis, hypertension, renal stones, band keratopathy, and dehydration.

53. **(D)** The most common cause of hypercalcemia is primary hyperparathyroidism. Surgical resection of the involved parathyroid adenoma is the treatment of choice. Other causes of hypercalcemia include: malignancy with bony metastasis, granulomatous disease, vitamin D intoxication, familial hypocalciuria hypercalcemia, and chronic renal insufficiency.

54. **(C)** When the serum calcium rises above 14.0 mg/dl and symptoms of mental status changes occur, acute lowering of the calcium level is crucial. The initial management of choice is rehydration with a rapid infusion of intravenous normal saline and subsequent calciuresis with intrave-

nous furosemide. The patient needs to be monitored closely with this aggressive treatment, and frequent serum calcium levels need to be drawn from the patient. An EKG (A) is needed, but not as urgently as intravenous normal saline. An electrocardiogram may show shortened Q-T intervals in hypercalcemia. Intravenous insulin (B) is the treatment of choice in severe hyperkalemia. Mithramycin (E) is the treatment of choice in chronic hypercalcemia that is refractory to hydration and diuresis. Hemodialysis (D) is the immediate treatment of choice in life-threatening hyperkalemia.

55. **(D)** The X-ray of the tibia and fibula shows periosteal elevation of hypertrophic osteoarthropathy, characterized by a faint radiolucent line along the shaft of the long bones (D). In early osteomyelitis, X-rays may be negative. In hematogenous infection, the lytic or osteopenic lesions may not appear for two to four weeks. Technetium bone scans are positive in 95% of cases in the first 24 hours (A). There is no evidence of metastatic lesions in these bones (B). In osteomalacia, there is decreased bone density, associated with trabecular loss and thinning of the cortices. A ground glass appearance may result from loss of trabeculae. Radiolucent bands, known as pseudofractures, typically perpendicular to the bone surface and ranging from a few millimeters to several centimeters in length, are characteristic of the disorder (C). Paget's disease is characterized by osteolytic activity in the skull or as a V-shaped advancing front in a long bone. In more advanced disease, there is evidence of sclerosis, thickening of the cortices, and enlargement of the long bones. Remodeling of the bone, which usually follows stress lines, accounts for the characteristic anterior bowing of the tibia and fibula (E).

56. **(E)** Tuberculin skin testing is not recommended for individuals with a history of compromised immune system. The U.S. Preventive Services Task Force on the Periodic Health Examination recommends that skin testing of asymptomatic persons should be performed on those at high risk of acquiring tuberculosis. Groups at risk include people recently arrived from economically deprived countries (A). Note that a positive skin test in immigrants may be due to the BCG vaccine (contains attenuated bacilli) rather than evidence of an active or dormant infection. A positive skin response to intradermal tuberculin administration should be followed by a chest X-ray, which

will confirm or rule out the existence of an active infection. All family members of a patient with TB (B) should be immediately screened for a possible exposure. Crowded conditions and increased susceptibility of hospitalized patients to infections are factors that may predispose to tuberculosis (C). Crowded conditions at schools make TB clearance mandatory for individuals who are planning to work at public schools, even on a voluntary basis. Since a positive skin test implies an intact (healthy) immune system, individuals with compromised T-cell deficiencies (e.g., as in DiGeorge's syndrome and HIV infection) most likely will not test positive in the presence of active tuberculosis. These individuals are not only at increased risk of contracting, but also of spreading, the disease. Therefore, any evidence of past or present history of T-cell immune deficiency in an individual mandates a radiological examination, if screening for TB is contemplated.

57. **(C)** All of the medications listed, except Captopril, have been used successfully to control hypertension in pregnancy. ACE inhibitors are not used in pregnant women since they are known to cause neonatal anuric renal failure.

58. **(A)** In addition to taking care of the child, you should notify the police since a hit-and-run incident is a criminal offense.

59. **(B)** A hydrocele is an accumulation of serous fluid which occurs congenitally in the cavity of the tunica vaginalitis or from infection or trauma. It presents as a non-tender testicular swelling.

60. **(E)** There is no need to auscultate a hydrocele. Inspection (A) reveals a large scrotum. Palpation (B) reveals a pear-shaped mass. Transillumination (C) shows the mass to be translucent. Pinching (D) the root of the scrotum indicates that the mass does not extend that high.

61. **(E)** Orchitis will usually present as tender testicular swelling. A hydrocele presents as a non-tender testicular swelling, as does a hematocele (A), a chylocele (B), a gumma (C), and tuberculosis (D).

62. **(B)** Usually the epididymis is behind the testis. In seven percent of males it is anterior to the testis.

63. **(D)** This patient has acute pancreatitis, which is inflammation of the pancreas secondary to a toxin or trauma, which releases pancreatic digestive enzymes and causes necrosis and inflammation of the pancreas. The amylase and lipase levels are elevated, which make the diagnosis of pancreatitis presumptively. Pancreatic cancer (A) would not present with acute abdominal pain. Jaundice, depression, and weight loss would be present initially. The lipase level is also not usually elevated. Chronic pancreatitis (B) can also present this way, but the beta cells in the pancreas would be destroyed and, thus, hypoglycemia or hyperglycemia would be present. This patient has a normal glucose level. In acute cholecystitis (C), there is inflammation of the gallbladder, most likely secondary to gallstones or alcohol. This patient does not have cholecystitis because there is no evidence of jaundice or right upper quadrant pain. The serum alkaline phosphatase level would be elevated in cholecystitis instead of the serum lipase and amylase. This patient had no evidence of trauma or hemorrhage and, therefore, bowel perforation (E) is not the correct answer.

64. **(B)** A CT of the abdomen would show parapancreatic inflammation and edema suggestive of pancreatitis. Laparoscopy (A) is an invasive surgical procedure, which is not useful in making the diagnosis of pancreatitis. It is useful to treat and make the diagnosis of appendicitis and abdominal obstruction secondary to adhesions. An ultrasound of the abdomen (C) is a good test, but it is not very useful in obese patients who have a lot of subcutaneous tissue because a deep, retroperitoneal organ, such as the pancreas, cannot be visualized. X-rays of the abdomen (D) are useful only to make the diagnosis of chronic pancreatitis because of visualization of calcification within the fibrosed pancreas. Abdominal X-rays are not useful in making the diagnosis of acute pancreatitis. Appendicitis, cholecystitis, and abdominal obstruction can all mimic the signs of pancreatitis on the clinical exam (E). A periumbilical hematoma called Cullen's sign is, however, suggestive of acute pancreatitis.

65. **(C)** The most common cause of acute, recurrent pancreatitis is alcohol use. This patient is an alcoholic and thus it is the most likely cause of this disorder. Biliary sludge (A) occurs in five percent of cases of pancreatitis, and nobody really knows the exact reason why sludge occurs and

causes pancreatic inflammation. Medications such as Lasix, AZT, DDI, and allupurinol can all cause acute pancreatitis (B). This patient is on no medications. Cholelithiasis is the number two cause of acute pancreatitis in the elderly population. Gallstones (D) cause obstruction of the common bile duct, which in turn causes a back-up of bile in the pancreatic duct and subsequent inflammation. A bite of a certain species of spiders can cause pancreatitis, but this is rare. Cytomegalovirus can also on rare occasions cause pancreatitis and cholangitis. It is unusual for bacterial and fungal pathogens to affect the pancreas (E).

66. **(E)** This patient has acute pancreatitis, for which the treatment of choice is supportive management such as intravenous fluids and nasogastric tube insertion if the patient is vomiting. This can prevent aspiration. Intravenous antibiotics (A) are indicated in sepsis, which this patient does not have. Oxygenation alone (B) is not helpful unless the patient is hypoxemic and other treatment modalities are also used. Morphine sulfate (C) can cause spasm of the sphincter of Oddi, which in turn can exacerbate pancreatitis. Thus, Demoral is often used for pain management in acute pancreatitis. Peritoneal lavage (D) has not been shown to change the outcome in pancreatitis according to multiple clinical studies in the literature.

67. **(C)** This patient could have pneumonia, pulmonary tuberculosis, or lung cancer. To initially work this patient up, a chest X-ray has to be performed to see if there are infiltrates, effusions, mass lesions, or bronchiectasis. If the chest X-ray suggests lung cancer, then a CT scan of the lungs and bronchoscopy can be performed. If the chest X-ray shows bilateral upper lobe of tuberculosis, then sputum for acid-fast bacilli can be sent. A PPD skin test (A) should be performed on all individuals suspected of having been exposed to tuberculosis. This test does not inform us if active tuberculosis is present even if the test is positive. A chest X-ray has to be performed first. A smear and culture of sputum for acid-fast bacilli (B) can be sent three times on three consecutive days if the chest X-ray is suspicious for pulmonary tuberculosis. Bronchoscopy (D) with biopsy or culture is the gold standard for obtaining tissue samples in the lung to make the diagnosis of cancer, tuberculosis, or pneumonia. This test can be performed only after an initial chest X-ray is done to guide the bronchoscopist to the tissue sample site. Empiric treatment (E) for presumed bronchitis is not satisfactory since a more serious disease, such as cancer or tuberculosis, can be missed.

68. **(C)** Acute chest syndrome in patients with sickle cell disease is often very difficult to distinguish from bacterial pneumonia (D).

69. **(E)** All of the choices are correct. This is a patient who appears septic with mental status. Head CT (B) needs to be done to rule out brain abscess, and the patient should be pan-cultured, including her cerebrospinal fluid [(A), (C), and (D)]. Lumbar puncture is done after the CT is evaluated for risk of herniation.

70. **(A)** The studies are consistent with a bacterial meningitis, most likely a *Streptococcus* meningitis. The elevation of nucleated cells, with a neutrophil predominance, makes a bacterial meningitis most likely, and the Gram-positive cocci in chains makes *Streptococcus* most likely (most likely *Streptococcus* pneumonia).

71. **(C)** It has commonly been described that patients will have a pneumonia that can seed the bloodstream, leading to meningitis. This has particularly been noted in pneumococcal pneumonias. The treatment is antibiotics effective against the particular organism.

72. **(E)** Ceftriaxone has good CNS coverage and covers *Streptococcus pneumoniae* very well. However, about 10% of pneumococcus is resistant to ceftriaxone, and vancomycin should be added as well.

73. **(A)** Acute management of seizures includes benzodiazepines. Antiepileptics should be started once seizures are controlled for prophylaxis.

74. **(C)** Rhabdomyolysis may be causing intrinsic acute renal failure. With creatinine phosphokinase levels reaching upward toward 100,000, the pigment from the myoglobin can often cause acute renal failure. Antibiotic causes (D) are unlikely, as vancomycin alone does not usually cause renal failure; its nephrotoxicity is only noted when combined with an aminoglycoside.

75. **(E)** Treatment for rhabdomyolysis includes stopping the seizures. Treatment for the

renal complications include hydration, sodium bicarbonate to maintain a urine pH greater than 6.5, and intravenous mannitol.

76. **(C)** Calcification of a congenital bicuspid aortic valve is the most common cause of aortic stenosis, the condition described in this case study. Rheumatic heart disease (A) and arteriosclerotic degeneration (B) are less common causes of this condition. Ankylosing spondylitis (D) and syphilis (E) are causes of aortic regurgitation, rather than aortic stenosis.

77. **(C)** Left-heart catheterization allows for precise determination of the pressure gradient across the aortic valve and is used to determine the appropriate treatment plan. Endomyocardial biopsy (A) is useful for the evaluation of myocarditis. Thallium stress test (B) is useful for the evaluation of coronary disease. Swan-Ganz catheterization (D) allows for the determination of right-heart pressures and the pulmonary wedge pressure, but does not allow for the determination of the pressure gradient across the aortic valve. Coronary arteriography (E) is often performed in patients with aortic stenosis to assess the need for coronary artery bypass at the time of aortic valve replacement. However, coronary arteriography does not help to determine the severity of aortic stenosis.

78. **(D)** Beta blockers are contraindicated in patients with advanced aortic stenosis, as the already compromised cardiac output can be dangerously reduced by beta blockade. Prosthetic valve replacement (A) or porcine valve replacement (B) are acceptable surgical options. Valvuloplasty (C) is not commonly used, but may be a useful therapy in patients unlikely to survive an open surgical procedure.

79. **(D)** Nitrates induce a venous vasodilation, thus reducing cardiac preload. Patients with aortic stenosis have a reduced cardiac output, which is dependent on an adequate preload. It is true that tachyphylaxes does develop with these agents, however, this is not the reason that they are avoided in severe aortic stenosis (A). The vasodilatory effects related to these agents will reduce afterload to a small degree, rather than increasing preload (B). Nitrate therapy is effective in a variety of cardiac and noncardiac conditions in addition to those related to coronary artery occlusion, such as coronary vasospasm and esophageal spasm (C). Sublingual nitroglycerin therapy has a greater bioavailability than oral agents due to the large first-pass effect of nitrates which are administered orally (E).

80. **(C)** Vomiting is not a common symptom associated with acute hemolytic transfusion reactions. Back pain (A) is a common presenting symptom. Fever (B) is an indication of immune activation, although its occurrence during a transfusion is not specific for an RBC transfusion reaction. Hypotension and hemolysis [(D) and (E)] are indications of severe reactions and may continue to renal failure and death.

81. **(D)** Further blood transfusion should be avoided during the acute episode. Management should focus on the maintenance of adequate hemodynamic status and renal function [(A) and (C)]. A sample of fresh blood should be sent to the blood bank to determine the antigen responsible for the reaction and the patient's proper blood type (B). Hemolysis commonly results in hyperkalemia (E), which must be monitored closely to avoid further cardiac complications.

82. **(D)** The Lewis antigen is not associated with hemolytic transfusion reactions. ABO (A) reactivate the compliment cascade and result in intravascular hemolysis. The Kell antigen (B) more commonly results in extravascular hemolysis. The Duffy antigen (C) is less common than ABO or Rhesus, but may also result in reactions. The Rhesus antigen (E) is a common blood-group antigen and may also occur in transmission from mother to child.

83. **(B)** Delayed reactions commonly occur five to ten days after transfusion. The reaction is more common in previously transfused patients (A). Alloantibody screen is often initially negative but becomes positive at the time of reaction (C). There is no association with the transmission of hepatitis C (D). Arterial ammonia levels (E) are not used in the diagnosis of acute or delayed transfusion reactions.

84. **(D)** Henoch-Schonlein purpura (HSP) is an autoimmune vasculitis of the small vessels which usually occurs in children, causing the clinical tetrad of arthritis, abdominal pain, hematuria, and nonthrombocytopenic purpura. This disorder is self-limiting and usually resolves in an

average of four weeks. However, two percent of patients progress to end-stage renal failure. DIC (B), heart disease (A), and septic arthritis (C) are not associated with HSP.

85.   **(D)**   Diabetics must have their diet closely observed. The most appropriate diet for an in-house diabetic patient is an 1,800 calorie ADA diet. There is usually no need to restrict the sodium [(A) and (B)] nor the cholesterol (C), although it may not be a bad idea. Diabetics should also have their serum and fingerstick glucose levels checked frequently while in the hospital.

86.   **(A)**   The signs of gonadal dysgenesis, or Turner's syndrome, include a webbed neck (B), shieldlike chest (C), delayed pubic hair growth (D), extremity lymphedema (E), and short stature.

87.   **(C)**   The current high rate of incidence of syphilis, gonorrhea, HBV, and rubella during pregnancy makes routine screening for these conditions mandatory. Screening for other conditions, such as cytomegalovirus, herpes simplex virus, parvovirus infections, and toxoplasmosis is indicated if sufficient clinical suspicion exists. Due to the higher-than-normal incidence of morbidity and mortality from toxoplasmosis and CMV, maternal testing for these conditions before pregnancy may be useful.

88.   **(B)**   A trial of sublingual nitroglycerine can be both therapeutic and diagnostic for angina pectoris. His discomfort is not severe enough at present to warrant morphine (A). A CPK (C) or an electrocardiogram (D) are appropriate maneuvers after you have tended to his symptoms. An emergency call to cardiology is not indicated at this time (E).

89.   **(E)**   Sedatives are not indicated in this setting.

90.   **(A)**   These new findings are consistent with acute ischemia in the inferior portion of the heart. An inferior infarction (B) would be associated with Q waves in these leads. This may subsequently develop in this patient. Anterolateral lesions would be evident in the leads 1 and AVL and/or the lateral precordium. A remote MI would not demonstrate acute ST elevations (D). You cannot diagnose hypertension from the electrocardiogram (E).

91.   **(B)**   This patient has new onset unstable angina and thus is at risk for an acute myocardial infarction. His cardiogram is changing while he is in the emergency room and the most prudent course is to admit him to a telemetry unit or a coronary care unit for observation. His condition is not critical (A), but he should not be sent home yet either, (C). He does not need an emergency heart catheterization (D) or a surgical consult for bypass (E) at this point.

92.   **(D)**   The administration of beta-blocking agents to asthmatic patients may lead to broncho-constriction mediated by beta-2 adrenergic mechanisms. Of the agents listed, Metoprolol is the most beta-1 selective agent and would thus be the agent of choice.

93.   **(C)**   When one person tests positive for a disease, the actual chance that he now has the disease depends on the sensitivity and specificity of the test and the prevalence of the disease. These together make up the positive-predictive value of the test.

94.   **(A)**   Sensitivity of a test is the percentage of patients who have the disease that will test positive on the test.

95.   **(E)**   In order to determine the positive-predictive value (the chance that a patient who tests positive for a disease will actually have the disease), you need to know the incidence of the disease in that population.

96.   **(C)**   In this case, you wish to know what the chances are that she has no coronary artery disease, based on the negative test. That is a definition of the positive-predictive value.

97.   **(D)**   A panorex view shows the entire mandible in one view on the radiograph. It is the single best view for diagnosing a mandible fracture. The Water's view (A) is a sinus view that is also good for looking at the orbits. The lateral (B) and anterior (C) skull films show the entire skull, yet the view of the mandible is limited. A submentovertex (E) or "jughandle" view is good for examining the zygomatic arches.

98.   **(C)**   This patient has absolute neutropenia secondary to reaching a nadir from chemotherapy

for her breast cancer. She is extremely immuno-suppressed and has a very low white blood cell count to fight off infection. She is at risk of acquiring infection from others and not transmitting infection. Thus, respiratory isolation is not needed for this patient. On the contrary, a mask and gloves would be prudent for visitors who come near her in order to prevent transmission of any viral or bacterial infection from the visitor to the patient. A full set of blood, urine, and sputum culture (A) is necessary in order to rule out sepsis. Granulocyte colony stimulating factor (Neupogen) (B) is an immunomodulating agent, which stimulates the bone marrow to produce granulocytes and thus increase the white blood cell count in this patient. Empiric treatment with antipseudomonal and anti-staphylococcus antibiotics (D) is a medical emergency whenever a neutropenic patient spikes a temperature. This rapid institution of antibiotics can prevent disseminated sepsis. Reverse isolation precautions (E) include strict hand-washing, no fresh fruits and vegetables, no fresh flowers, no rectal temperatures, and even gloves and masks for visitors. These reverse isolation precautions would prevent the patient from being exposed to a possible infectious source. These precautions should be maintained until the white blood cell count is over 500 cells.

99. **(B)** A brain tumor near the midline could produce headaches, abnormal smells, and decreased vision.

100. **(D)** Pseudohyperkalemia may occur when potassium is released from cells during blood sample clotting in the presence of thrombocytosis or leukocytosis [(A) and (B)]. It may also occur if there is red blood cell hemolysis due to drawing blood through too small a needle or if the tourniquet is excessively tight and the fists are repeatedly clenched [(C) and (E)]. Acidosis results in hyperkalemia by producing a redistribution of potassium from the intracellular fluid to the extracellular fluid (D).

101. **(B)** Most community-acquired pneumonia in this age group is due to *S. pneumoniae* and, because of the patient's history of mild chronic obstructive pulmonary disease, *H. influenzae* should also be considered. However, amoxicillin/clavulanate should be active against most strains

of these pathogens, so other organisms should be considered. The patient's recent return from a convention suggests that he spent time in buildings (convention centers, hotels) with large air-handling systems which can occasionally be contaminated with *Legionella pneumophila*. His underlying lung disease would also predispose him to disease after an exposure that might not lead to illness in others. Erythromycin would also cover *Mycoplasma pneumoniae*, another common cause of community-acquired pneumonia, although usually in a younger population. The coverage of trimethoprim/sulfamethoxazole (A) significantly overlaps that of amoxicillin/clavulanate and is unlikely to include other important organisms. Tobramycin (C) and aztreonam (E) are both excellent agents against a variety of moderately resistant Gram-negative bacilli, but these organisms are unlikely to be involved in this case. Amantadine (D) is an anti-influenza drug but the patient is not reported as having other influenza-like symptoms.

102. **(A)** Known left main coronary artery disease is a contraindication for performing an exercise stress test. A patient with hypotension is at risk for sudden death. In patients with a negative electrocardiogram response to a workload above 6 METS on stress testing performed three weeks after a heart attack, the one-year mortality rate is below two percent (B). If a patient has been placed on beta-blockers after a heart attack, exercise stress testing can determine if the sympathetic nervous system has been adequately suppressed to prevent another ischemic episode (C). Exercise stress testing is indicated for most patients with uncomplicated myocardial infarction. If a patient has ventricular arrhythmias during a stress test, the one-year mortality rate can exceed 25% (D). Post-myocardial infarction exercise tolerance testing is a valuable and cost-effective tool for predicting the risk of adverse cardiac events (E).

103. **(B)** The absence of fever along with a normal ESR and WBC is indicative of transient synovitis of the hip, a benign, self-limiting condition that must be differentiated from septic arthritis (C)—which would be characterized by an exam with severe pain with short arc motion, fever, and elevated ESR and WBC. A normal hip (A) should not have an effusion or pain. Perthes' disease (D) and DDH (E) would be obvious.

104. **(C)** At this point, a complete physical examination, including a thorough musculoskeletal evaluation, is important.

105. **(D)** Antinuclear antibody testing would not be useful in this patient at this time.

106. **(B)** Q waves in leads 2, 3, and AVF are consistent with a recent MI. Clinically, the patient does not appear to have a new MI, as indicated in (D). He has not had an anterolateral MI [(A) and (C)]. He has a normal heart and rhythm, making bigeminy unlikely (E).

107. **(C)** The increased sweating in this setting is suggestive of some form of autonomic dysfunction.

108. **(A)** The patient's clinical syndrome, with burning hand pain and some shoulder discomfort occurring a month after a myocardial infarction, is most consistent with the shoulder-hand syndrome, a form of reflex sympathetic dystrophy. Dressler's syndrome (B) is pericarditis following a myocardial infarction. Shy-Drager syndrome (C) is a cause of orthostatic hypotension. The clinical findings are not consistent with diabetic neuropathy (D) or multiple sclerosis (E).

109. **(C)** Prednisone can be very beneficial in early shoulder-hand syndrome.

110. **(D)** Physical therapy for the shoulder and hand, especially early in the course, as this is, can be very helpful in preventing further complications.

111. **(C)** There is no reason to anticipate ST segment elevation. However, radiography (A) at a later stage of this condition often shows an irregular osteopenia, called Sudeck's atrophy. A bone scan (B) often shows increased uptake in the affected part. Flexion contracture of the hand (D) and adhesive capsulitis of the shoulder (E) can occur.

112. **(B)** Skin testing is not appropriate because she was likely treated with the BCG vaccine, which will cause a false-positive reading on the skin testing. Appropriate screening for this patient would be chest radiographs.

113. **(C)** The abdominal film demonstrates nephrocalcinosis, with an abundance of stones in the renal papilla. The arrows indicate stone fragments present in the ureters (C). Conditions predisposing to nephrocalcinosis include hyperparathyroidism, vitamin D intoxication, and medullary sponge kidney. In this case, there is no reason to invoke a second diagnosis [(B) and (D)]. Gouty nephropathy is a tubulointerstitial disorder (E). Radiolucency is characteristic of uric acid nephrolithiasis. Although renal cell carcinoma may present with flank pain and hematuria, calcification, if present, is intrarenal (A).

114. **(A)** The patient's symptoms of rebound tenderness are very worrisome, and appendicitis needs to be ruled out with a surgical consult and surgery if necessary.

115. **(A)** The patient's symptoms are classic for unstable angina, a new change in the amount of angina, and the amount of exertion to cause it. In spite of the normal EKG, which can be normal in the periods between angina, he needs to be admitted for a possible stress test or cardiac catheterization.

116. **(D)** Her symptoms are classic for right lower lobe pneumonia. Since she is young and has no other co-morbidities, she can be treated as an outpatient with oral antibiotics and close follow-up.

117. **(A)** The patient's symptoms and laboratory results are consistent with acute pancreatitis, and the patient should be admitted for IV hydration, pain control, and bowel rest.

118. **(C)** A wheal is caused by edema of the skin, such as urticaria and insect bites.

119. **(E)** A vesicle is caused by accumulation of fluid between the upper layers of the skin, such as caused by a second-degree burn.

120. **(B)** A nodule is a solid and elevated lesion extending into the dermis, such as a gouty tophus.

121. **(A)** A macule is a localized change in skin color, such as vitiligo. A pustule (D) is a pus-filled vesicle or bullae, such as a furuncle.

122. **(D)** An angiogram is the radiographic test of choice prior to revascularization procedures or bypass procedures in a patient.

123. **(B)** An MRI of the cervical, thoracic, lumbar, or sacral region is the radiographic test of choice in a patient with a herniated disc to identify the extent and location of injury.

124. **(C)** An ultrasound is the radiographic test of choice in a patient with a kidney cyst or with a cyst in other organs. It can give you an idea of flow and density.

125. **(E)** Plain radiographs with appropriate views remain the radiographic test of choice with fractured bones in the body of any patient.

126. **(A)** In a patient with a facial fracture, where you are concerned with ocular involvement, a plain film may not give you enough resolution. Therefore, a CAT scan may be indicated as the radiographic test of choice. It will also reveal some soft tissue structures in the surrounding area that can aid in diagnosis.

127. **(D)** Routine screening of adolescents for suicidal intent is not recommended. It is performed only in adolescents presenting with depression (B). Clinicians should explore the underlying causes of their depression and ask if they use illicit drugs (E). Conversely, adolescents with a history of drug abuse need a further workup for a suicidal intent. A suicidal attempt (A) is not to be confused with suicidal gesture, which is made for a secondary gain and is not life-threatening (C).

128. **(D)** Ondansetron, a recently developed serotonin antagonist, is the recommended antiemetic agent of choice in identifying the cause of the pain (A), preventing it from recurring, and maintaining a clear sensorium. Fear and anxiety (B) are among factors that lower pain threshold. Other factors include depression, sadness, insomnia, and isolation. Conversely, anxiolytic and antidepressant therapy, rest, and empathy are known to raise pain threshold. Narcotic-produced confusion and drowsiness should be treated by adding methylphenidate to the treatment plan (C). The subcutaneous, not intravenous, route is used for patients who, due to intractable vomiting, are unable to take narcotic analgesics by mouth (E).

129. **(C)** A physician or other health-care worker is not obligated to tell everyone about his condition, but he is obligated to protect others from exposure by using universal precautions, as should all health-care workers.

130. **(E)** Patient-physician confidentiality necessitates that you obtain the patient's written consent before you can give anyone his medical or psychiatric information.

131. **(E)** ASCUS is defined as squamous cell abnormalities not attributable to reactive changes alone, but not characteristic of an SIL (squamous intraepithelial lesion). It is not a cancerous lesion. ASCUS has been shown to be associated with CIN (cervical intraepithelial neoplasia) and HPV infection. ASCUS associated with severe inflammation and an identifiable cause of infection can be managed by treating the underlying infection and repeating the Pap in four to six months. If ASCUS persists, colposcopy should be performed.

132. **(C)** Rabies is caused by the neurotropic virus transmitted by the bite of infected mammals. There is decreased appetite associated with rabies, not increased appetite. The symptoms that may occur include radiating dysesthesias (A), malaise (B), nausea (D), and restlessness (E).

133. **(D)** Deep tendon reflexes are hyperactive. In addition, there can be nuchal rigidity, flaccid paralysis, Babinski's sign, and even death.

134. **(B)** Because of the effects of the rabies virus, the pattern of breathing is shallow and irregular.

135. **(D)** The diagnosis of rabies is made by microscopic examination of the brain (B) or spinal cord (C) of the animal, not the tongue. Observation of the animal (A) as well as analysis of the saliva (E) may also make the diagnosis.

136. **(B)** Hemophilia A, one of the most frequently encountered serious coagulation disorders, may present shortly after birth due an extensive cephalhematoma or profuse bleeding following circumcision. In males with more moderate disease, the disease may not present until the child begins to crawl or walk. Characteristically, hemarthrosis occurs in a large, weight-bearing joint. Typically, these patients have a prolonged

PTT and a normal PT. The bleeding time is usually normal or only slightly elevated (A). The platelet count is normal (C). Definitive diagnosis for hemophilia A is confirmed with a Factor VIII assay (B). Clinically similar, although considerably less common, is hemophilia B, diagnosed by Factor IX assay. Deficiencies of Factor V and X are exceedingly rare autosomal recessive disorders, which usually present as musculoskeletal bleeding or menorrhagia. In these conditions, hemarthrosis is uncommon. Both the PT and PTT are elevated in these deficiency diseases [(D) and (E)].

137. **(C)** Colonoscopy is the best way to confirm the diagnosis of ulcerative colitis because it will allow direct examination of the colon. Rectal examination (A), ultrasound (B), and flat plate of the abdomen (D) would be too limited. Deep palpation of the abdomen (E) would be essentially non-specific.

138. **(E)** Ulcerative colitis can frequently lead to perforation (A), sepsis and infection (B), hemorrhage (C), and toxemia (D). All of these can be severe enough to lead to death. If electrolyte imbalance does occur, it is rarely a cause of death.

139. **(D)** The treatment of complicated ulcerative colitis must be fast and aggressive. Common treatment modalities include surgery (A) to remove the involved colon, IV fluids (B) to restore hydration, a nasogastric tube (C) to rest the bowel, and antibiotics (E) to prevent or treat infection. A low-fat diet is not part of the routine treatment protocol.

140. **(D)** There is a high risk of cancer developing in the colon of patients with ulcerative colitis and, as such, a prophylactic colectomy is often recommended in suggested individuals. Colonic bleeding (A), perforation (B), infection (C), and adhesions (E) often necessitate the removal of a portion of the colon, but rarely the entire colon.

141. **(B)** Herpes zoster virus is the pathogen responsible for the Ramsey-Hunt syndrome. An RNA virus from the Rhabdovirus (A) family is responsible for rabies and travels through nerves similar to the herpes zoster virus. A cause of the common cold is the Coronavirus (C). Influenza virus (D) is a seasonal pulmonary pathogen. Hepatitis C virus (E) is the most common cause of chronic hepatitis.

142. **(D)** In Ramsey-Hunt Syndrome, herpes zoster affects the geniculate ganglion of the seventh cranial nerve (facial nerve). The vagus nerve (B) (tenth cranial nerve) is responsible for motor function of the gastrointestinal tract, pharynx, and posterior tongue, and is not involved in this syndrome. Palsies of the accessory nerve (C) (eleventh cranial nerve) result in difficulties in neck and shoulder movement. The vestibulocochlear nerve (E) (eighth cranial nerve) is affected by tumors in the cerebello-pontine angle and is responsible for hearing and balance.

143. **(E)** Hyperparathyroidism is common in middle-aged women. It is usually secondary to a parathyroid adenomas, which can be removed, or parathyroid hyperplasia. Hyperparathyroidism causes hypercalcemia from excessive bone resorption and hypercalciuria, which can cause development of kidney stones. This patient has symptoms of nephrolithiasis—kidney stones. Hyperparathyroid patients usually have osteopenia if the disorder is long-standing. Hyperparathyroidism can also be associated with multiple endocrine neoplasia Type I.

144. **(D)** This female has symptoms of a malignancy. In this case, the cancer is medullary cell carcinoma of the thyroid gland, which is associated with an elevated calcitonin level and also associated with multiple endocrine neoplasia Type II.

145. **(A)** This patient has symptoms of Zollinger-Ellison syndrome, which is associated with diarrhea secondary to very high gastrin levels, large ulcers, and high gastric acidity. H2 blockers such as cimetidine or Zantac would not relieve the symptoms because of the very high acid levels in the gastric region. The proton-pump inhibitor omeprazole is the current treatment of choice for Zollinger-Ellison syndrome. This syndrome is also associated in some cases with multiple endocrine neoplasia Type II. In the past, surgery would have been the only option in these cases.

146. **(C)** Chronic active gastritis is the diagnosis in this executive. *Helicobacter pylori* is the Gram-negative organism, which causes these symptoms of epigastric tenderness. Treatment of choice is triple-antibiotic therapy for 14-21 days and also a proton-pump inhibitor. Once the organism is eradicated by therapy with antibiotics,

the symptoms of gastritis should not be recurrent. Diagnosis of *H. pylori* infection is by culturing the gastric fluid via endoscopy or performing a C14 labeled breath test.

147. **(D)** Because the wound is dirty, and there is uncertainty about the patient's prior immunizations, he has to receive both tetanus toxoid and tetanus immunoglobulin.

148. **(D)** Maternal prenatal surveillance requires measurements of blood pressure and the extent of its change as well as measurements of weight and the amount of its change. Additionally, symptoms such as headache and altered vision should be examined to rule out preeclampsia.

149. **(C)** Late benign syphilis, or gumma, is now rare, but was the most common presentation of untreated syphilis in the prepenicillin era. Gummas develop 1-10 years following the initial infection and may occur in any part of the body. They may be solitary or multiple, ranging in size from microscopic to several centimeters in diameter. They are typically slowly progressive indolent, and rapidly responsive to treatment. Primary syphilis (A) typically presents as a chancre, which occurs at any site of potential inoculation by direct contact. Manifestations of secondary syphilis (B) are protean, most often including localized or diffuse symmetric mucocutaneous lesions and generalized nontender lymphadenopathy. Acute meningitis occurs in approximately one percent of affected persons, although increased cells and protein are present in the CSF of approximately 30% of affected persons. *T. pallidum* may be recovered from the CSF of more than 30% of affected persons. In addition to the acute meningovascular syphilis (D) associated with acute infection (vide supra), late meningovascular syphilis also occurs. In this condition, there is diffuse inflammation of the pia and arachnoid, associated with focal or widespread arterial involvement. It most commonly presents as a stroke. Tabes dorsalis (E) is a slowly progressive degenerative disease of the posterior columns and posterior roots of the spinal cord.

150. **(E)** Herpes simplex encephalitis is characterized by hemorrhagic necrosis. Gingivostomatitis and pharyngitis are the most frequent clinical manifestations of the first episode of HSV-l. Genital lesions, including vesicles, pustules, and painful erythematous ulcers are the initial manifestations of HSV-2 (E). Syphilitic gummas may resemble other chronic granulomatous conditions, including tuberculosis, sarcoidosis, leprosy, and deep fungal infections [(A), (B), (C), and (D)].

151. **(A)** In approximately one percent of persons with secondary syphilis, the VDRL may be nonreactive in undiluted serum due to the presence of an actual high titer. Testing at higher dilutions of the serum paradoxically produces positive results. This is known as the prozone phenomenon (A). Mothers with a reactive VDRL deliver infants with a reactive VDRL due to passive transfer of the IgG antibodies (C). Because the antigen used in the nontreponemal tests are found in other tissues, false-positive reactions may occur. In these cases, titers rarely exceed 1:8. Such false-positive tests also occur in persons over age 70 [(B) and (E)]. The VDRL becomes positive one to two weeks following the onset of the chancre (D).

152. **(D)** False-positive reactions for syphilis are classified as acute if they become negative within six months. Conditions producing such reactions include mycoplasma pneumonia, malaria, and other viral or bacterial infections. False-positive tests may also occur following some immunizations (D). Chronic false-positive VDRLs, which persist for more than six months, are common in autoimmune disease, intravenous drug abusers, persons over age 70, and persons with leprosy [(A), (B), (C), and (E)].

153. **(D)** The history and physical examination suggest carpal tunnel syndrome, which is confirmed by the nerve conduction studies. This syndrome, which results from compression of the median nerve, may occur in a variety of conditions, including pregnancy, rheumatoid arthritis, hypothyroidism, and amyloidosis. Fibromyalgia (A) is diagnosed clinically and is characterized by diffuse musculoskeletal pain, stiffness, paresthesias, nonrestorative sleep, and easy fatigability. Patients with psychogenic rheumatism (B) have severe joint pain. The patient is often emotionally labile. Neuropathic joint disease (C) is associated with loss of pain sensation and/or proprioception. A decrease in the protective muscular reflexes results in repeated joint trauma. Reflex sympathetic dystrophy (E) is characterized by pain and tenderness, associated with signs and

symptoms of vasomotor instability, trophic skin changes, and the rapid development of bony demineralization.

154. **(E)** This patient has calcium pyrophosphate dihydrate deposition disease characterized by synovial fluid, which shows weakly positive, birefringent crystals. This disorder is also called chondrocalcinosis and occurs most frequently in the elderly. X-ray films would show linear calcifications in the joint space. Treatment is with nonsteroidal anti-inflammatory agents and steroids if the symptoms are very severe. Acute gouty arthritis (A) usually presents in the first metatarsophalangeal joint space, but it can occur in the knee joint if another underlying illness is present—such as diabetes. The synovial fluid would reveal needle-shaped, strongly negatively birefringent crystals under the polarizing microscope. In septic arthritis (B), the synovial fluid of the affected joint would reveal an elevated white blood cell count and cultures, which are positive for the offending organism. In septic arthritis, steroids are contraindicated. This patient does not have osteoarthritis (C) because there is no physical sign of crepitus present in the knee joint. This patient does not have rheumatoid arthritis (D); patients with rheumatoid arthritis usually have involvement of the wrist and metacarpal joint. The juxtaarticular joints are involved, not large joints such as the knee.

155. **(C)** You should begin your consultation by reviewing the patient's diet. Your next step should be advising on a diet based on recommendations of the American Heart Association (A). For the elderly with cardiovascular disorders, the most reasonable and safest exercise is walking in fresh air (B). Prescribing treatment against the patient's will or without his or her approval is not going to work. If after your explanations of the disease process and recommendations for a trial of nonpharmacological treatment, the patient insists on starting with medication-based treatment, you should respect that choice and act accordingly (C).

156. **(A)** Patients with sickle cell disease can become infected with parvovirus B10 and get aplastic anemia.

157. **(C)** The few nucleated cells, all of them being lymphocytes, makes bacterial meningitis

unlikely. Subarachnoid hemorrhage (D) would be associated with xanthochromia. This is consistent with aseptic meningitis, most commonly from viral meningitis, such as enterovirus, and coxsackievirus.

158. **(B)** This patient has the signs and symptoms of a tension pneumothorax and requires immediate care. To treat this, a needle is inserted into the chest on the side of tension pneumothorax. This will convert it to a regular phenumothorax which can be treated by placement of a chest tube (A). A chest X-ray (D) is used for diagnosis only. A tracheotomy (C) or intubation (E) would be used only for purposes of establishing an airway and, currently, that is something this patient does not need.

159. **(A)** The most common cause of painless lower gastrointestinal bleed is diverticulosis. Colon cancer (C) usually presents as occult lower GI bleeding, and hemorrhoids (D) usually present as streaks of blood in the stool. Aorto-enteric fistula (E) usually presents as a massive lower GI bleed and more commonly occurs in patients who have had an aortic graft placed. Although upper GI bleeds, such as peptic ulcer disease (B), can cause bright red blood per rectum, it usually causes melena, unless in situations of very brisk bleeding.

160. **(D)** This patient has stage IV primary biliary cirrhosis. This is a chronic disease of the liver manifested by cholestasis. The disease is progressive, and treatment is symptomatic with cholestyramine to alleviate the pruritus and calcium supplementation to prevent osteoporosis. Antimitochondrial antibodies are present in 95% of patients. Females are more commonly affected by this disorder. Liver transplantation for advanced primary biliary cirrhosis has become one of the major success stories for this disorder in recent times.

161. **(B)** This patient has acute pancreatitis with volume depletion, elevated lipase levels, and vomiting. The treatment of choice is symptomatic only with bed rest, oxygen, intravenous fluids, and a nasogastric tube for suctioning to give the bowel some rest. This patient should be given nothing orally in order to rest the intestines and decrease the inflammation and necrosis of the pancreas gradually over time. Gallstones and alcohol are the

two most common causes of acute pancreatitis. Endoscopic retrograde cholangiopancreatography is an invasive procedure, which can actually precipitate acute pancreatitis.

162. **(E)** Screening flexible sigmoidoscopy is recommended by the American Cancer Society every five years, beginning at age 50, to detect polyps, adenomas, and carcinoma of the descending colon. Patients with adenomatous polyps should undergo colonoscopy to remove these polyps and to look for synchronous polyps in the proximal colon. Fecal occult blood testing is also recommended for all men and women on an annual basis. This patient, who is a physician himself, should have a rectal examination and be scheduled for a screening flexible sigmoidoscopy.

163. **(A)** This female has chronic hepatitis B, which is the cause of her portal hypertension and liver cirrhosis. She has all the signs and symptoms of chronic cirrhosis. The subsequent abdominal pain associated with ascites is suggestive of spontaneous bacterial peritonitis. Paracentesis is the diagnostic procedure of choice to make the definitive diagnosis of SBP. The ascites fluid would reveal a white blood cell count over 300 cells/uL, neutrophils over 250/uL, and an elevated protein level if spontaneous bacterial peritonitis is present. *E. coli* is usually the most common bacterial organism cultured in the ascites fluid. The mortality is very high if this patient is not treated with intravenous antibiotics. A liver transplant is out of the question if this patient has an acute infectious process going on.

164. **(C)** This "scout" film for a computed tomographic scan of the head demonstrates a nail in the brain (A). The intracranial position is obvious on the frontal projection [(C) and (D)]. The patient reported that he had attempted suicide 12 years previously (B). If the patient is not able to give a history, this lesion is most appropriately evaluated with a computed tomographic scan. Contraindications to the use of magnetic resonance imaging include cardiac pacemakers and defibrillators, cerebral aneurysm clips, and magnetically activated implants or foreign bodies (E).

165. **(E)** Acute bronchitis is associated with a 57-year-old man with a productive cough and known COPD.

166. **(C)** Migraine headaches are associated with a 33-year-old woman who has right hemifacial congestion, photophobia, and a severe right-sided headache.

167. **(D)** Pneumonia is associated with a 37-year-old alcoholic male with a productive cough.

168. **(B)** Sinusitis is associated with a 22-year-old woman with bifrontal headaches and purulent postnasal drainage.

169. **(A)** *Enterobius vermicularis* (pinworm) is usually an asymptomatic infection. Perianal pruritus is the cardinal symptom. Due to nocturnal migration of the female worms, with deposition of eggs on the perianal skin, the itching is usually worse at night. Sometimes this leads to perianal excoriation, with superimposed bacterial infection. Infection, which occurs via the fecal-oral route, is common in conditions in which person-to-person contact is frequent (A). *Trichuris trichiura* (whipworm) infection is limited to the gastrointestinal tract. It is common in overcrowded conditions, especially those with poor sanitation. Mild infection may be asymptomatic; heavy infection in children causes bloody or mucoid diarrhea, growth retardation, and rectal prolapse. Infection is diagnosed by identifying lemon- or football-shaped eggs in fecal smears (B). In uncomplicated *Strongyloides stercoralis*, most immunocompetent persons are asymptomatic or have only mild abdominal symptoms. Gastrointestinal disease manifests as abdominal bloating, vague pain, and diarrhea with nausea. Recurrent urticaria, especially of the buttocks, may occur (C). *Ascaris lumbricoides* presents either as gastrointestinal or pulmonary disease. Pulmonary symptoms result from larval migration in the small blood vessels. Intestinal signs/symptoms result either from obstruction due to an unusually large number of parasites in the small intestine or from migration of adult worms to aberrant sites (D). *Necator americanus* (hookworm) infections are usually asymptomatic. A maculopapular dermatitis may occur at the site of skin penetration (E).

170. **(C)** As long as the agents are benign and the patient only takes one or two in small doses, they probably will not do any harm but are unlikely to help either. Larger doses of any may be toxic. Taking all of them together may be toxic.

171. **(C)** This lady's symptoms and findings are consistent with menopause.

172. **(B)** These symptoms are consistent with diabetes. If this woman has diabetes, it must be controlled or her pregnancy will be compromised.

173. **(D)** Cigarette smoking (A), use of phenacetin (B), cyclophosphamide (C), and even *schistosomiasis* (E) are all correlated with an increased risk of developing transitional cell carcinoma of the urinary bladder. Alcohol abuse (D) is not.

174. **(E)** An otherwise healthy child with otitis media is not likely to have thrush. The patients in (A), (C), and (D) are immunocompromised and thus at risk for thrush. Diabetics with poorly controlled disease (B) are also at risk.

175. **(B)** In vitamin B12 deficiency, the homocysteine level is elevated. Methylmalonic acid levels (A) would also be elevated 96% of the time in cobalamin deficiency. Anti-parietal cell antibody (C) and anti-intrinsic factor antibody levels would be elevated in pernicious anemia. This would decrease the absorption of vitamin B12 in the ileum. Mean corpuscular volume (D) greater than 100 fL is considered elevated and is associated with macrocytic anemia, from either B12 or folate deficiency and certain drugs. A normal cobalamin level (E) is presented 20-30% of the time in vitamin B12 deficiency. Vitamin B12 deficiency can cause serious neurological deficits if left untreated.

176. **(D)** Most bleeding following pelvic fractures is venous bleeding and will respond to external fixation. However, the bleeding occasionally is arterial, and this may require arterial embolization to control bleeding. Transfusion of FFP (A) would not be indicated, considering the normal coagulation parameters and fibrin split products. Removing the external fixator (B) would worsen any venous component of the bleeding. Open reduction (C) is not indicated in the acute setting, as this would release any tamponade pressure from the hematoma. Observation (E) is not indicated in the face of hemodynamic instability.

177. **(A)** Heterosexuals who have multiple sexual encounters with different partners, usually in unprotected settings, are susceptible to HIV infection.

178. **(C)** The leading diagnoses for this woman are brain tumor or leaking/ruptured aneurysm. Her symptoms are not typical of migraines (A). If she has a mass lesion, a lumbar puncture could cause herniation (B).

179. **(B)** This patient has classic hypothyroidism, the most common cause of which is Hashimoto's thyroiditis. If one suspects hypothyroidism, then a serum TSH assay should be performed as well as free thyroxine level. If the TSH is elevated (secondary to the negative-feedback loop), then hypothyroidism is present. Hypothyroid patients usually have elevated cholesterol levels, and this disorder is more common in women. Thyroid scanning with radionucleotide labeled technetium (A) provides useful data in evaluating if the thyroid nodule is functioning or non-functioning. Serum calcitonin levels (C) are elevated in medullary thyroid carcinoma. This test is not useful to screen for hypothyroidism. Sonography (D) accurately distinguishes solid, cystic, and mixed lesions within the thyroid gland. It can guide the endocrinologist in performing a fine-needle aspiration biopsy to evaluate a nodule in the thyroid gland. The thyroid-releasing hormone stimulation test (E) is a very useful procedure in diagnosing equivocal cases of thyrotoxicosis.

180. **(D)** IV gammaglobulin (A) has been demonstrated to decrease the incidence of coronary artery abnormalities in children with Kawasaki syndrome. Aspirin (B) prevents the thrombotic complications. An echo (C) is need to assess the coronary artery involvement of the syndrome. Corticosteroids (D) are presently contraindicated in the treatment of Kawasaki syndrome.

USMLE Step 3 – Practice Test 1
Day Two – Morning Session

1. **(A)** Your first priority in the management in this unconscious patient should be cardiopulmonary resuscitation (CPR). It starts with assessing the patient for ABCs: establishing airway, proper breathing (ventilation), and circulation.

2. **(B)** The next step in the management of acetaminophen (Tylenol) intoxication after proper measures of CPR and decontamination of the patient with ipecac is to prevent the systemic effects of acetaminophen overdose. This is achieved by N-acetylcysteine.

3. **(B)** Likewise, the antidote to prevent the systemic effects of benzodiazepine intoxication (e.g., flurazepam) is flumazenil.

4. **(A)** This 73-year-old comatose patient with aspirin overdose should be evaluated for his vital signs first. Decontamination is the next step and is usually enhanced with pH-dependent diuresis for substances with acidic properties (aspirin is a weak acid).

5. **(B)** The flexor carpi ulnaris flexes the wrist and deviates it ulnarly. It is located on the ulnar aspect of the forearm. The palmaris longus (A) also flexes the wrist but is more centrally located. The flexor carpi radialis (C) flexes the wrist and deviates it radially. It is located more radially. Pronator teres (D) is not located in the site of the injury, and there is no flexor indicis propius tendon (E). There is an extensor indicis propius, but this is on the dorsum of the wrist and extends the index finger.

6. **(C)** The ulnar nerve is located in the area of the region, and it gives sensation to the little finger and the ulnar half of the ring finger.

7. **(B)** With the flexor carpi ulnaris lacerated, there is unopposed flexion by the palmaris and flexor carpi radialis. Therefore, the wrist will flex with radial deviation (B).

8. **(C)** Guyon's canal, or ulnar tunnel, is formed by the transverse carpel ligament, the volar carpel ligament, and the pisiform. The cubital tunnel (A) is higher up in the arm around the olecranon of the elbow. The carpel tunnel (B) is located in the wrist under the transverse carpel ligament. Allen (D) is not a canal, but rather a test of arterial supply to the hand. Brachial (E) is not a canal either, but an area higher up in the arm.

9. **(A)** Treatment of hemodynamically stable ventricular tachycardia is initially treated with lidocaine.

10. **(B)** Classically, procainamide and quinidine are the medical mainstays for pharmacologic cardioversion.

11. **(C)** Amiodarone should be used for cases of sudden death or unstable ventricular tachycardia.

12. **(D)** In a narrow complex tachycardia that is hemodynamically stable, the first choice of medications should be adenosine.

13. **(A)** Serum alcohol level is associated with an agitated, confused, combative 34-year-old man who has been brought in by a friend who then left.

14. **(C)** Lumbar puncture is associated with a febrile, crying eight-month-old boy with no focal findings.

15. **(B)** Chest radiograph is associated with a 58-year-old male with fever, chills, and a productive cough.

16. **(D)** CPK is associated with a 69-year-old man with lesions on his knuckles.

17. **(A)** This patient is suffering from chronic bronchitis. Abnormalities observed on pulmonary function testing include the changes listed in choices [(B), (C), (D), and (E)], and increased residual volume.

18. **(D)** Simulated melena (black tarry stools with negative guaiac) is seen with the ingestion of cherries. Epistaxis (A), gastric ulcer (B), esophageal varices (C), and hemoptysis (E) all will lead to the digestion of blood, giving you a positive guaiac. Swallowing 50-60 ml of blood will produce a tarry stool.

19. **(D)** Spider angiomatous can be found with cirrhosis of the liver, but aren't classically seen with bacterial endocarditis. Classic physical findings with subacute bacterial endocarditis include Osler's nodes (painful nodules on the palms) (A), splinter hemorrhage (B), splenomegaly (C), hematuria (E), Janeway lesions, and Roth spots (in the retina).

20. **(A)** *Enterococcus* or *Streptococcus viridans* can cause SBE. *Staphylococcus* (B) usually will cause acute endocarditis and is more common in intravenous drug abusers. The *Haemophilus spp.* (C), *Eikenella spp.* (D), and fungal organisms (E) are much less common etiologies of SBE.

21. **(C)** SBE most commonly affects the mitral valve in normal patients. The tricuspid valve (A) is most commonly affected in intravenous drug users.

22. **(B)** History of intravenous drug abuse makes acute bacterial endocarditis with *Staphylococcus aureus* infection of particular concern.

23. **(C)** We know that this patient is hypovolemic by his vital signs, and his history of melena and hematemesis is concerning for a gastrointestinal bleed.

24. **(E)** All of the choices are appropriate. In a gastrointestinal bleed, the patient should be typed and crossed (A), have two large-bore intravenous lines placed (B), and get admission labs (D), including hematocrit and coagulation studies. Electrocardiogram (C) should be obtained to assess for ischemia secondary to anemia.

25. **(C)** Initiation of wide open crystalloids is the appropriate intervention. Although the patient is becoming hypotensive, it is because of hypovolemia, and not because of decreased peripheral vascular resistance. Volume resuscitation should be the most important treatment. In fact, these patients are often vasoconstricted already, so va-

sopressors often are not very helpful. There is no evidence for pericardial tamponade in this patient requiring pericardiocentesis (E).

26. **(A)** If crystalloids, such as normal saline or lactated Ringer's solution, are not adequate, you can try colloids, such as hetastarch solution or albumin solution. Any fluid less concentrated than serum, such as half-normal saline (E) and sterile water (B), will likely be quickly shunted to the extravascular spaces and should be avoided.

27. **(B)** In patients with an ongoing upper gastrointestinal bleed, the most important and appropriate initial intervention is an esophago-gastroduodenoscopy.

28. **(B)** In severe hypovolemic shock, the largest bore intravenous line (cordis) should be placed for the fastest fluid administration.

29. **(E)** The indications for intubation are for ventilation, oxygenation, and airway protection. The patient has no reason not to be ventilating (C) or oxygenating (D). However, due to his hypotension, his mental status is poor and it may be difficult for him to protect his airway.

30. **(C)** The erythrocyte sedimentation rate is an extremely nonspecific test. However, the only disease that it can reliably rule out with a normal value is temporal arteritis. Although in all of the other answer choices the ESR can be elevated, it is not always elevated.

31. **(B)** This patient has AIDS and *Candida esophagitis*. The most common cause of dysphagia and painful swallowing in a HIV patient with oral thrush is *Candida albicans* esophagitis. This is, in fact, so common, that empiric treatment with ketoconazole or fluconazole is given first to see if the symptoms resolve in two to three days after treatment has begun. Acyclovir (A) is given to patients with herpes esophagitis, which is not as common as *Candida esophagitis*. These lesions are shallow and vesicular in nature and determined by biopsy alone. Upper endoscopy with biopsy (C) is usually done only after the patient has failed treatment with antifungal agents. The biopsy of the esophageal lesion can then determine the exact cause of the dysphagia (infectious versus tumor). A barium swallow test (D) or esophagram can only tell us if there is a stricture or

reflux disorder. It should not be done initially until after the patient has had a trial of antifungal agents. Ganciclovir (E) is the treatment for cytomegalovirus infection. The CMV infection usually occurs in immunocompromised patients with a CD4 count less than 75. CMV esophagitis can be superimposed on candidal esophagitis, but the CD4 count has to be low. In this patient, it is only 204.

32. **(C)** The nurse has included you in her confidence. You have no right to tell anyone else, but it is appropriate to remind her to take the universal precautions that everyone is supposed to use. As long as she does this, she is really no more of a risk to anyone than is someone whose HIV status is unknown.

33. **(B)** Carcinoid syndrome is characterized by valvular heart disease, flushing, diarrhea and, less frequently, wheezing and paroxysmal hypotension. Liver involvement suggests that carcinoid tumors are located in the foregut, in which case flushing is intense and long-lasting. These tumors release serotonin, which triggers diarrhea and cardiac abnormalities. Serotonin is metabolized to 5-hydroxyindoleacetic acid, which is excreted excessively in urine and, in that way, serves as a diagnostic marker for this disorder. Pheochromocytoma (A) is associated with hypertension, not hypotension. It usually presents with headaches, diaphoresis, and palpitations secondary to excess catacholamine production by the adrenal glands. Mastocytosis (C) is associated with urticaria pigmentosa. There is an abnormal increase in mast cells in the bone marrow, liver, spleen, lymph nodes, skin, and gastrointestinal tract. Patients who have mastocytosis do not excrete excessive amounts of 5-hydroxyindoleacetic acid. Thyrotoxic patients (D) usually have hypertension and palpitations. Flushing is unusual. 5-hydroxyindoleacetic acid production is normal. Urticaria (E) is associated with symptomatic pruritic wheals and hives on the skin secondary to an allergic event. Liver enlargement is not common.

34. **(C)** Lateral deviation of the great toe is hallux valgus. Hammer toe (A) is fixation of a smaller toe in flexion. Hallux rigidus (B) is a stiffened great toe. Hallux varus (D) is medial deviation of the great toe. Gout (E) is an inflammatory disease that will often affect the great toe.

35. **(C)** Paranoid individuals (A) manifest an extreme mistrust of others. They constantly doubt others because they believe that others are out to betray them. As a result, they are quick to defend themselves in what they believe to be a "counterattack." Schizoid personalities (B), similarly, find difficulty in establishing close relationships. However, schizoid individuals do not demonstrate distrust of social relationships. Rather, they demonstrate apathy. Schizotypal individuals (C) are also loathe to make friends, owing to odd and socially anxious behavior. Histrionic individuals (D) are quite the opposite of paranoid individuals in that they are constantly attention-seeking. They often do this by dramatizing themselves. Finally, antisocial personalities (E) are those who cannot make close relationships because of a guiltless and irresponsible conscience. They often have trouble with the law.

36. **(B)** Barrier contraceptives protect against all forms of PID including those that are caused by chlamydial STDs. A concomitant genital infection with *Chlamydia* is present in as many as 45% of patients with gonococcal PID (D). Oral contraceptives interfere with the menstrual cycle and result in a decreased blood flow. They also contribute to decreased cervical dilatation and a decreased permeability of cervical mucus to microorganisms (A).

37. **(B)** In an emergency situation such as this, with no next-of-kin known or available, it is justifiable to proceed with medically necessary interventions.

38. **(A)** The patient has been abandoned and it will be appropriate to make him a ward of the court.

39. **(C)** You should try to obtain information regarding this child and his past history.

40. **(D)** The child's bruises and untreated fracture are very suspicious of child abuse.

41. **(C)** Painful swallowing, decreased oral intake and chills and fever should alert you to the possibility of pharyngitis, which ties all the symptoms together. The neck (A) should be examined for adenopathy. The oropharynx (B) should be observed to examine the throat. The lungs (D)

should be auscultated for the presence of any URI, and the abdomen (E) should be examined for any organomegaly. There is no reason here to examine the cranial nerves (C), which will test normally.

42. **(B)** A screening test should be inexpensive and easy to perform, and it should give you high sensitivity and specificity. Since you are expecting pharyngitis, a rapid Strep test (B) meets this criteria. All the other tests—a CBC (A), liver function tests (C), chest X-ray (D), and an electrocardiogram (E)—would not be useful as screening tests.

43. **(C)** Classically, rheumatoid arthritis presents as morning stiffness which improves with use. It affects multiple joints, particularly the proximal interphalangeal joints. Gout (B) and pseudogout (A) classically affect single joints and are excruciatingly painful. Septic arthritis (E) classically affects single joints and is associated with constitutional symptoms. Osteoarthritis (D) is a polyarticular arthritis, but classically worsens with use.

44. **(A)** Gastritis is not a concern here. The extra-articular manifestations of rheumatoid arthritis that are not uncommon are pulmonary fibrosis (B), vasculitis (C), serositis (D), and rheumatoid nodules (E).

45. **(E)** Aspirin does not cause toxicity to the pancreas. However, in supratherapeutic amounts, aspirin can cause an iron-deficiency anemia (via gastrointestinal bleed), acute renal failure, liver failure, and hepatitis.

46. **(A)** NSAIDs and systemic glucocorticoids are the mainstay for the symptomatic treatment of rheumatoid arthritis. It is still controversial whether or not glucocorticoids actually slow down the progression of the disease.

47. **(D)** There is no place for bleomycin in the treatment of rheumatoid arthritis. However, the other medications—gold (B), methotrexate (A), penicillamine (C), and hydroxychloroquine (E)—all have been shown to slow down the progression of the disease and joint destruction in patients who can tolerate the medications.

48. **(A)** In a patient with known rheumatoid arthritis, a single joint that is worse and more symptomatic is concerning for septic joint, which occurs with more frequency in patients with rheumatoid arthritis.

49. **(D)** Renal toxicity is not a side effect. Side effects of methotrexate include gastrointestinal toxicity (nausea and vomiting) (A), bone marrow toxicity (pancytopenia) (B), hepatitis (elevation in the transaminases) (C), and hypersensitivity pneumonitis (E).

50. **(A)** In a patient with rheumatoid arthritis, disabling joint destruction such as in the hips or knees can be treated with surgery and replacement.

51. **(A)** Vision screening of adults is not a component of a routine physical check-up. It may be appropriate in the elderly. All middle-aged men should be screened for hypercholesterolemia (B). Regular measurements of blood pressure should be performed in persons aged three and older (C). Body mass index (height and weight) determination is a part of the periodic health assessment and also helps to screen for obesity [(D) and (E)].

52. **(E)** Anorexia is seen with hypercalcemia. Perioral paresthesias (A), lethargy (B), irritability (C), and prolonged QT intervals (D) are all seen with hypocalcemia.

53. **(C)** Calcification of a congenital bicuspid aortic valve is the most common cause of aortic stenosis, the condition described in this case study. Rheumatic heart disease (A) and arteriosclerotic degeneration (B) are less common causes of this condition. Ankylosing spondylitis (D) and syphilis (E) are causes of aortic regurgitation, rather than aortic stenosis.

54. **(C)** Left-heart catheterization allows for precise determination of the pressure gradient across the aortic valve and is useful to determine the appropriate treatment plan. Endomyocardial biopsy (A) is useful for the evaluation of myocarditis. Thallium stress (B) test is useful for the evaluation of coronary disease. Swan-Ganz catheterization (D) allows for the determination of right-heart pressures and the pulmonary wedge pressure, but does not allow for the determination of the pressure gradient across the aortic valve. Coronary arteriography (E) is often performed in patients with aortic stenosis to assess the need for coronary artery bypass at the time of aortic valve replacement.

However, coronary arteriography does not help to determine the severity of aortic stenosis.

55. **(D)** Beta blockers are contraindicated in patients with advanced aortic stenosis, as the already compromised cardiac output can be dangerously reduced by beta blockade. Prosthetic valve replacement (A) or porcine valve replacement (B) are acceptable surgical options. Valvuloplasty is not commonly used, but may be a useful therapy in patients unlikely to survive an open surgical procedure (C).

56. **(D)** Nitrates induce a venous vasodilation, thus reducing cardiac preload. Patients with aortic stenosis have a reduced cardiac output, which is dependent on an adequate preload. It is true that tachyphylaxis does develop with these agents; however, this is not the reason that they are avoided in severe aortic stenosis (A). The vasodilatory effects related to these agents will reduce afterload to a small degree, rather than increasing preload (B). Nitrate therapy is effective in a variety of cardiac and noncardiac conditions in addition to those related to coronary artery occlusion, such as coronary vasospasm and esophageal spasm (C). Sublingual nitroglycerin therapy has a greater bioavailability than oral agents due to the large first-pass effect of nitrates which are administered orally (E).

57. **(A)** This patient has Kaposi's sarcoma, which is an HIV-related tumor. Kaposi's sarcoma is derived from pluripotent mesenchymal cells, and herpes-like virus 8 is believed to be involved with the etiology. This tumor occurs only in HIV individuals. The most common sites of involvement include the skin, mucous membranes, and visceral lymph nodes. The GI tract and lungs can also be involved in extensive disease. The gold standard for the diagnosis of Kaposi's sarcoma is biopsy. Once the diagnosis is established, then treatment with interferon, cytotoxic agents, and topical liquid nitrogen can be initiated. CT of the chest and abdomen (B) is very helpful in establishing the diagnosis, but these imaging tests are not very specific. Bone marrow aspiration and biopsy (C) is useful in making the diagnosis of mycobacterium avium cellulare (MAC) and lymphoma. It is not useful in making the diagnosis of KS. A lumbar puncture (D) is useful in making the diagnosis of cryptococcal meningitis or CNS lymphoma, but not Kaposi's sarcoma. KS lesions are not found in the brain and cerebral spinal fluid. Bronchoscopy (E) with biopsy can be done, but KS lesions are very friable and thus there is a risk of bleeding. Biopsy of the KS skin lesions are more appropriate.

58. **(D)** Patients with this disorder progress to end-stage renal disease, uremia, and have a "moth-eaten" appearance on the intravenous pyelogram. Kidney stones, hypertension, chronic infections, and hematuria are associated with this disorder. Nephritis (A) is associated with red blood cell casts in the urine. Polycystic kidney disease is not associated with red blood cell casts. Liver cysts are found in 33% of patients with polycystic kidney disease. They have no functional significance. Hepatomas (B) are rare. Proximal renal tubular acidosis (type II) (C) is associated with a urine pH greater than 7.0 and decreased capacity of the proximal tubule to reabsorb bicarbonate. It is not associated with polycystic kidney disease. Bladder cancer (E) is more common in males in a 3:1 ratio. It initially presents as microhematuria. Some of the risk factors are exposure to aniline dyes, tobacco, and schistosomiasis. It is not associated with polycystic kidney disease.

59. **(C)** Once a patient has gotten three tetanus immune globulins, he should get booster toxoid every ten years, or five if any injury is noted.

60. **(C)** A breast lump that changes with the menstrual period is more suggestive of fibrocystic breast disease. All of the other choices are concerning physical findings for breast cancer.

61. **(C)** The proper approach at this point in time is to make the patient comfortable. There are numerous cases in the courts arguing the merits of physician-assisted suicide and/or euthanasia, but at this time these are not legally sanctioned approaches.

62. **(C)** The aspirin should be stopped two weeks before surgery. This will allow the antiplatelet effects of aspirin to wear off. In addition to aspirin-containing products, medications that prolong bleeding, such as nonsteroidal, anti-inflammatory drugs, should be stopped, as well.

63. **(D)** One unit of transfused packed red blood cells is equivalent to about 500 cc of whole

blood, in terms of oxygen-carrying capacity and osmotic properties. Thus, from a 1,900 cc blood loss, 1,500 cc have been replenished by blood product transfusion. Since 3 cc of crystalloid are required for each cc of blood loss, the additional 400 cc of blood loss that has been unaccounted for would require 1,200 cc of crystalloid replacement.

64. **(C)** The approximate blood volume of an adult is 70 ml/kg. A 175-lb (80 kg) male should thus have an approximate blood volume of 5,600 ml.

65. **(C)**, 66. **(A)**, 67. **(B)**, and 68. **(D)** Although gout (A) is most common in the big toe, it may affect any joint. It is usually monarticular and joint fluid microscopy reveals needle-shaped crystals which are negatively birefringent. Osteoarthritis (B) is a common condition which generally affects weight-bearing or heavily used joints. Heberden's nodes are found on the distal interphalangeal joints and Bouchard's nodes are seen on the proximal interphalangeal joints. Classic radiographic findings include joint space narrowing, osteophytes, and cysts. Rheumatoid arthritis (C) generally occurs in a symmetrical distribution involving large and small joints. Constitutional symptoms, such as fever, are common in severe cases. In pseudogout (D), microscopy of joint fluid aspirate reveals positively birefringent crystals which are rhomboid-shaped. These are calcium pyrophosphate dihydrate crystals. Infective arthritis (E) can be caused by numerous organisms, most commonly *Staphylococcus aureus*. Joint fluid aspiration is useful to make the diagnosis based on cell count and culture.

69. **(D)** This patient has temporal arteritis, which is a vasculitis of the medium and large-size arteries. This is most common in the elderly and can masquerade as a routine tension or migraine headache. The immediate treatment of choice is high-dose prednisone to prevent blindness. This can occur because of involvement of the ophthalmic branch of the carotid artery. Temporal artery biopsy (A) is the diagnostic gold standard to make the definitive diagnosis, but this procedure would not be performed right away and, thus, blindness may ensue. Nonsteroidal anti-inflammatory agents (B) are used for migraines and tension headaches, which are usually bilateral. This patient's headache is unilateral and associated with a fever. Antibiotics (C) are needed if this patient has meningitis, which would present with neck stiffness and mental status changes. A lumbar puncture would be needed to make the diagnosis of meningitis. A CT of the brain (E) would be necessary if one suspects an acute stroke or hemorrhage in the brain. This patient has no neurologic findings suggestive of a bleed or stroke.

70. **(C)** The antidepressant drugs, TCA (D), SSRI (C), and MAOI (B) are all equally effective in alleviating depressive symptoms. However, SSRIs are considered the first-line therapy for depression because of their significantly better tolerability and side-effect profile compared to MAOs and TCAs. Phenothiazines (E) are used for the treatment of schizophrenia.

71. **(D)** This patient has shingles or herpes zoster. The lesions are self-limiting over time but very painful. A Tzanck prep is obtained by taking a swab from the vesicular fluid off the lesion and looking under the microscope. In herpes zoster, multinucleated giant cells and ballooning of the epidermal cells are seen under the Tzanck prep slide. Biopsy of the skin vesicles (A) would not give a very quick diagnosis. The procedure would also be invasive and painful to the patient. Topical steroids (B) applied to the dermatomal lesions would exacerbate the shingles and cause replication of the virus. Acyclovir (C) is the treatment of choice in immunocompromised individuals to prevent dissemination. It has also been shown to prevent post-herpetic neuralgia pain in zoster patients. An electrocardiogram (E) is not necessary because the cause of the thoracic pain is not related to the cardiovascular system, but to nerve root involvement by the herpes virus.

72. **(D)** This patient has been exposed to tuberculosis but does not have active pulmonary infection. Thus, watchful waiting is the prudent thing to do and a follow-up chest X-ray is indicated if symptoms of weight loss, sweating, fever, and anorexia occur suggestive of active tuberculosis. Isoniazid and B12 prophylaxis (A) are indicated if the patient is younger than 35 years old and has a positive PPD status. If the patient is older than 35 years old, then the American Thoracic Society recommends no prophylaxis against TB because of the higher risk of liver toxicity. Obtaining sputum for acid-fast bacilli is not needed because this patient has no symptoms of cough

and has a normal chest X-ray (B). Thus, the yield would be negligible. A CT of the chest (C) would most likely be normal if the chest X-ray is normal and the patient is asymptomatic. This test would be useless and certainly not indicated in the management of this patient. A repeat PPD test is indicated only if the initial testing is negative (E). In this case, the PPD skin test was positive to 10 mm induration, and, thus, another skin test is not necessary, not even in the future.

73. **(E)** You need to explain your thinking and plans to the patient, but it is appropriate to regulate his analgesic intake.

74. **(B)** Again, explaining your reasoning is the correct thing to do.

75. **(A)** If a patient is not happy with your care of him or if you find you cannot deal with a patient, you should give him the names of four other physicians in the area whom he can see instead of you.

76. **(B)** Someone appears to have forged the prescription. At this point, telling the pharmacist you did not write the prescription is the correct thing to do.

77. **(A)** In diarrhea, potassium levels are 35 mEq/L. In sweat (B), pancreatic juices (C), and bile (E), the level is 5 mEq/L. In gastric juice (D), the level is 10 mEq/L.

78. **(E)** The first and immediate management would be to lower the temperature with either cold compresses, tepid bath, or antipyretics such as children's Tylenol. This would prevent another febrile seizure attack. After doing this, one should identify the source of the fever (otitis media, pneumonia, sinus, urinary tract) and treat any infection found with antibiotics. Clinically important intracranial structural abnormalities are uncommon in infants and toddlers and, therefore, CT and MRI of the brain (A) are not recommended unless focal neurological findings are present on physical exam. For children older than 18 months, a lumbar puncture (B) is not warranted unless meningeal signs such as neck stiffness, Kernig's sign, and a prolonged postictal state is present. In a child with a first febrile seizure in whom the temperature and infection can be controlled by

outpatient antibiotics, immediate hospitalization (C) is not necessary. As long as the patient is medically stable, there is no need to keep the patient for observation overnight. No evidence exists that an EEG (D) can predict recurrent febrile seizures or the onset of epilepsy. The American Academy of Pediatrics does not recommend an EEG for a neurologically healthy child with a first febrile seizure.

79. **(D)** In a witnessed cardiac arrest, when a defibrillator is not available, a precordial thump is the first initial treatment, then followed by cardiopulmonary resuscitation and calling for help.

80. **(B)** It does not matter if this is your patient; you can enroll him only after obtaining appropriate informed consent. Furthermore, it is unethical to threaten the patient with withdrawal of your care (D) if he does not participate.

81. **(C)** The IRB reviews all protocols for their safety to protect study subjects from harm.

82. **(E)** Infected pressure sore secondary to bed rest may occur in sedentary hospitalized patients, however, they are less likely to develop in patients who are alert and able to move all extremities. This is the least likely possibility of fever in this patient. Thrombophlebitis secondary to an intravenous catheter (A) which has not been changed is a common cause of nosocomial fever. Aspiration pneumonia (B) is a standard complication of upper endoscopy, especially in patients with active GI bleeding. Urinary tract infection secondary to indwelling Foley catheter (C) is also a common cause of nonsocomial infections, often with resistant Gram-negative organisms. Drug fever (D) may occur secondary to nearly any medication, although H_2 blockers and antibiotics are common culprits.

83. **(D)** Diagnostic peritoneal lavage is utilized in the evaluation of intra-abdominal trauma. A WBC >500 cells/cc is indicative of trauma. So are the following: hematocrit >2%, RBC >50,000 cells/cc, amylase >100 units, and the presence of bile, bacteria, or food fibers.

84. **(E)** Pneumothorax is not a complication of peritoneal lavage because you are performing the procedure in the abdomen, not the chest.

Infection (A), perforation (B), bleeding (C), and death (D) are, however, possible complications from the procedure.

85. **(C)** Xanthoma disseminatum are generalized skin deposits associated with hypercholesterolemia. Juvenile xanthoma (A) are systemic deposits associated with a familial type of disordered fat metabolism. Xeroderma pigmentosa (B) is a developmental disease of the skin with sensitivity to sunlight. Xanthelesma (D) are localized deposits in the eyelids that are usually associated with hypercholesterolemia. Hyperkeratosis (E) presents as skin lesions characterized by a thickened layer of skin and histologic evidence of increased keratin.

86. **(A)** The skin deposits of xanthoma disseminatum do not occur on the oral mucosa. They occur on the face (B), trunk (C), axillae (D), flexor surfaces of the limbs (E), and the scalp.

87. **(E)** Appropriate initial treatments for a patient who is not responsive, but is breathing and having an adequate blood pressure, are naloxone (A) and thiamine (C). An intravenous line should also be inserted (D) to assist in quick administration of medications. Once labs are drawn, and if the patient is hyperglycemic, insulin can be started, but shouldn't be started any earlier.

88. **(C)** This patient probably has missed her menstrual cycles because of stress. If her endometrium is primed and ready for menstruation, then administering oral progesterone (10 mg) will result in withdrawal bleeding. If withdrawal bleeding does not occur, then further work-up is necessary. An endometrial biopsy (A) is needed only if administering oral progesterone does not result in withdrawal bleeding. Colposcopy (B) is an invasive procedure that involves taking a biopsy and scraping from the cervix. This procedure is done only after a Pap smear comes back with abnormal cells on cytopathology. Oral estrogen administration (D) alone will not result in withdrawal bleeding and thus will not aid in the management of this patient. An elevated serum prolactin level can also result in oligomenorrhea (E), but this patient has no signs of lactation or cranial adenomas. Obtaining a serum prolactin level would be useful only if the progesterone withdrawal test did not happen.

89. **(A)**, 90. **(B)**, 91. **(D)**, and 92. **(C)** Fatty liver (steatosis) occurs when increased amounts of triglycerides reach the liver, either via the bloodstream or lymphatics, if there is increased synthesis or decreased oxidation of lipids in the liver, or if there is decreased export of very low density lipoproteins from the liver. Macrovesicular steatosis (A) is the most common form. It is seen in persons with alcoholism, diabetes mellitus, obesity, and those who undergo prolonged parenteral nutrition. Microvesicular steatosis occurs in Reye's syndrome, acute fatty liver of pregnancy, and with drugs, such as valproic acid and tetracycline.

Primary biliary cirrhosis is characterized by four stages. Stage I shows marked periductular inflammation and injury to both septal and interlobular bile ducts. The primarily mononuclear cell inflammation may be associated with granuloma formation. The second stage (B) is characterized by bile ductular proliferation, early cholestasis, and periportal inflammation. In stage III, there is marked fibrosis, with distortion of the normal architecture. Cholestasis may appear. Cirrhosis characterizes stage IV. It may be associated with absence of bile ducts.

In hepatocellular carcinoma, tumor cells may closely resemble normal hepatocytes. Under a higher power magnification, tumor cells may have pleomorphic nuclei, prominent nucleoli, and abundant granular eosinophilic cytoplasm. Mitotic figures and necrosis may also be apparent. The fibrolanmelar subtype (D) is an uncommon variety.

A Masson trichrome-stained normal liver biopsy (C) is shown for comparison with the pathologic specimens.

93. **(B)** To determine the percentage of body burn in adults, the "rule of nines" is used: Head 9%, Chest 9%, Abdomen 9%, Upper back 9%, Lower back 9%, Arm 9%, each Upper leg 9%, each Lower leg 9%, and each Perineum 1%.
Therefore, a 50% burn over each arm is 50% x 2 x 9% = 9%, which is closest to 10%.

94. **(B)** To determine fluid requirements, the Parkland formula is used. The total fluid requirement during the first 24 hours = % body burn x body weight (kg) x 4 cc. Replace with lactated Ringer's solution over the first 24 hours.
1/2 of fluids in first 8 hours
1/4 of fluids in second 8 hours
1/4 of fluids in third 8 hours

Therefore, this patient requires 10% x 4 cc x 70 kg = 2,800 cc for the first 24 hours.

95. **(E)** The magnetic resonance imaging study of the brain demonstrates a left parietal arteriovenous malformation. The cerebral angiogram confirms the presence of the arteriovenous malformation. Several interventional therapeutic options are available, depending on the age of the patient, degree of neurologic dysfunction, and location of the lesion. These options include surgical resection of the lesion (A), embolization of arterial feeders (B), or radiation-induced thrombosis with either focused gamma rays (C) or proton beam therapy (D). BCNU is used in the management of malignant astrocytomas (E).

96. **(D)** Under no circumstances should the mobility of the neck be assessed in a trauma patient. It should remain in a cervical collar and be immobilized. Inspection of the skull and face for fractures (A), the pupils (B) for reaction and size, the ears and nose for otorrhea and rhinorrhea (C), and position of the trachea (E) for deviation should all be part of the head and neck survey.

97. **(C)** A tension pneumothorax is suspected with a rapid heart rate, absent breath sounds, and a deviated trachea. It is an emergency and needle thoracostomy is urgently required. An esophageal intubation (A) should be suspected with the absence of breath sounds and gastric sounds on auscultation. A right main stem (B) bronchus may be detected by the presence of unequal breath sounds. A hemothorax (D) should be suspected by a decrease in breath sounds and dullness on percussion. Atelectasis (E) will not be associated with a deviated trachea or absent breath sounds.

98. **(C)** A tension pneumothorax is a surgical emergency. It needs urgent needle thoracotomy to convert it to a simple pneumothorax. With the simple pneumothorax, standard tube thoracotomy is then indicated. There is no time to get a chest X-ray (A). Repositioning the tube (B) will not correct the problem. A chest tube (D) takes more time and needle thoracotomy must be performed first. Positive pressure (E) will not correct the problem, either.

99. **(B)** Cullen's sign is faint ecchymosis around the umbilicus as a result of hemoperitoneum. Grey-Turner's sign (A) is ecchymosis on the abdomen and flanks as a result of infiltration of the extraperitoneal tissues with blood. Murphy's sign (C) is inspiratory arrest secondary to acute cholecystitis. McBurney's sign (D) is tenderness over McBurney's point midway between the umbilicus and anterior superior iliac spine in acute appendicitis. There is no such sign as Cushing's sign (E).

100. **(A)** A skull film is rarely ordered because with skull trauma, a CT of the head and brain is ordered, and it will usually reveal skull fractures better than plain film. In the evaluation of the trauma patient, the lateral C-spine (C), chest X-ray (D), and pelvis (E) films are almost routine. A mandible film (B) is usually ordered with facial fracture.

101. **(B)** With a fractured femur it is possible to have associated vascular damage and, thus, with a fractured left femur you could lose the peripheral pulses of the left foot. It is unlikely to have warm toes (A) with absent pulses. A popliteal pulse (D) would be distal to the femur and not be absent. The brachial pulse (E) is in the arm and is unrelated to the lower extremities.

102. **(B)** The Glasgow coma scale is the sum of a number from 1 to 4 for best eye opening, 1 to 6 for best motor response, and 1 to 5 for best verbal response. The score is, therefore, from 3 to 15 and correlates somewhat with prognosis of the patient.

Eye Opening		Best motor response		Best verbal response	
Spontaneous	4	Obeys	6	Oriented	5
To speech	3	Localizes	5	Confused conversation	4
To pain	2	Withdraws	4	Inappropriate words	3
Nil	1	Abnormal flexion	3	Incomprehensible sounds	2
		Extension response	2	Nil	1
		Nil	1		

This patient receives 2 + 1 + 1, and this equals 4.

103. **(B)** The respiratory pattern of midbrain compression is hyperventilatory. Deep sighs and yawns (C) are seen with early diencephalon compression. Cheyne-Stokes (E) respiration is seen with late diencephalon compression.

104. **(B)** Left homonymous hemianopsia involves loss of the left temporal and right nasal fields and is the result of a lesion of the right optic tract. A left optic tract lesion (A) would produce the opposite. A left optic nerve lesion (C) would produce a blind left eye, and a right optic nerve

lesion (D) would produce a blind right eye. A lesion of the optic chiasm (E) would produce a bitemporal hemianopsia.

105. **(C)** Drooping of the upper eyelids is known as ptosis. It may be congenital, acquired, or neurogenic in origin. An outfolding of the eyelid is an ectropion (A). An infolding of the eyelid is an entropion (B). Enophthalmos (D) is an eyeball that is retrusive, and exophthalmos (E) is an eyeball that is protrusive.

106. **(C)** A myocardial infarction must be excluded in a 50-year-old male with the additional risk factors of hypertension and hyperlipidemia and this clinical history (C). In this clinical setting, it is inappropriate to administer medications until a history and examination have been performed (A). In persons with myocardial infarction, time from onset of symptoms until the administration of thrombolytics is critical. Therefore, examination should be undertaken immediately to exclude this cause of symptoms (B). This patient has a scheduled appointment. Presumably, insurance coverage issues were addressed at the time the appointment was verified (E).

107. **(A)** The electrocardiogram is of only fair technical quality, with significant baseline artifact in the precordial leads. Despite this, dramatic changes of acute inferolateral injury and the probable infarction are visible. The ST segments are markedly elevated in the inferior leads, culminating in hyperacute T waves. Hyperacute changes are probably also present in V4-V6 since the T waves are broadened and peaked. Mirror-image reciprocal changes are seen in lead aVL and the anterior precordial leads. In the absence of contraindications, thrombolytic therapy is the treatment of choice in persons with an acute myocardial infarction (A). It is indicated for persons with ischemic symptoms persisting for more than 30 minutes in the presence of new ST segment elevation of at least 0.1 mV in at least two inferior, anterior, or lateral leads. Chewable aspirin, 160 mg, is administered simultaneously with fibrinolytic therapy (B). Oral use of beta-adrenergic blockers following acute myocardial infarction is supported by well-conducted clinical trials (C). An upper gastrointestinal endoscopy is contraindicated in this clinical setting (D). There is no clinical indication to perform a lung scan (E).

108. **(E)** In the primary prevention of lipid disorders (adults without coronary artery disease or other evidence of atherosclerosis), a cholesterol level less than 200 mg/dL is considered desirable (B). Risk factors for coronary artery disease include males older than 45 years, females older than 55 years, premature menopause, smoking, hypertension, diabetes, family history of premature coronary artery disease, and an HDL cholesterol less than 35 mg/dL (D). An HDL cholesterol greater than 50 mg/dL is considered a negative risk factor for coronary artery disease (C). In secondary prevention of lipid disorders (adults with evidence of coronary artery disease or other evidence of atherosclerosis), the optimal LDL cholesterol is 100 mg/dL or lower (A). Both serum total cholesterol and HDL cholesterol levels can be measured at any time of the day. Fasting is not essential, since a fat-containing meal does not significantly affect these tests (E).

109. **(A)** The angiogram shows a proximal stenosis of the left anterior descending coronary artery [(A) and (C)]. No aneurysms are evident on this study (B). In polyarteritis nodosa, there is a segmental, spotty distribution of arterial lesions. Necrotizing inflammation affects the small and medium-sized muscular arteries (D). No stent is evident on this study (E).

110. **(E)** Troponin I and T, in concert with troponin C, regulate the calcium-dependent interactions between myosin and actin (C). The differences in the amino acid sequences between troponin I and T in cardiac muscle from those in skeletal muscle permitted the development of monoclonal antibodies with very little cross-reactivity (A). In several clinical studies, levels of troponin I and T have been shown to be sensitive and specific markers of myocardial cell injury (D). A quantitative relationship has also been reported between cardiac troponin T levels and long-term clinical outcome for persons with either unstable angina or non-Q wave myocardial infarction (B). The cost-effectiveness of measuring these proteins remains to be established (E).

111. **(A)** The arteriogram demonstrates complete occlusion of the right common iliac artery. Revascularization procedures (both operative and nonoperative) are usually reserved for persons with disabling symptoms or rest pain. Percutaneous transluminal angioplasty is successful in over

90% of cases of iliac artery lesions, with three-year patency rates exceeding 75% (B). Rotational atherectomy is useful when lesions are fibrotic or calcified. Although clinical trials are still to be done, this procedure is thought to be particularly useful in smaller vessels (C). An intravascular stent is a wire-mesh collar, which is crimped on a deflated balloon. The stent, after being placed across the atherosclerotic lesion, is expanded by inflating the balloon. Patency rates exceeding 90% at one year have been reported for iliac artery lesions (D). Surgical approaches include endarterectomy of the stenotic artery or a bypass procedure. Immediate postoperative graft patency rates approach 99% for aortofemoral bypass procedures (E). Pentoxifylline, 400 mg orally TID, which acts by increasing red cell membrane deformability and thereby decreasing effective blood viscosity, prolongs the duration of exercise and the distance the patient can walk before the onset of claudication occurs. Pentoxifylline is most commonly used in occlusive disease of the arteries in the lower leg and foot (A).

112. **(A)** Brain imaging is an important test to evaluate focal neurologic dysfunction. Because contrast-enhancing agents carry a small risk of neurotoxicity and the potential to obscure a small hypodense infarct, noncontrast studies are preferred initially. The noncontrast computed tomographic scans shown here demonstrate early characteristic changes of an infarct in the distribution of the right middle cerebral artery. In Panel A, the normal gray-white differentiation is seen at the insular cortex on the left, but is absent on the right ("insular ribbon sign"). The right sylvian fissure is effaced when compared to the left. In Panel B, the left-sided sulci are better seen. The cortical gyri have a preserved gray-white differentiation when compared to the right. There is also a slightly diminished density in the distribution of the right middle cerebral artery, which is best demonstrated in the frontal and occipital regions (A). The lateral medullary syndrome, one cause of which is occlusion of the posterior inferior cerebellar artery, presents with a clinical syndrome of severe vertigo, nausea, vomiting, nystagmus, ipsilateral ataxia, and ipsilateral Horner's syndrome (B). Basilar artery occlusion produces massive brain stem dysfunction. The locked-in state is one of the most severe clinical manifestations (C). Occlusion of the posterior cerebral artery presents with loss

of all or part of the visual field, depending on site of occlusion. Memory deficits, visual hallucinations, and dyslexia may also occur (D). A transient ischemic attack (TIA) is a neurologic deficit caused by decreased blood flow in a particular artery supplying the brain. Although it has been arbitrarily defined as a deficit lasting less than 24 hours, most TIAs resolve within an hour (E).

113. **(A)** Compared to the computerized tomographic scans obtained at the time of admission, these scans demonstrate severe hypodensity in the distribution of the right middle cerebral artery, consistent with a right cerebral infarction. These hypodense infarcts develop increasingly well-demarcated margins as edema peaks between three and five days [(C) and (E)]. Also demonstrated here is a shift in the midline from right to left [(A) and (B)]. A mass effect on the ventricular system is evident (D).

114. **(E)** He has a substance abuse problem and needs medical help.

115. **(A)** Asymptomatic osteoporosis is extremely common and is of high prevalence in postmenopausal females. Osteoporosis (B) is the most common underlying disorder in fracture of the neck of the femur in the elderly and may lead to ischemic necrosis of the femoral head. Back pain (C) is the most common complaint in patients with osteoporosis and occurs secondary to fractures and collapse of weakened vertebrae. Blood levels of calcium, phosphate, and alkaline phosphatase are normal in osteoporosis (D) unlike other bone diseases such as Paget's disease or metastatic bone involvement. Long-term heparin use (E) predisposes toward the development of osteoporosis, as does glucocorticoid use and renal failure.

116. **(B)** All of the answer choices are possible complications from placement of a central line, but the symptoms of acute onset of shortness of breath, chest pain, and tachycardia, occasionally with hypotension, are concerns for tension pneumothorax. The diagnosis is made clinically with decreased breath sounds on the ipsilateral side and deviation of the trachea to the contralateral side.

117. **(A)** Although poorly controlled diabetics are susceptible to numerous infections, the history and physical examination are suggestive of

rhinocerebral mucomycosis, a medical emergency. The classic black necrotic turbinates are often mistaken for a "dried blood appearance" on the nasal mucosa. The CAT scan shows involvement of the paranasal sinuses and periorbital soft tissues. Immediate admission to the hospital for further diagnostic and therapeutic measures is most appropriate [(A) and (D)]. Therapy with penicillin, antihistamines, other broad spectrum antibiotics, and acyclovir are inappropriate [(B), (C), and (E)].

118. **(E)** Regardless of its financial impact on the study, you must report the adverse reaction. It is unethical to withhold such information. The purpose of adverse reports is to inform the pharmaceutical company and the FDA and ultimately to protect the public from any adverse events. There is nothing to discuss with your colleagues, except if they are interested in the study, and you do not need a lawyer, since the liability, if any, is with the company, if you do what you are responsible for, i.e., reporting the side effect.

119. **(B)** Dysentery occurs secondary to mucosal invasion of the pathogenic organism. Common causes include *Shigella* and enteroinvasive *E. coli*. Ulcerative erosions into arterial vessels are a mechanism of GI bleeding from peptic ulcer disease (A). Dysentery is not generally associated with a systemic coagulopathy unless sepsis and disseminated intravascular coagulation develop (C). Thrombosis of submucosal capillaries does not occur in dysentery (D). Bowel necrosis is a cause of bleeding in ischemic bowel disease, but is not common in infectious dysentery (E).

120. **(A)** The Centers for Disease Control functions to promote disease control and health-education programs, and to promote immunization.

121. **(B)** The Environmental Protection Agency (EPA) is a federally funded agency that is in charge for protection and promotion of environmental quality. The EPA issues rules and regulations for hazardous waste control, for solid waste disposal, and for recovery of resources from wastes.

122. **(C)** The American Cancer Society is a nonprofit voluntary agency. It has been organized in an attempt to increase cancer awareness.

123. **(E)** Formerly known as Professional Standards Review Organizations, Professional Review Organizations (PROs) is a nonprofit association that works closely with businesses as well as the Department of Health and Human Services to ensure quality medical care and hospital utilization. Their responsibilities include reviewing the quality of medical care provided to Medicaid and Medicare patients.

124. **(E)** Screening asymptomatic patients for lung cancer by either sputum cytology (A) or chest X ray (B) is not recommended. There is insufficient evidence for routine performance of tonometry to screen for glaucoma (C) or endoscopy to detect laryngeal cancer (D).

125. **(A)** This woman has clinical sinusitis. The most appropriate thing to do initially is to prescribe antibiotics. If this were a chronic condition, or kept recurring, a further work-up may be indicated, such as ordering plain films (B) or a CAT scan (C). Aspiration of the sinus (D) or exenteration (E) would be more radical and may be indicated in more extreme cases of chronic sinusitis.

126. **(C)** Breast cancer is the most likely cancer to metastasize to bone of the choices given. Other cancers that commonly metastasize to bone include thyroid, prostate, kidney, and lung. The other cancers mentioned (ovary, uterus, colon, and stomach) are less likely to metastasize to bone [(A), (B), (D), and (E)].

127. **(D)** She is not infected, but should change her lifestyle. The HIV antibody test is composed of an ELISA test which is extremely sensitive, but lacks 100% specificity. There is a two percent false-positive rate. Therefore, each positive ELISA test is confirmed by a Western blot, which, if negative, means that someone is not infected with HIV and has a false-positive on the ELISA test.

128. **(B)** Tobacco smoking will give a patient a burning tongue without a visible lesion. Oral cancer (A) initially will not give a patient a burning tongue, but later may produce ulceration. Odontalgia (C) is a toothache, and will not usually affect the tongue. Myxedema (D) leads to tongue enlargement. Thyrotoxicosis (E) will lead to a tongue tremor.

129. (B) Increased plasma iron is consistent with the diagnosis of hemochromatosis, an autosomal recessive disease characterized by liver disease and diabetes and, occasionally, by autosomal and joint manifestations. Transferrin saturation (A) is increased in genetic hemochromatosis, usually greater than 50%. Iron binding capacity (C) is usually mildly decreased in hemochromatosis. Serum ferritin (D) is increased in hemochromatosis.

130. (A) The diagnosis of somatization disorder (A) must be made before an individual turns 30 years old. Three criteria must be met before the diagnosis can be made: first, there must be complaints of pain in four different bodily sites; second, there must exist two different gastrointestinal complaints; and third, there must be a history of sexual dysfunction or decrease in libido. Undifferentiated somatoform disorder (B) refers to a condition in which only one symptom is complained about for greater than one-half year. It is also a disease with an unidentifiable organic cause. Conversion disorder (C) is a disease in which a patient claims loss of motor or sensory power in a hysterical manner. Pain disorder (D) is a disease in which patients complain about pain without any organic basis. Hypochondriasis (E) is a disorder in which a patient becomes fixated on the apprehension of contracting a serious disease. The disorder is characterized by a non-delusional state and the patient is not relaxed by reassurance from medical personnel. It also exists for more than six months.

131. (D) The recurrent crampy nature of the pain is consistent with biliary colic. A right upper quadrant ultrasound should be done to rule out cholelithiasis.

132. (D) The antithyroid microsomal antibody test is elevated not only in autoimmune Grave's disease but also in Hashimoto's thyroiditis. Grave's disease is associated with thyrotoxicosis, and Hashimoto's thyroiditis is associated with hypothyroidism. The serum thyroglobulin concentrations (A) are increased in all forms of hyperthyroidism. The thyroid radionucleotide uptake and scan (B) are usually increased in thyrotoxicosis. The thyroid-stimulating hormone assay (C) would be below 1.0 in any form of thyrotoxicosis. The

free thyroxine level (E) would be elevated in hyperthyroidism.

133. (D) The bone-mineral density would be decreased, not increased, in Grave's disease secondary to increased bone turnover from elevated metabolic activity. Grave's disease is an autoimmune disease associated with an increase in catabolic activity and excessive sympathomimetic activity. The serum antithyroglobulin antibody level (A) is usually elevated in Grave's disease. Anemia (B), mild hypercalcemia, mild elevations of liver function tests, and tachycardia (C) are detectable in Grave's disease. There is an increased uptake on the thyroid scan (E) in Grave's disease.

134. (C) Therapy of hyperthyroidism depends on the etiology of the problem. Currently, permanent radioactive iodine ablation is the treatment of choice for Grave's disease. If subsequent hypothyroidism occurs after ablation, then only one pill needs to be taken (Synthroid) instead of multiple antithyroid medications. L-thyroxine (A) is the treatment of choice for any cause of hypothyroidism. Prednisone (B) is the treatment of choice for self-limited thyroiditis that is very painful. Nonsteroidal anti-inflammatory agents (D) are also useful to alleviate the pain and inflammation in subacute thyroiditis secondary to a viral infection or iodide-induced thyroiditis. Tapazole (E) and Propylthiouracil (PTU) are antithyroid drugs that are used to suppress thyroxine production. They both have side effects and have to be taken multiple times a day. Thyroid ablation is the current treatment of choice for Grave's disease.

135. (A) All dirty wounds and dog bites, if not checked at the hospital, should be checked the following day. It is not uncommon to have a wound become infected within 24 hours. Checking the wound early will give you the opportunity to catch an infection before it worsens.

136. (B) The most likely cause of conjunctivitis in a child is bacterial. It will almost always lead to a clinical "pink eye." Viral conjunctivitis (A) is less common. Patients with upper respiratory infection (C) will have watery eyes, but they won't be pink. Blepharitis (D) is an infection of the eyelid and lashes with the presence of a matted exudate.

137. (A) The mother of the infected child should be treated all of the time.

138. **(A)** Alpha-adrenergic blockers such as phentolamine are helpful in mild cases of stress incontinence. The patient in question, however, has been diagnosed with mixed incontinence which involves overflow incontinence (due to obstruction) and neurogenic incontinence (secondary to conditions such as diabetic neuropathy). Biofeedback therapy (B) in conjunction with pelvic muscle exercises can help patients control pelvic muscles and reduce incontinence. Anticholinergic agents (C), such as oxybutynin and propantheline, can help patients with urge incontinence by relaxing sphincter muscles. Bladder training (D) requires the patient to resist or inhibit the sensation of urgency, to postpone voiding, and to urinate according to a timetable rather than according to urge. Routine and scheduled toilet assistance (E) is used to empty the bladder regularly to prevent leaking.

139. **(B)** *Gardnerella vaginalitis* or *Hemophilus vaginalitis* is the causative agent here. Treatment is with metronidazole. With *Trichomonas* infection (A), one usually observes a frothy vaginal discharge and trichomonads on saline wet mount. HPV (C) causes genital warts (condyloma acuminata) and can cause dysplasia and cancer of the cervix. *Candida albicans* (D) causes vaginal yeast infections characterized by cottage cheese-like discharge, and hyphae and buds observed on KOH wet mount. Chlamydial infection (E) can cause a urethritis and salpingitis.

140. **(A)** Ingestion of acetaminophen (Tylenol) is one of the leading causes of drug overdose in the United States. Toxicity may occur with a minimum acute ingestion of 140 mg/kg (approximately 10 grams). In persons who present within four hours of ingestion, activated charcoal should be administered. In an adult, activated charcoal is administered in a dose of 50-100 grams (C). Syrup of ipecac, although less effective than activated charcoal, is indicated for home use of poisonings. The usual dose is 30 ml in an adult (D). Sodium bicarbonate is indicated as intravenous treatment of life-threatening arrhythmias due to tricyclic overdose (B). Forced diuresis is effective for overdose with phenobarbital or salicylates (E). Due to the potential fatal nature of this overdose, the most appropriate advice is to call the emergency medical service (A).

141. **(D)** Acute toxicity of acetaminophen is hepatic, usually appearing 24-48 hours following overdose [(A), (B), and (E)]. In overdose, ingestion of two or more drugs is common. In all cases, it is important to query the family and friends, as well as to evaluate pill bottles and other supporting materials. Screening of blood, urine, and gastric aspirates for drugs is also necessary (C). Nomograms have been established for monitoring plasma or serum concentrations following overdose. These nomograms are used prognostically and therapeutically (D).

142. **(B)** Based on the nomogram, the plasma acetaminophen level is clearly in the toxic range, assuming that the level was drawn when the patient arrived, which was at least eight hours post ingestion. Acetylcysteine (Mucomyst), 140 mg/kg orally or by gastric tube, administered as an initial load, followed by 70 mg/kg q4H for a total of 17 doses, is the definitive treatment. It is preferably administered within eight hours post ingestion, but may be effective if administered up to 24 hours post ingestion (B). Activated charcoal, 50-100 grams orally, is appropriate if the patient presents within four hours post ingestion. If administered less than one hour prior to acetylcysteine, any residual charcoal should be removed by gastric lavage (A). Phytonadione (vitamin K1), 10 mg, administered intramuscularly or subcutaneously, is an antidote for overdose with warfarin. At this point, there is no evidence of a coagulopathy (C). Dimercaprol (BAL), 2.5-5.0 mg/kg IM q4-6H, is an antidote for heavy metal poisonings (D). Deferoxamine mesylate, 1 gram IM q8H or 10-15 mg/Kg/h IV infusion, is an antidote for iron overdose (E).

143. **(A)** Acetylcysteine is the definitive treatment for acetaminophen overdose, when toxic levels are present. The drug is thought to act by providing a reservoir of sulfhydryl groups, which bind to toxic metabolites (A). Alternatively, the drug may stimulate the synthesis and repletion of hepatic glutathione [(B) and (C)]. In ethylene glycol poisoning, pyridoxine may be administered to promote the conversion of glyoxylate to glycine (D). In organophosphate poisoning, pralidoxime reactivates cholinesterase, thereby counteracting clinical signs of weakness, muscle fasciculations, and respiratory depression (E).

144. **(C)** In this setting, the most likely diagnosis is acetaminophen toxicity. Nausea, vomiting,

diarrhea, and abdominal pain are characteristic complaints occurring 4-12 hours post ingestion. In view of potential hepatotoxicity, monitoring liver function is critical (C). It is too early for hepatic disease to be evident on liver spleen scans (B). Extrahepatic disease is also unlikely in a previously healthy woman (A). Acetaminophen is not toxic to the gastrointestinal tract (D). In this previously healthy female, the likelihood of an infectious agent causing the clinical picture is remote (E).

145. **(B)** The typical early symptoms of acetaminophen hepatotoxicity are usually followed by a 12-24 hour period of relative quiescence [(C) and (D)]. As the initial symptoms resolve, the hepatic damage becomes manifest. Maximal damage may not be evident for four to six days following ingestion (B). Because of the massive dose of acetaminophen ingested, hepatic damage is expected in this case. Discharge during the period of risk is not appropriate [(A) and (E)].

146. **(B)** Survivors of acute acetaminophen toxicity usually recover completely, without evidence of residual liver disease (B). Serum aminotransferase levels (ALT, AST) commonly exceed 5,000 U/L. Hypoglycemia, lactic acidosis, and coagulopathy may also be present (D). Hepatic disease may take up to six days to peak before resolution begins.

147. **(C)** Acetaminophen, phenacetin, and aspirin may all be nephrotoxic when consumed in large quantities for prolonged periods. Analgesic nephropathy is characterized by tubulointerstitial damage and papillary necrosis. More than half of these patients have pyuria, which may be either sterile or associated with pyelonephritis (A). Proteinuria is typically mild, with less than 1-2 grams of protein excreted each day (C). A "ring sign," representing a radiolucent sloughed papilla on an intravenous pyelogram, is pathognomonic of papillary necrosis (B). Progression to end-stage renal failure occurs over several years (D). Transitional cell carcinoma of the urinary pelvis or ureters may develop as a late complication of analgesic abuse (E).

148. **(A)** The proper location for the tip of a Swan-Ganz, or pulmonary artery catheter, is in the pulmonary artery or in one of the main branches,

usually the right. Choice (A) is the only one that would meet this criterion.

149. **(A)** The anion gap in this patient is elevated and the bicarbonate suggests metabolic by subtracting $(CL + HCO_3)$ from NA. Type IV renal tubular acidosis results in a normal anion gap with metabolic acidosis and is, therefore, not consistent with this patient. Renal failure (B) is associated with a rise in organic acids, while diabetic ketoacidosis is associated with elevated ketoacids, both of which are non-chloride anions. Sepsis (D) is associated with elevated lactic acid, and ethylene glycol ingestion (E) is associated with elevated glycolic acids.

150. **(A)** Classically, GN will present with hematuria with the red cell casts. Sometimes, patients will complain of urinary frequency and dysuria, as well.

151. **(D)** In a routine cystitis, evidenced by urine dipstick positive for nitrite and leukocyte esterase, routine cultures usually are not necessary, and appropriate empiric antibiotics can be begun.

152. **(A)** In uncomplicated cystitis, the appropriate treatment is a short term (three days) of oral medications such as sulfa drugs, fluoroquinolones, or first-generation cephalosporins.

153. **(E)** Pelvic inflammatory disease presents with symptoms similar to this woman's. On examination, a friable cervical mucosa is often seen. Patients classically complain of cervical motion tenderness and often have adnexal tenderness as well. The presence of genital warts shows that previous unprotected sexual activity has occurred and that the patient has potentially been exposed to other sexually transmitted diseases, as well.

154. **(B)** These cells are infected epithelial cells and are called clue cells. The pear-shaped organisms are classic for trichomoniasis. Hyphae are present in yeast infections. White cells are usually not present in bacterial vaginosis because the infection is a superficial infection.

155. **(C)** In the absence of another diagnosis, bladder spasm must be considered. Commonly, patients will complain of suprapubic tenderness and irritative voiding symptoms.

156. **(B)** The appropriate treatment for bladder spasm is an anti-spasmodic, such as phenazopyridine.

157. **(C)** Hematuria of unknown etiology must always be followed up. If it doesn't clear, it should be followed up by cystogram or cystoscopy.

158 **(C)** Vertigo may be either physiologic or pathologic. Physiologic vertigo results from a mismatch of the three stabilizing sensory systems (vestibular, visual, and somatosensory). Motion sickness is exacerbated by sitting in a closed space or by reading, which gives the visual system the miscue that the environment is stationary (A). Height vertigo results from a mismatch between the sensation of normal body sway and lack of its visual detection (B). Seasickness results from maladaptation of the vestibular system when it is subjected to unfamiliar head movements (E). Benign positional vertigo (BPV) is the most common cause of pathologic vertigo (C). It can result from head injury, viral labyrinthitis, vascular occlusion, or for unknown reasons. It is thought to be produced from free-floating calcium carbonate crystals that inadvertently enter the long arm of the posterior semicircular canal (D).

159. **(B)** Antinuclear antibodies are one of the best screening tests for systemic lupus erythematosis (SLE). If they are negative, there is a less than one percent chance that the disease will develop (A). More than 95% of persons with SLE will manifest a positive ANA if the test substrate contains human nuclei, such as WIL-2 or HEP-2 cells (B). ANAs may be present in low titer in normal persons (D). The frequency of positivity increases with age (C). Many drugs induce ANA positivity. Between 50-75% of persons taking procainamide for several months will develop ANA positivity (E).

160. **(E)** The diagnosis of systemic lupus erythematosus (SLE) is confirmed by the presence of characteristic antibodies. The specificity of antibodies to double-stranded DNA and to Sm exceed 95% (A). Antibodies to double-stranded DNA are more specific for SLE than antibodies to single-stranded DNA (E). High serum levels of anti-dsDNA usually correlate with disease activity, especially renal disease (C). Anti-Ro (SSA) is associated with Sjögren's syndrome and is also common in ANA-negative SLE (D).

161. **(E)** Hypocomplementemia is common in patients with immune complex disease. The most commonly used assays for diagnosis and management of these diseases are CH50, C3, and C4. Low levels of complement usually reflect disease activity, especially renal involvement (A). Total functional hemolytic complement levels are the most sensitive measure of complement activation, but also the most subject to laboratory error [(B) and (C)]. Very low levels of CH50 with normal levels of C3 suggest an inherited deficiency of a complement component (D). C1q, C1r, C1s, C4, and C2 deficiencies have all been associated with SLE, SLE-like syndromes, discoid lupus, glomerulonephritis, and vasculitis. C1 INH deficiency is associated with angioneurotic edema (E).

162. **(E)** The American Rheumatism Association developed criteria for the classification of SLE, rather than the diagnosis of SLE. However, if at least four of the overall criteria are present, the sensitivity and specificity for SLE is approximately 96%. The hematologic criteria are one component of these overall criteria. Anemia occurs in at least half of patients with active disease. Although chronic disease anemia is the most common, a Coombs'-positive anemia with reticulocytosis (A) also occurs (E). Leukopenia, thought to be due to immune mechanisms, is common, but rarely associated with infection (B). Lymphopenia, also thought to be secondary to immune mechanisms, may occur with active disease (C). Mild, but not severe, thrombocytopenia also occurs commonly (D).

163. **(B)** The lupus anticoagulant (LA) is a member of the family of antiphospholipid antibodies. The LA is recognized by a prolonged thromboplastin time (B), which does not correct with the addition of normal plasma [(C) and (A)]. More sensitive tests are the Russell viper venom time and the rabbit brain neutral phospholipid test [(D) and (E)].

164. **(C)** Laboratory tests help to distinguish drug-induced lupus from the idiopathic form of the disease. In both conditions, ANA positivity exceeds 95% (C). In the drug-induced form, antibodies to double-stranded DNA are rare (A). Hypocomplementemia is also rare (B). Anti-histone

antibodies are very common in the drug-induced form, but rare in SLE (D). Persons who are slow acetylatora or positive for HLA-DR4 are at increased risk for developing drug-induced lupus (E).

165. **(B)** Spontaneous stillbirths and miscarriages occur in SLE, with overall fetal losses approaching 50%. Women with antiphospholipid antibodies are predisposed to recurrent mid-trimester fetal loss (A). Fetal mortality increases in the presence of major organ involvement, especially renal disease (B). Neonatal lupus is a rare condition. Transmission of maternal anti-Ro antibodies across the placenta predisposes to neonatal lupus (C). Transient neonatal thrombocytopenia is thought to result from maternal antiplatelet antibodies (D). Congenital heart block is associated with anti-Ro antibodies (E).

166. **(A)** Approximately half of patients with SLE develop clinical lupus nephritis. Minimal or mesangial nephritis, which has a very good prognosis, is characterized by a minimally active urinary sediment and mild-to-moderate proteinuria (B). Approximately one quarter of those with focal proliferative nephritis develop the nephrotic syndrome (E). Diffuse proliferative glomerulonephritis is associated with an active urinary sediment, proteinuria (which may be in the nephrotic range), decreased glomerular clearance, hypocomplementemia, and elevations in immune complexes (C). In membranous glomerulonephritis, there is marked proteinuria, but a relatively benign sediment (D). Berger's disease (IgA nephropathy) is characterized by deposition of IgA in the glomeruli (A).

167. **(C)** A history of peptic ulcers is not associated with any particular etiology of dysphagia. The etiology of dysphagia can usually be determined by a careful history. Solid-food dysphagia is more common in structural lesions of the esophagus, while liquid-food dysphagia is more common with neuromuscular dysphagia (A). A prolonged duration of symptoms suggests non-malignant process, while new-onset dysphagia is more worrisome for malignancy (B). A history of heartburn suggests the possibility of a reflux-associated peptic stricture (D). Associated weight loss is often seen with dysphagia related to esophageal carcinoma (E).

168. **(E)** The classic finding of achalasia on barium swallow includes the "bird's beak esophagus," a gradual tapering of a dilated esophagus to a narrowed gastroesophageal junction. Esophageal cancer usually appears as a stricture or asymmetrical narrowing in the esophagus on barium swallow (A). A Schatzki's ring appears immediately above the gastroesophageal junction as a fixed, symmetrical "shelf-like" irregularity (B). Barium swallow in patients with diffuse esophageal spasm shows aperistaltic contractions and is often described as a "cork-screw esophagus" (C). Peptic stricture is difficult to differentiate from other causes of structural dysphagia by barium swallow alone, but does not show an aperistaltic, dilated esophagus (D).

169. **(A)** Esophageal manometry is the gold standard for the diagnosis of achalasia. Twenty-four-hour pH probe is the gold standard for the diagnosis of gastroesophageal reflux disease (B). Proton pump inhibitors are useful in the treatment of peptic ulcer disease and gastroesophageal reflux disease, but are generally not useful in patients with achalasia (C). Full thickness esophageal biopsy cannot be performed through an endoscope and would not be useful in attempting to diagnose achalasia (D). Pneumatic balloon dilation is usually the treatment of choice for achalasia; however, due to the associated risk of esophageal perforation, this procedure is generally not performed unless the diagnosis of achalasia is confirmed (E).

170. **(C)** Esophageal cancers in the distal esophagus most commonly arise from Barrett's mucosa, a metaplastic transformation of the normal esophageal squamous mucosa into a specialized columnar epithelium (SCE). SCE can progress to dysplasia and subsequently into adenocarcinoma. Squamous cell cancers are also common in the esophagus, but occur more commonly in the proximal esophagus (B). Sarcomas are rare in the esophagus (B). Unfortunately, patients with esophageal cancer rarely develop symptoms until the tumor has progressed beyond the stage of carcinoma-in-situ (D). As discussed, Barrett's mucosa is a metaplastic transformation of the esophagus, which is a preneoplastic lesion (E).

171. **(B)** The first step is always the history and examination. This patient has an acute septic arthritis with an effusion. Aspirating this will help

guide your management by sending for leukocyte count, Gram stain, and cultures. A CBC (A) may be reasonable, especially if the patient has a fever; however, the rest will not help in the diagnosis. A radiograph of the knee (C) will typically show only soft tissue swelling. MRI (D) is not indicated. Blood cultures (E) should be done along with other fluids and may help guide the source from which this infection disseminated.

172. **(D)** Antibiotics are administered intravenously, typically for two to four weeks. Drainage is facilitated by daily joint aspirations until fluid no longer accumulates. There is no reason for bed rest (B). The affected joint should be at rest when acutely inflamed; however, mobilization is essential to prevent atrophy when the acute inflammation has diminished.

173. **(E)** Risk factors for septic arthritis include immunosuppression, previous joint damage (rheumatoid arthritis and joint surgery), trauma, penetrating wounds, and prosthetic joint replacement. There is also a risk for septic arthritis in very young patients. His recent surgery is most likely his highest risk. Choice (A) only may aggravate his arthritis. Diabetes (B) may provide a risk if he is severely debilitated, especially with the other mentioned predisposing conditions. Choice (C) is a possibility, but not as likely as his recent surgery. Choice (D) may predispose if he had a septicemia in view of his concomitant problems (recent joint surgery and arthritis).

174. **(E)** With a patient in an asthma attack, it is important to quickly assess the patient and give treatment. Registering the patient (A) is not a good option. You should institute treatment based on the clinical presentation rather than waiting for a blood gas (B) or a chest X-ray (C). Intubation (D) may be necessary later, based on the results of treatment.

175. **(C)** Answering this question requires knowledge of the hemoglobin oxygen saturation curve. An oxygen saturation of 90% corresponds to an arterial oxygen tension of 60 mm Hg. Below this point, rapid arterial desaturation occurs. A saturation of 89% corresponds to a PaO_2 of about 57 mm Hg.

176. **(A)** Small cell carcinoma pulmonary malignancy is not associated with rheumatoid arthritis. Pulmonary nodules are associated with rheumatoid arthritis (B). In Caplan's syndrome, patients with rheumatoid arthritis who are exposed to industrial agents develop pulmonary nodules. Obliterative bronchiolitis and fibrosing alveolitis may develop in rheumatoid arthritis in a manner similar to lupus or scleroderma [(C) and (E)]. Pleural effusions are common in rheumatoid arthritis and other connective tissue diseases (D).

177. **(E)** There are numerous extra-articular manifestations of rheumatoid arthritis. However, urethral discharge is not associated with rheumatoid arthritis; rather it is a manifestation of the rheumatoid factor negative arthropathy, Reiter's syndrome. Episcleritis occurs in approximately one percent of patients with rheumatoid arthritis (B). Felty's syndrome is a condition consisting of rheumatoid arthritis, splenomegaly, leukopenia, and thrombocytopenia (C). Pericarditis is often seen in patients with rheumatoid arthritis, although it is usually asymptomatic (D).

178. **(A)** Your first step in any diagnosis is a complete history and physical exam. There is no substitute for this. The adjunctive radiological exams offered in the answer choices may be ordered, but only after a thorough clinical examination. The exams may then be ordered more judiciously based on the clinical exam.

179. **(E)** In a herniated disc, the gelatinous substance around the spinal cord, the nucleus propulses, herniates and causes impingement of the nerves. Depending on the history and examination, there is a wide variety of treatment. Conservative measures such as traction (A), nonsteroidal anti-inflammatory drugs (C), and muscle relaxants (D) may be given, or surgery (B) may be the treatment of choice. In no circumstance would neck exercises be instituted, because it could only worsen the acute situation.

180. **(C)** Bacterial meningitis is the least likely cause of such prolonged fevers of undetermined origin, as this infection is almost always fatal if not treated rapidly. Diverticulitis (A) and other intra-abdominal infections are a common cause of

fever of unknown origin (FUO). Hodgkin's disease (B), as well as other hematological malignancies, such as leukemia, are another common cause. Factitious fever (D) can be very difficult to diagnose, but also must be considered in the differential diagnosis. Temporal arteritis (E) should be considered in middle-aged and elderly patients with FUO and nonspecific symptoms. Biopsy may be necessary to make the diagnosis.

USMLE Step 3 – Practice Test 1
Day Two – Afternoon Session

1. **(D)** Pearly margin, telangiectatic vessels, and central ulceration are classic findings of BCC, although some tumors may be multifocal. Tumors are locally invasive but they are rarely metastatic (A). Tumors are generally slow growing (B). Hemorrhage from the lesion (C) is not a common presentation of BCC.

2. **(D)** Deep venous thrombosis is a common cause of unilateral leg swelling; however, the occurrence of bilateral DVT is unusual. Right-heart failure (A) is a common cause of pedal edema secondary to passive congestion. Obstruction of the inferior vena cava (B) secondary to malignancy can also cause bilateral pedal edema. Constrictive pericarditis (C) secondary to pericardial infiltration or infusion is another possibility. Liver failure (E) with subsequent volume expansion and hypoalbuminemia is also a common cause.

3. **(D)** Poststreptococcal glomerulopathy is a cause of nephritis rather than nephrotic syndrome. Diabetes mellitus (A), in its advanced stages, may cause nephrotic range proteinuria. Amyloidosis (B) is another cause of nephrotic syndrome. Minimal change disease (C) is the most common cause of childhood nephrotic syndrome. Focal and segmental glomerulosclerosis (E) may be idiopathic or secondary to heroin abuse and is a cause of nephrotic syndrome in 10-20% of cases.

4. **(B)** Cholesterol is elevated in nephrotic syndrome secondary to increased hepatic synthesis. Compliment levels (A) are usually normal in nephrotic syndrome. Creatinine (C), potassium (D), and blood urea nitrogen (E) are unlikely to be normal until, and only if, the patient develops some degree of renal failure secondary to nephrotic syndrome.

5. **(C)** Multiple myeloma may have many renal manifestations, including amyloidosis, light chain nephropathy, and calcium nephropathy. Lung cancer (A) and other carcinomas are associated with membranous nephropathy. Systemic lupus erythematosus (B) has several renal manifestations, including membranous nephropathy, although it more commonly causes nephritis. Chronic hepatitis B infection (D) and gold therapy (E) are also associated with membranous nephropathy.

6. **(C)** Increased tubular secretion of albumin is not the cause of hypoalbuminemia and albuminuria in the nephrotic syndrome, rather it is a loss of albumin during filtration in the glomeruli. Activation of renin-angiotensin syndrome (A) and renal sodium retention (B) account for the hypervolemic state. Fluid migration into the interstitium (D) occurs as a result of hypoalbuminemia. Increased hepatic lipoprotein synthesis (E) through an unclear mechanism is also present in the nephrotic syndrome and accounts for the increased cholesterol.

7. **(A)** Thirty to fifty percent of patients with membranous nephropathy will progress to end-stage renal disease in 10 years. Unlike minimal change disease, patients with his condition will not have a uniform remission with steroid therapy and its role is controversial (B). Although it is true that all patients do not receive therapy, this is because there are no outstanding therapies available (C). A significant proportion of patients will develop renal failure. There is an increase in the risk of bacterial infections, likely related to losses in the urine of low molecular-weight compliment and immunoglobulin (D).

8. **(B)** Ultrasound/Doppler study of renal veins is the correct answer, as it will allow for the determination of renal vein thrombosis, a common complication of nephrotic syndrome, which presents with an acute deterioration of renal function and often with hematuria. Repeat renal biopsy to evaluate disease progression (A) is not indicated as it would be unlikely to be useful or to change patient management. Therapy with intravenous Cytoxan (C) is also not indicated in membranous nephropathy. Listing for renal transplantation (D) is also not indicated at this time. An acute deterioration of renal function is unlikely to

be secondary to the underlying renal disease in this patient and, therefore, other causes should be sought, such as renal vein thrombosis or interstitial nephritis.

9. **(E)** All of the tests indicated are likely to be elevated concomitant with a reduction in glomerular filtration. Secondary to reduced excretion, potassium (A), phosphorus (B), magnesium (C), and uric acid (D) are all commonly elevated in renal failure. Treatment for removal requires hemodialysis and phosphate binders.

10. **(A)** This patient has thiamine or vitamin B1 deficiency. Early thiamine deficiency presents as anorexia and weight loss. It is very common in alcoholics. Advanced thiamine deficiency presents as beriberi or high-output congestive heart failure. Wernicke-Korsakoff syndrome also is a manifestation of thiamine deficiency in alcoholics. It is associated with progressive mental impairment, nystagmus, gait ataxia, and ophthalmoplegia. The Korsakoff syndrome has memory and confabulation as prominent features.

11. **(C)** This elderly nursing home patient has vitamin C deficiency from lack of intake of citrus fruits, tomatoes, or leafy vegetables. She has symptoms and signs of scurvy, which include capillary fragility, poor wound healing, and swollen and bleeding gums. Joints, muscle, and subcutaneous tissues may become sites of hemorrhage. As little as 10 mg of ascorbic acid a day can completely prevent the clinical manifestations of scurvy.

12. **(B)** Vitamin A is a retinoid. It is fat soluble. Vitamin A has a pivotal role in the differentiation of epithelial tissues, and some researchers say that long-term vitamin A deficiency can lead to an increased risk of cancer. Night blindness is an early manifestation of vitamin A deficiency. This patient has frequent traffic accidents from night blindness.

13. **(E)** Vitamin K deficiency occurs frequently in newborns and manifests clinically as increased tendency to hemorrhage. Fetal stores of vitamin K tend to be low and, thus, newborns lack a supply of vitamin K that can be provided by normal intestinal flora. Deficiency generally does not develop unless there is an abnormality of intestinal

function or an antibiotic therapy is given. The best sources of vitamin K are green, leafy vegetables. Vitamin K is lipid soluble, and a vitamin K deficiency responds rapidly to vitamin K administration, either orally or intramuscularly.

14. **(B)** The cinefluoroscopy study demonstrates an intact aortic valve prosthesis and a ruptured mitral valve prosthesis [(A) and (B)]. The severed minor mitral valve strut had broken off (C). Both the free floating disk and the defective mitral valve prosthesis are visible in this frame [(D) and (E)].

15. **(A)** Sputum should be sent for direct fluorescent antibody for PCP. A culture (B) can take several days to come back, and PCP does not stain on the Gram stain (C). There are no serum antibody tests (D) or urine antigen tests (E) for pneumocystis carinii. Less than 50% of AIDS patients with pneumocystosis will have positive methenamine silver sputum stains.

16. **(E)** Trimethoprim/sulfamethoxazole for 21 days is the first-line therapy, and the other ones should only be considered if someone is not tolerant to sulfa drugs.

17. **(E)** Room air PaO^2 or <75 mm Hg is the indication. Corticosteroids have been shown to be beneficial to these circumstances in decreasing mortality.

18. **(C)** Trimethoprim/sulfamethoxazole is the first-line of therapy for prophylaxis for PCP in HIV-positive patients with a CD4 count less than 200 or in patients who have had a previous PCP infection. Dapsone and aerosolized pentamidine are second-line therapies if the patients cannot tolerate sulfa drugs.

19. **(A)** There is a 5-10% cross-reactivity between the penicillins and the cephalosporins. Therefore, patients with a documented penicillin allergy should avoid the cephalosporins.

20. **(A)** The patient should shift his weight every two hours. Shifting weight is essential to controlling pressure sores and is done by rotating the patient. The patient can also sleep on special air mattresses to avoid pressure.

21. **(C)** The history and physical examination suggest an acute process (pneumonia), superimposed on a chronic condition (emphysema). The chest radiograph demonstrates hyperlucency of the lung fields, which are increased. A large bulla is apparent in the right lung field. The right heart border is obliterated by the right lower lobe pneumonia [(C), (A), and (B)]. In dextrocardia, the heart appears as a "mirror" image on the roentgenogram. There may be an associated situs inversus. The cardiac structures on this film are in the normal position (D). A roentgenologic diagnosis of pneumothorax requires the identification of the visceral pleural line. There is no evidence of either a rib fracture or pneumothorax on this film (E).

22. **(B)** With infection, fluid levels may develop within a bulla. This follow-up chest radiograph demonstrates such an air fluid within a bulla. The thinness of the wall of a bulla usually helps to distinguish it from true cavitation (B). An encapsulated hydropneumothorax is in the differential diagnosis of this lesion (A). Both diaphragms are clearly visible on this film. A subdiaphragmatic effusion, when unilateral, occurs more commonly on the right. It is often associated with elevation of the diaphragm. In this film, the left costophrenic angle is sharp, but the right angle is blunted (C). No endotracheal tube is apparent on this film (D). Pulmonary markings are visible throughout the left lung field. In tension pneumothorax, the mediastinum shifts away from the side of the pneumothorax (E).

23. **(A)** This chest X-ray shows resolution of the right lower lobe infiltrate. The right border of the chest is no longer obscured by the infiltrative process (A). The lesion is in an atypical location for tuberculosis. If testing was indicated, it should have been performed when the cavitary lesion was first noted two months ago. The improved clinical status also speaks against tuberculosis (B). In view of the improvement, both roentgenographically as well as clinically, a period of "watchful waiting" of this peripherally located lesion is indicated [(C) and (D)]. Although there is some hyperlucency at the left lower base, lung markings can be distinguished. The area of hyperlucency is not significantly changed from the film taken two months previously, which would be extremely unusual for a pneumothorax (E).

24. **(B)** Based on the clinical history and the sequential radiographic films, the most likely diagnosis is a resolving parapneumonic effusion within a bulla adjacent to an area of pneumonia (B). It would be extremely unusual for a squamous cell carcinoma to appear this suddenly in someone who is clinically improving. The peripheral location is also somewhat atypical for a squamous cell carcinoma, which typically presents as a central mass with endobronchial growth (A). Pulmonary hamartomas occur more commonly in men, with a peak incidence at age 60. They are benign, peripherally located, clinically silent lesions that contain the normally present pulmonary components (smooth muscle, collagen) but in a disorganized fashion. The absence of this lesion on previous films makes this diagnosis less likely (E). A history of asbestos exposure can be obtained in over 80% of persons with malignant mesotheliomas. The first radiographic manifestation may be a local scalloping or an irregular mass related to the pleura (C). When thromboembolism is complicated by pulmonary infarction, the oligemia is usually replaced by parenchymal consolidation. The ipsilateral hemidiaphragm may also be elevated. The classic wedge-shaped consolidation in the lung periphery, also known as "Hampton's hump," is a very rare finding in pulmonary infarction (D).

25. **(C)** If persistent hypoxemia (PaO_2 less than 55 mm Hg) is documented in persons with chronic lung disease, survival can be improved with continuous supplemental home oxygen therapy. Persons with a PaO_2 of less than 59 mm Hg in the presence of cor pulmonale, polycythemia, or congestive heart failure also require continuous home oxygen therapy (C). The goal of treatment is to achieve an oxygen saturation of more than 90%. Acute increases in $PaCO_2$ cause somnolence and confusion and require immediate diagnostic evaluation and therapy. Oxygen therapy should be instituted with extreme caution in persons with chronic hypercapnia, since hypoxemia may be the primary stimulus to respiration [(D) and (E)].

26. **(B)** The history and physical examination suggest an acute infectious process. The chest X-ray shows improvement from his previous film, with only a small pleural-based scar evident on this film. In this clinical setting, a 7-10-day course of broad spectrum antibiotics is indicated.

Although viral infections are often the cause of clinical decompensation, clinical studies have documented that such regimens decrease both the duration and severity of infective episodes, even in the absence of positive bacterial cultures [(B) and (A)]. The clinical picture does not suggest a pulmonary embolus. In a clinical setting such as this, ventilation-perfusion scans can be difficult to interpret. [(C) and (D)]. The use of systemic corticosteroids is controversial. However, either the inhalational or oral route would be indicated prior to the use of intravenous therapy (E).

27. **(C)** Alpha₁antitrypsin deficiency is a hereditary disorder, which may present with emphysema in young nonsmokers. Alpha₁antitrypsin is an antiprotease that protects the lower respiratory tract against neutrophil elastase (C). Serum IgA, either alone or in concert with other immunoglobulins, may be altered in several disease states. Chronic infections increase IgA nonspecifically (A). C'1 esterase deficiency is associated with both angioedema and severe abdominal pain (B). A decreased serum ceruloplasmin is one of the criteria for the diagnosis of Wilson's disease (D). Although the serum angiotensin-converting enzyme is elevated in approximately two-thirds of persons with sarcoidosis, there are a significant number of both false-positive and false-negative results (E).

28. **(D)** Physician-patient confidentiality makes it unacceptable for you to give information to anyone about a patient unless you have the patient's specific permission. Proof that the caller is who she says she is would also be important to obtain.

29. **(A)** Fibrocystic breast disease is the most common breast lesion, both benign and malignant.

30. **(E)** A history of fibrocystic disease has not been shown to increase the incidence of breast cancer. Risk factors include nulliparity (D), family history (C), female gender (A), and age (B).

31. **(E)** The diagnosis of each of the answer choices is made on the basis of pathology, not by history, physical examination, mammogram, or aspirate.

32. **(E)** Please see the explanation for question number 31.

33. **(E)** A mammogram can only increase or decrease the suspicion for cancer. The only way to make the diagnosis is with pathology.

34. **(A)** Biopsy and pathology is the only way to make a diagnosis. Unless physical examination, aspirate, and mammogram are all negative for malignancy, then it should be biopsied.

35. **(A)** About nine percent of all women will be diagnosed with breast cancer—about one in eleven.

36. **(C)** They should be used in postmenopausal patients with positive axillary nodes and receptors. Anti-estrogen medications should not be used in premenopausal woman.

37. **(C)** This patient has suffered a fracture of his orbit and mandible. The left eye is swollen and he has paresthesia and ocular findings. This is characteristic of an orbital fracture. The malocclusion results from a fracture to the mandible, causing the teeth to shift, throwing the bite out of alignment with a resulting malocclusion. There is no evidence to suggest any nasal [(A) and (B)], maxillary (D), or frontal bone (E) fracture.

38. **(A)** Entrapment is the inability of the eyeball to move. With an orbital floor fracture, the inferior rectus muscle is trapped and the eyeball is prohibited from looking upward. There will therefore be diplopia, or double vision, on upward gaze. Ectropion (B) is outfolding of the eyelid. Entropion (C) is infolding of the eyelid. Ptosis (D) is a resting eyelid that droops due to either paralysis or disruption of the eyelid opening mechanism.

39. **(A)** The inferior rectus (A) allows the eye to look upward. When it gets trapped, the eyeball cannot look upward. Although the other muscles do insert onto the eyeball, they are not involved with this problem; they may also be entrapped by fractures, though. The medial wall of the orbit is another place where entrapment sometimes occurs with entrapment of the medial rectus muscle.

40. **(A)** Surgery will correct a muscle that is entrapped. It is important to make sure the problem is not caused by swelling, and that can be determined by a "forced duction test." One grasps the muscle with a fine instrument and pulls on it.

If the problem is swelling, then the eyeball should move. If it is entrapped, then it won't. Exploration (B), therefore, should be done on entrapped muscles. A repair (C) of the fracture would be indicated. One would reconstruct the orbital defect. Antibiotics (D) should be used with any open fracture. Elevating the head of the bed (E) will reduce swelling. Observation may help initially, but usually won't solve the problem.

41. **(E)** Bleeding is not a long-term problem. The bleeding that occurs early will solve quickly. Infection (A) is a complication of any open fracture. Antibiotics will lessen this. Diplopia (B) can result if the entrapped muscle is not adequately taken care of. Malocclusion (C) will result if the mandible fracture is not adequately taken care of. Paresthesias (D) result from the fracture. As long as the nerve is intact, then resolution should occur. The condition of an intact nerve that is damaged or bruised with ability to return to normal is known as neuropraxia.

42. **(D)** These patients should recover in the hospital postoperatively. They should not be discharged after surgery (A) because they have undergone extensive surgery and should be monitored. They should be on a soft or liquid diet, and not a regular diet, (B) because of the mandible fracture. Activity should be light, not full (C), because exertion may delay or harm the healing process. Anticoagulation (E) is not needed and will only lead to potentially dangerous bleeding.

43. **(C)** Uncomplicated bone healing in an adult takes approximately six weeks. It is less in a child. It may take longer in the elderly or the sick.

44. **(C)** The most likely diagnosis with the short course is acute bacterial bronchitis. This antibiotic choice is good for both streptococcus species and for the common Gram-negative species in this smoker.

45. **(C)** The patient's presentation is most consistent with appendicitis. An ectopic pregnancy (A) would usually not present with evidence of peritoneal irritation. The patient is too young for a ruptured diverticulum (E) to be high in your differential diagnosis. The other conditions do not commonly present in this fashion.

46. **(D)** In a poorly controlled insulin-dependent diabetic with a superimposed acute process, the most likely diagnosis is diabetic ketoacidosis. Consistent with this diagnosis is the anion gap, hyperglycemia, and metabolic acidosis (D). The hyponatremia is artifactual. Each 100 mg/dL increase in glucose concentration causes a 1.6 mEq/L decrease in the sodium (B). Redistribution of potassium from the intracellular fluid to the extracellular fluid can result from acidosis. As the diabetic ketoacidosis is treated, the potassium will shift into the cells (C). Superimposed hyperglycemia may be seen as part of diabetic ketoacidosis if an adequate glomerular filtration rate is maintained, thereby allowing exchange of ketoacid anions for chloride in the kidneys. Although lactic acidosis must be considered in the differential diagnosis, it occurs most commonly in clinical situations characterized by inadequate tissue oxygenation, such as shock and hypoxemia, which are not evident in this patient (A). Hyperchloremic acidosis, caused by conditions such as renal tubular dysfunction, loss of alkali, or production of hydrochloric acid, is a normal anion gap acidosis (E).

47. **(B)** Iron-deficiency anemia is the leading cause of anemia in infants and children in the United States.

48. **(D)** Environmental intervention is recommended for children with blood lead levels between 10-24 micrograms/dl. Patients with blood lead levels of 25-45 micrograms/dl need aggressive environmental intervention. Chelation therapy is not routinely given. Patients with lead levels between 45-70 micrograms/dl and no neurological symptoms of encephalopathy can receive oral chelation therapy. They may need hospitalization for initiation of therapy and for environmental intervention to be made. Children with lead levels greater than 70 micrograms/dl or with symptoms of encephalopathy require inpatient chelation therapy.

49. **(C)** All signs in this child lead to child abuse. Isolating the child from abusive parent(s) and ensuring her safety should be your first priority in any child-abuse case. Dealing with resisting parents is not an uncommon occurrence when hospitalization of an abused child is being considered. Acting in the child's best interest provides the best legal and ethical grounds for your action and eliminates the necessity for a

third-party intervention. Getting legal advice, however, is always helpful and prudent.

50. **(C)** People with stable hypertension can have worsening conditions. The most important first step is controlling the elevated blood pressure. Further workup should then be undertaken as indicated.

51. **(A)** The first step in evaluating a new breast lesion should be mammography.

52. **(D)** This new lesion must be considered malignant until proven otherwise. Despite his cessation of cigarettes, he remains at risk for lung cancer. Metastatic cancer (E) does not usually present as a solitary lung lesion.

53. **(E)** Before treatment is begun, a throat culture should be obtained to determine if the patient has Strep throat. If so, she should be treated with penicillin, since there is no age limit for Strep infections or the risk of rheumatic disease. Antibiotics can be started after the culture is obtained and before the results are back. Prophylactic nocturnal treatment (B) is not adequate for an acute infection. There is as yet no vaccine (C) available for Strep throats.

54. **(B)** Desensitization is appropriate for such a patient.

55. **(D)** Blackouts such as these may be the first indication that a "closet" alcoholic drinks too much.

56. **(B)** The most common cause of new-onset seizures in an adult is a brain tumor. Epilepsy (D) does not usually present for the first time at this age.

57. **(C)** Sjögren's syndrome requires two of the following three symptoms: dry eyes (which can be manifested as a sense of itchiness or grittiness), dry mouth, and a connective tissue disease.

58. **(D)** Barrier methods of contraception, such as condoms, sponges, diaphragms, and spermicides, protect against sexually transmitted diseases (STDs). Since cervical HPV and HSV-2 infections have been implicated in the pathogenesis of cervical cancer, there may be protection from development of cervical neoplasia.

59. **(B)** Vecuronium (A) is a paralyzing agent whose specific role is to provide skeletal muscle relaxation. Lidocaine (C) and bupivicaine (D) are local anesthetics that will provide a moderate degree of skeletal muscle relaxation. Midazolam (B) is a benzodiazepine and has no muscle relaxant properties.

60. **(A)** Pneumococcal pneumonia is the most common bacterial pneumonia. It is usually lobar and reaches the lungs through the respiratory passages. Staphylococcal (B), streptococcal (C), and klebsiella (D) pneumonia are not as common. Herpetic infections (E) are viral, not bacterial.

61. **(D)** The mental foramen is located in the mandible below the apices of the premolar teeth. It allows passage of the mental nerve, which gives sensation to the chin and lower lip.

62. **(C)** The mental nerve gives sensation to the lower lip and chin on the ipsilateral side. There is some occasional cross-innervation to the other side.

63. **(D)** The vaccine is widely recommended for the elderly. It consists of 23 types of pneumococci, which are responsible for 87% of the pneumococcal bacteremia [(A) and (B)]. Its effectiveness in children (C) for therapeutic or prophylactic purposes is not supported by current research data. The current wide use of the pneumococcal vaccine contradicts (E).

64. **(D)** Pesticide exposure in farmers is suggested to contribute to the development of malignant melanoma (A), cancer of the prostate (B), Hodgkin's disease (C), leukemia, and cancer of the lip (E). There is no supporting evidence for a possible linkage between pesticides and pancreatic cancer.

65. **(C)** Measles-mumps-rubella vaccine should be administered twice, at 12-15 months and at 4-6 years.

66. **(B)** All children should receive periodic height and weight measurements as screening for growth retardation and obesity. The other choices need to have sufficient grounds to be performed in pediatric population.

67. **(D)** Beta-blockers have been shown to reduce portal pressures and thus portal hypertension. This can alleviate pressure on the esophageal varices and an upper GI bleed can be prevented. Any insult to an already compromised liver can result in fulminant liver failure, as in this case. Viral hepatitis (A) can infect the hepatocytes in the liver and result in acute liver decompensation. Nyquil (B) is an over-the-counter sleep and cold medication which contains alcohol, and thus this drug can precipitate acute liver failure in an already compromised individual. Acetaminophen is metabolized in the liver and ingestion in large quantities can result in liver failure in an already compromised individual. Bacterial peritonitis (C) can present as fever and abdominal pain in a patient with ascites. The most common organism involved is *E. coli*. This infection can also precipitate fulminant liver failure in an alcoholic with cirrhosis. Diuretics (E) are prescribed for individuals with ascites, but volume depletion can occur, leading to changes in the portal pressures and, thus, acute variceal bleeding. Excessive diuresis can also result in the hepatorenal syndrome.

68. **(E)** Congenital hyposplenism occurs in Fanconi's syndrome (E). Splenomegaly may result from infiltration of the organ by neoplastic cells or by lipid-laden macrophages, as occurs in lymphoma (A), leukemias, or metastatic tumors. Splenic intrasinusoidal extramedullary hematopoiesis involving all three myeloid cell lines associated with dilated and distended pulp sinuses occurs in myelosclerosis with myeloid metaplasia (C). Infiltrative diseases, such as Gaucher's (B) or Niemann-Pick disease, produce splenic enlargement by increasing the number of splenic red pulp histiocytes. In hemolytic diseases, such as hereditary spherocytosis (D), there is pooling of abnormal red blood cells in sinuses and pulp cords because of increased red cell rigidity. Such cells have decreased ability to traverse the red pulp sinusoidal endothelium.

69. **(E)** Despite the massive increase in bone turnover, extracellular calcium homeostasis is usually normal. The plasma levels are thought to be regulated by reutilization of calcium ions as well as by feedback control of parathyroid secretion (E). Due to the marked proliferation of blood vessels in pagetic bone, blood flow to the affected areas may be significantly increased. When the disease affects more than one-third of the skeleton, this increased blood flow may be associated with high output cardiac failure (A). Pathologic fractures may occur during the destructive phase of the disease and is particularly common in persons with bowing (B). Urolithiasis probably results from increased urinary calcium excretion during the periods of bone resorption (C). Hearing loss may result from direct involvement of the ossicles of the inner ear or of bone in the region of the cochlea. Impingement by bone on the 8th cranial nerve as it passes through the auditory foramen may also result in hearing loss (D).

70. **(D)** Partial simple seizure (A) is seen in association with focal muscle twitching, usually involving either the arm or the leg. It is often preceded by a lesion in the cranium, such as an infarct or tumor. Partial simple seizures are seen most often in adults. Partial complex seizures (B) are seen in children, and often are associated with lip-smacking and staring. Patients with partial complex seizures demonstrate semi-purposeful actions, and their seizures are often preceded by sensory delusions, such as a deja vu experience or smelling abnormal odors. Generalized absence seizures (C) are also known as petit mal seizures. They are also seen in children, and often are only recordable by a brief episode of staring. Generalized tonic-clonic seizure are also known as grand-mal seizures. They are characterized by jerking of the extremities and muscle contraction. Sometimes there can be loss of consciousness and biting of the tongue. Finally, alcohol withdrawal seizures (E) are manifested between one and four days after cessation of alcohol consumption. These are typically isolated seizures and are characterized as grand-mal seizures.

71. **(C)** Hemoglobin electrophoresis would not be particularly helpful in this patient's evaluation at this point. All of the other tests would be useful.

72. **(D)** A family history of nephrolithiasis in this setting would be helpful.

73. **(B)** Nephrolithiasis is the most likely diagnosis in this patient. The absence of abnormal findings on the abdominal radiograph does not lessen its likelihood since many stones are radiolucent.

74. **(E)** Even if this patient has uric acid stones, administration of allopurinol in the acute situation would not be beneficial.

75. **(A)** The clinical history is classic for temporal arteritis and polymyalgia rheumatica. A patient with a high suspicion of TA should be started on high-dose corticosteroids as soon as possible to avoid permanent eye damage and blindness. If the clinical features are classic and the ESR is consistent, treatment can be initiated as the lesion can be patchy and can be missed on biopsy (B). Biopsy should not delay the initiation of treatment significantly. This condition usually affects middle-aged and older patients, not younger patients (C). Additional symptoms may include jaw claudication and scalp tenderness, not delirium or psychosis (D).

76. **(C)** The symptoms of unilateral pain with renal failure make either obstruction or a unilateral vascular compromise a concern. A renal ultrasound with Doppler would be able to rule out hydronephrosis, making obstruction much less likely. The Doppler would show the arterial flow and would be able to rule out renal artery thrombosis.

77. **(B)** The patient's spouse has the right to know that he is HIV-positive, especially if they are not practicing protected sex.

78. **(A)** You should strongly advise him to use condoms to protect all sexual partners.

79. **(C)** The wife's life is in danger from unprotected sex. As a physician, it is your duty to inform someone whose life is at risk. This is one situation in which patient-physician confidentiality is superseded by the rights of another.

80. **(B)** This is essentially the same situation as the patient who threatens to kill someone and has the means to do so.

81. **(E)** Normal $PaCO_2$ is about 40 mm Hg, so this is not failure. Tachypnea >35 breaths per minute (A), pH <7.25 indicating acidosis (B), a vital capacity <15 ml/kg (C), and a PaO_2 <70 mm Hg on 50% O_2 (D) all indicate impending or frank failure and are indications for mechanical ventilation.

82. **(D)** A chest tube should not be performed unless you suspect a pneumothorax or hempothorax. A chest X-ray (A) should be performed to locate the position of the tube and detect any problems such as a pneumothorax. Auscultation of bilateral breath sounds (B) should be performed and should be equal to assure adequate placement of the endotracheal tube. An arterial blood gas (C) should be performed to allow you to set appropriate ventilatory settings. Securing of the tube is important (E) to prevent accidental extubation or movement of the tube.

83. **(E)** This patient has myasthenia gravis, which is an autoimmune disease associated with weakness and easy fatigability of skeletal muscles. Many patients present with ocular motor disturbances and oropharyngeal weakness secondary to the immune-mediated disease of the acetacholine receptor complex and autoantibodies, which bind to the receptor and reduce their number. This, in turn, decreases the effectiveness of the postsynaptic muscle membrane. Anticholinesterase drugs such as mestinon or pyridostigmine are the ones most commonly used in the treatment, and not the diagnosis, of myasthenia gravis. Anticholinesterase receptor antibodies (A) are highly specific for myasthenia gravis, and they are virtually never present in healthy individuals. EMG studies are highly sensitive to diagnose myasthenia gravis. It would show increased jitter in some muscles in these patients. It would show abnormal neuromuscular transmission. Weakness caused by abnormal neuromuscular transmission characteristically improves with administration of the edrophonium chloride test (C). This is an excellent pharmacologic test to diagnose myasthenia gravis. A CT of the anterior mediastinum (D) is useful to search for a thymoma. Thymectomy has been shown to induce remission in myasthenia gravis patients.

84. **(C)** You should inform your colleague that he has done something you disagree with and

why. Since this is the first time, it is probably not appropriate to inform the chief. You may decide not to have him cover your service again, but you should tell him why.

85.   **(D)**   Tetanus is a neurological disorder, characterized by increased muscle tone and spasms, caused by the toxin, tetanospasmin. Neonatal tetanus, which occurs primarily in developing countries, follows infection with contaminated materials, such as application of animal dung to the umbilical stump of children born to inadequately immunized women (A). In the United States, most cases of tetanus occur in inadequately immunized persons (B). "Cephalic tetanus" is a rare form of localized tetanus, which follows either head injury or ear infection. Typically, dysfunction of one or more cranial nerves, especially the seventh, is observed (E). Conditions conducive to infection, including a change in the oxidation-reduction potential at the site of injury, must be present. This altered redox state allows spores to revert to a vegetative form, which produces tetanospasmin (C). At the presynaptic terminal, tetanospasmin blocks the release of glycine and gamma-aminobutyric acid (GABA), inhibitory neurotransmitters (D). This increases the firing rate, resulting in rigidity.

86.   **(E)**   Screening for breast cancer is not recommended at this time. However, teaching self-examination techniques for breast lumps may be prudent. Regular Pap testing (A) is performed for all women who are or have been sexually active. Evaluating this patient for gonorrhea (B) is indicated by her presenting symptom (purulent discharge). Screening for gonorrhea is recommended for persons at high risk. Periodic screening for HIV infection (C) should be offered to all patients that present with sexually transmitted diseases. Measurements of urine hCG levels (D) have become a routine practice for sexually active women of reproductive age.

87.   **(D)**   Surgical wounds are most commonly infected by *Staphylococcus spp.* A nosocomial wound infection can be caused by methicillin-resistant staphylococcal species and should be treated initially with vancomycin until sensitivities come back.

88.   **(A)**   The antibiotic choice gives good coverage for pneumococcus, but also covers Gram-negative organisms, which are a concern for pneumonia in patients with chronic obstructive pulmonary disease.

89.   **(C)**   This patient is exhibiting the classic triad of right and upper quadrant pain, fever, and jaundice consistent with ascending cholangitis. These patients should be treated aggressively for Gram-negative organisms with aminoglycosides and possibly anti-pseudomonal penicillins. Appropriate treatment also includes decompression with percutaneous drainage or ERCP.

90.   **(E)**   An uncomplicated cystitis can be treated with three days of sulfamethoxazole.

91.   **(D)**   Osteopenia and hypercalcemia are part of the differential diagnostic picture for several conditions, including T-cell lymphoma, metastatic solid tumors to the bone, sarcoidosis, and Addison's disease. Chronic renal failure would cause osteopenia with osteolytic lesions because of secondary hyperparathyroidism, but hypocalcemia would occur, not hypercalcemia. In thyrotoxicosis (A), the bone shows increased rates of resorption because of the effect of the thyroxine. The increased resorption leads to elevations in serum calcium. Approximately 15-20% of patients with multiple myeloma (B) would have hypercalcemia. The tumor produces lymphotoxins which cause hypercalcemia secondary to osteolytic lesions of the bone. Compression fractures are common, along with bone pain and anemia. Plasma cells are found in abundance in the bone marrow. In primary hyperparathyroidism (C), serum calcium elevation is accompanied by elevated levels of intact parathyroid hormone. In thyrotoxicosis, the parathyroid hormone level would be decreased. Solid tumors (E) may produce such osteolytic factors as parathyroid hormone-related protein and cause osteopenia and hypercalcemia. Breast cancer should be in the differential diagnosis for a 38-year-old female with compression fractures and hypercalcemia.

92.   **(C)**   A tendon rupture is likely along with fractures and ligament avulsions present with acute bone pain. Staphylococcal infection (A), osteosarcoma (B), Paget's disease of bone (D), and hyperparathyroidism (E) all present with chronic bone pain.

93. **(D)** This patient has trichinosis from ingestion of infected pork meat. The meat contains encysted larvae of trichinella spiralis. Seven days after ingestion, the patient can have pulmonary and abdominal symptoms. Serologic testing is useful and treatment is with thiabendazole. L-tryptophan (A) has been in the news for causing marked eosinophilia and myalgias. The cpk level would not be elevated. Thrombolytic therapy (B) would be indicated if this patient has an acute myocardial infarction within four to six hours of presentation. He does not present with chest pain, and the elevated cpk level is from skeletal muscle involvement. Intravenous hydration (C) would be indicated in rhabdomyolosis, which involves a very high cpk level and skeletal muscle breakdown with release of myoglobin. Eosinophilia would not be associated with rhabdomyolosis. Steroids (E) can sometimes cause dissemination of trichinosis infection, but it can be used in severe inflammatory involvement of the central nervous system and myocardium. This patient presents with gastrointestinal symptoms.

94. **(D)** An EEG that remains flat-line over a period of 24-48 hours in a patient requiring total life support is considered evidence of brain death, and should be obtained before you decide what to do.

95. **(A)** You can tell the family that the patient will probably never recover higher functions at this point. You should discuss the situation with the family, if at all possible.

96. **(D)** In this situation, even though the wife is truly the next-of-kin, the best solution would be a ruling from the Ethics Committee of your hospital.

97. **(C)** Since it has been agreed that the patient is not viable, which is why you have turned off the respirator, you would not do anything to resuscitate him at this point.

98. **(C)** This patient has de Quervain's thyroiditis, or subacute granulomatous thyroiditis, which is characterized by a tender, enlarged, assymetrical thyroid gland and giant cells on the biopsy. This disorder is more common in females, and it is thought that a prior viral infection may predispose to this self-limited illness. The radio-active iodine uptake is low and the thyroid gland is poorly visualized on the thyroid scan. Hashimoto's thyroiditis (A) is an autoimmune disease that presents with an enlarged, non-tender thyroid gland. Biopsy may reveal fibrosis and plasma cells. This disorder does not usually manifest acutely. Graves' disease (B) is also an autoimmune disorder characterized by hyperthyroid symptoms. The radioactive iodine uptake is usually elevated and the thyroid gland would be strongly visualized on the thyroid scan. Subacute lymphocytic thyroiditis (D) is associated with a painless thyroid gland and absence of giant cells on the biopsy. Medullary cell carcinoma of the thyroid gland (E) is associated with an elevated thyrocalcitonin level and a family history of disease. Biopsy of the thyroid gland reveals sheets of tumor cells separated by a hyaline-amyloid containing stroma.

99. **(A)** Her symptoms sound like a viral syndrome without any bacterial infections. Treatment is supportive and it should resolve on its own.

100. **(A)** The appropriate immediate treatment for ongoing seizures is a benzodiazepine diazepam. The anti-epileptics, such as phenytoin (C) and phenobarbital (B), are for prophylaxis of additional seizures. Medications such as pentobarbital (D) and Vecuronium (E) are used to stop musculoskeletal activity to avoid the complications of seizures.

101. **(C)** Hypercalcemia is not a common cause. Common causes of decreasing the seizure threshold include hyponatremia (A), hypoglycemia (B), hypocalcemia, hyperosmolar non-ketotic state (D), and sub-therapeutic medication levels (E).

102. **(A)** Intravenous loading of phenytoin must be pushed slowly or hypotension will result.

103. **(D)** Ventricular arrhythmias are not a common complication. Common complications of seizures include aspiration (A), rhabdomyolysis (B), myoglobinuria (C), and hyperthermia (E). Electrolyte disturbances and stress on the heart can cause ventricular arrhythmias, but not seizures alone.

104. **(C)** In any severe pain requiring narcotics, it's difficult to assess a patient you don't know over the telephone. If a patient requires narcotics, it's probably wise to send them to the emergency room to make sure that no life-threatening illnesses are present.

105. **(D)** This patient has a deep-puncture laceration secondary to a dog bite and infection with *Pasteurella mulocida, Staph. aureaus,* and streptococci is of primary concern. Primary closure of the wound is usually not performed until after a few days because if one closes the wound prematurely, then the infection may not be able to drain on its own and will subsequently spread to the tendon sheaths in the hand. Tetanus prophylaxis (A) is important for any wound or trauma. 0.1 cc I.M. is given as a booster if the patient cannot remember his last tetanus shot. Rabies prophylaxis (B) with immunoglobulin is important after a dog bite because one does not know if the dog was infected with rabies or not. Augmentin (C) is an excellent choice of antibiotics for a hand bite because it covers anaerobes and Gram-positive organisms. It is given orally. Good irrigation with saline (E) and debridement is necessary in deep puncture-type wounds to wash out the bacteria and to sterilize the wound.

106. **(A)** Immediately administering aspirin during a myocardial infarction has been shown to decrease mortality and increase survival in cardiac patients. This is because of the antiplatelet effect of aspirin, which reduces further thrombosis in the coronary artery. While administering aspirin during a myocardial infarction is the best first step, it should be noted that TPA is considered the best therapy choice in acute coronary thrombosis. Intravenous nitroglycerin (B) is important to administer to decrease the propagation of clot formation, but it should be started only after thrombolytic therapy (streptokinase or TPA) has been given within the first four to six hours after chest pain has occurred. Beta-blockers (C) are also given during a myocardial infarction to decrease the heart rate and to subsequently decrease the catecholamines load on the heart. But in this case, beta-blockers are contraindicated because the pulse is already very low and further reduction of the heart rate can result in a cardiac arrest. Diuretics (D), such as Lasix (loop-diuretic), are indicated during a myocardial infarction when congestive heart failure is also present. But in this case, Lasix can make the hypotension worse, resulting in further clinical deterioration. Defibrillation (E) is indicated only when the patient has no palpable pulse and ventricular fibrillation is present on the heart monitor. This patient with severe bradycardia and hypotension probably needs a pacemaker.

107. **(D)** The Canadian Task Force on the Periodic Health Examination recommends that all pregnant women should receive at least one ultrasound. HIV testing (A) is offered only to pregnant women who are at increased risk of the infection. All pregnant women, regardless of prior history, should be screened for preeclampsia and eclampsia at the first prenatal visit and periodically throughout pregnancy (B). Rh (D) immune globulin is given to unsensitized Rh-negative women at 28-29 weeks' gestation and 72 hours of delivery (C). All pregnant women over 35 years of age and older should undergo amniocentesis (E).

108. **(D)** The appropriate next step is to call a surgical consult on an emergency basis (D). The likeliest diagnosis is appendicitis with peritonitis, which is a surgical emergency. A radiograph (A) is appropriate later, as is paracentesis (B). Antibiotic therapy (C) should await the surgical evaluation. A nasogastric tube (E) might be necessary, but not before a surgical evaluation.

109. **(B)** This patient must be considered to have pneumonia, probably pneumococcal, and treated accordingly, until and unless it is ruled out by cultures. Heavy drinkers are especially prone to pneumonia, especially pneumococcal, which can be rapidly fatal if not treated. This individual may develop DTs (A), but this cannot be assumed at this point. Asthma (C), atelectasis (D), and bronchitis (E) would not cause a presentation such as this.

110. **(D)** This presentation is most consistent with bowel obstruction, which, in this age group, is most likely secondary to colon cancer.

111. **(C)** An abdominal CT is not one of the first tests that is necessary in this setting. The other tests listed would help assess the severity (e.g., leukocytosis, level of amylase) or origin (e.g., lipase, amylase consistent with pancreatic disease, urinalysis in evaluation of renal disease) of the patient's condition.

112. **(A)** Individuals with nasal polyps who take nonsteroidal anti-inflammatory agents, the major active ingredient in over-the-counter agents for menstrual cramps, are more susceptible to asthma than are other people.

113. **(D)** Diabetic peripheral neuropathy is the most common cause of Charcot arthropathy, which can present with a severe painless deformity such as this.

114. **(C)** When hypercalcemia is noted as an incidental finding in the output setting, the most common etiology is primary hyperparathyroidism. In the inpatient setting, hypercalcemia is most commonly caused by malignancy such as breast cancer (A), myeloma (D), etc. Sarcoidosis (E) can cause hypercalcemia because of a decrease in vitamin D levels.

115. **(B)** Patients usually are male and overweight and have numerous occurrences each night of upper airway obstruction causing numerous awakenings that the patient is often not aware of. Diagnosis can be confirmed by a sleep study showing numerous episodes of desaturation. Primary pulmonary hypertension (A) classically presents with increasing shortness of breath on exertion and is much more common in middle-aged women. Pneumonia (C) presents with fevers, chills, and cough, and uremia (D) presents with other symptoms of nausea and vomiting, as well. Multi-infarct dementia (E) presents with other neurological complaints.

116. **(D)** The first choice for perioperative antibiotic coverage in this patient would be vancomycin. Cefazolin (E) is incorrect because of the small (0.3%) incidence of cross-reactivity between cephalosporins and penicillins. Administration of this drug would be contraindicated in a person with a known history of anaphylaxis to penicillin. Gentamicin (A) and cefotetan (C) have a different coverage spectrum, while imipenem (B) has too broad a coverage and its common intra-operative use may lead to the development of resistant organisms.

117. **(C)** Flow through a catheter is inversely proportional to length and directly proportional to the fourth power of the radius. A 10-gauge cath-

eter is twice as wide as a 20-gauge catheter, and will thus provide 16x more flow. Since the length of the larger catheter is twice that of the smaller, flow will be reduced by one-half on the basis of length alone. The overall flow will thus be 8x greater in the 10-gauge catheter.

118. **(B)** A platelet count of 50,000 is generally regarded as adequate for surgical hemostasis.

119. **(D)** Except for insulin, all the other hormones listed are stress hormones and are released by surgical stimulation. Glucagon, and not insulin, is released by surgical stimulation.

120. **(E)** Neither chemotherapy nor radiation therapy alone have had a significant impact on the overall rates of cancer mortality. However, a combination therapy of the two modalities, when used aggressively, may produce increased long-term survival rates.

121. **(E)** The focusing of an object on the retina is known as refraction. Correction of refractive errors is possible with spectacles, contact lenses, or surgical procedures. Light entering the eye is initially focused by the cornea and then by the lens. In myopia, the eye is too large for its refractive power and the image of a distant object focuses in front of the retina (A). In hyperopia, the eye is too small and the image focuses behind the retina (B). In the aging eye, the lens becomes less malleable and it can no longer focus on near objects. This accommodative loss is known as presbyopia (C). In young persons, accommodation is able to compensate for minor degrees of hyperopia (D). A large, uncorrected refractive error is known as ametropia. A major difference in the refractive error between the two eyes is known as anisometropia. (E).

122. **(A)** In addition to septic and mechanical complications, total peripheral nutrition also has metabolic complications. Hypophosphatemia is one of them and may cause 2,3-DPG decrease and the shift of the oxygen dissociation curve to the right, muscle weakness, neurologic symptoms, and convulsions.

One of the complications of PEEP is a decrease in venous return to the heart and a corresponding decrease in cardiac output. To avoid this, PEEP should be increased slowly until acceptable PaO_2 is achieved. In the critically ill patient, available arterial oxygen has to be determined by measuring PaO_2, cardiac output, hemoglobin, and hemoglobin saturation.

123. **(C)** Markedly increased CO_2 production results from the metabolism of infused glucose during parenteral nutrition and leads to metabolic hypercarbia. The problem can usually be resolved by reducing the glucose and adding more fat and amino acid to the infusion.

124. **(A)** Among the medical complications of CPR, cardiac complications include congestive heart failure, hypotension, and ventricular tachyrhythmia. All of them occur within the first 48 hours of resuscitation. Noncardiac post-CPR complications are neurologic, metabolic, hematologic, and traumatic in origin.

125. **(E)** Bronchopulmonary dysplasia is one of the most unfortunate complications of successful intensive respiratory care in the neonate. This is a relatively new iatrogenic entity and is associated with the advent of highly sophisticated technology.

126. **(B)** Hematuria is blood in the urine and may result from trauma, neoplasia, infection, coagulopathy, or kidney stone. Hemoptysis (A) is the process of coughing up blood. Hemetemesis (C) is the vomiting of blood. Epistaxis (D) is bleeding from the nose. Hemothorax (E) is blood within the pleural cavity.

127. **(E)** A workup of hematuria would include all of the things that could cause it, as mentioned in the previous answer. Therefore, one would perform a detailed history and physical (A), order lab tests looking for any coagulopathy (B), order a urinalysis (C) to study the urine, and perform a cystoscopy (D) to endoscopically examine the urinary tract. An MRI of the kidneys (E) would more likely be done later on in the workup and not initially.

128. **(E)** Diabetes mellitus usually will not cause hematuria, but glycosuria. The more likely reasons are trauma (A), coagulopathy (B), tumor (C), and kidney stones or nephrolithiasis (D). All of these will cause bleeding in the GU tract, which

will then pass through the urethra and present as clinical hematuria.

129. **(E)** Doxycycline is the appropriate antibiotic for urethritis, as well as prostatitis. The other antibiotics listed do not work as well and will not be as effective in eradicating the infection.

130. **(C)** CMV retinitis is a dreaded complication of HIV infection that can cause blindness.

131. **(B)** Allopurinol would not be useful in this patient. All of the other modalities are necessary.

132. **(C)** Erythromycin, 500 mg per oral route every 6 hours for 10 to 14 days, is the treatment of choice for this young patient with *Mycoplasma pneumoniae* pneumonia. This pneumonia is an atypical pneumonia, most commonly treated with erythromycin. The patients usually afflicted with this particular type of pneumonia are young and live in closed quarters such as dormitories or military facilities. The chest X-ray is usually worse than the clinical exam appears. Serum cold-agglutinin titers are usually elevated, and occasionally ear involvement occurs.

133. **(D)** This elderly patient has been in the intensive care setting and probably has been colonized and subsequently infected with a nosocomial Gram-negative organism such as *Pseudomonas aeruginosa*. The therapy of choice for this virulent organism is the third-generation cephalosporin antibiotic ceftazadime. This patient should receive immediate intravenous treatment for her pneumonia.

134. **(B)** This immunocompromised patient has *Pneumocystis carinii* pneumonia, which is diagnosed by history and clinical examination as well as by silver-staining of the sputum on bronchoalveolar lavage. This pneumonia is treated by the first-line agent trimethoprim-sulfamethoxazole. If this patient is allergic to the sulfa moiety, then dapsone, atovaquone, or trimetrexate can be used. The A-a gradient is usually widened in PCP pneumonia, and the LDH is usually elevated, as well.

135. **(A)** Most osteomyelitis cases are caused by *Staphylococcus aureus*, which can be resistant to

penicillin by the beta-lactamases. Vancomycin generally has excellent bone penetration and is widely used as therapy for staphylococcus osteomyelitis. Resistance hardly develops. Renal function must be monitored, as well as serum vancomycin levels.

136. **(D)** Interval CPK screening is not useful in detection of susceptible persons. Malignant hyperthermia consists of a group of inherited disorders characterized by a rapid temperature elevation in response to inhalational anesthetics or muscle relaxants. Triggering anesthetics release calcium from the membrane of the muscle cell's sarcoplasmic reticulum, which is defective in storing this ion (E). This results in a sudden increase in myoplasmic calcium, which activates myosin ATPase. Ultimately, sudden massive muscle contraction occurs, leading to a rapid rise in body temperature (A). A linkage to mutations in the skeletal muscle ryanodine receptor (RYR1) has been observed in some families with the autosomal dominant disorder (B). In individuals with one form of autosomally dominant inherited disease, biopsied muscle contracts on exposure to caffeine or halothane at concentrations that do not alter normal muscle contraction (C).

137. **(B)** Pain localized to the jaw and jaw joint is most often temporomandibular joint (TMJ) disease. It is related to stress and the clenching and bruxism that go along with that. This puts excessive stress on the joint. Myocardial infarction pain (A) won't usually go to the joint. Peptic ulcer pain (C) also classically doesn't go to the jaw or joint. Osteoarthritis (D) and rheumatoid arthritis (E) can certainly affect the jaw and jaw joint, but won't occur as it does in this executive under a lot of stress.

138.. **(D)** For the patient with an acute TMJ disorder, it is best to rest the joint. This is done acutely with a soft diet (A) to ease mastication, analgesics (B) to relieve pain, rest (C) to ease the joint, and a period of two weeks to reevaluate the situation (E). In the acute period, an MRI (D) is not indicated. It may be necessary if more treatment is contemplated, such as surgery.

139. **(B)** Herpes zoster virus is the pathogen responsible for the Ramsey-Hunt syndrome. An RNA virus from the Rhabdovirus (A) family is re-

sponsible for rabies and travels through nerves similar to the herpes zoster virus. A cause of the common cold is the Coronavirus (C). Influenza virus (D) is a seasonal pulmonary pathogen. Hepatitis C virus is the most common cause of chronic hepatitis (E).

140. **(D)** In Ramsey-Hunt Syndrome, herpes zoster affects the geniculate ganglion of the seventh cranial nerve (facial nerve). The vagus nerve (tenth cranial nerve) is responsible for motor function of the gastrointestinal tract, pharynx, and posterior tongue, and is not involved in this syndrome (B). Palsies of the accessory nerve (eleventh cranial nerve) result in difficulties in neck and shoulder movement (C). The vestibulocochlear nerve (eighth cranial nerve) is affected by tumors in the cerebello-pontine angle and is responsible for hearing and balance (E).

141. **(D)** The clinical complications of sleep apnea arise from the physiologic changes brought about by the apneic episodes. Hypoxia, hypercarbia, and acidosis result from these apneic episodes. Neuropsychiatric and behavioral disturbances probably arise from the fragmented sleep and the loss of slow-wave sleep (C). Some affected persons develop nonsustained ventricular tachycardia or severe bradycardia with asystole, suggesting this as the cause of nocturnal death (E). The combined effects of increased left ventricular afterload, recurrent nocturnal hypoxemia, and increased sympathoadrenal activity is thought to explain the exacerbation of left-heart failure in persons with underlying cardiac disease (A). Chronic hypoxemia, particularly in obese persons, is considered a risk factor for pulmonary hypertension (B). Epidemiologic studies have implicated sleep apnea as a risk factor for systemic hypertension (D).

142. **(B)** The patient is competent and his permission is required before you can obtain an HIV test.

143. **(C)** The patient is an adult who has made a decision regarding a medical treatment that you must honor.

144. **(A)** The courts have ruled that a physician may give transfusions in life-threatening circumstances to minors, even if this is contrary to the parents' religious beliefs.

145. **(B)** You must perform emergency procedures even in the absence of consent.

146. **(D)** Only the child's guardian(s), in this case the parents, can approve the use of experimental agents in a minor.

147. **(E)** This patient's kidneys are failing because of his primary disease, end-stage cardiomyopathy. Only replacing his heart can save his life.

148. **(B)** There is a national waiting list for all organs. Patients who meet certain medical criteria are placed on this list.

149. **(A)** Organ transplantation should be independent of a patient's personal wealth.

150. **(D)** He does not appear to be an alcoholic, but any alcohol is not good for transplant patients, in part because of the possibility of hepatotoxicity from the drugs used to prevent rejection.

151. **(B)** The length of time a patient must wait varies with his tissue type, the severity of his condition, etc.

152. **(A)** Any intercurrent problem should be treated in such patients.

153. **(B)** If the patient develops severe, recurrent arrhythmias that are difficult to treat, his condition may be considered so severe as to advance him to a higher place on the waiting list.

154. **(A)** He will need monitoring in the CCU setting until transplantation.

155. **(E)** This patient most likely has emphysema or COPD (chronic obstructive pulmonary disease). It results from loss of recoil of the alveoli, and the patient is constantly gasping for air.

156. **(D)** This patient has an infection of his epiglottis. There will be a high fever and a sore throat. You must be aware of possible impending airway obstruction and the emergent need for intubation.

157. **(B)** Bronchitis is an infection of the bronchioles. Smokers lose the protective cilia mechanism that would normally ward off this infection. Antibiotics will usually cure this. Smokers are also

strongly advised to cease smoking, as well.

158. **(A)** Asthma attacks the bronchioles and leads to constriction. Treatment is aimed at dilating them. The patient will classically tell you that breathing is as difficult as "sucking air though a straw."

159. **(A)** The patient described is classic for gonorrhea infection. Single-dose therapy with intramuscular penicillin is an effective therapy, although other regimens are also effective, including cephalosporins and ofloxacin. The pathogenic organism *Hemophilus ducreyi* (B) is responsible for chancroid, a sexually transmitted disease characterized by painful genital warts. Positive VDRL (C) is sensitive for syphilis, although not specific. The human papillomavirus (D) is a common cause of genital warts. Gonorrhea requires treatment and does not generally resolve spontaneously (E). Untreated cases may result in blood-borne spread to the joints and, in women, to pelvic inflammatory disease.

160. **(A)** The symptoms of inability to swallow and a deviated uvula are consistent with peritonsillar abscess, which needs to be drained surgically.

161. **(D)** Metastatic lung cancer is unlikely in this otherwise asymptomatic patient. However, HIV-positive individuals are at increased risk for lymphoma (A) and fungal infections (E). They also can develop reactive lymphadenopathy (B) or lymphadenitis (C).

162. **(E)** Fine-needle aspiration is the best way to diagnose this problem.

163. **(B)** The likeliest diagnosis in this patient is CMV retinitis, which is usually found in patients with low CD4 counts. An ophthalmologist would be most likely to make this diagnosis definitively.

164. **(E)** HIV positivity and an opportunistic infection indicate the presence of full-blown AIDS.

165. **(D)** This patient has chronic obstructive pulmonary disease with an exacerbation of bronchitis. He is a long-term smoker and he has hypoxia with PCO_2 retention. The initial treatment of choice would be nebulizer beta-adrendergic agonists such as albuterol and antibiotics if necessary. This would

alleviate his immediate symptoms. This patient does not have a pulmonary embolism because he is retaining PCO_2 and not hyperventilating with a respiratory alkalosis. The chest X-ray in pulmonary embolism would usually be normal or show an effusion (A). Bronchoscopy (B) would eventually be needed if the patient's symptoms are not alleviated with empiric treatment. This invasive procedure would allow the physician to biopsy the lung parenchyma and obtain a definitive diagnosis. It is not the initial management of choice. If tuberculosis is suspected, then the patient should be placed in isolation and sputum for acid-fast bacilli should be obtained for smear (C). Cultures of AFB take six to eight weeks to come back. A PPD panel can be done later in the course of the admission. Diuretics (E) should be given to a patient with congestive heart failure. This patient does not have congestive heart failure because he has a low-grade fever and purulent sputum production.

166. **(B)** You may order or perform procedures that are acutely necessary in patients whose guardians are not immediately available.

167. **(D)** It is appropriate to treat her symptomatically for now and have her return if she worsens.

168. **(C)** You can only enroll this patient with her guardian's consent and only if the IRB has already agreed to permit mentally impaired individuals to participate in the trial.

169. **(C)** Emergency evaluation and treatment is medically necessary and you do not need the guardian's consent.

170. **(A)** Again, a medically necessary emergency procedure can be performed in the absence of the guardians.

171. **(E)** You have taken care of this patient in the proper fashion.

172. **(A)** Life-threatening emergencies supersede permission from unavailable guardians.

173. **(E)** There are other ways to manage this patient. Mentally impaired individuals are usually included in trials, with appropriate permission by guardians and IRB, only when the condition being treated is one for which they are at particularly high risk and there are few or no other treatments.

174. **(A)** Pregnancy, oral contraceptive use, biliary cirrhosis, and chronic active hepatitis are all associated with increased thyroid binding globulin (TBG). Although this results in an increase in serum T4, the free T4 and metabolic state are normal. Although T3 is less strongly protein-bound than T4, the total T3 is also increased in conditions in which the TBG is increased.

175. **(B)** Synthetic Levothyroxine therapy is usually administered to persons with thyroid hypofunction to sustain serum T4 slightly above the normal range. In this situation, normal or nearly normal T3 concentrations are maintained.

176. **(C)** Radiographic contrast agents, particularly ipodate and iopanoate, inhibit 5' deiodinase, resulting in decreased peripheral conversion of T4 to T3.

177. **(D)** Thyroid hormone resistance syndrome may be due to either pituitary or peripheral factors. It is characterized by decreased responsiveness to elevated levels of thyroid hormone. It is associated with elevated levels of T3 and free T4 and elevated levels of TSH.

178. **(D)** Migraine headaches usually occur with periorbital pain. There is also associated photophobia.

179. **(A)** Headaches from stress and eyestrain typically occur in the occipital region.

180. **(C)** Temporal arteritis usually occurs in the elderly. The pain is along the temporal region. It must be treated aggressively, otherwise it could lead to blindness. Steroids are indicated initially.

USMLE STEP 3

Practice Test 2

NOTE:
The following practice test contains more questions than the actual USMLE Step 3 computer-based examination. This is necessary to provide a score that is roughly comparable to the computer-based exam which contains Computer-based Case Simulations (CCS) questions. Due to the interactive nature of CCS questions, it would be impossible to present them in book form. Although the format is different, this test will give you an accurate idea of your strengths and weaknesses, and provide guidance for further study.

USMLE STEP 3 PRACTICE TEST 2

Day One – Morning Session

(Answer sheets appear in the back of this book.)

TIME: 3 Hours
180 Questions

> **DIRECTIONS**: Each of the following numbered items or incomplete sentences is followed by an answer or a completion of the statement. Choose the **ONE** choice that **BEST** answers the question or completes the sentence.

1. Which one of the following is NOT true of infection with influenza virus?

    (A) Transmission is primarily via small particle aerosol.

    (B) Viral replication destroys respiratory ciliated epithelium.

    (C) The quantity of virus in the respiratory tract correlates with the severity of illness.

    (D) Viremia is common.

    (E) Immunity appears to be subtype-specific.

2. Most newborns have elevated levels of

    (A) hemoglobin A.

    (B) hemoglobin A1C.

    (C) hemoglobin C.

    (D) hemoglobin F.

    (E) hemoglobin S.

3. An 18-year-old male develops enteric hepatitis two-and-a-half weeks after eating at a diner. Which one of the following represents the viral agent most likely to have caused this disease?

    (A) Hepatitis A

    (B) Hepatitis B

    (C) Hepatitis C

    (D) Hepatitis D

    (E) Hepatitis E

4. A 56-year-old male is diagnosed with colonic carcinoma. It is suspected the patient is colonized by an infectious agent important in the initiation of the neoplasm. Which one of the following represents the most likely infectious agent?

    (A) *Streptococcus pyogenes*

    (B) *Staphylococcus aureus*

    (C) *Streptococcus bovis*

    (D) *Staphylococcus epidermidis*

    (E) *Streptococcus agalactiae*

5. A 35-year-old man with AIDS presents to the emergency room complaining of right-sided weakness and a headache over the course of several days. He also has a low-grade fever. His only other opportunistic infection in the past was oral thrush. On exam, he was found to have 2/5 motor strength on the right lower

and upper extremity and no nuchal rigidity. His blood pressure was 130/80 mm/hg. His T-cell count was 35. His CMV titers were positive and so were his serum toxoplasmosis titers. The CT scan of the brain revealed ring-enhancing lesions of the left parietal lobe. What would be the next step in management of this patient's condition?

(A) Stereotactic brain biopsy

(B) Empiric treatment with sulfadiazine and pyrimethamine

(C) Radiation therapy to the brain

(D) Amphotericin

(E) Antihypertensive therapy

6. A six-year-old white male with Angelman's syndrome presents to your office for follow-up. You started him on phenytoin two weeks ago for recurrent tonic-clonic seizures. Which effect is LEAST commonly associated with phenytoin?

(A) Nystagmus on lateral gaze

(B) Morbilliform rash

(C) Liver dysfunction

(D) Gingival hypertrophy

7. During your hospital rounds, you see a 17-year-old patient of yours who is hospitalized for malnutrition. Your psychiatric consultant indicates to you that the patient has a "morbid fear of becoming fat." Which one of the following statements is true regarding this patient?

(A) This condition is a common cause of amenorrhea in the teenage group.

(B) Refeeding should be initiated by the administration of large quantities of calories rapidly by nasogastric tube.

(C) Depression is an uncommon associated feature.

(D) Death from this condition is rare.

Questions 8-11 refer to the following:

During your emergency room shift, the paramedics bring in a patient with status epilepticus. No history is available. Physical examination reveals a 30-year-old female who is unable to communicate. Temperature is 99.9°F, pulse is 120, and blood pressure is 200/100.

8. Immediate management includes all of the following EXCEPT

(A) establishment of airway and venous access.

(B) administration of intravenous diazepam.

(C) administration of 50 ml of 50% glucose.

(D) an electroencephalography.

(E) oxygen by face mask.

9. Which one of the following is true with regard to grand-mal seizures?

(A) Patients rarely loose sphincter control.

(B) Episodes are characterized by a blank stare often accompanied by mild blinking of the eyelids.

(C) Prodromal warnings rarely occur.

(D) In adults, these seizures are commonly associated with febrile episodes.

(E) The postictal phase may continue for several hours.

10. All of the following help to distinguish seizures from syncope EXCEPT

(A) EEG results.

(B) pulse rate at the time of occurrence.

(C) presence of motor activity during episode.

(D) presence of warning symptoms.

(E) loss of awareness.

11. Which one of the following blood chemistry abnormalities most commonly results in epileptic activity?

    (A) Hypocalcemia

    (B) Hypokalemia

    (C) Hypercalcemia

    (D) Hyperkalemia

    (E) Hypophosphatemia

12. The 78-year-old woman you just admitted to the nursing home spikes a temperature to 104.1°F. All of the following would be appropriate EXCEPT

    (A) blood cultures.

    (B) chest X-ray.

    (C) sputum.

    (D) complete blood count.

    (E) electrocardiogram.

13. With lead poisoning, a "lead line" may be seen in

    (A) the skin.

    (B) the gingiva.

    (C) the teeth.

    (D) the nails.

    (E) the tongue.

14. During your morning hospital rounds, the laboratory calls to inform you that the serum NA+ on one of your patients is 129. Other values are not yet available. NA+ was 135 yesterday. The patient is an insulin-dependent diabetic who was admitted the day prior with bacterial pneumonia. Which one of the following is the most likely cause of the reduced sodium?

    (A) Hyperglycemia

    (B) Nephrogenic diabetes insipidus

    (C) SIADH

    (D) Psychogenic polydypsia

    (E) None of the above.

For Questions 15-18, select the cranial nerve that is being tested.

    (A) The trigeminal nerve

    (B) The facial nerve

    (C) The acoustic nerve

    (D) The vagus nerve

    (E) The accessory nerve

15. Have the patient open his mouth and say "ah" while you look for elevation of the uvula.

16. Have the patient show you his lower teeth.

17. Have the patient clench his teeth and test the strength of the temporalis and masseter muscles.

18. Have the patient raise his shoulders while palpating the upper border of the trapezii.

19. A 40-year-old woman presents with joint pain in her hands, which has been worsening over the last several months. She notes that the stiffness and pain is worse in the morning and seems to get better as the day progresses. Her physical exam is notable for some erythema around her proximal interphalangeal joints. Besides nonsteroidal anti-inflammatory agents, you tell the patient an alternative treatment for symptomatic flare-ups would be

    (A) gold salts.

    (B) methotrexate.

    (C) penicillamine.

    (D) glucocorticoids.

    (E) hydroxychloroquine.

20. The most appropriate treatment for the patient above would be to

    (A) begin the patient on oral iron supplementation.

    (B) begin monthly vitamin B12 injections.

    (C) begin a course of chemotherapy.

(D) begin monthly blood transfusions.

(E) begin weekly erythropoietin injections.

21. You are reviewing the X-rays, shown in the figures below, of a 20-year-old male. X-ray B was taken three years after X-ray A. Your clinical considerations include all of the following EXCEPT

Panel A

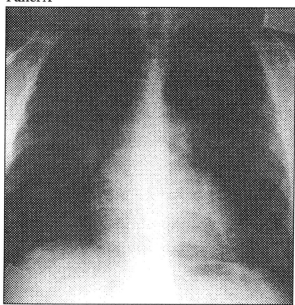

Panel B

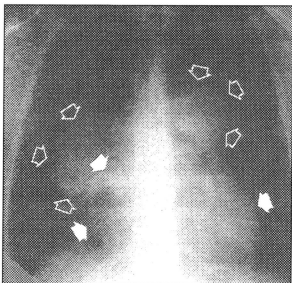

(A) primary pulmonary hypertension.

(B) congenital heart disease.

(C) pulmonary thromboembolic disease.

(D) right-to-left cardiac shunt.

(E) pulmonary veno-occlusive disease.

22. A 45-year-old man whom you follow occasionally for mild hypertension comes to your office demanding that you schedule a vasectomy for him because he does not want his wife to have any more children. He smells of alcohol. You

(A) schedule the procedure.

(B) try to talk him out of it.

(C) tell him he is too young.

(D) explain to him calmly that he should return when he has not had anything to drink.

(E) call his wife.

23. On weekend rounds, you are called to see one of your colleague's patients who had been admitted for alcoholic pancreatitis. He is a 45-year-old man who has become very agitated and uncooperative. He is tachycardiac and hypertensive. You order

(A) an electroencephalogram.

(B) sedation for presumptive delirium tremens.

(C) emergency brain MRI.

(D) lumbar puncture.

(E) blood cultures.

24. A 57-year-old male who has been transferred to your service after a bowel resection a few days earlier has developed an acute painful left great toe. He has a history of gout. All of his routine medications had been stopped prior to surgery, and not all have been restarted yet. All of the following tests should be ordered EXCEPT

(A) serum uric acid.

(B) aspiration of toe.

(C) CBC.

(D) radiograph of the foot.

(E) bone scan.

25. A 59-year-old man is followed for the management of essential hypertension. All of the following are sequelae of essential hypertension EXCEPT

    (A) left ventricular hypertrophy.

    (B) retinal hemorrhage.

    (C) chronic glomerulonephritis.

    (D) atheromatous plaque formation in coronary arteries.

    (E) cerebrovascular disease.

26. A 59-year-old man comes to the emergency room with severe pain in the right large toe for the past 12 hours. Physical exam reveals a swollen, erythematous toe, sensitive to the touch. Synovial fluid examination suggests acute gout. Serum uric acid is 12.5. Which one of the following modalities has no role in the acute management of this patient?

    (A) Oral colchicine

    (B) Oral indomethacin

    (C) Intra-articular triamcinolone

    (D) Oral allopurinol

    (E) Intravenous colchicine

27. A 60-year-old male complains of weakness, fatigue, and bleeding from the oronasal area. He also has blurred vision, dyspnea, and pallor. Physical exam shows lymphadenopathy, hepatosplenomegaly, and sensorimotor peripheral neuropathy. Bone marrow aspirate revealed hypercellular infiltration with lymphoid cells and plasma cells. Serum electrophoresis showed a large number of high-molecular-weight monoclonal IgM proteins (greater than 3 gm/dl). What is the correct diagnosis?

    (A) Multiple myeloma

    (B) Waldenstrom's macroglobulinemia

    (C) Solitary plasmacytoma of bone

    (D) Chronic lymphocytic leukemia

    (E) Hyperviscocity syndrome

Questions 28-35 refer to the following:

A 67-year-old male with coronary artery disease, who is a long-standing patient of yours, complains of progressive shortness of breath, diaphoresis, and chest pain. On physical examination in your office, the patient is afebrile. Blood pressure is 140/98 and pulse is 108. Respirations are 28. Cardiac exam reveals tachycardia and a soft systolic murmur not previously noted. The rest of the examination is unremarkable.

28. All of the following conditions are included in your differential diagnosis EXCEPT

    (A) pulmonary embolus.

    (B) unstable angina.

    (C) primary pulmonary hypertension.

    (D) aortic dissection.

    (E) aortic stenosis.

29. You order an electrocardiogram immediately, based upon which the diagnosis of pulmonary embolism becomes your greatest concern. All of the following are electrocardiographic findings consistent with pulmonary embolism EXCEPT

    (A) rsR' pattern in Lead V1.

    (B) sinus tachycardia.

    (C) right ventricular strain pattern.

    (D) small Q-wave in Lead III.

    (E) nonspecific T-wave changes in multiple leads.

30. Chest X-ray reveals atelectasis in the right lung base. Which one of the following tests would be the next test that you would attempt to obtain?

    (A) Pulmonary angiogram

    (B) Lower extremity Doppler study

    (C) Impedance plethysmography

    (D) Lower extremity venogram

    (E) Ventilation-perfusion scan

31. Your diagnostic evaluation confirms your suspected diagnosis of pulmonary embolism. Your treatment regimen would be which one of the following?

    (A) Intravenous heparin by continuous infusion, followed by oral anticoagulation therapy for 6-12 weeks

    (B) Immediate initiation of high-dose Coumadin therapy to maintain a PT of 1.5-2 times normal

    (C) Subcutaneous heparin at a dose of 5,000 U BID

    (D) Fibrinolytic therapy with urokinase

    (E) None of the above.

32. All of the following factors predispose to pulmonary thromboemboli EXCEPT

    (A) bed rest.

    (B) pancreatic cancer.

    (C) total hip replacement.

    (D) pregnancy.

    (E) chronic liver disease.

33. The most common source of pulmonary thromboembolic material is

    (A) iliofemoral vein.

    (B) popliteal vein.

    (C) superficial femoral vein.

    (D) aortic thrombus.

    (E) None of the above.

34. Which one of the following tests is the most sensitive for the diagnosis of deep venous thrombosis?

    (A) Nuclide venography

    (B) Radionuclide fibrinogen scan

    (C) Doppler ultrasound

    (D) Impedance plethysmography

    (E) Contrast venograpy

35. All of the following are potential pathophysiologic occurrences that are associated with pulmonary embolism EXCEPT

    (A) reduced cardiac output.

    (B) pulmonary vasoconstriction.

    (C) irritation of the pleural surface.

    (D) inflammation of the visceral surface of the pericardium.

    (E) right-sided heart failure.

Questions 36-39 refer to the following:

The urologist in your hospital is ill and you must cover for him. You are asked to make a diagnosis of a patient's illness based on the color of the urine. Match the disease with the following colors.

    (A) Colorless

    (B) Cloudy white

    (C) Yellow

    (D) Blue-green

    (E) Red

36. Hyperbilirubinemia

37. Tetracycline ingestion

38. Urinary tract infection

39. Excessive fluid intake

40. You sutured a facial laceration on an 18-year-old girl in the emergency room. You ask her to come in for suture removal in how many days?

    (A) 1-2

    (B) 3-5

    (C) 7-10

    (D) 10-14

    (E) 14-21

41. Each of the following diseases is highly associated with the HLA B27 antigen EXCEPT

    (A) ankylosing spondylitis.

    (B) systemic lupus erythematosus.

(C) Reiter's syndrome.

(D) juvenile rheumatoid arthritis.

(E) psoriatic arthritis.

42. In the cardiac surgical patient, cardiopulmonary bypass is associated with all of the following EXCEPT

  (A) hemodilution.

  (B) hyperthermia.

  (C) hypernatremia.

  (D) platelet dysfunction.

  (E) non-pulsatile blood flow.

For Questions 43-46, match the following burn depths with the appropriate treatment.

  (A) First-degree burn

  (B) Second-degree burn

  (C) Third-degree burn

  (D) Fourth-degree burn

43. Treatment of this burn normally involves surgical removal or amputation.

44. This burn can usually be treated with topical antibiotics.

45. This burn can be treated with excision and skin grafting.

46. This burn may be treated with topical antibiotics, but sometimes may require excision and skin grafting.

47. A 19-year-old white female presents to the physician's office with complaints of arthralgias, malaise, headaches, pleuritis, and a malar rash on the face. Her urine analysis showed red blood casts. Her lab tests revealed leukopenia. All of the following serologic tests are useful to determine systemic lupus erythematosus as the diagnosis EXCEPT

  (A) antinuclear antibody.

  (B) anti-double stranded DNA antibody.

  (C) false-positive VDRL titer.

  (D) anti-sm antibody.

  (E) antinuclear ribonucleoprotein antibody.

Questions 48-50 refer to the following:

A 54-year-old patient is concerned over a pigmented lesion on the back of her arm that has been slowly growing. There is no axillary lymphadenopathy and no systemic signs.

48. Your next step is

  (A) reassure the patient that there is nothing to worry about.

  (B) smear the lesion and send off for a culture and sensitivity.

  (C) perform a biopsy.

  (D) take an arm X-ray.

  (E) treat it with topical steroids.

49. After a work-up is performed, the diagnosis is malignant melanoma. The lesion is 5 x 5 millimeters and invades into the papillary dermis. Your recommendation is

  (A) follow-up in one year.

  (B) wide local excision.

  (C) wide local excision with axillary lymph node resection.

  (D) radiation therapy.

  (E) chemotherapy.

50. The patient has now been free of disease for seven years and asks you what she should do when she goes outside. You tell her

  (A) not to worry since she is cured.

  (B) to wear clothes that fully cover exposed body parts.

  (C) to avoid the sunlight totally at all times.

  (D) to smear topical steroids over the entire surface of her arms.

  (E) None of the above.

51. A 30-year-old man with AIDS was exploring caves in the Mississippi river valley during a recent vacation. He was just admitted with complaints of a cough, fever, malaise, and increasing shortness of breath. His chest X-ray is shown in the figure, as is the methenamine silver stained smear from his bronchoalveolar lavage. Based on these findings, you begin treatment for

Panel A

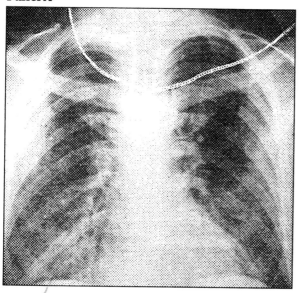

Panel B

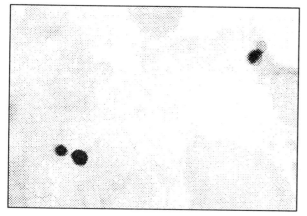

    (A) *Pneumocystis carinii.*

    (B) *Herpes simplex.*

    (C) *Candida albicans.*

    (D) *Histoplasma capsulatum.*

    (E) *Streptococcus pneumoniae.*

52. Indications for endotracheal intubation in a 45-year-old female who is two days post-emergent cholecystectomy for ascending cholangitis include all of the following EXCEPT

    (A) respiratory rate of 52.

    (B) Glasgow coma scale of 5.

    (C) arterial pH of 7.07.

    (D) heart rate of 137.

    (E) arterial PaO2 of 32.

53. Your 44-year-old female patient reports a mass felt on breast self-examination. You advise her to

    (A) ignore it and feel for it again in one week.

    (B) schedule a mammogram.

    (C) make an appointment right away to your clinic.

    (D) call the surgeon and schedule a mastectomy.

    (E) have the surgeon perform a biopsy.

54. A 34-year-old female has been trying to get pregnant for the last six years, without being able to conceive. She has symptoms of amenorrhea and excessive hair on her upper lip. On exam, she is obese, with hirsutism. Lab data reveal an elevated luteinizing hormone and normal follicular stimulating hormone. Serum testosterone levels were mildly elevated. What is the most likely diagnosis?

    (A) Prolactin-secreting tumor of the pituitary gland

    (B) Stein-Leventhal syndrome

    (C) Hypothalamic hypothyroidism

    (D) Cushing's syndrome

    (E) Premature ovarian failure

For Questions 55-58, match the most likely diagnosis with the symptoms presented.

    (A)   Pulmonary tuberculosis

    (B)   Chronic obstructive pulmonary disease

    (C)   Reactive airway disease

    (D)   Bacterial pneumonia

    (E)   Acute bronchitis

55. A 24-year-old man presents with four years of intermittent episodes of shortness of breath. He notes no exacerbating factors or associated symptoms of fever or chills. His pulmonary function testing reveals a normal DLCO and decreased FEV1, which reverses to normal after bronchodilator treatment. TLC and RV are normal.

56. A 33-year-old woman presents with three days of cough productive of rusty-brown sputum. Three days ago, she noted the onset of rigors and since then has had feelings of chills and fevers, but never took her temperature. She also complains of right-sided sharp chest pain with deep inspiration.

57. A 50-year-old woman presents with three months of shortness of breath with exertion. She denies any fevers, chills, or chest pain. Her past medical history is significant for hypertension and a 40-pack-year smoking history. Physical examination reveals slightly decreased breath sounds throughout. Chest X-ray reveals normal cardiac silhouette and slightly flattened diaphragms.

58. A 38-year-old man presents with one week of cough productive of yellow-green sputum. He complains of generalized malaise, but denies fevers, chills, night sweats, and chest pain. Physical examination reveals normal lung sounds diffusely.

59. An 18-year-old white female presents to her allergist with symptoms of frequent sneezing, watery and itchy eyes, pruritic upper palate, and watery, clear rhinorrhea. On exam, she has blue, boggy nasal turbinates and an elevation of eosinophils on a nasal discharge smear. She has a family history of similar symptoms. All of the following are treatment options for this patient EXCEPT

    (A)   inhaled nasal corticosteroids.

    (B)   oral non-sedating antihistamine agents.

    (C)   air-conditioning.

    (D)   normal saline drops to each nostril.

    (E)   avoiding alcohol use with antihistamines.

60. A 25-year-old male contacts you upon his return from a trip to China. Some of his travel companions have recently been diagnosed with acute hepatitis A. He is currently asymptomatic. Physical examination is normal. Concerning infection with hepatitis A, you explain all of the following EXCEPT

    (A)   fecal shedding of hepatitis A virus ends with the appearance of anti-HAV in the serum.

    (B)   fecal shedding of the virus declines as serum transaminases reach peak levels.

    (C)   an HAV carrier state occurs in 50% of exposed persons.

    (D)   IgG anti-HAV persists in the serum for many years.

    (E)   serum IgM anti-HAV usually indicates that an infection has occurred within the past few months.

61. A 45-year-old male presents with symptoms of severe epigastric pain, diarrhea, and weight loss. He obtains no relief with H2 blockers. His serum gastrin level is elevated to over 800 ng/L. By upper endoscopy, a lesion was located in the postbulbar duodenum. What is the most likely diagnosis?

    (A)   Pancreatitis

    (B)   Zollinger-Ellison syndrome

    (C)   *H. pylori*-induced duodenal ulcer

(D)   MEN type II

(E)   Celiac sprue

62.   A 39-year-old high school teacher is seen for a four-year history of low back pain, generalized bone and muscle pain, dyspareunia, and fatigue. On physical examination, she looks very apprehensive, helpless, and tearful. Her left eye is swollen and hyperemic. She denies spousal abuse and attributes all her symptoms to recurrent viral infections. Concerning her condition, which one of the following statements is true?

(A)   Domestic violence is unusual in middle-class families.

(B)   Anxiolytics are integral components of the treatment plan in all cases.

(C)   The estimated prevalence rate of spousal abuse in North America is 10%.

(D)   The patient most likely will establish a new life on her own.

(E)   Individual psychotherapy is the treatment of choice for abusers.

63.   A 20-year-old man presents to your office with 10 days of listlessness, a cough that is dry, and low-grade fevers. Chest examination reveals bilateral inspiratory dry rales. Chest radiograph reveals bilateral fluffy infiltrates. The most likely organism to cause this syndrome is

(A)   *Streptococcus pneumoniae.*

(B)   *Haemophilus influenzae.*

(C)   *Legionella.*

(D)   *Mycobacterium tuberculosis.*

(E)   *Mycoplasma pneumoniae.*

64.   Screening of obstetrical patients for gestational diabetes should be scheduled at

(A)   6 weeks.

(B)   18 weeks.

(C)   20 weeks.

(D)   28 weeks.

(E)   36 weeks.

65.   A 25-year-old man with AIDS comes in with *Pneumocystis carinii* pneumonia. He is quite tachypneic and his oxygen saturation by ear oximetry is 89% on room air. He was previously in good health. You

(A)   tell the patient that he needs to be intubated.

(B)   tell the patient he is going to die imminently and nothing should be done except to make him comfortable.

(C)   give him high-dose morphine.

(D)   begin intravenous pentamidine.

(E)   call a full code.

66.   An 82-year-old male with osteoarthritis presented with a history of diarrhea, steatorrhea, and a 20-kg weight loss. He has been undergoing a diagnostic evaluation. An upper gastroduodenoscopy and a computed tomographic scan of the abdomen were normal. He was lost to follow-up for several months, but returns now for the results of his upper gastrointestinal barium X-ray studies, shown in the figure. You recommend

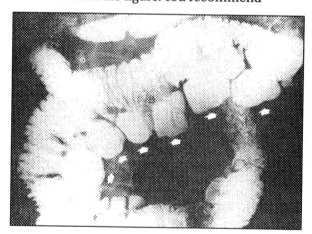

(A)   oral antibiotics.

(B)   surgical consultation.

(C)   oncologic consultation.

(D)   low-fiber diet.

(E)   pancreatic supplements.

Questions 67-74 refer to the following:

A 30-year-old male presents to your office complaining of fatigue and low-grade fevers for the past week. He also notes recent onset of generalized arthralgias and headache.

67. All of the following conditions should be considered in your differential diagnosis EXCEPT

    (A) bacterial meningitis.

    (B) Lyme disease.

    (C) leptospirosis.

    (D) influenza.

    (E) Epstein-Barr virus.

68. Physical examination reveals a large erythematous, annular lesion on the right buttock. You order a Lyme antibody titer, which is positive. Which one of the following conditions may also result in a positive Lyme antibody titer?

    (A) Secondary syphilis

    (B) Mycobacterial pneumonia

    (C) Psittacosis

    (D) Herpes encephalitis

    (E) None of the above.

69. Based on the clinical history and the positive antibody titer, you decide that a course of treatment for Lyme disease is warranted. What is the name of the annular skin lesion noted on this patient?

    (A) Erythema nodosum

    (B) Erythema chronicum migrans

    (C) Erythema multiforme

    (D) Erythema marginatum

    (E) None of the above.

70. Which one of the following is the pathogenic organism that requires treatment in Lyme disease?

    (A) *Chlamydia trachomatis*

    (B) *Ureaplasma urealyticum*

    (C) *Rickettsia prowazekii*

    (D) *Blastomyces dermatitidis*

    (E) None of the above.

71. All of the following antibiotics are effective as therapy for Lyme disease EXCEPT

    (A) amoxicillin.

    (B) tetracycline.

    (C) erythromycin.

    (D) streptomycin.

    (E) ceftriaxone.

72. Upon returning for follow-up and initiation of antibiotic therapy, you note that the patient has a drooping of the right corner of the mouth and inability to completely close the left eye. The cause of these neurologic syndromes is

    (A) vasculitis stroke.

    (B) Lyme encephalitis.

    (C) cranial neuritis.

    (D) transverse myelitis.

    (E) sensory radiculopathy.

73. All of the following are additional complications that may potentially develop in this patient EXCEPT

    (A) first-degree A-V block.

    (B) lymphadenopathy.

    (C) jaundice.

    (D) knee swelling.

    (E) acrodermatitis.

74. Which one of the following is appropriate advice to give to the patient's family?

    (A) Obtain prophylactic vaccination against Lyme disease.

    (B) Avoid exposure to ticks.

    (C) Use prophylactic antibiotics prior to camping trips.

    (D) Avoid skin contact with the patient.

(E) Avoid close contact with house pets.

75. You are consulted to see a patient on the psychiatry service for polydipsia. He is a 38-year-old man with bipolar disorder being treated with lithium. He is on no other medications and his physical examination is without abnormalities. He is alert and oriented to name, place, and time. Urine studies reveal an osmolality of 130 and a volume of 22 liters in 24 hours. Serum studies reveal a sodium level of 148, a serum creatinine of 0.5, and a glucose of 100. Urine osmolality after water deprivation is 150. The most likely etiology of the patient's symptoms is

(A) Type I diabetes mellitus.

(B) Type II diabetes mellitus.

(C) diabetes insipidus.

(D) psychogenic polydipsia.

(E) None of the above.

76. A 58-year-old woman presents to your office with questions regarding estrogen replacement therapy. You tell her that the benefits include all of the following EXCEPT

(A) decreased incidence of myocardial infarction.

(B) decreased incidence of stroke.

(C) decreased incidence of osteoporosis.

(D) decreased incidence of endometrial cancer.

(E) decreased death rate of all causes.

77. A 28-year-old man presents to the emergency room with four episodes of severe headaches. He states that they are behind his right eye and are very sharp and severe and associated with lacrimation in that eye. He states that he has never had similar headaches to this previously. The most likely etiology of this patient's headaches is

(A) migraine headache.

(B) tension headache.

(C) subdural hematoma.

(D) subarachnoid hemorrhage.

(E) cluster headache.

78. Classifying a patient as anuretic requires a urine output less than what volume per day?

(A) 100 cc

(B) 250 cc

(C) 500 cc

(D) 1,000 cc

(E) 2,000 cc

79. A 54-year-old man reports to you that his surroundings seem to be spinning when his eyes are open. This describes

(A) syncope.

(B) dizziness.

(C) vertigo.

(D) presbycusis.

(E) entrapment.

For Questions 80–83, match the most likely diagnosis with each numbered question.

(A) Muddy, brown casts in the urine

(B) Red blood cell casts in the urine

(C) Myoglobin in the urine

(D) Gross hematuria

(E) Sterile pyuria

80. A 40-year-old man was in the intensive care unit for septic shock. His urine output was very low and he was hypotensive.

81. A 24-year-old bodybuilder was exercising vigorously and suddenly felt sudden pain and weakness in his thighs bilaterally. His creatinine phosphokinase level was 2,000 mg/dl.

82. A 26-year-old female with a positive antinuclear antibody test and positive anti-double stranded DNA antibody test presents with a malar rash.

83. A 50-year-old homeless, alcoholic male who lives in a shelter presents with fever, weight loss, purulent sputum production, and bilateral upper lobe cavities on the chest X-ray.

84. A 48-year-old man with a history of mild hypertension presents to your office and asks about the efficacy of medications for prevention of coronary artery disease. You tell him that

   (A) there are no medications that have been shown effective in decreasing the incidence of coronary artery disease and that smoking cessation and a low cholesterol diet are the only things that you can offer.

   (B) there has been some evidence to support that some lipid-lowering medications can decrease the incidence of coronary artery disease.

   (C) there has been evidence that has shown that one aspirin each day can decrease the incidence of coronary artery disease.

   (D) there has been no evidence to support that management of mild hypertension will decrease the incidence of coronary artery disease.

   (E) None of the above.

Questions 85-88 refer to the following:

You refer your 73-year-old patient to a cardiologist because of an abnormal echocardiogram, and he wants to localize the disease process to an anatomic region. Match the following abnormal heart sounds with the respective disease process that you would encounter while auscultating the heart.

   (A) Basal systolic murmur

   (B) Midprecordial systolic murmur

   (C) Apical systolic murmur

   (D) Basal diastolic murmur

   (E) Apical diastolic murmur

85. Pulmonic regurgitation

86. Mitral stenosis

87. Ventricular septal defect

88. Aortic stenosis

89. The signs of pulmonary emphysema include all of the following EXCEPT

   (A) barrel chest.

   (B) hyporesonant lungs.

   (C) hyperresonant lungs.

   (D) rales.

   (E) decreased breath sounds.

Questions 90-97 refer to the following:

A 21-year-old single female with three children comes into the emergency department for the first time. She has noticed aching in her joints for about a week, some low-grade fevers, and a swollen left knee for two days. She is not married and lives with her boyfriend who often works nights.

90. Your brief initial history should include all of the following EXCEPT

   (A) sexual history.

   (B) recent trauma.

   (C) use of intravenous drugs.

   (D) recent surgery.

   (E) childhood vaccinations.

91. The first procedure you should perform on this patient is

   (A) urinalysis.

   (B) vaginal culture.

   (C) knee aspiration.

   (D) rectal culture.

   (E) throat culture.

92. Which one of the following statements is true?

   (A) No special handling is required for the sample you obtained in the last question.

(B) Some of the sample should be sent for virologic studies.

(C) Some of the sample should be sent for cytology.

(D) The sample requires special handling on its way to the laboratory.

(E) Some of the sample should be sent for cryptococcal antigen.

93. On physical examination you notice several small erythematous papules on the patient's arms. They are not tender and she had not even noticed them. Your primary diagnosis now is

(A) staphylococcal sepsis.

(B) disseminated gonococcal infection.

(C) meningococcemia.

(D) Rocky Mountain spotted fever.

(E) rubella.

94. All of the following tests should be obtained EXCEPT

(A) CBC.

(B) vaginal culture.

(C) rectal culture.

(D) skin culture.

(E) throat culture.

95. The appropriate management of this patient is

(A) a shot of bicillin and discharge to home.

(B) hospitalization for intravenous antibiotics and drainage of the knee.

(C) oral ampicillin and discharge to home.

(D) intravenous penicillin with a 23-hour observation period in the emergency department and discharge to home.

(E) knee drainage.

96. Which one of the following will need to be done?

(A) You will have to call the patient's boyfriend and tell him what is wrong with her.

(B) You will need to see the patient's boyfriend and treat him.

(C) You will need to trace all of the patient's sexual contacts.

(D) You will need to notify the Department of Health regarding this infection.

(E) You will need to tell the patient's employer about the disease so all of her co-workers can be examined.

97. The patient's knee symptoms resolve in 48 hours. Which one of the following courses is most likely for her skin lesions?

(A) She will be left with atrophic spots.

(B) She will be left with scars.

(C) They will resolve completely.

(D) She will need subcutaneous steroid injections.

(E) She will need systemic steroids.

98. A 24-year-old man presents with increasing shortness of breath for three weeks. He denies any fevers, night sweats, weight loss, chills, cough, or chest pain. He denies any other medical problems. He smokes a few cigarettes a day and is a social drinker. He is sexually active and he denies history of illicit drug use. Physical examination reveals his temperature to be 99.7°F, and his respiratory rate to be 24. Lungs are clear. Chest radiograph reveals bilateral interstitial infiltrates. The most likely diagnosis is

(A) *Pneumocystis carinii* pneumonia.

(B) acute bacterial bronchitis.

(C) viral bronchitis.

(D) bacterial pneumonia.

(E) congestive heart failure.

Questions 99-102 refer to the following:

A 53-year-old woman is brought to the walk-in clinic by her husband because she has been somnolent and lethargic lately. He is especially surprised because he says she has been on "a health kick" lately and has been taking a lot of vitamins and eating lots of vegetables. She had been walking two miles a day until she started to feel poorly about a week ago. On examination she is lethargic but arousable. She has no focal signs. She appears well-nourished.

99. Her electrocardiogram shows a short Q-T interval. You are not surprised when the laboratory tests show

    (A) hyperkalemia.

    (B) hypokalemia.

    (C) hypocalcemia.

    (D) hypercalcemia.

    (E) hyponatremia.

100. The chest radiograph shows a calcified left upper lobe nodule. The notation on the radiology folder indicates that this radiograph is unchanged from one a few years ago, but you cannot find the old films. You decide to

    (A) order a chest CT scan.

    (B) proceed in your workup, assuming that the radiograph is unchanged.

    (C) order a fine needle biopsy of the nodule.

    (D) tell the husband the patient probably has a paraneoplastic syndrome.

    (E) call a thoracic surgeon.

101. You decide that you need to ask the patient's husband

    (A) which vitamins the patient has been taking.

    (B) where she has traveled recently.

    (C) what her parents died from.

    (D) how many siblings she has.

    (E) how many children she has.

102. You are not surprised to discover that the patient has been taking a lot of

    (A) vitamin E.

    (B) iron.

    (C) vitamin C.

    (D) vitamin D.

    (E) vitamin B.

103. A preoperative patient asks you about the use of spinal anesthesia for her surgery. Spinal anesthesia can be utilized for all of the following operations EXCEPT

    (A) open reduction, internal fixation of a tibial fracture.

    (B) tubal ligation.

    (C) ventral hernia repair.

    (D) cesarean section.

    (E) repair of forearm tendon laceration.

Questions 104 and 105 refer to the following:

A 33-year-old gravida 2 para 1 is tested for gestational diabetes with an oral glucose challenge at 24-weeks gestational age. The results are found to be high.

104. How will you manage this patient?

    (A) Perform a three-hour oral glucose tolerance test.

    (B) Start the patient on insulin therapy immediately, as she has gestational diabetes mellitus.

    (C) Start the patient on an oral hypoglycemic medication.

    (D) Place the patient on a strict 1,800-calorie ADA diet and have her monitor her fingersticks.

    (E) Do nothing. It is normal for pregnant women to have elevated blood sugars during the second trimester.

105. The single greatest risk for the fetus that is associated with diabetic pregnancies is

    (A) congenital anomalies.

    (B) spontaneous abortion.

    (C) intrauterine death.

    (D) macrosomia.

    (E) growth retardation.

Questions 106-113 refer to the following:

A 40-year-old woman has been admitted to your inpatient service because of fever, weight loss, lymphadenopathy, and leukopenia. She has a history of transient rashes and sometimes gets chest pain. She has had some vague muscle and joint pains. She says she had pneumonia about 10 years ago. Her admitting lab results are as follows

    HGB 11.1
    HCT 30
    WBC 1,500
    Platelets 110,000
    Urinalysis 4+ protein
    Electrolytes normal
    Chemistry normal except total
    protein 8.3

106. You examine the patient on morning rounds. She has cervical, axillary, and inguinal lymphadenopathy and an erythematous, slightly raised rash on her cheeks. Her lungs are clear. You order all of the following tests EXCEPT

    (A) antinuclear antibodies.

    (B) bone marrow aspirate.

    (C) intravenous pyelogram.

    (D) sedimentation rate.

    (E) chest radiograph.

107. You ask about her family history. The most helpful information you learn is that

    (A) her uncle had prostate cancer.

    (B) her sister has breast cancer.

    (C) her aunt had lupus.

    (D) her father had a myocardial infarction.

    (E) her mother had a stroke.

108. Your working diagnosis at this point is

    (A) lymphoma.

    (B) leukemia.

    (C) glomerulonephritis.

    (D) systemic lupus.

    (E) subacute bacterial endocarditis.

109. A 24-hour urine collections reveals greater than 2 gms. of protein. This is consistent with

    (A) glomerulonephritis.

    (B) nephrotic syndrome.

    (C) interstitial nephritis.

    (D) polycystic kidney disease.

    (E) urinary tract infection.

110. The ANA is positive with a titer of 1:640. You anticipate that the patient will also have

    (A) elevated complement levels.

    (B) normal sedimentation rate.

    (C) elevated CPK.

    (D) positive antibodies to DNA.

    (E) no other autoantibodies.

111. The nurses call you during the day to tell you that the patient is having a grand-mal seizure. She has never had a seizure before. This is most consistent with

    (A) a brain tumor.

    (B) a subdural hematoma.

    (C) meningitis.

    (D) a stroke.

    (E) cerebritis.

112. You order anti-epileptic medication and decide to begin treatment with

    (A) high-dose prednisone.

    (B) a nonsteroidal anti-inflammatory agent.

    (C) cyclosporine.

(D) low-dose prednisone.

(E) cyclophosphamide.

113. As you expected, the chest radiograph shows

    (A) an infiltrate.

    (B) cardiomegaly.

    (C) no abnormalities.

    (D) a pleural-based mass.

    (E) aortic calcification.

114. A 34-year-old man with cirrhosis and ascites is hospitalized for nausea, vomiting, and increased lethargy for three days. His vital signs reveal that he is febrile with a temperature of 102°F; he has a heart rate of 90, a respiratory rate of 14, and a blood pressure of 110/70. His lungs are clear and his heart is without murmurs or gallops. His abdominal exam reveals decreased bowel sounds throughout and distension with shifting dullness. The most likely cause of the patient's symptoms is

    (A) spontaneous bacterial peritonitis.

    (B) pneumonias.

    (C) urosepsis.

    (D) bacterial meningitis.

    (E) metastatic hepatocellular carcinoma.

115. A 52-year-old man who has had a recent upper respiratory tract infection presents with weakness in the lower extremities which he feels is progressively getting worse. On exam, he has diminished deep-tendon reflexes. He is taking no medications, has no known allergies, and no significant family or past medical history. A few days later, he develops paralysis of both proximal and distal muscles of both extremities. His cerebral spinal fluid protein concentration is elevated to 108 mg/dl. What is the correct diagnosis?

    (A) Myasthenia gravis

    (B) Multiple sclerosis

    (C) Shy-Drager syndrome

    (D) Guillain-Barre syndrome

    (E) Amyotrophic lateral sclerosis

Questions 116 and 117 are together.

116. A 24-year-old first-time mother asks you when she can expect the first teeth to erupt in her infant's mouth. You tell her at

    (A) one month.

    (B) three months.

    (C) six months.

    (D) three year.

    (E) two years.

117. The location of these teeth will be in the

    (A) anterior mandible.

    (B) anterior maxilla.

    (C) posterior mandible.

    (D) posterior maxilla.

    (E) None of the above.

118. A 42-year-old woman complains of chest pain that is worsened when she breathes. All of the following may be a reason for this EXCEPT

    (A) rib fracture.

    (B) myocardial infarct.

    (C) costochondritis.

    (D) intercostal myositis.

    (E) shingles.

119. The most common kind of urinary stone is comprised of

    (A) calcium.

    (B) struvite.

    (C) cystine.

    (D) uric acid.

    (E) cholesterol.

120. A 28-year-old woman with a history of cystic fibrosis presents to the emergency room

with fever, chills, and cough productive of green sputum for two days. The most likely causative organism is

- (A) *Pseudomonas aeruginosa.*
- (B) *Streptococcus pneumonia.*
- (C) *Staphylococcus aureus.*
- (D) *Haemophilus influenzae.*
- (E) *Mycobacterium tuberculosis.*

121. Red blood cell characteristics in hereditary spherocytosis include all of the following EXCEPT

- (A) the life span of the red blood cell is reduced to 150 days.
- (B) the degree of spectrin/ankyrin deficiency correlates with the degree of spherocytosis, as measured by osmotic fragility.
- (C) defects in protein 3 are present only in the dominant form of the disease.
- (D) as red blood cells age, they slowly lose portions of the lipid bilayer.
- (E) "splenic conditioning" accentuates the membrane loss.

122. During morning rounds, you find that one of your patients with diffusely metastatic pancreatic cancer has developed a fever. He is unarousable and does not appear to be in pain. The family and patient have previously agreed that he should not be resuscitated if he arrests. You do not think that workup and treatment of his fever is in his best interest at this point. You

- (A) call the family to discuss your opinion with them.
- (B) call the priest.
- (C) call the Ethics Committee.
- (D) do nothing.
- (E) start antibiotics.

Questions 123-126 refer to the following:

You are asked to examine the knees of a 17-year-old high school student who presents to your office for his school physical. You note lateral deviation of the leg from midline.

123. This is known as

- (A) genu varum.
- (B) genu valgum.
- (C) genu recurvatum.
- (D) genu medialis.
- (E) genu lateralis.

124. The cause of the above deformity is

- (A) lateral femoral growth.
- (B) medial femoral growth.
- (C) prominent development of the medial femoral condyles.
- (D) prominent development of the lateral femoral condyles.
- (E) underdevelopment of the medial femoral condyles.

125. The patient is also noted to have fluid in the knee joint. All of the following may cause this fluid EXCEPT

- (A) gout.
- (B) pseudogout.
- (C) trauma.
- (D) arthritis.
- (E) tumor.

126. On examination of the patient's right knee, there is a medial knee mass. This may represent

- (A) anserine bursitis.
- (B) Morrant-Baker's cyst.
- (C) semimembranous bursitis.
- (D) popliteal abscess.
- (E) infrapatellar bursitis.

127. A 53-year-old man with severe hypertension has a blood pressure of 220/150 in your office at his routine visit. You recommend that he go to the emergency room for acute man-

agement because you do not have the appropriate drugs and facilities in your office. He refuses and insists on going to work. You should

(A)　call the police to take him to the hospital.

(B)　call a psychiatrist to get him committed.

(C)　refuse to ever see him again.

(D)　document his refusal in your notes and try to get him to sign a statement saying he refused your advice.

(E)　give him a return appointment in a year.

Questions 128 and 129 refer to the following:

Your 45-year-old receptionist presents with positive Tinel's and Phalen's signs.

128. You diagnose

(A)　cubital tunnel syndrome.

(B)　carpal tunnel syndrome.

(C)　de Quervain's disease.

(D)　Dupuytren's disease.

(E)　wrist fracture.

129. All of the following would be appropriate for this patient EXCEPT

(A)　splint.

(B)　steroid injections.

(C)　surgery.

(D)　observation.

(E)　rest.

130. A 12-year-old girl is seen at your clinic for fever (104°F), irritability, malaise, conjunctivitis, and photophobia. She remembers that one of her classmates had similar complaints four days ago. Her blood pressure is 115/75. The next day, her mother calls to tell you that the daughter's temperature is 101°F, and she developed a red maculopapular rash on the forehead. The girl's condition would

have been prevented if she had been immunized by

(A)　gamma globulin.

(B)　serum products.

(C)　anti-toxin.

(D)　live attenuated virus.

(E)　toxoid.

131. A 32-year-old baseball player suddenly collapses during a game. On exam, he is disproportionately tall with long arms and legs. He had a mid-systolic click on cardiac auscultation, as well as a diastolic murmur. His past medical history is significant for severe myopia and multiple joint dislocations. Which of the following is the most likely cause of his syncopal attack?

(A)　Mitral valve prolapse

(B)　Aortic dissection

(C)　Spntaneous pneumothorax

(D)　Pulmonary emboli

(E)　Ventricular arrhythmia

132. A 20-year-old nursing student who was PPD-negative before entering nursing school is found to be PPD-positive after her first ward rotation. The first action the Student Health physician who sees her should take is

(A)　repeat the PPD.

(B)　check her liver functions.

(C)　obtain a sputum sample for culture.

(D)　order a chest radiograph.

(E)　obtain a urine culture.

133. A 35-year-old man with a long history of alcohol intake comes to the physician's office complaining of painful breasts which are enlarged. All of the following are causes of gynecomastia EXCEPT

(A)　cirrhosis of the liver.

(B)　spironolactone.

(C)　thyrotoxicosis.

(D)　carcinoma of the prostrate.

(E)　germ-cell testicular tumors.

134. A 78-year-old female presents with weakness, fatigue, anorexia, and symptoms of salt craving. On exam, her blood pressure was 80/60 mmHg and she had hyperpigmentation. Lab data reveals hyperkalemia. What is the most likely diagnosis?

   (A) Chronic primary adrenocortical insufficiency

   (B) Hyporeninemic hypoaldosteronism

   (C) Cushing's disease

   (D) Conn's syndrome

   (E) Secondary adrenal insufficiency

Questions 135-142 refer to the following:

A 40-year-old alcoholic male is brought in by the Emergency Medical Service after being found sleeping in front of an elegant residential building. He responds appropriately to your questions. There is no focal neurologic deficit. He is not clinically intoxicated. Blood alcohol level is 300 mg.

135. This phenomenon is known as

   (A) alcohol withdrawal.

   (B) Wernicke's syndrome.

   (C) tolerance.

   (D) acetaldehyde syndrome.

   (E) blackouts.

136. The temperature recorded with the rectal probe is 28°C. Care must be exercised during rewarming because there is

   (A) increased cardiac susceptibility to ventricular fibrillation between 28-30°C.

   (B) increased risk of asystole between 35-37°C.

   (C) increased risk for pulmonary embolism between 28-30°C.

   (D) increased risk for hyperkalemia.

   (E) increased risk for rebound hyperglycemia.

137. All of the following laboratory abnormalities may occur in hypothermic patients EXCEPT

   (A) hyperkalemia.

   (B) disseminated intravascular coagulation.

   (C) metabolic acidosis.

   (D) increased urine specific gravity.

   (E) hyperamylasemia.

138. A 23-year-old intravenous drug user presents to the emergency room with complaints of sudden onset of fever, nocturnal diaphoresis, arthralgias, and myalgias. Physical examination reveals a critically ill-appearing young male with a temperature of 104°F, blood pressure 100/70, pulse of 110, and respiration of 24. Skin shows multiple recent injection sites, some purulent; lungs have few bibasilar rales; coronary exam reveals grade II/VI blowing, high-pitched decrescendo diastolic murmur, best heard in the third left intercostal space; abdomen has hepatosplenomegaly. Transesophageal echocardiographic imaging of the aortic valve and root are shown in the figure. You begin treatment for

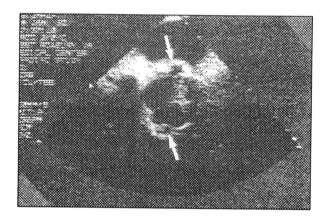

   (A) Libman-Sacks endocarditis.

   (B) acute bacterial endocarditis.

   (C) septic pulmonary emboli.

   (D) HACEK endocarditis.

   (E) marantic endocarditis.

139. The organism most likely to be isolated from blood cultures is

   (A) *Streptococcus bovis.*

   (B) *Candida albicans.*

(C)   *Pseudomonas aeruginosa.*

(D)   *Staphylococcus aureus.*

(E)   *Staphylococcus epidermidis.*

140. Which one of the following is NOT true regarding blood cultures in endocarditis?

   (A)   Arterial blood offers no advantages over antecubital vein blood samples.

   (B)   They should be spaced 60 minutes apart to demonstrate continuous bacteremia.

   (C)   The rate of positivity is increased by observing them over three weeks with periodic sampling for Gram stain and subculture even in the absence of turbidity.

   (D)   Bacteremia is maximum just prior to the temperature peak.

   (E)   Only one culture should be obtained from each venipuncture site.

141. Two days later, gross hematuria develops. As part of the diagnostic evaluation, a contrast-enhanced computed axial tomographic scan of the abdomen, shown in the figure below, was performed. You diagnose

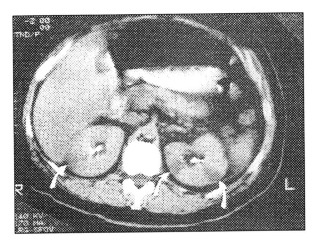

   (A)   interstitial nephritis secondary to antibiotic therapy.

   (B)   acute tubular necrosis secondary to antibiotic therapy.

(C)   bilateral papillary necrosis.

(D)   embolic renal infarction.

(E)   incidental polycystic disease.

142. A 57-year-old man is being treated for hypertension. The physician seeks to use a diuretic agents which directly modifies water absorption rather than one that affects salt excretion. Which of the following pharmacologic agents can be utilized?

   (A)   carbonic anhydrase inhibitors (e.g., acetazolamide).

   (B)   loop diuretics (e.g., furosemide).

   (C)   thiazides (e.g., hyrochlorothiazide).

   (D)   anti-diuretic hormone (ADH) antagonists (e.g., democlocycline).

   (E)   potassium-sparing diuretics (e.g., spironolactone).

143. Your wife, a school nurse, reports that many of the children in the first grade have been scratching their heads for the past two days. Parents of some of the children have observed small white capsules firmly attached to the hair. Microscopic examination of one of these capsules is illustrated in Panels A and B. Your diagnosis is

Panel A

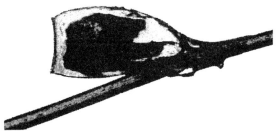

Panel B

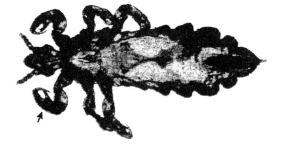

(A) *Pulex irritans.*

(B) *Dirofilaria immitis.*

(C) *Pediculus capitis.*

(D) *Cimex lectularius.*

(E) *Latrodectus mactans.*

144. A 41-year-old male with psoriasis complains of right foot pain. On examination, there is swelling and tenderness of the first phalanx. X-ray findings (shown in the figure below), which are consistent with psoriatic arthritis, include all of the following abnormalities EXCEPT

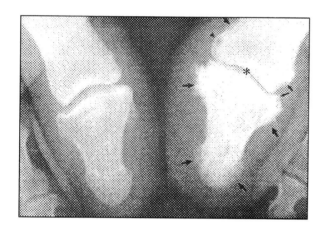

(A) asymmetric distribution.

(B) subchondral cysts.

(C) soft tissue swelling, confined to the joint distribution.

(D) new periosteal bone formation.

(E) marginal erosions.

145. A decline in a mortality rate of coronary artery disease in the U.S. has been mostly attributed to

(A) the use of pacemakers.

(B) anti-smoker programs.

(C) the better diet of control groups at risk.

(D) advanced technology.

(E) anti-stress programs.

146. A 61-year-old female presents to your office with bloody sputum, dyspnea, cough, weight loss, and malaise. A complete physical and laboratory assessment reveal a mass in the left lung. The patient has been a heavy smoker and lives in an old house. The most likely diagnosis in this patient is

(A) laryngeal carcinoma.

(B) COPD.

(C) bronchogenic carcinoma.

(D) pleural mesothelioma.

(E) rupture of a preexisting tuberculosis.

147. An 11-year-old female is referred to you for evaluation of a positive tuberculin reaction. Based on the chest X-ray, shown below, you discuss all of the following with the mother EXCEPT

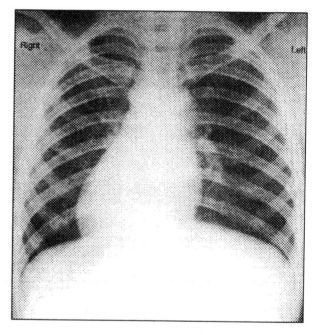

(A) longevity is normal.

(B) pain due to acute appendicitis occurs in the left lower quadrant.

(C) pain due to biliary colic presents with symptoms/signs in the left upper quadrant.

(D) the child requires extensive cardiac evaluation.

(E) there is no evidence of tuberculosis on this X-ray.

148. While performing examination of the testes, all of the following should be determined EXCEPT

(A) shape.

(B) size.

(C) consistency.

(D) sensitivity to pressure.

(E) weight.

149. Subclavian compression may arise from all of the following EXCEPT

(A) scalenus anticus syndrome.

(B) subclavian steal syndrome.

(C) cervical rib.

(D) costoclavicular syndrome.

(E) hyperelevation of the arm.

150. A 64-year-old man presents with a long history of nocturia. He now has some trouble initiating a urinary stream. Your initial diagnostic test is

(A) a PSA.

(B) a digital rectal exam.

(C) a pelvic ultrasound.

(D) a cystoscopy.

(E) a glucose tolerance test.

151. During your hospital rounds, you are called with the laboratory value of one of your partner's patients. The lab informs you that the platelet count in this patient is 850,000. All of the following conditions can result in this laboratory abnormality EXCEPT

(A) chronic liver disease.

(B) myeloproliferative disease.

(C) postsplenectomy.

(D) inflammatory bowel disease.

(E) adenocarcinoma of the lung.

152. A 20-year-old male presents to your office with symptoms of polyuria and polydipsia. He's noted that he drinks gallons of water each day and is almost always feeling thirsty. Physical examination is unremarkable. Laboratory values reveal a serum sodium of 140, glucose of 87, and osmolality of 280. Urine osmolality is 150. The most likely diagnosis is

(A) diabetes insipidus.

(B) diabetes mellitus.

(C) psychogenic polydipsia.

(D) normal healthy behavior.

(E) None of the above.

153. A 38-year-old Hispanic male was admitted to the hospital because of severe weakness and lower extremity thigh pain. He was a previously healthy male with no prior past medical history except for a recent viral syndrome. Lab data revealed a CPK level that was elevated to 12,000 mg/dl, elevation in BUN and creatinine, and a urine test positive for myoglobin. The urine was strongly positive for occult blood, but microscopic examination revealed only two erythrocytes per high-powered field. What would be the initial treatment plan in this particular patient?

(A) Steroids

(B) Antiviral therapy

(C) Vigorous intravenous hydration

(D) Antibiotics

(E) Dialysis

Question 154-157 refer to the following:

A 67-year-old man comes to your office complaining of difficulty in swallowing.

154. Which one of the following is LEAST helpful in determining the etiology of his symptoms?

(A) Symptoms related to solids versus liquids

(B) Duration of symptoms

(C) History of peptic ulcers

(D) Associated heartburn

(E) Weight loss

155. A barium swallow is obtained, which reveals a dilated esophagus and a narrowing at the gastroesophageal junction. Which one of the following diagnoses is most likely based on this finding?

(A) Esophageal cancer

(B) Schatzki's ring

(C) Diffuse esophageal spasm

(D) Peptic stricture

(E) Achalasia

156. The best test to confirm this diagnosis is

(A) esophageal manometry.

(B) 24-hour pH probe.

(C) therapeutic trial with a proton pump inhibitor.

(D) upper endoscopy with full-thickness esophageal biopsy.

(E) pneumatic balloon dilation of the gastroesophageal junction.

157. If this patient was found to have dysphagia secondary to an esophageal cancer at the gastroesophageal junction, the most likely histopathology of the tumor would be

(A) squamous cell carcinoma.

(B) smooth muscle sarcoma.

(C) adenocarcinoma.

(D) carcinoma-in-situ.

(E) Barrett's mucosa.

158. You are treating a patient in the emergency room who suffered a gunshot to the leg, nicking the femoral artery. The patient is hemorrhaging badly and requires a blood transfusion. Although there is inadequate time for blood typing, in the patient's wallet there is a card indicating that the patient's blood type is AB positive. Which one of the following types of blood are acceptable for transfusion?

(A) AB negative

(B) O positive

(C) B negative

(D) A positive

(E) All of the above.

Questions 159-166 refer to the following:

A 48-year-old previously healthy man presents to your office with symptoms of pruritus. He has no previous medical conditions and has had no previous surgeries. He is not taking any medications. Physical examination reveals a slightly jaundiced white male in no acute distress. Lungs are clear and cardiac examination is benign. Abdominal examination reveals normoactive bowel sounds. The abdomen is not tender or distended, and no masses or hepatosplenomegaly is noted.

159. All of the following diseases need to be high on the differential diagnosis EXCEPT

(A) cholelithiasis.

(B) pancreatic cancer.

(C) primary sclerosing cholangitis.

(D) cholangiocarcinoma.

(E) ampullary carcinoma.

160. Other pertinent things that should be asked about in this patient are all of the following EXCEPT

(A) color of stools.

(B) history of headaches.

(C) color of urine.

(D) history of melena.

(E) None of the above.

161. Blood is sent off for laboratory examination. Pertinent values include a sodium of 140, potassium of 4.3, chloride of 110, CO_2 of 28, serum creatinine of 0.7, and a glucose of 120. His white count is 7.8 with a normal differential, a platelet count of 330 K, and a hematocrit of 45%. His serum bilirubin is 8.7 mg/

dl, alkaline phosphatase is 560 IU/l, SGPT is 560 IU/L, and SGOT is 53 IU/L. These laboratory findings are most consistent with

(A) viral hepatitis.

(B) cholestatic liver disease.

(C) hepatocellular carcinoma.

(D) cirrhosis of the liver.

(E) hemolytic anemia.

162. A blood test to confirm the etiology of the elevation in alkaline phosphatase would be

(A) elevation of acidphosphatase.

(B) elevation of amylase.

(C) elevation of gamma-glutamyl transpeptidase.

(D) elevation of the prothrombin time.

(E) elevation of urine urobilinogen.

163. You order a CT scan of the abdomen and it reveals no masses, no evidence of hepatitis, no evidence of cirrhosis, and biliary tracts that are not well visualized. The next appropriate test to order would be

(A) right upper quadrant ultrasound.

(B) esophagogastroduodenoscopy.

(C) endoscopic retrograde cholangiopancreatography.

(D) HIDA scan.

(E) open liver biopsy.

164. The tests performed confirm the diagnosis of primary sclerosing cholangitis. The patient asks you about treatment options. You tell him that the most effective form of treatment you can offer him is

(A) liver transplantation.

(B) cyclosporine.

(C) systemic corticosteroids.

(D) plasmapheresis.

(E) chemotherapy.

165. Of the following, the most appropriate medication for the symptomatic treatment of his pruritus is

(A) cholestyramine.

(B) tetracycline.

(C) corticosteroids.

(D) antihistamines.

(E) phenothiazines.

166. Before he undergoes treatment, you tell him that further testing needs to be done. This will include

(A) cerebral angiogram to rule out cerebral aneurysms.

(B) colonoscopy to rule out inflammatory bowel disease.

(C) renal ultrasound to rule out polycystic kidney disease.

(D) endomyocardial biopsy to rule out amyloidosis.

(E) alpha-1-antitrypsin levels to rule out deficiency as an etiology.

167. A sample of 100 medical students was found to have a mean serum cholesterol level of 198 mg/dL with a variance of 25 mg/dL. If the data is normally distributed, the cholesterol levels of 95% of the medical students will be in the range (mg/dL)

(A) 173-223.

(B) 188-208.

(C) 148-248.

(D) 193-203.

(E) 198-203.

For Questions 168-171, match the etiology of hypoglycemia with its characteristic signs.

You are preparing to meet a lawyer to discuss a murder case involving the possibility of death by injection of insulin. You want to explain to the lawyer how various etiologies of hypoglycemia can be distinguished from one another by using the following illustrations

	Plasma insulin	C-peptide	Insulin antibodies	Proinsulin
(A)	increased	increased	absent	in creased
(B)	very high	normal/low	may be present	normal/low
(C)	increased	increased	absent	normal
(D)	low	low	absent	____

168. Exogenous insulin

169. Insulinoma

170. Hypoglycemia secondary to sulfonylureas

171. Hypoglycemia secondary to extrapancreatic sarcoma

For Questions 172-175, choose the best lettered answer for each numbered question. Each answer may be used once, more than once, or not at all.

(A) Heart transplant

(B) No transplant

(C) Liver transplant

(D) Renal transplant

172. Patient with alcoholic cirrhosis who is still drinking heavily

173. Patient with end-stage renal disease due to severe hypertension

174. Patient with dilated cardiomyopathy due to coxsackievirus, with ejection fraction of less than 20%

175. Patient with lupus and creatinine clearance of 75 cc

176. A 45-year-old male, previously in excellent health, complains of fever, rigors, headache, myalgias, and arthralgias. One month ago he was camping in the western national parks and stayed in the rustic cabins. Approximately two weeks ago he had a similar illness. His companion is also ill. Your laboratory technician asks you to confirm her findings on the Wright's stained peripheral smear, shown in the figure in the next column. You indicate that

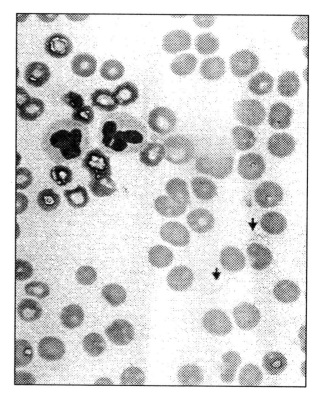

(A) the abnormality is an artifact.

(B) treatment for relapsing fever should be initiated.

(C) an FTA-ABS should be ordered immediately.

(D) quarantine measures should be immediately instituted.

(E) treatment for Rocky Mountain spotted fever should be initiated without delay.

177. A 20-year-old woman presents with acute onset of shortness of breath and a sharp right-sided chest pain with deep inspiration. She says this began one day ago after her final exam week in college. She denies any fevers, chills, cough, or other medical

problems, and is only taking oral contraceptives. Physical examination reveals that she is afebrile and has a respiratory rate of 24. Lungs are clear. Chest radiograph reveals no infiltrates or effusions. Complete blood count reveals a white blood count of 9,000 and a hematocrit of 38%. Arterial blood gas reveals a pH of 7.30, pCO_2 of 28, and a pO_2 of 74. A ventilation-perfusion scan is done, which is read as low probability for pulmonary embolism. The next appropriate step would be to

(A) discharge the patient to home with a prescription for NSAIDs.

(B) order a pulmonary arteriogram.

(C) begin anti-coagulation empirically.

(D) plan for a bronchoscopy.

(E) order a CT of the chest.

178. Which one of the following statements regarding screening for carcinoma in men is true?

(A) Occult blood testing or sigmoidoscopy should be performed for all men aged 50 or older to screen for colorectal cancer.

(B) Digital rectal examination is an effective screening tool for prostate cancer in asymptomatic men.

(C) Adolescent and young males with insidious-onset testicular pain, swelling, or heaviness should be screened for testicular carcinoma.

(D) A history of orchiopexy is not an indication for testicular cancer screening.

(E) Routine screening for oral cancer in asymptomatic males who use tobacco or excessive amounts of alcohol is mandatory.

179. A 57-year-old female with peripheral vascular disease returns for evaluation of her blood pressure, which has been difficult to control for the past month. Today she also

complains of muscle weakness and polyuria. Physical examination reveals blood pressure of 180/110, pulse of 90, respiration of 12; a high-pitched epigastric bruit; and laboratory values of K 3.1 mEq/L, HCO_3- 40 mEq/L, Cr 2.5 mg/dL, and Chol 300 mg/dL. As part of her work-up, a renal arteriogram, shown in the figure, was performed. You now recommend

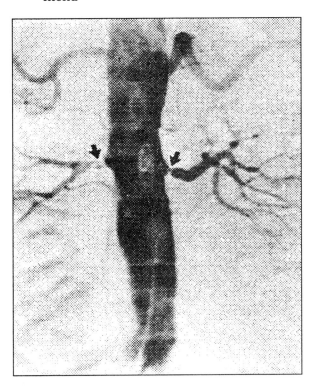

(A) Captopril renal scintigram.

(B) three-dimensional phase-contrast MRI.

(C) percutaneous transluminal angioplasty.

(D) renal vein renin assays.

(E) addition of Captopril 50 mg ID to the current medical regimen.

180. A 44-year-old woman presents to your clinic with chills and colicky pain. You diagnose cholangitis. You would expect the lab tests to reveal

    (A) decreased hematocrit.

    (B) elevated BUN.

    (C) elevated liver function tests.

    (D) normal urinalysis.

    (E) elevated glucose.

USMLE STEP 3
PRACTICE TEST 2

Day One – Afternoon Session

(Answer sheets appear in the back of this book.)

TIME: 3 Hours
180 Questions

DIRECTIONS: Each of the following numbered items or incomplete sentences is followed by an answer or a completion of the statement. Choose the **ONE** choice that **BEST** answers the question or completes the sentence.

---

1. Regarding counseling HIV-positive patients, which one of the following statements is true?

    (A) Yearly immunization with influenza vaccine is recommended for older patients with HIV.

    (B) TB testing should be optional for patients with HIV seropositivity.

    (C) Positive HIV seropositivity is a contraindication for most vaccinations.

    (D) OPV should be administered to all HIV-positive patients every 10 years.

    (E) Tetanus toxoid should be given to all HIV-positive patients every 10 years.

Questions 2-9 refer to the following:

A 64-year-old man comes to the emergency room complaining of bright red blood per rectum for the past 20 minutes. The bleeding is painless and not associated with stool mixed with blood. Other past history is negative. Medications include ibuprofen 800 mg TID for low back pain for the past eight days. Physical examination reveals BP of 90/60 with pulse of 110, respirations of 12, and afebrile. Rectal exam reveals blood in the rectal vault. Recent blood test results from the office from two weeks prior are normal.

2. All the following should be done in the initial management of this patient EXCEPT

    (A) type and cross four units of blood.

    (B) hydrate with normal saline.

    (C) monitor blood pressure and pulse.

    (D) contact gastroenterologic and surgical consultants.

    (E) maintain patient on clear-liquid diet.

3. All of the following are diagnostic tests of potential utility in this patient EXCEPT

    (A) CAT scan of the abdomen.

    (B) flexible sigmoidoscopy.

    (C) tagged red blood cell scan.

    (D) angiogram.

    (E) upper endoscopy.

4. Blood tests are ordered. The hematocrit and MCV in this patient are most likely to indicate which one of the following?

   (A) Microcytic anemia

   (B) Normocytic anemia

   (C) Macrocytic anemia

   (D) Reduced hematocrit with mixed population of microcytic and macrocytic cells

   (E) Normal hematocrit with normocytic cells

5. The most likely diagnosis in this patient based on the history is

   (A) diverticulosis.

   (B) diverticulitis.

   (C) hemorrhagic esophagitis.

   (D) inflammatory bowel disease.

   (E) small bowel lymphoma.

6. After further diagnostic evaluation, diagnosis of angiodysplasia is confirmed and immediate surgical intervention is decided upon. As the patient's internist you are concerned about the patient's recent use of ibuprofen. Which one of the following hematological tests would you suspect may be abnormal after this patient's use of ibuprofen?

   (A) PT

   (B) PTT

   (C) Platelet count

   (D) Bleeding time

   (E) Factor VIII level

7. Which one of the following would you recommend because of the use of ibuprofen in this patient?

   (A) Delay surgery until the hematological effects of the ibuprofen wear off.

   (B) Administer fresh frozen plasma at the time of surgery.

   (C) Administer platelet infusion at the time of surgery.

   (D) Proceed with surgery without any changes in management based on the ibuprofen use.

   (E) Obtain a hematological consultation.

8. Which one of the following statements is true regarding angiodysplasia?

   (A) Angiodysplasia is an uncommon cause of GI bleeding in elderly patients.

   (B) Angiodysplastic lesions are seen only in the colon.

   (C) Most cases of angiodysplasia are associated with mitral stenosis.

   (D) Endoscopic therapy can be effective for isolated angiodysplastic lesions.

   (E) Angiodysplasia is a premalignant condition.

9. The patient undergoes right hemicolectomy. However, two days postoperatively he develops fever to 102°F. All of the following are potential causes of postoperative fever EXCEPT

   (A) wound infection.

   (B) atelectasis.

   (C) pneumonia.

   (D) urinary tract infection.

   (E) infectious gastroenteritis.

10. A 42-year-old man comes in because of increasing nocturia. His urinary stream is good. He has noted that his mouth seems dry, and he drinks a lot of water to compensate. The first test you order is

   (A) prostate ultrasound.

   (B) hemoccult.

   (C) fasting blood glucose.

   (D) PSA.

   (E) urinalysis.

Questions 11-18 refer to the following:

A 23-year-old man with a 12-year history of diabetes mellitus comes to the ER because of a productive cough and low-grade fever. He also has been having some nausea and vomiting and has been sleeping a lot. His serum glucose is 52.

11. The first thing you should do is

    (A) get blood cultures.

    (B) get sputum cultures.

    (C) order a chest radiograph.

    (D) give the patient glucagon.

    (E) give the patient intravenous D50.

12. The likeliest cause of this patient's hypoglycemia is

    (A) an insulinoma.

    (B) improvement of his diabetes.

    (C) he has continued to take his insulin despite poor oral intake.

    (D) he has pneumonia.

    (E) he has not been taking his insulin.

13. You now proceed to evaluate the patient's cough. All of the following should be done now EXCEPT

    (A) a chest radiograph.

    (B) a CBC.

    (C) a blood culture.

    (D) a sputum culture.

    (E) a V/Q scan.

14. You should now give the patient all of the following EXCEPT

    (A) insulin injections on a sliding scale.

    (B) continuous insulin infusion.

    (C) antibiotics.

    (D) intravenous hydration with a glucose-containing solution.

    (E) acetaminophen.

15. This patient is likely to have all of the following associated conditions EXCEPT

    (A) nephropathy.

    (B) retinopathy.

    (C) hypertension.

    (D) methicillin-resistant staphylococci.

    (E) diarrhea.

16. This patient is likely to have a history of

    (A) diabetic ketoacidosis.

    (B) influenza.

    (C) chlamydial infections.

    (D) migraines.

    (E) arthritis.

17. The appropriate disposition of this patient is

    (A) discharge to home after a 23-hour observation period.

    (B) admission to the ICU.

    (C) admission to the ward.

    (D) transfer to a nursing home.

    (E) admission to a telemetered bed.

18. The patient's radiograph has demonstrated left upper lobe pneumonia. The most likely responsible organism is

    (A) *Staphylococcus aureus.*

    (B) *Chlamydia trachomatis.*

    (C) *Haemophilus influenzae.*

    (D) *Streptococcus pneumoniae.*

    (E) *Candida albicans.*

For Questions 19-22, match the numbered condition with the best answer. Each answer may be used once, more than once, or not at all.

19. Vesicular lesion

20. Painless papule

21. Wart

22. Chancroid

(A) *H. ducreyi*

(B) *H. simplex*

(C) *N. gonorrhoea*

(D) *Papillomavirus*

23. A 23-year-old woman presents to the walk-in clinic with vaginal dysesthesia. She has been sexually active with multiple partners. On pelvic exam you find

   (A) purulent discharge.

   (B) a prolapsed uterus.

   (C) an ovarian cyst.

   (D) vesicular vaginal lesions.

   (E) an impacted tampon.

24. A 73-year-old man with a remote history of alcoholism, who is hospitalized for a chole-cystectomy, becomes acutely confused one evening. He is somewhat combative. The patient is most likely to respond to

   (A) haloperidol.

   (B) ativan.

   (C) benzodiazepine.

   (D) oxygen.

   (E) antibiotics.

25. A 52-year-old woman comes to see you because, during a recent job physical, her PPD was positive. She does not remember ever having a PPD before. Her chest radiograph is negative. She does not know anyone who has had tuberculosis. You recommend

   (A) INH.

   (B) INH, ethambutol, and rifampin.

   (C) a rest cure.

   (D) no intervention.

   (E) hospitalization.

26. A 33-year-old woman had an uncomplicated vaginal delivery two days ago. On the morning of the day of discharge, she complains of urinary burning and frequency. A urinalysis shows 20-30 wbc/HPF. You send her urine for culture. You decide to

   (A) keep her in the hospital and treat with intravenous antibiotics.

   (B) keep her in the hospital and treat with oral antibiotics.

   (C) get an IVP.

   (D) let her go home with a prescription for oral antibiotics and follow-up in a week.

   (E) let her go home on Pyridium.

27. A 35-year-old man who is known to be HIV-positive comes to see you because of a sore throat. You find that he has thrush. You now diagnose him as having

   (A) AIDS.

   (B) lymphoma.

   (C) Sjögren's syndrome.

   (D) carious teeth.

   (E) xerostomia.

Questions 28-35 refer to the following:

A 47-year-old woman presents to your office with complaints of fatigue, myalgias, and arthralgias. She has noticed that she does not feel like doing anything when she gets home from work or on weekends and no longer participates in activities that she used to enjoy, such as bridge, knitting, and playing tennis. She admits to feeling "low" at times, but has no trouble falling asleep. She takes no medications except occasional acetaminophen for her achiness. She has no other medical complaints.

28. You order some screening tests, including

   (A) rheumatoid factor.

   (B) EKG.

   (C) complete blood count.

(D) antinuclear antibody titer.

(E) chest radiograph.

29. You ask the patient about her family history. Which one of the following is the most likely response?

(A) Her mother and sister have rheumatoid arthritis.

(B) No one in her family has anything like her problems.

(C) Her aunt and sister have lupus.

(D) Diabetes runs in her family.

(E) Her mother and maternal aunts and grandmother all had erosive osteoarthritis of the hands.

30. On physical examination, which one of the following findings is most likely to be encountered?

(A) Polyarthritis

(B) Trigger points

(C) Septic bursitis

(D) Fever

(E) Rash

31. This patient is likely to have as an association to her condition

(A) vasculitis.

(B) abdominal pain.

(C) chills.

(D) weight loss.

(E) mild to moderate depression.

32. You inquire about the patient's sleeping habits. Which one of the following is the likeliest description of her sleep?

(A) Severe insomnia

(B) Snoring

(C) Day-night reversal

(D) Narcolepsy

(E) Falls asleep quickly but does not feel rested in the morning.

33. This condition is often associated with

(A) high fevers.

(B) quick recovery.

(C) rapid progression.

(D) loss of time from work.

(E) diabetes.

34. The drug of choice in the initial treatment of this condition is

(A) prednisone.

(B) low-dose amitriptyline at bedtime.

(C) cytotoxic agents.

(D) flurazepam.

(E) benzodiazepine.

35. This patient's diagnosis is

(A) fibromyalgia.

(B) chronic fatigue syndrome.

(C) Ebstein-Barr virus infection.

(D) mononucleosis.

(E) osteoarthritis.

36. A 72-year-old man on your service who was admitted for evaluation of weight loss develops a severe right-sided headache over his temple and has some blurring of his vision. You begin empiric treatment and start evaluating him for

(A) migraines.

(B) temporal arteritis.

(C) CVA.

(D) ruptured berry aneurysm.

(E) cataracts.

37. A 45-year-old man, who is HIV-positive and whom you have been following for several years, comes in for his routine appointment. He complains of the recent onset of blurred vision in his left eye. You obtain a CD4 count and find that it is less than 50. A likely explanation for his visual symptoms is

    (A) lymphoma.

    (B) CMV retinitis.

    (C) temporal arteritis.

    (D) cataract.

    (E) *Chlamydia trachomatis.*

38. A 21-year-old woman comes in because of a scaling, pruritic rash on her elbows and behind her ears. She has noticed a few lesions on her scalp, too. Your working diagnosis is

    (A) erythroderma.

    (B) atopic dermatitis.

    (C) psoriasis.

    (D) erythema multiforme.

    (E) urticaria.

39. A 37-year-old woman of Swedish ancestry comes in because of progressively worsening tingling of her feet. She has a history of anemia. Her father has atrophic gastritis. A peripheral smear of her blood shows macrocytic red cells. You order

    (A) a Schilling test.

    (B) a bone marrow biopsy.

    (C) a bone marrow aspirate.

    (D) CD4 counts.

    (E) an antiphospholipid antibody titer.

40. You are on an airplane on your way to a much-deserved vacation in Hawaii, relaxing after dinner, when the crew asks for a doctor over the intercom system. You wait for someone else to volunteer, but, since no one does, you push your call light. The cabin crew comes and tells you a patient in the back is choking. You go to see the patient and find a middle-aged man who is turning blue, trying to cough. His wife tells you he

just finished his dinner, too. Your first action is to

    (A) try to do a tracheostomy.

    (B) tell the pilot to land immediately.

    (C) try a Heimlich maneuver.

    (D) try mouth-to-mouth resuscitation.

    (E) reassure the wife and cabin crew that the man will be all right.

41. Respiratory syncytial virus can cause all of the following conditions in children EXCEPT

    (A) pneumonia.

    (B) bronchiolitis.

    (C) sinusitis.

    (D) bronchitis.

    (E) croup.

42. A seven-year-old child presents with an earache of two days' duration and a fever of 101°F. The organism you want to make sure you treat with empiric antibiotics is

    (A) *Staphylococcus aureus.*

    (B) *Neisseria meningitidis.*

    (C) *Histoplasma capsulatum.*

    (D) *Streptococcus pneumoniae.*

    (E) *Pseudomonas aeruginosa.*

Questions 43-46 refer to the following:

A five-year-old boy is brought to the neighborhood walk-in clinic because of increased irritability, abdominal pain, and vomiting. He lives in an old apartment house that was built before World War II. His mother says he has been symptomatic for a while, but she thought he had a viral illness until the last few days.

43. You should ask the mother all of the following EXCEPT

    (A) Does the patient have pica?

    (B) Does he spend most of his time in buildings like his own?

(C) Has she seen him put things from the environment into his mouth?

(D) Does anyone beat him?

(E) Has he had any siblings with similar problems?

44. The likeliest cause of this boy's symptoms is

    (A) lead poisoning.

    (B) acetaminophen overdose.

    (C) salicylate ingestion.

    (D) Reyes' syndrome.

    (E) ethylene glycol ingestion.

45. Which one of the following tests should be obtained to confirm your diagnosis?

    (A) Serum iron level

    (B) Serum salicylate level

    (C) Serum lead level

    (D) Toxicology screen

    (E) Urinary mercury concentration

46. If this patient remains untreated, he may develop all of the following EXCEPT

    (A) papilledema.

    (B) coma.

    (C) seizures.

    (D) meningitis.

    (E) ataxia.

47. A 72-year-old woman is brought in by her family because of complaints of worsening headaches, weakness, and occasional blurring of vision for the last week. Your neurologic examination shows no focal findings. She has no papilledema. She has no loss of memory. You order

    (A) blood cultures.

    (B) an MRI of the brain.

    (C) an antinuclear antibody titer.

    (D) a toxicology screen.

    (E) a Westergren sedimentation rate.

48. An 18-year-old male with sickle cell anemia comes in because of bone pain for several days. The bone pain itself has not been too severe, but it has been associated with severe fatigue. His peripheral smear shows many sickled cells, but very few of any other kind of cell. His CBC is pending. You suspect

    (A) acute leukemia.

    (B) aplastic crisis.

    (C) HIV infection.

    (D) sepsis.

    (E) lymphoma.

49. A 14-year-old girl is brought in because of severe neck pain, headache, and photophobia. Which one of the following is most critical to do early in the evaluation?

    (A) EEG

    (B) Skull films

    (C) Arterial blood gases

    (D) Lumbar puncture

    (E) Somatosensory evoked potentials

Questions 50-57 refer to the following:

You admit a 52-year-old female to the hospital with symptoms of shortness of breath, weight loss, and recurrent fevers. Physical examination at the time of admission is unremarkable. A chest X-ray is obtained, the findings of which make you suspicious for a diagnosis of sarcoidosis.

50. Which one of the following is LEAST commonly observed on chest X-rays in patients with sarcoidosis?

    (A) Bilateral hilar adenopathy

    (B) Diffuse parenchymal changes

    (C) "Eggshell calcifications"

    (D) Isolated coin lesion with pleural effusion

    (E) Bilateral hilar adenopathy and diffuse parenchymal changes

You wish to confirm the diagnosis of pulmonary sarcoidosis.

51. Which one of the following tests is NOT useful in helping to make the diagnosis of pulmonary sarcoidosis?

(A) Bronchoalveolar lavage

(B) Pulmonary function testing

(C) Gallium 67 lung scan

(D) Fiber-optic bronchoscopic biopsy

(E) Swan-Ganz catheterization

52. On closer physical examination, you note that the patient has bilateral tender red nodules on the anterior surface of her legs. The cause of this rash is likely to be

(A) lupus pernio.

(B) erythema gangrenosum.

(C) erythema nodosum.

(D) fungal infection.

(E) cryoglobulinemia.

53. In addition to this patient's pulmonary and skin involvement, which one of the following additional sites is most likely to be involved?

(A) Stomach

(B) Pancreas

(C) Eye

(D) Facial nerve

(E) Heart

54. Which one of the following statements is true regarding the epidemiology of sarcoidosis?

(A) The majority of patients present with sarcoidosis after the first decade of life.

(B) In the United States, the majority of patients are black.

(C) Rare cases of sexual transmission have been reported.

(D) Males are more susceptible to the disease than females.

(E) None of the above.

55. Which one of the following statements is NOT true regarding the pathogenesis and pathophysiology of sarcoidosis?

(A) Granuloma formation is common in affected sites.

(B) Large numbers of activated T-cells accumulate in affected organs.

(C) Antibody-mediated processes are extremely important in the immunopathogenesis of the disease.

(D) T-cell proliferation is maintained by the release of IL-2 by activated T-cells in affected areas.

(E) The fibrotic response seen in some individuals is mediated through the release of growth factors by macrophage.

56. The patient wishes to know more about the prognosis and treatment of her condition. Which one of the following statements is true regarding the prognosis of sarcoidosis?

(A) Seventy percent of patients with sarcoidosis will die of this condition.

(B) Ninety percent of patients with sarcoidosis will remit spontaneously.

(C) Five to ten percent of patients with sarcoidosis will develop lymphoma in the future.

(D) Eye involvement may lead to blindness.

(E) None of the above.

57. You decide to treat your patient with corticosteroids. Which one of the following statements is true regarding the treatment of sarcoidosis with corticosteroids?

(A)   Lymph node involvement is an indication for treatment with corticosteroids.

(B)   Treatment is generally life-long.

(C)   Inhaled glucocorticoids are useful for pulmonary disease.

(D)   Treatment should be dictated by levels of angiotensin-converting enzyme.

(E)   None of the above.

Questions 58-61 refer to the following:

A 39-year-old male comes to the emergency room complaining of severe pain in the right flank which radiates to the testicle. Physical exam reveals a man in significant discomfort with a temperature of 101.9°F, pulse of 120, and blood pressure of 170/100. There is marked tenderness in the right flank. Urinalysis reveals microhematuria.

58.   Which one of the following statements is true regarding the evaluation of this patient?

(A)   The majority of renal stones will not be seen on X-ray.

(B)   IVP is not necessary if a stone is visualized on plain radiograph.

(C)   Urgent urological consultation is indicated.

(D)   Most ureteral stones require interventional therapy.

(E)   None of the above.

Prior to initiating the evaluation, the patient's pain markedly subsides. Straining of the urine reveals a stone.

59.   Which one of the following is NOT true regarding types of kidney stones?

(A)   Calcium stones are most common.

(B)   Uric acid stone formation is associated with alkaline urine.

(C)   Cystine stones are usually seen in younger patients.

(D)   Urea-splitting organisms in the urine may result in stones.

(E)   Cystine stones are formed only by patients with cystinuria.

60.   Urine Gram stain of the ER specimen reveals Gram-negative rods. Which one of the following antibiotics is most likely to be effective in the treatment of this patient?

(A)   Vancomycin

(B)   Penicillin

(C)   Oxacillin

(D)   Ceftriaxone

(E)   None of the above.

61.   The patient is admitted to the hospital and treated with antibiotics and soon discharged. You see him in your office one week later for follow up. Analysis of the stone reveals that it is a calcium stone. The patient informs you that he has had similar episodes of pain twice in the past which remitted spontaneously. Which one of the following agents is LEAST likely to reduce the risk of a recurrent stone in this patient?

(A)   Hydrochlorothiazide

(B)   Sodium citrate therapy

(C)   Triamterene

(D)   Inorganic phosphates

(E)   Cellulose phosphate

62.   A 52-year-old female presented to her physician with symptoms of polyuria, polydipsia, weakness, and malaise. Her fasting blood glucose level was 379 mg/dl. Which of the following treatment options lowers blood sugar by interfering with intestinal absorption of complex carbohydrates?

(A)   Metformin

(B)   NPH insulin

(C)   Sulfonylurea

(D)   Acarbose

(E)   Regular insulin

Questions 63 and 64 refer to the following:

A 24-day-old infant is brought into your office by his mother who says that the baby has had a fever for one day and does not want to take his formula. The baby has not been vomiting.

63. Physical signs and symptoms suggestive of a toxic infant include all of the following EXCEPT

    (A) poor or delayed capillary refill.

    (B) tachycardia.

    (C) a slow irregular or decreasing respiratory rate.

    (D) stridor.

    (E) diarrhea.

64. The baby's temperature is found to be 102°F. How will you manage this patient's symptoms?

    (A) Give Tylenol and send the baby home.

    (B) Observe the baby over the next two to three hours for signs of sepsis and send him home if none appear.

    (C) Treat empirically with oral antibiotics for otitis media, as this is the most likely source of his fever.

    (D) Obtain a CBC and blood cultures and send the baby home, noting you will call the mother if there are any abnormalities.

    (E) Arrange for hospital admission and full evaluation for sepsis to be performed.

65. A comatose child who has been struck by a hit-and-run driver is brought into the ER. He was on his way to school by himself when he was struck. You must

    (A) wait for his parents to come and give permission.

    (B) treat him immediately and worry about contacting his parents later.

    (C) treat him immediately and have someone try to track down his parents.

    (D) call the police immediately.

    (E) get a court order to permit you to treat him.

66. A 47-year-old woman complains of dyspnea and awakening at night with a choking sensation. She was discharged from the hospital three weeks ago, following a complicated course, which included prolonged mechanical ventilation. The helical computed tomographic study, shown in the figure, confirms your diagnosis of

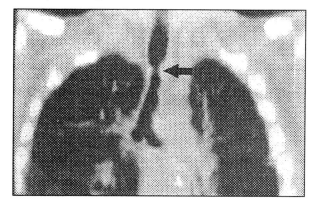

    (A) esophageal web.

    (B) foreign body.

    (C) midtracheal stricture.

    (D) tracheal compression by a substernal thyroid.

    (E) laryngeal carcinoma.

67. A 54-year-old male is hospitalized with a urinary tract infection and is on intravenous antibiotics. On the fifth hospital day, he has a change of mental status and his fever is elevated to 103°F. His chest X-ray shows diffuse bilateral alveolar infiltrates consistent with adult respiratory distress syndrome. Arterial blood gas reveals pH of 7.29, pCO_2 of 30, and pO_2 of 50. Blood cultures are positive for *E. coli*. This patient's blood pressure is 70/40

mm/hg. All of the following should be included in the management plan for this patient EXCEPT

(A) intubation and central line placement.

(B) intravenous hydration.

(C) intravenous corticosteroids.

(D) aminoglycosides.

(E) positive end expiratory pressure on the ventilator (PEEP).

68. After having been transferred from the intensive care unit to a regular floor, a patient complains of dysuria, urinary frequency, hesitancy, and fever. Urine analysis reveals 50-100 white blood cells and the leukocyte esterase is positive. This patient has a foley catheter in place to monitor the urine output. What would be the next step in management?

(A) Intravenous pyelography

(B) Intravenous normal saline to flush the kidneys

(C) Empiric treatment with penicillin

(D) Remove the foley catheter and treat with trimethoprim-sulfamethoxazole

(E) Find out the results of urine and blood cultures prior to initiating antibiotic therapy

69. Select the correct statement about formation of the cardia septa.

(A) The endocardial cushions form the intraventricular septum.

(B) The opening between the septum primum and the septum secundum is the ostium primum.

(C) The septum secundum can completely separate the atria if there is an endocardial cushion defect.

(D) The opening left by the ostium secundum is the foramen ovaie.

(E) In 20% of people, the septum primum and septum secundum does not completely fuse.

70. Two months ago you treated a five-year-old child for a dermatitis of the fingers and volar wrists and the elbows. The mother now returns with the child's cousin, who has a similar dermatologic condition. Based on skin scrapings, shown in the photo, you confirm the diagnosis of

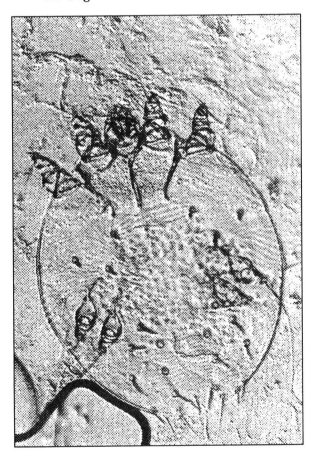

(A) scabies.

(B) lice.

(C) fleas.

(D) bedbugs.

(E) myiasis.

Questions 71-74 refer to the following:

As a clinician, you are asked to interpret the following hypothetical epidemiological relationship between stroke and regular measurements of hypercholesterolemia that is used to screen for the disease.

Test	Stroke	
	Present	Absent
Positive	25	35
Negative	15	60

71. What is the specificity of the test for developing stroke?

    (A) 28.6%

    (B) 26.6%

    (C) 4.9%

    (D) 41.7%

    (E) 63%

72. What is the positive predictive value of the test in the diagnostic evaluation of the stroke?

    (A) 28.6%

    (B) 26.6%

    (C) 4.9%

    (D) 41.7%

    (E) 63%

73. Given the data from the above table, what is the odds ratio for stroke?

    (A) 28.6%

    (B) 26.6%

    (C) 4.9 %

    (D) 41.7%

    (E) 63%

74. Attributable risk of hypercholesterolemia to developing a stroke is

    (A) 28.6%.

    (B) 26.6%.

    (C) 4.9%.

    (D) 41.7%.

    (E) 63%.

75. All of the following diseases are associated with smoking, EXCEPT

    (A) bacterial pneumonia.

    (B) COPD.

    (C) asthma.

    (D) asbestosis.

    (E) silicosis.

76. You are called to the clinic to see a 54-year-old fair-skinned woman who has a pigmented lesion on her back that has been bothering her because her bra strap rubs against it. She wants the lesion removed. She says her husband thinks it is bigger, but she cannot tell because she cannot see it. The lesion is about 1 cm in width, with irregular margins, and irregular amounts of pigment. Instead of performing a quick office excision you arrange for a surgical removal because you suspect

    (A) basal cell carcinoma.

    (B) squamous cell carcinoma.

    (C) seborrheic keratosis.

    (D) melanoma.

    (E) hemangioma.

77. You are called to consult on a 34-year-old man who presents with weakness, fatigue, a blood urea nitrogen of 50, and a creatinine of 1.2. He has no history of renal problems. He recently lost his job and has been drinking a lot. He has been having some diarrhea but no vomiting. After obtaining a CBC, you order

    (A) a creatinine clearance.

    (B) a chest radiograph.

    (C) a stool hemoccult.

    (D) an electrocardiogram.

    (E) thyroid function tests.

For Questions 78 and 79, select the most appropriate test to order on the following clinic patients.

    (A)   Chest X-ray

    (B)   Electrocardiogram

    (C)   Arterial blood gas

    (D)   Upright film

    (E)   Complete blood count

78. A 27-year-old male with acute onset of sharp abdominal pain and distention

79. A 66-year-old male with acute onset of left jaw pain

80. A 62-year-old man with hypertension and congestive heart failure presents after a suicide attempt. He has taken one bottle of digitalis pills. Of the following possible arrhythmias, all can be seen EXCEPT

    (A)   first-degree atrioventricular block.

    (B)   third-degree atrioventricular block.

    (C)   multifocal atrial tachycardia.

    (D)   bidirectional ventricular tachycardia.

    (E)   All of the above can be seen.

81. An 82-year-old female with a history of stroke and mild dementia is found comatose in her unventilated apartment during a heat wave. Her core temperature was 105°. Cardiopulmonary resuscitation measures, along with ice packs and cold intravenous saline solution, could not revive her and she expired. All of the following are associated with the diagnosis of heatstroke and hyperthermia EXCEPT

    (A)   in classic heatstroke, the underlying pathophysiologic mechanism of the disorder is impaired heat dissipation.

    (B)   risk factors for heatstroke include dehydration, obesity, and neurologic and cardiovascular disease.

    (C)   the posterior hypothalamus is the body's thermostat.

    (D)   leukocytosis, renal dysfunction, and depressed fibrinogen levels are lab abnormalities that can occur in heatstroke.

    (E)   diuretics, neuroleptics, alcohol, and anticholinergics can all predispose the patient to heatstroke.

82. A 38-year-old homemaker with insulin-dependent diabetes mellitus for 10 years presents with inability to walk on her heels. On exam, she had bilateral weakness and atrophy of the intrinsic foot muscles and absent ankle jerks. Pinprick and temperature sensation were diminished below her upper thighs and upper arms. Nerve conduction studies revealed a moderately severe sensorimotor polyneuropathy. All of the following are true regarding diabetic neuropathy EXCEPT

    (A)   distal symmetric diabetic polyneuropathy is the most common type of neuropathy.

    (B)   diabetic proximal motor neuropathy is vascular in origin.

    (C)   tight control of blood glucose levels can cure neuropathic pain.

    (D)   the most effective approach to diabetic polyneuropathy is prevention.

    (E)   painful diabetic neuropathy can sometimes be alleviated by phenytoin, amitriptyline, and topical capsaicin.

For Questions 83-86, select the most likely diagnosis.

    (A)   Alcoholic liver disease

    (B)   Viral hepatitis

    (C)   Cholangiocarcinoma

    (D)   Acute cholangitis

    (E)   Acute cholecystitis

83. A 60-year-old male presents with right upper quadrant pain for 15 hours. Physical examination reveals scleral icterus and a temperature of 102°F. Liver function tests show SGOT

of 147, SGPT of 150, total bilirubin of 4.5, and alkaline phosphatase of 350.

84. A 27-year-old female presents with right upper quadrant discomfort, nausea, fatigue, and muscle ache. Liver function tests show SGOT of 188, SGPT of 277, total bilirubin of 1.0, and alkaline phosphatase of 66.

85. A 68-year-old female presents with weight loss, anorexia, and fatigue. Physical examination reveals jaundice and muscle wasting and spider angiomata. Liver function tests show SGOT of 150, SGPT of 62, total bilirubin of 5.2, and alkaline phosphatase of 88.

86. A 50-year-old male presents with severe epigastric and right upper abdominal pain. On physical examination, temperature is 102°F. Liver function tests show SGOT of 41, SGPT of 36, total bilirubin of 1.0, and alkaline phosphatase of 61.

For Questions 87-91, match the symptoms with the diagnoses.

    (A)   Acute gout

    (B)   Suppurative arthritis

    (C)   Pseudogout

    (D)   Gonococcal arthritis

    (E)   Rheumatoid arthritis

87. A 32-year-old woman with temporomandibular joint pain and tingling warm joints with a normal uric acid level and no response to colchicine.

88. A 65-year-old man who is suddenly awakened in the night with a burning, tingling great toe.

89. An 18-year-old male with a history of soft tissue infection and a temperature of 102.4°F and a painful, tender, and swollen wrist.

90. A 32-year-old male with a sudden onset of a painful, warm, and swollen knee lasting for two to four days and gradually subsiding.

91. A 19-year-old male with warm and tender joints following a diagnosis of urethritis three weeks ago.

92. You have admitted a 70-year-old female patient from a nursing home with a suspected diagnosis of bacterial meningitis. Gram stain of the CSF shows Gam-negative organisms. Which one of the following is the most likely cause of this patient's meningitis?

    (A)   *S. pneumoniae*

    (B)   *H. influenzae*

    (C)   *L. monocytogenes*

    (D)   *S. aureus*

    (E)   *E. coli*

93. You are asked to come to the emergency room to repair a 4-cm laceration of the forearm of a 13-year-old student. You wish to perform a 2-layer closure. The deep layer may be

    (A)   silk.

    (B)   nylon.

    (C)   steel.

    (D)   chromic gut.

    (E)   cotton.

94. Moderate tenderness found with a peptic ulcer may be located

    (A)   just under the left costal margin.

    (B)   just under the right costal margin.

    (C)   between the scapulae.

    (D)   just below the xiphoid.

    (E)   3-6 cm below the xiphoid.

95. You are reviewing the spot film (shown in the figure on the next page) of an upper gastrointestinal study of an 85-year-old male resident of a nursing home. The patient has a mild dementia and is unable to give an adequate history. The nursing staff reports that he has lost 40 pounds over the past three months. They also report that he initially choked on solids. Now he chokes on liquids as well. You diagnose

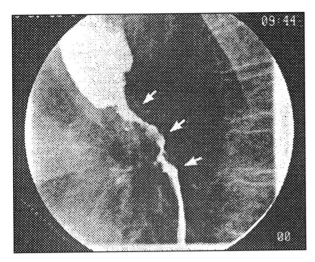

(A) achalasia.

(B) esophageal carcinoma.

(C) esophageal varices.

(D) diffuse esophageal spasm.

(E) Schatzki's ring.

For Questions 96-99, choose a lettered answer for each numbered question. Each answer may be used once, more than once, or not at all.

(A) Man without a weapon who threatens to kill his mother

(B) Man with a gun who confidentially threatens to kill his mother

(C) Physician who injects a terminal patient who wants to die with an overdose of morphine

(D) Employer asking for suicide patient's medical records

(E) Physician who charges for more injections than he performs

96. Duty to warn

97. Patient-physician confidentiality

98. Fraud

99. Physician-assisted suicide

100. A 35-year-old female with chronic asthma comes to the emergency room for the tenth time in three weeks. It is the general consensus of everyone involved in her care, including her family, that she does not take her medications as prescribed. Indeed, despite what should be a very adequate dose of theophylline, her theophylline level is very low. You

(A) refuse to take care of her because she is wasting medical resources.

(B) call her insurance company.

(C) discuss her management with her and her family in the presence of a psychiatric social worker.

(D) commit her.

(E) report her to the Board of Health.

Questions 101 and 102 refer to the following:

101. A 33-year-old male returns from a diving meet complaining of an earache. The most likely diagnosis is

(A) conductive hearing loss.

(B) sensorineural hearing loss.

(C) otitis externa.

(D) otitis media.

(E) migraine headache.

102. The most appropriate treatment is

(A) IV antibiotics.

(B) oral antibiotics.

(C) topical antibiotics.

(D) incision and drainage.

(E) tympanoplasty.

103. A 43-year-old woman with a history of peptic ulcer disease presents with three weeks of intermittent nausea and vomiting. She is now unable to keep down solids, but is able to swallow liquids well. She denies any abdominal pain or hematemesis or coffee-ground emesis. She denies any other medical illnesses and is only taking famotidine for ulcers. On physical examination, she is afebrile, her blood pressure is 120/70, heart rate is 80, and respiratory rate is 14. Her lungs are clear and her heart reveals no gallops or

murmurs. Her abdominal exam reveals no distension or tenderness. Obstructive series reveals a dilated stomach with an air-fluid level. Of the following, the most likely diagnosis is

(A) diabetic ketoacidosis.

(B) gastric outlet obstruction.

(C) diabetic gastroparesis.

(D) small bowel obstruction.

(E) large bowel obstruction.

104. You are called to the ER to see a 21-year-old pregnant woman who is experiencing a severe chest pain. The pain extends along the left arm and up to the left shoulder. Physical assessment shows a patient who is breathing fast and perspiring heavily. Laboratory tests indicate cocaine intoxication. The patient is nine months pregnant with her first child. Provided that the patient's condition is controlled and delivery is uneventful, the infant is at increased risk for which one of the following conditions?

(A) Cardiac septal defects

(B) Seizures

(C) Spina bifida occulta

(D) Cleft palate

(E) Gray baby syndrome

105. After having been transferred from the intensive care unit to a regular floor, a patient complains of dysuria, urinary frequency, hesitancy, and fever. Urine analysis reveals 50-100 white blood cells and the leukocyte esterase is positive. This patient has a foley catheter in place to monitor the urine output. What would be the next step in management?

(A) Intravenous pyelography

(B) Intravenous normal saline to flush the kidneys

(C) Empiric treatment with penicillin

(D) Remove foley catheter and treat with trimethoprim-sulfamethoxazole

(E) Find out the results of urine and blood cultures prior to initiating antibiotic therapy

Questions 106-108 refer to the following

106. You have just admitted a 17-year-old male with hematuria. Questions to ask include all of the following EXCEPT

(A) "Any associated pain?"

(B) "Amount of blood present?"

(C) "At what point of stream does it occur?"

(D) "Any associated smell?"

(E) "Any medication usage?"

107. The reasons for hematuria include all of the following EXCEPT

(A) trauma.

(B) infection.

(C) neoplasm.

(D) coagulopathy.

(E) aspirin use.

108. Which one of the following tests that you have ordered would help you the least?

(A) Blood glucose

(B) Urinalysis

(C) An intravenous pyelogram (IVP)

(D) Cystoscopy

(E) Prothrombin Time/Partial Thromboplastin Time (PT/PTT)

Questions 109-112 refer to the following:

Your pregnant 37-year-old wife calls your office. She is devastated by the news she just received from her obstetrician, indicating that a "triple screen," done at 17 weeks of gestation, was mildly abnormal.

109. You confirm the obstetrician's recommendation to

(A) repeat the test in six weeks.

(B) repeat the test in six months.

(C) undergo an amniocentesis.

(D) undergo an abortion.

(E) take folic acid, 0.4 mg daily.

110. The obstetrician discussed the problem of specificity and sensitivity of these tests. You explain that in an ideally specific test

(A) all persons with a positive test will manifest a predefined disease.

(B) all persons with a negative test will not manifest a predefined disease.

(C) no one with the disease will have a negative test.

(D) the results are used to confirm the absence of disease.

(E) the results are used to exclude the presence of a disease.

111. She also asks you to explain what is meant by the sensitivity of a test. You indicate that in an ideally sensitive test

(A) all persons with a predefined disease will have a positive test result.

(B) the results are used to confirm the presence of a disease.

(C) the results are used to exclude the absence of a disease.

(D) all persons with a positive test will have a predefined disease.

(E) no one without the disease will have a positive test.

112. Three weeks later, an amniocentesis is performed. The amniotic fluid alpha fetoprotein is normal. Cytogenetic analysis is also performed. Based on the karyotype, shown in the figure in the next column, you diagnose

(A) healthy female.

(B) healthy male.

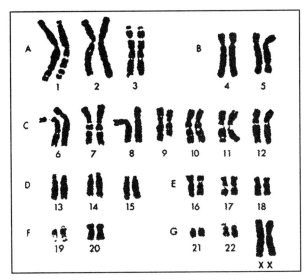

(C) Down's syndrome.

(D) Turner's syndrome.

(E) Klinefelter's syndrome.

113. A medical student sticks himself on a needle from a patient who is a known drug user and who refuses to let you obtain an HIV test. You

(A) draw the blood test anyway.

(B) draw baseline blood on the student for HIV and hepatitis.

(C) treat the patient empirically for AIDS.

(D) flunk the student.

(E) tell the student not to worry.

Questions 114-116 refer to the following:

A 42-year-old female with long-standing hypertension is admitted to the hospital directly from the nephrology clinic where she has been followed closely for chronic renal insufficiency. Her mental status has suddenly changed from baseline to being neither alert nor oriented to time, place, and person. Physical examination reveals clear lungs and a flat abdomen, and lab results indicate oliguria, BUN of 100 mg/LI, and creatinine of 10 mg/LI.

114. All of the following are some of the signs and symptoms of uremia EXCEPT

(A)　asterixis.

(B)　peripheral neuropathy.

(C)　nausea and vomiting.

(D)　Kussmaul's respirations.

(E)　alopecia.

115. What would be the immediate treatment of choice for this patient?

(A)　Plasmapheresis

(B)　Hemodialysis

(C)　Peritoneal dialysis

(D)　Diuresis

(E)　Foley catheter insertion

116. All of the following should be the appropriate advice given to a patient with chronic renal failure EXCEPT

(A)　high-protein diet.

(B)　avoidance of magnesium-containing products.

(C)　all over-the-counter medications should be discussed with the physician.

(D)　begin a low potassium and low sodium diet.

(E)　erythropoietin should be administered if the hemoglobin is below 7.0 g/dl.

117. All of the following are associated with brief intense perineal pain EXCEPT

(A)　it is the presenting symptom of proctalgia fugax.

(B)　it is more common in women than men.

(C)　the pain is near the coccyx or within the rectum.

(D)　the pain usually subsides within minutes.

(E)　the reason for the pain is spasm of the levator ani muscles.

Questions 118-121 refer to the following:

A 32-year-old man is admitted to your service because of acute shortness of breath. His chest radiograph shows a 50% pneumothorax on the right. He denies chest pain, trauma, and history of similar problems. He has not smoked in six years. He is otherwise healthy.

118. Your first therapeutic maneuver after beginning oxygen by face mask is

(A)　begin CPAP.

(B)　place an arterial line.

(C)　begin theophylline.

(D)　order a toxicology screen.

(E)　call for a surgical consultation.

119. The surgeon decides

(A)　to put a chest tube into the patient.

(B)　to perform a limited thoracotomy.

(C)　you should not have bothered him.

(D)　to do nothing.

(E)　to inject talc into the pleurae.

120. The likeliest diagnosis is

(A)　the patient had a puncture wound of the chest and is denying it because he doesn't want to deal with the police.

(B)　spontaneous pneumothorax.

(C)　tuberculosis.

(D)　aspergillosis.

(E)　emphysema.

121. The usual cause of this condition is

(A)　tuberculosis.

(B)　emphysema.

(C)　HIV/AIDS.

(D) mesothelioma.

(E) idiopathic.

Questions 122-125 refer to the following:

A 62-year-old female is referred to you for work-up of a murmur detected by her surgeon. You want to auscultate the heart sounds accordingly by listening to the correct anatomic area. Match the following heart ausculatory areas to their named valves.

(A) Left fifth interspace just medial to the midclavicular line

(B) Right fifth interspace just medial to the midclavicular line

(C) Just lateral to the lower edge of the sternum

(D) Left second interspace close to the sternum

(E) Right second interspace close to the sternum

122. Aortic area

123. Pulmonic area

124. Tricuspid area

125. Mitral area

126. A 42-year-old man presents to your office for the first time with shortness of breath, which has been increasing for the last four months. He denies any fevers, chills, or cough. His physical examination reveals a blood pressure of 102/74, a heart rate of 108, and a respiratory rate of 14. His cardiac exam reveals a point of maximal impulse 3 cm to the left and downward. Auscultation reveals a normal S1 and S2 with an S3 and S4 gallop. Lungs reveal minimal inspiratory. Appropriate focused questions on the patient's history should include all of the following EXCEPT

(A) past history of exposure to Adriamycin.

(B) past history of rheumatic heart disease.

(C) past history of an extended viral syndrome.

(D) past history of alcohol ingestion.

(E) past history of colon cancer.

Questions 127-133 refer to the following:

127. You are called to the emergency room to see a 48-year-old male who has had a decreased appetite for two months and has lost 15 pounds over this period as well. He has mild hypertension. He has had no surgeries. He smokes two packs per day and has an occasional drink. He takes a diuretic for his hypertension and has no allergies. Significant physical exam findings include a 3 x 3 centimeter ulcerated mass on his soft palate and a hard right cervical lymph node. Based on the history and physical examination you are highly suspicious for

(A) pharyngitis.

(B) oropharyngeal carcinoma.

(C) oral candidiasis.

(D) lymphoma.

(E) Kaposi's sarcoma.

128. You now wish a second opinion and ask for the services of a(n)

(A) dentist.

(B) head and neck surgeon.

(C) internist.

(D) oncologist.

(E) nutritionist.

129. All of the following would be appropriate in the work-up EXCEPT

(A) biopsy.

(B)　panendoscopy.

(C)　chest X-ray.

(D)　liver-function tests.

(E)　colonoscopy.

130.　In addition to the work-up, the patient needs to improve his nutritional status. You opt for

(A)　an increased oral diet.

(B)　placement of a nasogastric tube with increased caloric requirements.

(C)　initiation of TPN.

(D)　placement of a J-tube with increased caloric requirements.

(E)　placement of a G-tube with increased caloric requirements.

131.　The work-up is diagnostic for squamous cell carcinoma. The traditional treatment is likely to be

(A)　surgery.

(B)　radiation.

(C)　chemotherapy.

(D)　nothing, since this is untreatable.

(E)　None of the above.

132.　The patient is successfully treated and is discharged home. Your most important recommendation is.

(A)　improved nutrition.

(B)　smoking and alcohol cessation.

(C)　hypertension control.

(D)　potassium supplementation because of his being on a diuretic.

(E)　low cholesterol diet.

133.　You will need to see this patient for follow-up in

(A)　three months

(B)　six months

(C)　one year

(D)　three years

(E)　five years

Questions 134-138 refer to the following:

134.　You are asked to come to the emergency room to evaluate a 77-year-old woman who was found in her nursing home on the floor after "passing out." She comes into the emergency room and complains of left hip pain. Her vital signs are stable. Your physical examination reveals a carotid bruit, a heart murmur, decreased breath sounds, and pain of the hip on leg abduction. Your initial work-up should include all of the following studies EXCEPT

(A)　EKG.

(B)　chest X-ray.

(C)　hip films.

(D)　head CT.

(E)　MRI of the neck.

135.　An echocardiogram of the heart should be performed because

(A)　there is a murmur.

(B)　it could be a source of emboli leading to her syncope.

(C)　there may be a heart valve.

(D)　there may be an aneurysm.

(E)　it will test ejection fraction.

136.　The bruit should initially be evaluated with

(A)　ultrasound of the neck.

(B)　CAT scan of the neck.

(C)　MRI of the neck.

(D)　angiogram of carotid arteries.

(E)　plain films.

137.　The work-up is complete and the carotids are the source of her syncope. She is also deemed a surgical candidate. Prior to her surgery, which test must the vascular surgeon have to properly localize and treat the arteries?

(A)   Ultrasound of the neck

(B)   CAT scan of the neck

(C)   MRI of the neck

(D)   Angiogram of carotid arteries

(E)   Plain films

138. The procedure that the vascular surgeon will perform is

    (A)   angioplasty.

    (B)   carotid artery bypass.

    (C)   ligation of the carotid artery.

    (D)   carotid endarterectomy.

    (E)   None of the above.

Questions 139-142 refer to the following:

You are preparing a lecture for first-year medical residents on neurologic emergencies. Your first case, shown in the figure below, is a contrast-enhanced computed tomographic scan of the head.

139. The differential diagnosis includes all of the following EXCEPT

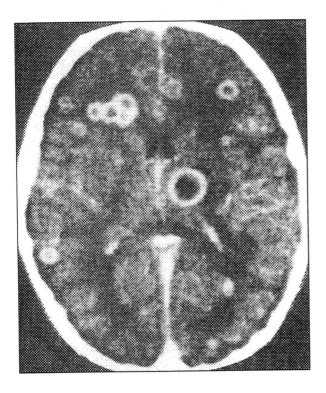

(A)   multiple brain abscesses.

(B)   metastatic cancer.

(C)   resolving cerebral infarcts.

(D)   granulomas.

(E)   early herpes simplex encephalitis.

140. Your second case illustrates pre- and post-treatment contrast-enhanced computed axial tomographic (CAT) scans of the brain of a person who was seropositive for HIV and toxoplasmosis. The post-treatment scan is shown in Panel B on the next page. The pre-treatment scan, shown in Panel A below, illustrates all of the following EXCEPT

Panel A

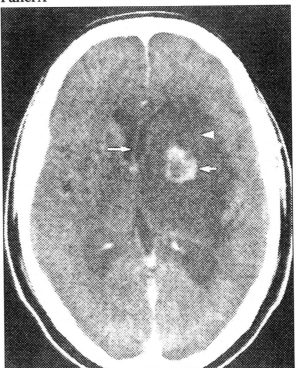

Panel B

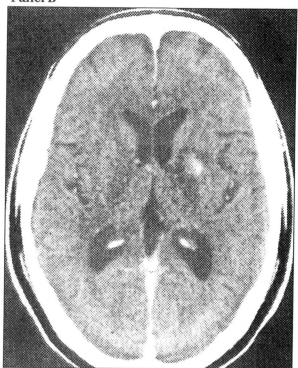

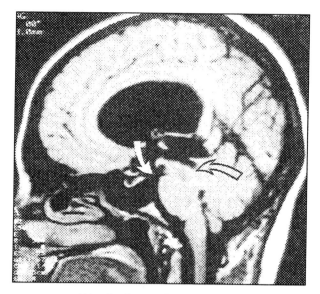

(A) ring-enhancing mass with irregular borders in the basal ganglia.

(B) compression of the left lateral ventricle.

(C) marked edema surrounding the mass.

(D) ventricular shift to the left.

(E) displacement of the falx cerebri to the right of midline.

141. Your third case is a magnetic resonance imaging (MRI) of the brain (shown in the right column), which illustrates a noncommunicating hydrocephalus due to stenosis of the caudal aqueduct of Sylvius. You discuss all of the following EXCEPT

(A) hydrocephalus refers to the net accumulation of CSF within the cerebral ventricles, which results in their enlargement.

(B) noncommunicating hydrocephalus results from lesions obstructing the intracerebral CSF circulation at or proximal to the foramina of Luschka and Magendie.

(C) communicating hydrocephalus results from obstruction of the basal cisterns or convexity subarachnoid space so that the ventricular system communicates with the spinal subarachnoid space, but CSF cannot drain through the arachnoid villi.

(D) communicating, but not noncommunicating, hydrocephalus is treated by shunting.

(E) both communicating and noncommunicating hydrocephalus are obstructive.

142. Your fourth case is an electroencephalogram (EEG), shown in Panel A, from a 13-year-old male with fever, altered sensorium, and sudden onset of seizures. For comparison, a normal, awake EEG is shown in Panel B. This boy's EEG illustrates which one of the following?

Panel A

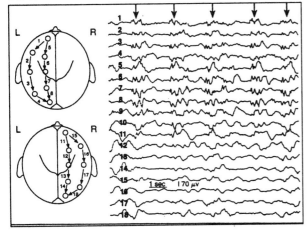

Panel B

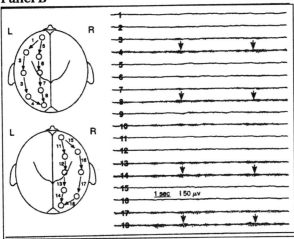

(A) Complex repetitive discharges composed of spiky elements mixed with slower waveforms bilaterally

(B) Complex repetitive discharges composed of spiky elements mixed with slower waveforms in the left hemisphere

(C) Complex repetitive discharges composed of spiky elements mixed with slower waveforms in the right hemisphere

(D) Normal alpha activity bilaterally

(E) Symmetric activity between the right and left hemispheres

143. A 74-year-old female with no past medical history presents to her dermatologist with discoloration and thickening of all the nails on her feet, which is causing embarrassing cosmetic problems for her. There is no associated pain. A potassium hydroxide preparation of the nail bed debris scrapings revealed hyphae, and cultures grew the dermatophyte *Trichophyton rubrum*. On examination, there was subungal debris present and friability of the nail plates. All of the following would be the recommended treatment of choice for this condition EXCEPT

(A) griseofulvin.

(B) amphotericin B.

(C) itraconazole.

(D) terbinafine.

(E) fluconazole.

144. Your 25-year-old male patient comes to your office complaining of headaches for the past several weeks. He describes the headaches as a bilateral, dull nagging pain in the temples. He describes the pain as band-like and worse at the end of the day. During the physical examination, the patient describes a throbbing sensation behind the eyes. The most likely diagnosis is

(A) tension headache.

(B) temporal arteritis.

(C) migraine headache.

(D) cluster headache.

(E) trigeminal neuralgia.

For Questions 145-148, match each case with the likeliest diagnosis.

(A) Sickle cell crisis

(B) Gastroesophageal reflux

(C) Costochondritis

(D) Angina

(E) Chronic bronchitis

145. A 54-year-old man presents with dyspnea and numbness in his left shoulder after a stressful presentation at a meeting.

146. A 35-year-old woman presents complaining of severe retrosternal discomfort, which was worsened by drinking a cup of coffee.

147. A 63-year-old woman comes in because of anterior chest pain that is worsened by movement.

148. A 23-year-old man comes in because of progressively worsening chest pain associated with right upper quadrant pain and shortness of breath.

149. During a routine physical examination of a 67-year-old male asymptomatic patient, you decide to screen him for stroke. He has been smoking for over 20 years and states to be a social drinker. Auscultation for carotid bruits is unrevealing. Your decision is justified by which one of the following statements?

    (A) Given the patient's age, it is a prudent decision.

    (B) This patient has more than one risk factor for stroke.

    (C) Most patients that claim to be social drinkers are, in fact, potential alcoholics and, therefore, have an increased risk for developing cardiovascular and cerebrovascular complications.

    (D) Any of the above alone or in combination.

    (E) None of the above.

For Questions 150-153, match the test results with the diagnosis.

You have set aside this afternoon to evaluate diagnostic tests for your patients with Cushing's syndrome. Match the following test results with the clinical diagnosis.

Overnight Dexamethasone Test	Plasma ACTH Dexamethasone	High dose of ACTH	CRH Stimulation
(A) Suppression	Normal	————	Normal
(B) No suppression	Normal/high	Suppression	Normal/increased
(C) No suppression	High/normal	No suppression	No response
(D) No suppression	Low	No suppression	No response

150. Normal

151. Pituitary adenoma

152. Ectopic production

153. Adrenal lesion

154. Your 47-year-old patient with hypertension and asthma comes to your office with an erythematous rash on sun-exposed distribution. Serologic tests reveal a positive ANA. All of the following agents have been strongly associated with a lupus-like syndrome EXCEPT

    (A) hydralazine.

    (B) isoniazid.

    (C) procainamide.

    (D) phenothiazine.

    (E) hydroxychloroquine.

155. A 10-year-old combative male is brought to the emergency room by the EMS. Their report indicated that the child had complained of a headache, malaise, myalgias, anorexia, nausea, and a sore throat. He also complained of a tingling sensation and jumping of the muscles of his right arm. His temperature is 105°F, respiration is 20, pulse 110, and blood pressure 90/60. On examination, the child is excited, agitated, and confused, with healed wounds on forearms and legs.

Opisthotonic posturing is present. Pupils are irregular and dilated. Salivation is present. DTRs are increased. Cardiorespiratory arrest occurs following a grand-mal seizure. Resuscitation efforts fail. A representative hematoxylin and eosin-stained slide of the cerebellum is shown in the figure. Your diagnosis is

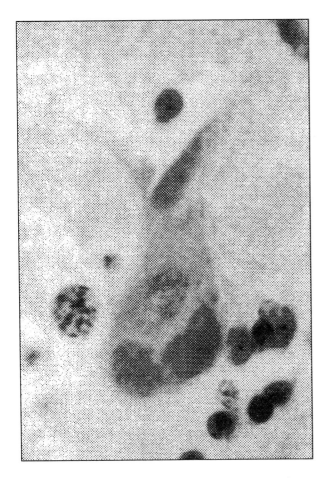

(A) subacute sclerosing panencephalitis.

(B) progressive multifocal leukoencephalopathy.

(C) Creutzfeldt-Jakob disease.

(D) rabies.

(E) Reye's syndrome.

156. A perforated duodenal ulcer will present as

    (A) acute RLQ pain.

    (B) acute RUQ pain.

(C) chronic RLQ pain.

(D) chronic RUQ pain.

(E) intermittent diffuse abdominal pain.

Questions 157-160 refer to the following:

A 20-year-old female patient comes to your office complaining of severe lower-back pain for the past two days. The pain began several hours after helping her friend move boxes. She denies symptoms of incontinence or fever. Physical examination reveals paraspinal tenderness in the lower back and normal neurologic exam. You determine that empirical therapy is warranted.

157. Treatment may include all of the following EXCEPT

    (A) bed rest.

    (B) nonsteroidal anti-inflammatory agents.

    (C) warm compresses.

    (D) initiation of back and abdominal strengthening exercises upon resolution of the acute exacerbation.

    (E) colchicine every four hours as needed.

158. The patient tells you that her friend had a similar experience and underwent an MRI exam. The patient asks you to pursue additional testing with an MRI exam. You should do which one of the following?

    (A) Tell the patient that you will order the MRI only if she is willing to pay for the exam herself.

    (B) Order a CT scan as a less expensive alternative.

    (C) Refer the patient to an orthopedic surgeon for a second opinion on the matter.

    (D) Explain to the patient that an MRI is not indicated at this time based on her symptomatology.

(E) Ask the patient to find another physician who may order the test for her.

159. Which one of the following diagnostic tests is most likely to reveal an abnormality in a patient with lumbosacral strain?

(A) Back X-rays

(B) EMG/nerve conduction studies

(C) CT scan of the back

(D) Myelogram

(E) None of the above.

160. All of the following predispose toward the development of lumbosacral strain EXCEPT

(A) leg-length discrepancy.

(B) occupation requiring lifting.

(C) history of ulcerative colitis.

(D) accentuated lordosis.

(E) obesity.

161. A 48-year-old female presents to the emergency room with fatigue, weakness, poor appetite, weight loss, and left upper quadrant abdominal discomfort. On exam, she appeared thin and pale with splenomegaly. Her white blood cell count was 54,000/uL. Blood and urine cultures were negative. The chest X-ray was negative. She was afebrile. Bone marrow biopsy revealed multiple blast cells. Which one of the following tests would assist us in the diagnosis?

(A) Alpha-fetoprotein

(B) Leukocyte alkaline phosphatase

(C) Angiotensin-converting enzyme level

(D) Serum ceruloplasmin

(E) CA-125

162. A 64-year-old man has been recalled following annual laboratory testing, which showed an isolated increase in his alkaline phosphatase level. He reports mild pain in his right lower extremity, which has been present for "years." The X-ray, shown in the figure, is consistent with

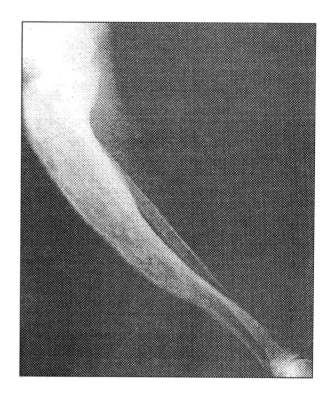

(A) old well-healed fracture.

(B) Paget's disease.

(C) metastatic disease.

(D) rickets.

(E) osteoporosis.

163. A 23-year-old male presents with symptoms of weight loss, abdominal pain, fever, and joint pain. On exam, he has peripheral lymphadenopathy, steatorrhea, nystagmus, and cranial nerve defects. Biopsy of the small bowel reveals a heavy infiltration of macrophages that stain positive for periodic acid-schiff (PAS) reagent. What is the most likely diagnosis?

(A) Small intestinal lymphoma

(B) Celiac sprue

(C) Isospora belli infection

(D) Lymphangiectasia

(E) Whipple's disease

164. All of the following present with painful palmar swelling EXCEPT

   (A) thenar space infection.

   (B) palmar abscess.

   (C) carpel tunnel syndrome.

   (D) ulnar bursa abscess.

   (E) acute tenosynovitis.

For Questions 165-168, match the following mechanisms of immunologically mediated inflammation with the appropriate patient and clinical setting.

   (A) Allergic (IgE mediated)

   (B) Cytotoxic (Type II) reaction

   (C) Immune complex formation (Type III)

   (D) Delayed-type hypersensitivity reaction (Type IV)

   (E) None of the above.

165. A 70-year-old undomiciled male with cough and fever. Sputum studies reveal acid-fast bacilli.

166. A 30-year-old female brought to the emergency room with anaphylactic shock after accidental ingestion of shellfish.

167. A 30-year-old female with photosensitivity and butterfly rash. Blood tests reveal positive antinuclear antibody.

168. A 57-year-old male, who recently traveled to Wisconsin, who now complains of cough. Sputum culture reveals blastomycosis.

For Questions 169-172, match the following toxic medications with the symptoms presented.

   (A) Digoxin

   (B) Acetaminophen

   (C) Ethylene glycol

   (D) Opioid

   (E) Benzodiazepine

169. A 23-year-old man presents with shortness of breath since this morning. Urinalysis reveals oxalate crystals.

170. A 59-year-old woman presents with nausea and vomiting for three days. She also has noted halos around lights that she looks at.

171. A 38-year-old woman presents by her family because she is more drowsy than usual. She quickly awakes upon treatment with flumazenil.

172. A 28-year-old man presents with drowsiness. Physical examination reveals that his pupils are constricted and his respiratory rate is 10.

Questions 173-176 refer to the following:

A one-month-old child presents to the emergency room with a two-day history of vomiting and diarrhea, as well as a low-grade temperature.

173. You would expect to see all of the following EXCEPT

   (A) decreased pulse.

   (B) increased pulse.

   (C) decreased blood pressure.

   (D) dry mucous membranes.

   (E) concentrated urine.

174. Of the following baseline questions to elicit from the parents, the LEAST important is

   (A) gestational age of the infant.

   (B) family history.

   (C) immunization status.

   (D) infant's diet.

   (E) recent travel.

175. Palpation of a 2-cm firm mass deep in the epigastrium on the right side along with a description of projectile vomiting would lead you to conclude that the patient suffers from

(A) duodenal obstruction.

(B) pyloric stenosis.

(C) large bowel obstruction.

(D) esophageal atresia.

(E) diaphragmatic hernia

176. Which one of the following would be appropriate for this infant?

(A) Send home with the parents with a follow-up appointment in clinic

(B) Intravenous fluid administration

(C) Increased oral fluid intake

(D) Anti-emetics

(E) Anti-diarrheals

Questions 177-180 refer to the following:

A 40-year-old man with a history of alcohol-induced cirrhosis presents with increasing abdominal girth associated with abdominal pain and nausea and vomiting. He denies any fevers, chills, diarrhea, or constipation. He denies any other medical illnesses and is not taking any medications. He denies any recent alcohol use or illicit drug use. On physical examination, he has a temperature of 100.0°F, a pulse of 90, a blood pressure of 110/70, and a respiratory rate of 16. His lungs are clear and his heart reveals no murmurs or gallops. His abdomen is distended with a fluid wave and mildly tender to palpation diffusely without rebound.

177. Of the following statements regarding spontaneous bacterial peritonitis (SBP), the true one is

(A) SBP can present without fever.

(B) SBP is not usually a cause of worsening hepatic encephalopathy.

(C) SBP always presents with abdominal pain.

(D) SBP is common in patients with small amounts of ascites.

(E) SBP is not fatal, even if not treated.

178. The way to diagnose SBP is

(A) ascites fluid culture positive for bacterial organisms.

(B) ascites fluid Gram-positive for bacterial organisms.

(C) ascites fluid Gram-positive for polymorphonuclear leukocytes.

(D) ascites fluid cell count with greater than 250 polymorphonuclear leukocytes/microliter.

(E) ascites fluid pH greater than 7.6.

179. The most common causative organism of SBP is

(A) *Streptococcus pneumoniae.*

(B) *Haemophilus influenzae.*

(C) *Escherichia coli.*

(D) *Klebsiella pneumoniae.*

(E) *Pseudomonas aeruginosa.*

180. Of the following antibiotics, all are appropriate choices for initial treatment EXCEPT

(A) gentamicin.

(B) ceftriaxone.

(C) ceftazidine.

(D) ampicillin/clavulanic acid.

(E) ticarcillin/clavulanic acid.

USMLE STEP 3
PRACTICE TEST 2

Day Two – Morning Session

(Answer sheets appear in the back of this book.)

TIME: 3 Hours
180 Questions

DIRECTIONS: Each of the following numbered items or incomplete sentences is followed by an answer or a completion of the statement. Choose the **ONE** choice that **BEST** answers the question or completes the sentence.

For Questions 1-4, match the form of Mendelian transmission associated with each of the disorders.

    (A)   Autosomal dominant

    (B)   Autosomal recessive

    (C)   X-linked

    (D)   None of the above.

1.   Color blindness

2.   Sickle cell anemia

3.   Cystic fibrosis

4.   Nonalcoholic steatohepatitis

5.   A 37-year-old female presents with symptoms of headache, weakness, fatigue, and gingival bleeding. She had signs of pallor on examination. There is no evidence of splenomegaly. The white blood cell count is greater than 100,000. Schistocytes and blast cells are seen on the peripheral smear. Her physician suspects disseminated intravascular coagulation. Which one of the following hematological malignancies is associated with DIC?

    (A)   Acute lymphocytic leukemia

    (B)   Chronic myelogenous leukemia

    (C)   Multiple myeloma

    (D)   Acute promyelocytic leukemia

    (E)   Chronic lymphocytic leukemia

6.   A 65-year-old female patient comes to the emergency room complaining of shortness of breath. Physical exam reveals decreased breath sounds in the right lung base. Chest X-ray reveals a right pleural effusion. Pleural fluid analysis is as follows: Protein: 4.0g/dl (serum protein is 7.2), LDH: 350 (serum LDH: 400). Which one of the following is the LEAST likely cause of this patient's effusion based on pleural fluid analysis?

    (A)   Nephrotic syndrome

    (B)   Systemic lupus erythematosus

    (C)   Bronchogenic carcinoma

    (D)   Parapneumonic effusion

    (E)   Metastatic breast cancer

7. A 60-year-old asymptomatic male was referred by his sister for evaluation. She was recently diagnosed with kidney disease that was reported "to run in families." Physical examination is significant for hepatomegaly and ballottable kidneys. Two sections from a contrast-enhanced abdominal computed tomographic study are shown in the figure. Based on these findings, you discuss all of the following EXCEPT

Panel A

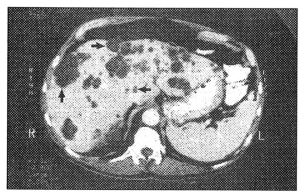

Panel B

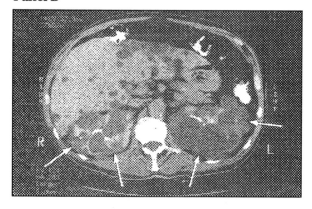

   (A) intracranial aneurysms occur in approximately 10% of affected persons.

   (B) the most common genetic defect is located on the short arm of chromosome 16.

   (C) gross hematuria occurs in 40% of affected persons at least once.

   (D) liver and kidney lesions improve with age.

   (E) hypertension develops in at least 60% of affected persons.

8. A pharmacy calls you because one of your patients has brought in four prescriptions for codeine from four different physicians in the last month. You

   (A) refuse to see the patient again.

   (B) tell the pharmacist not to bother you.

   (C) tell the pharmacist the patient must have a lot of pain.

   (D) tell the pharmacist to call the police.

   (E) discuss the situation with your patient.

9. You examine a 54-year-old farmer who presents with a slowly enlarging and discolored area of the skin around his left ear. Your clinical suspicion is confirmed by biopsy results; the farmer has a skin cancer. Which one of the following statements about this condition is FALSE?

   (A) It is prevalent in light-skinned populations.

   (B) It is the most common type of cancer in light-skinned populations.

   (C) Sensitivity and direct and prolonged exposure to UV radiation are the major risk factors in developing this form of skin cancer.

   (D) Squamous cell carcinoma accounts for over 65% of all cases of skin cancer in the United States.

   (E) This patient has basal cell carcinoma.

10. Intertrigo usually can be seen in

   (A) the hair roots.

   (B) the cornea.

   (C) the retina.

   (D) the skin.

   (E) the tympanic membrane.

11. You are covering a clinic for your partner, and his 45-year-old female patient comes in complaining of an abdominal pain. The first thing to do is

    (A) give her an IM pain medication.

    (B) order X-rays.

    (C) pass an NG tube and get a surgical consult.

    (D) perform a rectal examination.

    (E) review the old chart.

12. A lymphangiogram, obtained 30 minutes following injection of 99mTc-labeled human albumin (Panel B), and a coronal and transaxial section of a magnetic resonance imaging study (Panel C) were performed to evaluate the bilateral symmetric, nonpitting swelling of the legs of the woman shown in the figure (Panel A) below. All of the following are true EXCEPT

    (A) the lymphatic vessels and regional lymph nodes are normal.

    (B) the radionuclide migrates cephalad promptly.

    (C) the magnetic resonance imaging study demonstrates massive subcutaneous deposition of fat.

    (D) the magnetic resonance imaging study demonstrates massive fluid accumulation.

    (E) the irregular high-intensity subcutaneous signals on the coronal MRI studies represent venous varicosities.

Questions 13-16 refer to the following:

A 38-year-old man presents to your office with five days of increasing diarrhea. He states that previously, he had been on amoxicillin for sinusitis for two weeks, which he stopped taking three days ago. Five days ago, he noted the onset of diarrhea, which has

Panel A   **Panel B**   **Panel C**

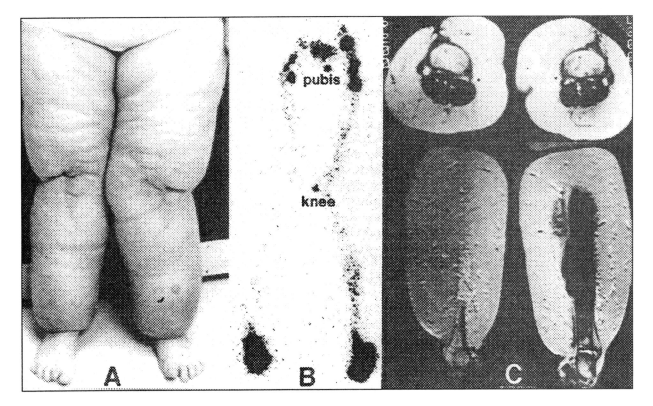

subsequently become blood-tinged and has had a mucus character. He also complains of low-grade fevers, chills, and diffuse abdominal pain. He denies this ever occurring before. On physical examination, his temperature is 100.3°F, blood pressure is 110/70, heart rate is 78, and respiratory rate is 16. His abdominal exam reveals normal bowel sounds and diffuse tenderness to palpation. He also complains of mild rebound tenderness. He does not have any abdominal masses, nor is he distended. Rectal examination reveals guaiac-positive stool.

13. Appropriate initial tests to order would be all of the following EXCEPT

   (A) flexible sigmoidoscopy.

   (B) abdominal flat plate X-ray.

   (C) complete blood count.

   (D) stool sample sent for *Clostridium difficile* toxin.

   (E) stool sample sent for culture.

14. If each of the previous tests were ordered, which one of the following results would lead you to admit the patient for observation?

   (A) Flexible sigmoidoscopy that showed blood and stool in the distal colon

   (B) Abdominal flat plate X-ray that showed a dilated colon to 5 ¹/₂ cm

   (C) Complete blood count that revealed a hematocrit of 33%

   (D) Stool sample results positive for *Clostridium difficile* toxin

   (E) Stool sample results positive for *Campylobacter spp.*

15. The most likely diagnosis, based on history and physical examination, is

   (A) inflammatory bowel disease.

   (B) irritable bowel syndrome.

   (C) *C. dif.* colitis.

   (D) ischemic bowel syndrome.

   (E) bacterial colitis.

16. The most appropriate initial treatment while awaiting laboratory results would be to

   (A) send home and begin oral metronidazole.

   (B) admit to the hospital for IV vancomycin.

   (C) begin oral steroids and sulfasalazine.

   (D) begin a low-dose antidepressant.

   (E) send home with an antimotility medication.

17. A 27-year-old gravida 2 para 1 at 16 weeks gestational age, with no prior prenatal care, comes to you for her initial prenatal visit. In addition to her routine labs, she consents to an HIV test. The result is positive. You advise her that

   (A) she will need to have a caesarean section to prevent transmission of the HIV virus to her baby.

   (B) she should breast feed her infant.

   (C) her baby will most likely be infected with the HIV virus, as well.

   (D) AZT has been shown to be beneficial in reducing transmission from mother to child if given in the second and third trimesters, intrapartum, and to her baby for the first six weeks of life.

   (E) the baby will be born with a chromosomal abnormality.

18. A 24-year-old female is brought into the emergency room comatose. Her friends found an empty bottle of sleeping pills next to her on the floor. The first therapeutic maneuver you perform is

   (A) gastric lavage.

   (B) administer ipecac.

   (C) begin peritoneal dialysis.

(D)   administer chelating agents.

(E)   administer naloxone.

19.   A 65-year-old man with emphysema who uses home oxygen comes to the emergency room because of a three-day history of a cough productive of greenish sputum. His chest radiograph is unchanged. You order nebulizers for him and

    (A)   schedule a bronchoscopy.

    (B)   begin pentamidine.

    (C)   teach his wife how to perform chest percussion for drainage.

    (D)   prescribe oral antibiotics.

    (E)   admit him to the hospital.

20.   A 1 x 1 centimeter non-healing wound is noted on the anterior tibia. Your next step is to

    (A)   biopsy it.

    (B)   culture it.

    (C)   educate the patient on the importance of wound care.

    (D)   anesthetize the area and attempt a primary closure.

    (E)   obtain a lower extremity angiogram.

21.   The simultaneous arterial (A) and left ventricular (LV) tracings, shown in the figure in the next column, were recorded in a patient with hypertrophic obstructive cardiomyopathy. Which one of the following is NOT true?

    (A)   The first three beats show a peak systolic gradient of approximately 25 mm Hg.

    (B)   On the first sinus beat after the premature ventricular contraction, the peak systolic gradient increases to over 100 mm Hg.

    (C)   On the first sinus beat after the premature ventricular contraction, the pulse pressure decreases.

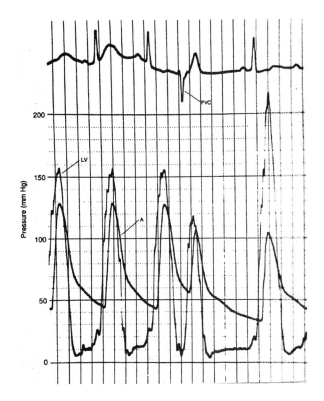

    (D)   The increased pulse pressure after a premature ventricular contraction results from a reduction of stroke volume.

    (E)   The phenomenon illustrated here is known as the Brockenbrough-Braunwald sign.

Questions 22-29 refer to the following:

A 22-year-old woman at 30 weeks of gestation presents to your office. She is complaining of painless vaginal bleeding. Her blood pressure is 100/60 mm Hg and her hematocrit is 30%. The fetal heart rate is 120 beats/min.

22.   With respect to this patient's condition, which one of the following statements is INCORRECT?

    (A)   Its incidence is 1 in 200 pregnancies.

    (B)   It may recur about five percent of the time in subsequent pregnancies.

(C)　Nulliparity is a risk factor.

(D)　Advanced maternal age is a risk factor.

(E)　Large placenta is a risk factor.

23.　Diagnosis is confirmed by

(A)　ultrasonography.

(B)　radioisotope scanning in the absence of ultrasound availability.

(C)　direct vaginal examination in about 20% of cases and in the presence of classic clinical presentation.

(D)　Both (A) and (B).

(E)　All of the above.

24.　When the exact location of placenta previa cannot be fully delineated by ultrasonography, which one of the following procedures should be performed?

(A)　Repeat ultrasonography after the patient is stabilized

(B)　Direct vaginal examination

(C)　Radioisotope scanning

(D)　Double setup

(E)　Any of the above.

25.　A double setup

(A)　refers to repeat ultrasound.

(B)　is a vaginal examination performed with the immediate capability of converting to C-section.

(C)　is elected only for hemodynamically unstable patients.

(D)　may be accomplished in an outpatient setting.

(E)　(B) and (C).

26.　Continuous fetal heart rate and uterine contraction pattern monitoring are used to ascertain fetal well-being. Regarding periodic changes that occur with uterine contractions, which one of the following statements is true?

(A)　Fetal heart and uterine contraction tracings are mirror images of one another.

(B)　Late deceleration patterns may be secondary to maternal hypotension.

(C)　Variable decelerations are thought to occur consequent to fetal head compression.

(D)　Early decelerations are thought to occur from vagal stimulation.

(E)　Beat-to-beat variability reflects intact neural pathways from the fetal cerebral cortex through the medulla, vagus nerves, and cardiac conduction system.

27.　Fetal scalp blood sampling

(A)　is indicated in all cases as an essential component of prenatal monitoring.

(B)　requires repeating 15 minutes after the first sampling results were between 7.28-7.30.

(C)　is indicated when the heart rate pattern on fetal monitoring appears ominous.

(D)　that shows a pH between 7.20 and 7.25 is normal.

(E)　that shows a pH ranging from 7.28 to 7.30 is menacing and requires immediate delivery of the fetus.

28.　Which of the following statements about abruptio placenta is correct?

(A)　It occurs in 0.2-2.4% of all deliveries.

(B)　In women who have experienced one abruptio placenta, the risk of recurrence is twice that of the normal population.

(C)   Cigarette smoking and cocaine abuse are not related risk factors.

(D)   Congenital hypofibrinogenemia appears to protect against placental abruption.

(E)   All of the above.

29.   Current guidelines from the American College of Obstetricians and Gynecologists state that the parturient who has had a previous C-section with a lower uterine segment transverse incision

(A)   can be permitted a trial of labor.

(B)   cannot be permitted a trial of labor.

(C)   should not be of any consideration since incision scars are associated with a high incidence of rupture and may not qualify for a trial of labor.

(D)   All of the above.

(E)   None of the above.

30.   A 16-year-old female comes to the emergency department complaining of severe lower abdominal pain and vaginal bleeding for one day. Upon further questioning, she notes that she is sexually active and that her LMP was seven weeks ago. What is the most likely potentially life-threatening cause of her symptoms?

(A)   Threatened abortion

(B)   Missed abortion

(C)   Ectopic pregnancy

(D)   Fibroids

(E)   Salpingitis

31.   A 32-year-old woman presents to your office with dysuria. The most likely cause is

(A)   vaginal wall carcinoma.

(B)   pregnancy.

(C)   uterine fibroid.

(D)   partial obstruction of the urethra.

(E)   bladder paralysis.

32.   A 55-year-old male with peptic ulcer disease refractory to cimetidine returns for the results of his endoscopic biopsy, shown in the figure below. He continues to smoke two packs of cigarettes daily. He is under increased stress at work due to downsizing as a result of corporate mergers. You recommend

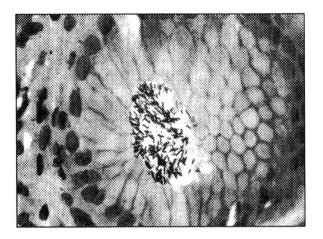

(A)   psychotherapy referral.

(B)   immediate oncology referral.

(C)   decreasing cigarette consumption to one pack per day.

(D)   a trial of famotidine, 80 mg with breakfast.

(E)   a trial of tetracycline, metronidazole, and bismuth.

Questions 33-39 refer to the following:

A 27-year-old primigravida in her third trimester of pregnancy comes in for her routine appointment. She has a blood pressure of 150/94, which is the first time it has been elevated during the pregnancy. She volunteers that her shoes have recently been feeling too tight.

33.   You order all of the following laboratory exams on an emergency basis EXCEPT

(A)   urinalysis.

(B)   serum electrolytes.

(C)   platelet count.

(D) prothrombin time.

(E) chest radiograph.

34. A dipstick test of the urine reveals proteinuria. Your working diagnosis is

(A) essential hypertension.

(B) acute renal failure.

(C) glomerulonephritis.

(D) preeclampsia.

(E) pheochromocytoma.

35. This patient is at significantly increased risk for all of the following EXCEPT

(A) a bleeding diathesis.

(B) a stroke.

(C) pancreatitis.

(D) seizures.

(E) headaches.

36. You prescribe all of the following EXCEPT

(A) diuretics.

(B) vasodilators.

(C) bed rest.

(D) quiet environment.

(E) time off from work.

37. The patient's husband calls a few days later to tell you she has developed a lot of bruises even though she swears she has stayed in bed except to go to the bathroom. You suspect

(A) spousal abuse.

(B) consumptive coagulopathy.

(C) hemophilia.

(D) idiopathic thrombocytopenic purpura.

(E) the husband is overly anxious.

38. The patient's symptoms are likely to completely resolve

(A) after a week of bed rest.

(B) never.

(C) following delivery.

(D) with administration of antihypertensives.

(E) with dialysis.

39. You can tell the husband that

(A) the patient will probably not be able to have more children.

(B) the patient's prognosis is very good.

(C) the baby is likely to have a congenital anomaly.

(D) the patient is likely to have chronic seizures.

(E) the patient is likely to have renal insufficiency.

Questions 40-46 refer to the following:

You are called to the emergency room to see a 37-year-old man with a traumatic injury to his left hand. It occurred several hours ago while he was slicing vegetables in his restaurant. His past medical history (PMH) is significant for hypertension and non-insulin-dependent diabetes mellitus, both of which are well controlled. Upon seeing him, his blood pressure is 160/100, pulse is 84, RR is 18, and temperature is 99.2°F. He has a bulky bandage around his left hand, and he is in a mild amount of pain.

40. The most likely cause for his elevated blood pressure is

(A) his essential hypertension is under poor control.

(B) undiagnosed pheochromocytoma.

(C) factitial reading.

(D) pain and apprehension.

(E) hypovolemia.

41. The least important question asked in your history data-gathering is

(A)   tetanus status.

(B)   hand dominance.

(C)   occupation.

(D)   previous hand trauma.

(E)   family history.

42.   On physical examination, the patient is unable to flex the distal interphalangeal joint of his ring finger. There is an injury of the

(A)   flexor digitorum superficialis of the ring finger.

(B)   flexor digitorum profundus of the ring finger.

(C)   extensor digiti communis of the ring finger.

(D)   flexor carpi ulnaris.

(E)   flexor carpi radialis.

43.   Appropriate management would include all of the following EXCEPT

(A)   tetanus toxoid administration.

(B)   irrigation and exploration of the wound.

(C)   closure of the skin.

(D)   repair of the tendon injury.

(E)   splinting of the hand and arm.

44.   Which test is used to test the arterial supply to the hand?

(A)   Trendelenburg

(B)   Allen

(C)   McMurray

(D)   Kocher

(E)   Kernig

45.   If this patient complained of numbness of his small finger, which of the following nerves would you suspect an injury to?

(A)   Radial

(B)   Median

(C)   Ulnar

(D)   Musculocutaneous

(E)   Hypothenar

46.   The patient is taken to the operating room, and the tendon and artery are repaired. The nerve is visualized and no laceration is seen. The most likely explanation for this finding is

(A)   an inexperienced examiner.

(B)   a neuropraxia.

(C)   a neurotmesis.

(D)   an axontmesis.

(E)   a laceration outside the field of exploration.

47.   A 47-year-old man, who is hospitalized with a pneumonia, was found by his physician to be jaundiced. On examination, he had hepatomegaly and scleral icterus. The prothrombin time was prolonged and his albumin level was low. His serum aminotransferase levels were elevated as well as serum alkaline phosphatase levels. This patient has had a history of blood transfusions in the past secondary to trauma. His second-generation hepatitis C antibody test was positive. All of the following instructions should be given to the patient EXCEPT

(A)   individuals should not donate blood, body organs, other tissue, or semen.

(B)   household articles such as toothbrushes and razors should not be shared.

(C)   treatment with interferon alpha-2b should be recommended if hepatitis C persists after six months.

(D) hepatitis C vaccine should be given right away.

(E) a liver biopsy is recommended if hepatitis C antibody and elevation of aminotransferases persist after six months.

48. A 70-year-old man with hypertension and diabetes mellitus is doing well seven days after suffering a large myocardial infarction. He has not had any conduction disturbances, hypotension, or congestive heart failure. However, on day eight, he becomes very short of breath and hypotensive. Chest radiograph reveals a boot-shaped heart that is much larger than previously, and electrocardiogram reveals no ischemic changes, but low voltages. The most likely etiology is

(A) myocardial rupture.

(B) papillary muscle rupture.

(C) flash pulmonary edema.

(D) pulmonary embolism.

(E) sepsis.

49. A 37-year-old healthy female comes to the emergency room complaining of headache, photophobia, and nausea. On physical exam, T = 101, P = 100, and blood pressure is 120/65. There is evidence of nuchal rigidity on examination. CSF examination is performed, which reveals yellow fluid with 670 cells (95% lymphocytes), glucose: 60, protein: 48. Gram stain of the fluid shows no organisms. Which one of the following diagnoses is most likely?

(A) Bacterial meningitis

(B) Aseptic meningitis

(C) Migraine headache

(D) Subarachnoid hemorrhage

(E) None of the above.

50. The area of splenic dullness is

(A) the left posterior axilla, not exceeding a vertical distance of 9 cm.

(B) the left mid axilla, not exceeding a vertical distance of 9 cm.

(C) the left anterior axilla, not exceeding a vertical distance of 9 cm.

(D) the left midclavicular line, not exceeding a vertical distance of 9 cm.

(E) Cannot be determined.

Questions 51-54 refer to the following:

A 73-year-old retired leather worker complains of back pain, exacerbated by movement. The pain does not occur at night. He also complains of fatigue and weakness for the past few weeks.

51. The Wright-Giemsa stained bone marrow aspirate confirms your diagnosis of

(A) metastatic prostate carcinoma.

(B) multiple myeloma.

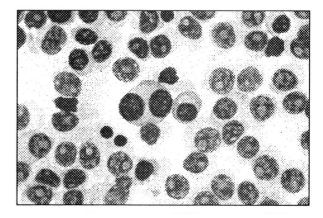

(C) chronic lymphocytic leukemia.

(D) myeloid metaplasia.

(E) metastatic lung cancer.

52. The most likely X-ray finding in this patient is

(A) blastic lesions of the vertebral spine.

(B) diffuse punched-out bony lytic lesions.

(C) normal.

(D) "fishmouth" deformity of the vertebrae.

(E) "bamboo spine."

53. The classic triad of myeloma consists of which one of the following?

(A) Marrow plasmacytosis greater than 10%, lytic bone lesions, serum and/or urine M-component

(B) Marrow plasmacytosis greater than 25%, lytic bone lesions, serum and/or urine A-component

(C) Marrow plasmacytosis greater than 10%, blastic bone lesions, anemia

(D) Marrow plasmacytosis greater than 10%, lytic bone lesions, Bence-Jones proteinuria

(E) Plasmacytoma, blastic bone lesions, hypercalcemia

54. The major causes of renal failure in multiple myeloma are hypercalcemia and "myeloma kidney." "Myeloma kidney" is characterized by

(A) large, wax, laminated casts in the distal and collecting tubules.

(B) precipitated monoclonal heavy chains.

(C) hyperuricemia.

(D) deposition of monoclonal heavy chains in the renal glomerulus.

(E) amyloid deposition in the renal glomerulus.

55. A 72-year-old male comes to your office for a pre-op physical and a mass is found on his chest X-ray measuring 2 x 2 centimeters. Your next step is to

(A) repeat the chest X-ray.

(B) look for old X-rays and compare.

(C) perform a biopsy.

(D) perform a CAT scan.

(E) schedule the patient for surgery.

56. Swollen gums may occur in all of the following EXCEPT

(A) Dilantin use.

(B) gingivitis.

(C) carcinoma of the soft palate.

(D) scurvy.

(E) odontogenic abscess.

For Questions 57-60, match the case with the correct diagnosis.

(A) Subacute bacterial endocarditis

(B) Atrial fibrillation

(C) Pericarditis

(D) Mitral valve prolapse

(E) Hypocalcemia

57. A 32-year-old drug addict with splinter hemorrhages on his fingers and exudates in his fundi

58. A 45-year-old woman admitted for elective hysterectomy who develops acute stabbing substernal chest pain when she coughs

59. A 56-year-old man with a prolonged Q-T interval on a routine electrocardiogram

60. A 67-year-old man with congestive heart failure who has developed an irregular heart rate

61. You suspect rickets in one of your patients. A lab value consistent with the diagnosis is

(A) elevated serum calcium.

(B) elevated serum phosphorus.

(C) decreased serum calcium.

(D) decreased serum alkaline phosphatase.

(E) elevated amylase.

62. With respect to primary and secondary prevention of tuberculosis, which one of the following statements is INCORRECT?

    (A) Isoniazid prophylaxis is indicated for all patients who test positive on skin testing.

    (B) BCG vaccination protects against tuberculous meningitis and disseminated TB in children over five years of age.

    (C) The primary form of TB in infants and children is highly contagious.

    (D) Every single case of TB should be reported to public health departments.

    (E) A prior BCG vaccination in people from developing countries may produce a false-positive result on tuberculin testing.

63. A 40-year-old woman presents to your office with two days of right temporal head pain. She also has noted that her vision has decreased on the right side, as well. She denies any other symptoms. Definitive diagnosis can be made by

    (A) erythrocyte sedimentation rate.

    (B) temporal artery biopsy.

    (C) CT of the head.

    (D) lumbar puncture.

    (E) None of the above.

64. James Brown visits a physician at his work site with a complaint of an enlarging area of skin discoloration. The lesion is confirmed to be squamous cell carcinoma. Given the fact that Mr. Brown is the second case discovered during the year, which one of the following actions is most appropriate for the physician?

    (A) Express his suspicions about a possible association between the patient's skin cancer and his present job and suggest that the patient quit.

    (B) Release information to enforcement agencies and request an immediate investigation for hazardous substances at the workplace.

    (C) Inform local health preventive agencies.

    (D) Release his findings to the management and other workers.

    (E) Inform neither workers nor management but search for possible carcinogens at the work site.

65. **An 85-year-old female who has been living alone in her apartment complains of symptoms of lethargy, weakness, and malaise. The physician tells her it is due to stress and does nothing. Three months later the patient has bleeding gums, perifollicular hemorrhages, and joint pain. X-rays of the bones revealed subperiosteal elevation. Which one of the following dietary deficiencies can lead to this disorder?**

    (A) **Ascorbic acid**

    (B) **Vitamin B12**

    (C) **Niacin**

    (D) **Thiamine**

    (E) **Vitamin A**

66. An 18-year-old female is brought in to her physician's office by her parents because of symptoms of fever, headache, malaise, weakness, and vomiting. She has had no prior medical history. These symptoms have lasted for one week prior to the visit. On examination, the patient appears toxic with a temperature of 102°F and a petechial rash on her lower extremities. She has neck stiffness. What would be the next immediate step in management of this patient?

    (A) CT of the head

    (B) Lumbar puncture

    (C) Skin biopsy

    (D) Blood cultures

    (E) Intravenous hydration

67. Which one of the following is the most potent narcotic analgesic?

    (A) Morphine

    (B) Meperidine

    (C) Hydromorphone

    (D) Fentanyl

    (E) Sufentanil

68. A 24-year-old woman presents to your office for the first time looking for a primary care physician. She denies any previous medical problems or surgeries. She smokes one pack of cigarettes per day and she is sexually active. Oral contraceptives are the only medications that she takes. Family history is negative for any cancers or heart disease. Initial vital signs are blood pressure of 160/80, heart rate of 90, temperature of 99°F, and respiratory rate of 16. The most appropriate management decision would be to

    (A) begin aggressive antihypertensive medications.

    (B) send off serum thyroid panels.

    (C) check the blood pressure at the next visit and, if still elevated, consider initiation of antihypertensive medications.

    (D) send off urine metanephrines and catecholamines.

    (E) order a renal ultrasound with Doppler.

69. All of the following statements are true of the polymerase chain reaction EXCEPT

    (A) it allows amplification of very specific pieces of DNA from extremely small samples.

    (B) it can be performed on archival samples.

    (C) it is vulnerable to minute contamination by any DNA.

    (D) it is vulnerable to infidelity during replication.

    (E) it requires DNA from living cells.

70. A 53-year-old woman whom you have seen once a year for several years for routine care comes to your clinic for an unscheduled visit. She has been going through a difficult divorce and has developed headaches. Her blood pressure is 150/96. It had previously been normal. You decide to

    (A) reassure her and tell her to come back for her annual visit in four months.

    (B) start her on antihypertensives.

    (C) give her a benzodiazepine.

    (D) tell her to return for a blood pressure check in a week.

    (E) give her a narcotic for her headaches.

71. A 72-year-old man with severe myopia presents for scleral buckle repair of a spontaneous retinal detachment. His past medical and surgical history are unremarkable. Physical examination is normal. Regarding retinal detachment and its repair, which one of the following statements is true?

    (A) Peripheral retinal and macular detachment exceeding 24 hours can be treated electively.

    (B) Macular retinal detachment exceeding 24 hours can be treated electively.

    (C) Recent or impending macular detachment requires urgent attention.

    (D) All of the above.

    (E) None of the above.

72. A 26-year-old previously healthy college student, home for vacation, complained to the triage nurse of the sudden onset today of a headache, myalgias, nausea, vomiting, and fever. He has a seizure while waiting to be examined. Blood cultures, performed as part of your diagnostic examination, were positive. Gram stain of the blood, shown on the next page, suggests

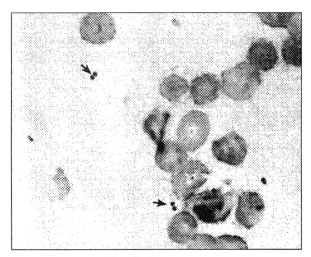

(A) *Staphylococcus aureus.*

(B) *Streptococcus bovis.*

(C) *Neisseria meningitidis.*

(D) *Streptococcus pneumoniae.*

(E) *Escherichia coli.*

73. While performing a Weber's test on a 22-year-old patient referred to you, there is lateralization to the left ear. This indicates

    (A) conductive loss of the right ear.

    (B) conductive loss of the left ear.

    (C) perceptive loss on the left side.

    (D) bilateral conductive loss.

    (E) bilateral perceptive loss.

74. A 21-year-old college student presents to the infirmary with symptoms of dry, hacking cough, fever, and shortness of breath. On exam, she has no rales or rhonchi, but the ear exam reveals bullous myringitis. Chest X-ray shows bilateral alveolar infiltrates. What would be the initial management plan for this patient?

    (A) CT scan of the chest

    (B) Steroids

    (C) Hospitalization with intravenous cephalosporin

(D) Oral erythromycin

(E) Beta-adrenergic agonist nebulizer treatments

75. A new diagnostic test is being studied and compared to the gold standard. Of 100 patients who don't have the disease, the new test is positive in eight patients and negative in 92 patients. Of 100 patients who do have the disease, the new test is positive in 98 patients and negative in two patients. Which of the following statements is correct regarding the test?

    (A) The sensitivity is 92%.

    (B) The sensitivity is 95%.

    (C) The specificity is 98%.

    (D) The specificity is 92%.

    (E) None of the above; it is impossible to determine the sensitivity or specificity without the pretest probability.

76. When performing a lung examination, tympany will replace resonance with

    (A) emphysema.

    (B) pneumothorax.

    (C) pleural effusion.

    (D) neoplasm.

    (E) atelectasis.

77. A 68-year-old man is hospitalized for ascending cholangitis and sepsis. He undergoes decompression with a percutaneous drainage, and he is placed on an antipseudomonal penicillin and an aminoglycoside and remains extremely ill. However, on the third day of treatment, his serum creatinine begins to rise. Of the following statements, which statement is true regarding the dosing of the aminoglycoside?

    (A) Twenty-four-hour urine studies should be sent each day to assess creatinine clearance.

(B) The serum creatinine should be used to re-calculate the creatinine clearance each day.

(C) The aminoglycoside should be stopped.

(D) Random levels of the aminoglycoside should be followed and redosed when it reaches the trough level.

(E) The dosing of the aminoglycoside should not change.

78. An 18-year-old white female presents to her allergist with symptoms of frequent sneezing, watery and itchy eyes, pruritic upper palate, and watery, clear rhinorrhea. On exam, she has blue, boggy nasal turbinates and an elevation of eosinophils on a nasal discharge smear. She has a family history of similar symptoms. All of the following are treatment options for this patient EXCEPT

(A) inhaled nasal corticosteroids.

(B) oral non-sedating antihistamine agents.

(C) air-conditioning.

(D) normal saline drops to each nostril.

(E) avoiding alcohol use with antihistamines.

Questions 79-85 refer to the following:

A 65-year-old male complains of bright red rectal bleeding since this morning. He denies pain, change in bowel pattern, or constitutional symptoms. He has been in good health and has not seen a physician for several years. Examination is significant for bleeding hemorrhoids. The spun hematocrit is 39%.

79. After controlling the bleeding, you advise

(A) a colonoscopy.

(B) a hemorrhoidectomy.

(C) injection of the hemorrhoids with sclerosing agents.

(D) banding of the hemorrhoids.

(E) a low-fiber diet.

80. The patient refuses all of your recommendations, but agrees to monitor his stool for subsequent bleeding during the next two weeks. You discuss all of the following, as they pertain to fecal occult blood screening for colorectal cancer, EXCEPT

(A) eating rare red meat may cause a false-positive result due to the presence of heme.

(B) peroxidase activity in turnips and horseradish may cause a false-positive result.

(C) ingestion of salicylates may produce false-positive results.

(D) ingestion of vitamin C may produce false-negative results.

(E) ingestion of iron supplements causes a false-negative result.

81. At his return appointment, two of the three cards are positive for occult blood. He indicates that he has followed your instructions meticulously. He refuses your recommendation for colonoscopy, but agrees to a barium enema, which is shown in the figure below. You now recommend

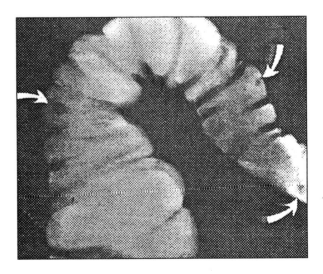

(A) colonoscopy.

(B) surgical consultation.

(C) CEA level.

(D) liver-spleen scan.

(E) chest X-ray.

82. In total, six lesions were found, all of which were excised. You are reviewing the histology (shown in the figure below) of a typical lesion. You now recommend

(A) CEA level.

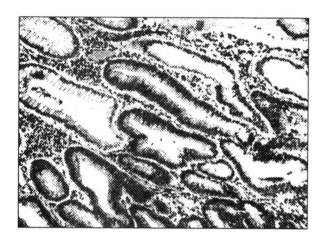

(B) oncology consultation.

(C) liver-spleen scan.

(D) repeat colonoscopy in three years.

(E) computed tomography of the abdomen/pelvis.

83. You also discuss his other laboratory tests: Chemistry multichannel: WNL; CBC: Hct 37%, Hgb 12 g/dL, WBC 5,000/mm³, MCV 70 micrometers³, MCHC 31 Hb/cell, serum ferritin 10 ng/mL. Based on these results, you recommend

(A) bone marrow aspiration and biopsy.

(B) ferrous sulfate, 325 mg daily.

(C) repeat CBC in two months.

(D) iron-containing vitamin cocktail.

(E) blood transfusion.

84. The man returns 10 years later. Following his retirement, he had relocated to Spain. He did not seek medical attention because he was feeling well. The histopathology of polypoid lesion, which was expected at colonoscopy, is shown in the figure below. You diagnose

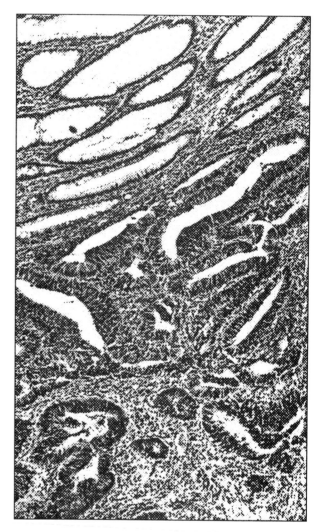

(A) recurrent adenomatous polyp.

(B) adenocarcinoma of the colon.

(C) villous adenoma.

(D) vascular ectasia of the colon.

(E) hamartoma of the colon.

85. Regarding the diagnostic usefulness of carcinoembryonic antigen in this condition, which one of the following is true?

(A) It has limited usefulness, since it is decreased in smokers.

(B) It is an excellent screening test for adenocarcinoma of the colon.

(C) It is specific for diseases of the colon.

(D) In persons undergoing therapy for metastases, a decline in levels suggests a favorable response to therapy.

(E) If routinely monitored postoperatively, it identifies curable from incurable colon cancer patients.

86. Which one of the following daily medications is usually withheld from a patient on the morning of a scheduled surgical operation?

    (A) Atenolal

    (B) Diazepam

    (C) Furosemide

    (D) Diltiazem

    (E) All should be held since the patient should be kept NPO.

For Questions 87-90, match the problems with the findings.

You are in the psychiatric ward, covering for one of your colleagues, and you must diagnose the problems below based on these pertinent findings

    (A) persecutory or grandiose delusions

    (B) tachycardia, sweating, fatigue, and muscle tenderness

    (C) emotional immaturity

    (D) insomnia and despondency

    (E) delirium

87. Paranoid reaction

88. Depression

89. Hysterical personality

90. Anxiety

91. Your patient is a 30-year-old woman. Her pulse is 120 beats/min and her blood pressure is 180/100 mm Hg. Her temperature measures 39.2°C. The medical records received from her family physician show that she has been on methimazole for hyperthyroidism. To prevent this patient from possible development of intraoperative thyrotoxic crisis, you should decide on a right dose of the antithyroid drug. To do so, which of the following laboratory tests should you order to evaluate this patient's thyroid problem?

    (A) Total plasma T4 and T3 levels

    (B) Thyroid resin uptake

    (C) Radioactive iodine uptake

    (D) Serum TSH

    (E) All of the above.

For Questions 92-95, select the most appropriate initial treatment for the patient with diabetes mellitus.

    (A) Dietary control

    (B) Oral hypoglycemics

    (C) Oral metformin

    (D) Sliding scale insulin

    (E) Daily insulin regimen

92. A 50-year-old obese man with hypertension and no previous history of diabetes mellitus who presents with a fasting glucose of 208

93. A 13-year-old girl who presents with fasting glucose levels of over 300

94. A 39-year-old woman, without significant past medical history, who has never previously been diagnosed with diabetes presents

after a hospitalization for non-ketotic hyper-osmolar coma

95. A 49-year-old man with type II diabetes mellitus that had been controlled with diet, but now presents with a fasting glucose of 300

96. A 45-year-old female, hospitalized for dehydration secondary to viral gastroenteritis, presents one morning with asymptomatic "spots" on both her lower extremities. She had been taking oral hypoglycemic agents for type II diabetes and oral quinidine for nocturnal leg cramps. On examination, she is afebrile with multiple, red-purple, non-palpable purpura on the dorsa of her feet and anterior tibia. What would be the next step in the management of this patient?

  (A) Administration of vitamin C

  (B) Prednisone

  (C) Intravenous penicillin

  (D) Discontinuing quinidine

  (E) Chemotherapy

97. A 12-year-old female comes to the office complaining of polyarthralgias. Upon reviewing her records, you find that she has a history of frequent streptococcal pharyngitis. Her mother notes that she had a cough and fever three weeks ago which resolved. You order an antistreptolysin antibody, which is positive at high titer. Which one of the following are NOT manifestations of this patient's disease?

  (A) Erythema marginatum

  (B) Subcutaneous nodules

  (C) Chorea

  (D) Glomerulonephritis

  (E) Carditis

98. A 67-year-old male with known hypertension comes in to his physician's office presenting with symptoms of urgency, urinary hesitancy, and frequent micturition at night. On examination, he has an enlarged prostate gland. Which one of the following antihypertensive medications is best suited for this particular patient?

  (A) Verapamil

  (B) Terazosin

  (C) Clonidine

  (D) Nifedipine

  (E) Hydrochlorothiazide

99. A 66-year-old nonsmoking male with benign prostatic hypertrophy, who is otherwise healthy, consults you regarding an elevated prostate specific antigen (PSA) level, done as part of his "annual executive health evaluation." Physical examination is normal except for mild prostatic hypertrophy. ESR, CBC, and chemistry panel are WNL; PSA is 5.0 ng/mL. You discuss all of the following EXCEPT

  (A) PSA normally increases with age.

  (B) PSA test accuracy increases if age adjustment is taken into consideration when interpreting test results.

  (C) the "normal age-adjusted range" for PSA should be reduced by 50% in persons treated with finasteride.

  (D) PSA levels may be elevated in benign prostatic hypertrophy and prostatitis.

  (E) early detection of prostate cancer by PSA screening improves survival by 75%.

100. Which component of MMR should a patient receive after the age 10?

  (A) Measles vaccine

  (B) Mumps vaccine

  (C) Rubella vaccine

  (D) All of the above

  (E) None of the above

101. A 29-year-old woman presents to your office with two weeks of breast discharge. She denies any other complaints. On physical examination, you note easily expressed galactorrhea. Of the following medications, which one can cause these symptoms?

(A) Beta-blockers

(B) Phenothiazines

(C) Salicylates

(D) Penicillins

(E) ACE inhibitors

102. A 27-year-old woman presents to your office with cough productive of green sputum and night sweats and chills for one week. She tells you that she has not had any recent sick contacts except a few months ago when she was exposed to her brother who is now taking six medications for tuberculosis. Her lungs reveal a right apical pleural rub. Of the following, the most appropriate intervention would be to

(A) place a purified protein derivative (PPD) and check the results in 48-72 hours.

(B) obtain a chest radiograph.

(C) begin treatment with a three-drug regimen for tuberculosis.

(D) begin treatment for acute pneumonia.

(E) admit into an isolation room until tuberculosis has been ruled out or treatment begun.

103. A 39-year-old female on oral contraceptives presents with a swollen, tender left calf. A venogram has been ordered, but before it is done she develops pleuritic chest pain associated with a cough. You decide to begin treatment before the venogram because you are very worried about her. You order

(A) high-dose salicylates.

(B) intravenous heparin.

(C) oral Coumadin.

(D) intravenous streptokinase.

(E) a surgical consult.

104. A 35-year-old male has been admitted because of new onset of chest pain. The pain is sharp, anterior, and somewhat alleviated by sitting forward. Your working diagnosis is

(A) acute myocardial infarction.

(B) angina pectoris.

(C) dyspepsia.

(D) pericarditis.

(E) costochondritis.

105. A 73-year-old woman who was admitted last week for a stroke and now has hemiplegia is noticed to have a cough on rounds and you hear rales in the left upper lobe. The cough is productive of greenish sputum. A likely diagnosis is

(A) viral upper respiratory infection.

(B) mycoplasma pneumonia.

(C) aspiration pneumonia.

(D) Legionnaire's disease.

(E) COPD.

106. A 23-year-old male who was admitted two days ago with pneumococcal pneumonia has been treated appropriately and has defervesced. He was feeling much better last night, according to the nursing notes, but on rounds this morning he is very agitated and combative and appears to be hallucinating. You suspect that he has

(A) sepsis.

(B) meningitis.

(C) a brain tumor.

(D) delirium tremens.

(E) a ruptured berry aneurysm.

107. A 43-year-old male alcoholic was admitted to you four days ago with pancreatitis and has been responding to treatment. He feels much better and wants to eat. However, on rounds you discover that he has some ascites. A paracentesis is performed to assess which one of the following possible diagnoses?

(A) Subacute bacterial peritonitis

(B) Congestive failure

(C) Fluid overload

(D) Hemorrhagic pancreatitis

(E) Ruptured appendix

108. A 57-year-old man with cirrhosis due to hepatitis B was admitted for increasing ascites. The nurses call you to tell you he has started vomiting blood. All of the following are likely causes EXCEPT

(A) esophageal varices.

(B) gastric varices.

(C) gastroesophageal reflux disease.

(D) Mallory-Weiss.

(E) gastric ulcer.

109. A 53-year-old male transferred to your service after undergoing a coronary artery bypass for angina. He has been doing well but develops a fever and complains of pain in his foot. You discover that the great toe is warm and red. Which one of the following is the most likely cause of this condition?

(A) Gout

(B) Osteomyelitis

(C) Osteoarthritis

(D) Rheumatoid arthritis

(E) Psoriatic arthritis

110. A 30-year-old man with leukemia is severely granulocytopenic after his first course of chemotherapy. He is receiving antibiotics as per protocol but develops a fever and no localizing symptoms or findings. He has no skin rash. You decide to

(A) add amphotericin.

(B) change all of his antibiotics.

(C) assume it is "granulocytopenic fever" and decide not to treat.

(D) give high-dose salicylates.

(E) give a nonsteroidal anti-inflammatory.

Questions 111-118 refer to the following:

You are asked to see a 45-year-old male hospitalized with a torn ligament around his elbow about to undergo exploration and repair. His orthopedic doctor asks you to perform a preoperative history and physical. The patient states that his health is good; he sees a doctor only when he has problems. On review of systems, he reports a constant cough that has recently been blood tinged. He also states that he loses his breath more than he used to. He has had no previous surgery. He has had no hospitalizations. He is on no medication and has no known drug allergies. He smokes two to three packs per day, and has for 30 years. He drinks socially. His family history is non-contributory.

111. Which one of the following areas of the physical exam will be LEAST revealing?

(A) Heart and lungs

(B) Peripheral pulses

(C) Extremities

(D) Fundoscopic

(E) Abdomen

112. Upon examination of the lungs, you hear some wheezing at the bases. The most appropriate next test to order is

(A) EKG.

(B) chest X-ray.

(C) CT of the chest with contrast.

(D) CT of the chest without contrast.

(E) incentive spirometry.

113. All of the following may be reasons for hemoptysis EXCEPT

(A) carcinoma.

(B) mitral stenosis.

(C) laryngitis.

(D) pulmonary infarct.

(E) chronic bronchitis.

114. The reason for the wheezing that is auscultated is due to

    (A) bronchial narrowing.

    (B) bronchial dilatation.

    (C) a series of tiny explosions produced when previously deflated airways are reinflated.

    (D) friction along the pleural surfaces.

    (E) alveoli filled with fluid

115. A chest X-ray shows a 3-cm nodule in the left lower base of the lung, and the sputum that was analyzed confirms malignant cells. You now highly suspect a lung carcinoma. All of the following are appropriate next steps EXCEPT

    (A) thoracic surgeon consultation.

    (B) CT of the chest.

    (C) metastatic survey of the body.

    (D) proceed with the orthopedic surgery.

    (E) pulmonary function tests.

116. Before the patient goes for his cancer treatment you question him more extensively, and the patient states that he occasionally gets flushed and has occasional diarrhea. You now suspect that

    (A) the patient is malingering.

    (B) he has a separate gastrointestinal problem occurring.

    (C) he has an oat-cell carcinoma.

    (D) he has a squamous cell carcinoma.

    (E) he has distant metastasis.

117. After successful surgery for both his carcinoma and elbow, the most important advice you can offer this man for a prolonged life expectancy is to

    (A) stretch before exercise to avoid tendon injury.

    (B) stop smoking.

    (C) visit a doctor more frequently.

    (D) eat health foods and take vitamins.

    (E) watch his cholesterol.

118. Which one of the following organ systems is least affected by cigarette smoking?

    (A) Skin

    (B) Oropharynx

    (C) Cardiac

    (D) Gastrointestinal

    (E) Bladder

119. Based on the India ink preparation shown in the figure below, you begin treatment for

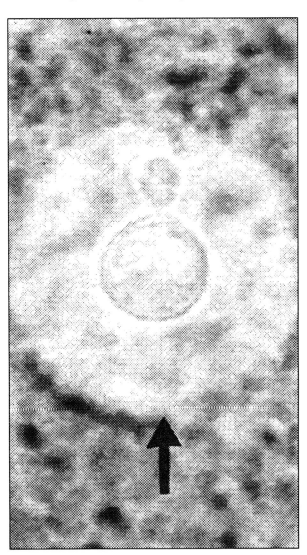

(A) *Toxoplasma gondii.*

(B) *Neisseria meningitides.*

(C) *Cryptococcus neoformans.*

(D) *Treponema pallidum.*

(E) *Streptococcus pneumoniae.*

120. A 23-year-old medical student presents to the emergency room hyperventilating while studying for her exams. She has perioral numbness and a headache. She is concerned that she may have muscular sclerosis. You obtain an arterial blood gas, after which you reassure her that she is having an anxiety reaction. Which one of the following is most likely to be this patient's blood gas?

   (A) pH = 7.58, pCO_2 = 20, pO_2 = 110, and HCO_3 = 18 O_2 Sat. = 99%

   (B) pH = 7.58, pCO_2 = 24, pO_2 = 62, and HCO_3 = 22 O_2 Sat. = 95%

   (C) pH = 7.39, pCO_2 = 25, pO_2 = 45, and HCO_3 = 15 O_2 Sat. = 72%

   (D) pH = 7.35, pCO_2 = 50, pO_2 = 55, and HCO_3 = 28 O_2 Sat. = 84%

121. Which one of the following statements regarding toxic shock syndrome (TSS) is FALSE?

   (A) Oliguria is a common symptom.

   (B) SGOT and SGPT levels are elevated.

   (C) Rash is macular, diffuse, and red.

   (D) IV antibiotics are the mainstay of therapy.

   (E) Reinfection is common with continuous use of tampons.

For Questions 122-125, match the diagrams with the conclusions in the next column.

Your new office manager has dropped onto the floor all the reports, including the diagrams, of the visual field tests that you recently performed. The patients will be arriving this afternoon for their test results, shown in the figures. Match the visual field diagram with your reported conclusions.

(A) Lesion of the optic chiasm

(B) Lesion of the temporal lobe

(C) Lesion of the parietal lobe

(D) Damage to the visual cortex

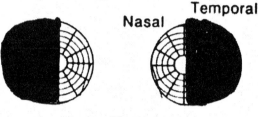

Figure 1

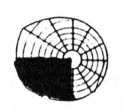 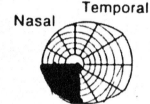

Figure 2

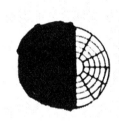 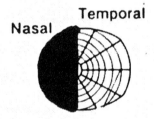

Figure 3

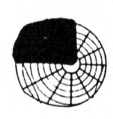 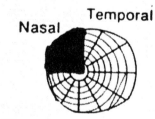

Figure 4

122. Figure 1

123. Figure 2

124. Figure 3

125. Figure 4

126. You are reviewing the intraoperative transesophageal echocardiogram (TEE) on a 40-year-old female shown below. Based on this study, which one of the clinical manifestations would NOT be predicted?

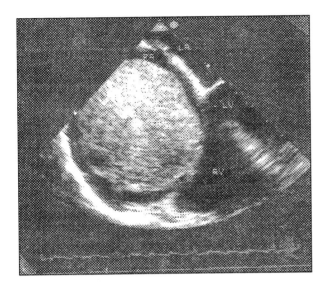

    (A) Hepatomegaly

    (B) Edema

    (C) Ascites

    (D) Systemic emboli

    (E) Cyanosis

127. Screening for anticardiolipin antibodies is appropriate in all of the following clinical settings EXCEPT

    (A) pregnancy-related thrombosis.

    (B) first pregnancy loss, if it occurs during the first trimester.

    (C) 45-year-old female with recurrent strokes.

    (D) 25-year-old female with systemic lupus erythematosus, complicated by an arterial thrombosis.

    (E) a 30-year-old female with thrombocytopenia.

128. A 45-year-old male who you have been seeing for over 20 years tells you he has been feeling nauseous and has had headaches, diarrhea, anorexia, and lassitude. This may represent

    (A) hydronephrosis.

    (B) hypocalcemia.

    (C) hypercalcemia.

    (D) hypotension.

    (E) hypertension.

129. The 71-year-old patient you admitted last evening for congestive heart failure has increasing shortness of breath and a worsening blood gas manifested with increasing CO_2. Your next step is

    (A) diuresis.

    (B) intubation and ventilatory support.

    (C) tracheotomy.

    (D) cardioversion.

    (E) pacemaker.

130. While on hospital rounds, you hear overhead that a code blue is called in one of your patient's rooms. You remember that he is a 68-year-old man with colon cancer who has expressed to you that he did not want to be resuscitated. Upon arrival, you realize that the code team has arrived and has begun resuscitation efforts. The most appropriate intervention would be to

    (A) call the family immediately and ask them if they would like to continue resuscitation efforts.

    (B) call the primary physician immediately and ask him if he would like to continue resuscitation efforts.

    (C) inform the code team of the patient's wishes and terminate efforts.

    (D) assist in resuscitation efforts but terminate efforts if no response is found in a few minutes.

    (E) None of the above.

131. Which one of the following is NOT true of electrical injuries?

    (A) It results from conversion of electrical energy into heat.

    (B) Severity of injury relates directly to voltage.

    (C) Local tissue destruction results if skin resistance is high.

    (D) Injury with direct current (DC) is more dangerous than injury with alternating current (AC).

    (E) Nervous tissue is highly susceptible to injury because of its low resistance.

132. A 47-year-old, markedly obese, black woman presents to your office for a periodic health examination. She has seen many doctors prior to this visit and is dissatisfied. She requests you to perform "all the tests known to man" since she believes "something is damn wrong" with her. You explain that there is very little evidence suggesting that the complete routine examination is effective. She insists on obtaining a complete physical. Which of the following statements regarding a routine complete physical examination is true?

    (A) This is a situation in which it may be reasonable to perform a complete checkup.

    (B) You should take as much time as needed to educate the patient until she understands the futility of her request.

    (C) The patient's request should always be a number-one priority in making your decision regarding their health even if it is not in the patient's best interest.

    (D) Any of the above.

    (E) All of the above.

133. A 31-year-old man presents to your emergency room after being bitten in the hand by another person. You note a superficial wound without penetration into the bone or joint. You clean it and place sutures. He has no other medical illnesses and is not taking any medications. He remembers that he has received three doses of tetanus immunization, but does not remember when he received his last one. Which one of the following is true regarding human bites?

    (A) Animal bites are worse than human bites.

    (B) The organisms involved in human bites are typically polymicrobial.

    (C) Close observation should be done to watch out for leptospirosis.

    (D) Antibiotic therapy is not warranted.

    (E) None of the above are true.

134. A 29-year-old female presents to your office for a periodic health examination. She is planning on making a business trip in two weeks to Central Africa. Physical examination is normal. At this time, you should

    (A) reassure her and wish her a good trip.

    (B) reassure her but advise her to show up for another check-up as soon as she returns.

    (C) advise her to reconsider her decision on making a trip to an area where malaria is well known to be endemic.

    (D) administer prophylactic mefloquine, the drug of choice for a travel to areas with chloroquine-resistant malaria.

    (E) urge her to show up next week for prophylaxis with mefloquine.

135. A 36-year-old gravida 2 para 1 at 16 weeks gestational age comes to the office for a routine visit. You order a maternal serum alpha fetoprotein (MSAFP) as part of her routine blood work. Elevations in MSAFP are associated with which fetal abnormality?

    (A) Clubfeet

    (B) Down's syndrome

(C)   Thalassemia major

(D)   Open neural defect

(E)   Tetralogy of Fallot

136. A 43-year-old man with a history of hypertension presents to you with the "worst headache of his life." He was in his usual state of health until earlier in the day. While having a bowel movement, he noted the acute onset of the headache. He's also noted nausea without emesis and some mild photophobia. He denies any fevers, chills, neck stiffness, or history of similar headaches. On physical examination, his vital signs are stable and he is afebrile. The remainder of his examination shows no abnormalities. A computed tomography scan (CT) of the head is ordered and reveals no evidence of intracranial bleed. Of the following, the most appropriate next intervention would be

(A)   lumbar puncture.

(B)   cerebralangiogram.

(C)   admission for observation with a repeat head CT in 24 hours.

(D)   discharge to home.

(E)   None of the above.

137. A 30-year-old woman presents with three days of right lower quadrant abdominal pain and diarrhea. She denies any nausea or vomiting. On physical examination, she has tenderness to palpation over her right lower quadrant without rebound tenderness. Rectal examination reveals guaiac-positive brown loose stool. Of the following, the most likely microorganism for this gastroenteritis is

(A)   rotavirus.

(B)   norwalk virus.

(C)   *Escherichia coli.*

(D)   *Yersinia enterolitica.*

(E)   *Vibrio cholerae.*

138. A 56-year-old foundry worker presents with difficulty breathing and dyspnea on exertion. There is no chest pain, fever, clubbing, or weight loss. Chest X-ray reveals multiple small nodules in the upper lobes and enlarged hilar lymph nodes that contain calcium on the outer rims (eggshell calcifications). Pulmonary function tests show an obstructive pattern with a decrease in lung volumes. What is the most likely diagnosis?

(A)   Tuberculosis

(B)   Histoplasmosis

(C)   *Mycobacterium avium intracellulare*

(D)   Silicosis

(E)   Byssinosis

139. Complications from a peptic ulcer can include all of the following EXCEPT

(A)   pyloric obstruction.

(B)   hemorrhage.

(C)   adenocarcinoma.

(D)   perforation.

140. A 54-year-old man with diabetes and hypertension underwent a cardiac catheterization with a percutaneous transluminal coronary angioplasty two days previously. His postprocedure course has been uneventful, and he has had no further chest pain. His medications are aspirin, nitroglycerin, and a betablocker. This morning, when planning to discharge him, his serum creatinine is noted to be elevated to 2.5 from his baseline of 1.6. The most appropriate intervention would be to

(A)   discharge him with follow-up in his physician's office in one week for repeat testing.

(B)   observe him for another 24 hours to ensure that his creatinine returns to normal.

(C)   give him a fluid bolus.

(D)   discontinue his aspirin.

(E)   order a renal ultrasound with Doppler.

141. A 47-year-old asthmatic patient with a history of hypertension and arthritis comes to your clinic complaining of wheezing despite

the use of her beta-agonist inhaler. Her medications include hydrochlorothiazide, indomethacin, diltiazem, methotrexate, and vitamin E. Which one of this patient's medications is most likely to be exacerbating her asthma?

(A) Hydrochlorothiazide

(B) Indomethacin

(C) Diltiazem

(D) Methotrexate

(E) Vitamin E

142. A 47-year-old black male with newly diagnosed small cell carcinoma of the lung is admitted to the hospital for chemotherapy. He will be receiving daunorubicin. What would be the initial test for the oncologist to order prior to initiating chemotherapy with daunorubicin?

(A) Pulmonary function tests

(B) Baseline renal function tests

(C) Bone marrow aspiration

(D) Echocardiogram

(E) Nerve conduction studies

143. You are preparing a lecture on *Herpes simplex* virus (HSV) infections for the staff of a drop-in clinic for sexually active adolescents. You plan to highlight your discussion with the slides shown in the figures. Panel A shows characteristic histologic changes of a vulvar HSV infection, including necrosis of the epidermis and dermis, acute inflammation, and nuclear debris and multinucleated giant cells. Panel B shows multinucleated cells with Cowdry type A intranuclear viral inclusions. In your presentation, you plan to discuss all of the following regarding *Herpes simplex* virus infection EXCEPT

(A) Histologic/cytologic methods do not differentiate between *Herpes simplex* and other viral infections, such as varicella zoster virus.

Panel A

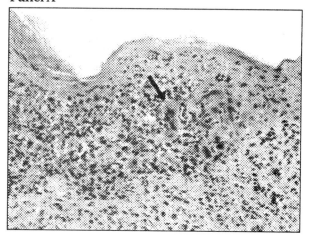

Panel B

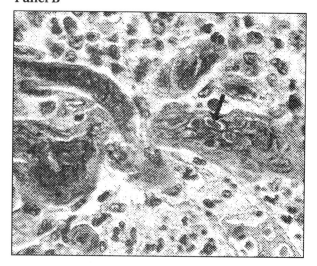

(B) Immunofluorescence and ELISA are as sensitive as viral isolation for detecting HSV in cervical secretions of asymptomatic carriers.

(C) The sensitivity of viral isolation techniques is higher in vesicular than in ulcerative lesions.

(D) The best method to confirm the diagnosis is isolation of the virus in tissue culture.

(E) Acute and convalescent serum can be useful for documenting seroconversion during primary HSV-2 infection.

144. You are scheduled to perform a laparoscopic tubal ligation on a divorced 36-year-old woman with two children. The day before her procedure, her ex-husband calls you and demands that you do not perform the operation on "his wife." You must

    (A) do as he asks.

    (B) proceed as your patient has instructed.

    (C) call the police.

    (D) call a lawyer.

    (E) tell the ex-husband what you think of him.

145. A 28-year-old Asian female hospitalized for a work-up of heart palpitations is found on examination to have a tender thyroid gland on palpation. She has a sore throat, elevated ESR, low-grade temperature, and a decreased 24-hour radioactive iodine uptake. There is no evidence for exophthalmos or pretibial myxedema. What would be the immediate initial recommended treatment?

    (A) Prednisone

    (B) Propylthiouracil (PTU)

    (C) Radioactive iodine therapy to the thyroid gland

    (D) Antibiotics

    (E) Fine needle aspiration of the thyroid nodule

For Questions 146-149, select the appropriate diagnosis for each patient.

    (A) Kaposi's sarcoma

    (B) Poison ivy

    (C) Urticaria

    (D) Psoriasis

    (E) Discoid lupus

146. A 30-year-old woman with alopecia and a scarring rash on her face

147. A 42-year-old male with a nontender, purplish, elevated lesion on his forearm

148. A nine-year-old boy who has been hunting insects in the woods

149. A 67-year-old male with scaling erythematous lesions on his scalp and arms

For Questions 150-153, select the most appropriate decision regarding triage.

    (A) Ask the patient to call to schedule an elective appointment within two to three weeks.

    (B) Ask the patient to call to schedule an urgent appointment in two to three days.

    (C) Ask the patient to come to the office the same day.

    (D) Ask the patient to come to the emergency room.

    (E) Ask the patient to be directly admitted to the hospital.

150. A 60-year-old man calls your office with 30 minutes of crushing substernal chest pain.

151. A 30-year-old woman calls your office with two hours of severe lower abdominal pain. Her last menstrual period was eight weeks previously.

152. A 25-year-old man calls your office after having noted a rash on his trunk. He has been taking amoxicillin for three days for sinusitis. He denies any shortness of breath.

153. A 33-year-old woman calls your office after having noted some nausea without vomiting over the previous two days. She has been taking erythromycin for five days for a community-acquired pneumonia, which has been improving.

154. A 34-year-old black male presents to the emergency room with complaints of shortness of breath, fever, weight loss, and pleuritic chest pain. The CD4 count was 50 cells. Chest X-ray reveals bilateral interstitial infiltrates, and the LDH was elevated to 450 mg/dl. What would be the next step in treating this patient?

    (A) IV penicillin

(B) IV trimethoprim-sulfamethox-azole

(C) Transbronchial biopsy

(D) IV Ganciclovir

(E) Corticosteroids only

155. A 72-year-old woman with a history of hypercholesterolemia, hypertension, and diabetes mellitus presents to your emergency room with an acutely painful right foot. She was well until one hour previously, when she noted the acute onset of her right foot pain. She is taking insulin and enalapril for her medical problems. Her vital signs are stable and she is afebrile. On physical examination, her right foot is noted to be mottled and cool to touch compared to the left side. Her dorsalis pedis pulse and posterior tibial pulse are noted to be diminished on the right compared to the left side. The most appropriate immediate intervention is

    (A) initiation of intravenous heparin.

    (B) initiation of thrombolytic therapy.

    (C) initiation of aspirin therapy.

    (D) immediate angiogram.

    (E) immediate magnetic resonance imaging of her right foot.

156. A 35-year-old man presents for elective resection of a 5-cm infrarenal abdominal aortic aneurysm. His past medical history is significant for systemic hypertension, inferior myocardial infarction, and stable angina. The patient also reports heavy smoking for over 15 years. What is the significance of abdominal aortic aneurysm in this preoperative patient?

    (A) The risk of rupture approximates 20%.

    (B) The probability of the rupture without surgery is almost 50%.

    (C) Abdominal pain, back pain, and leg ischemia can be symptoms of an aneurysm of this size.

    (D) The mortality rate associated with elective surgery is about five percent.

    (E) The mortality rate of repairing a ruptured aneurysm is 10%.

Questions 157-160 refer to the following:

You are performing a full neurologic workup on a patient complaining of lower extremity weakness and you want to test nerves. Match the following nerve root to the cutaneous sensation in the anterior aspect of the body.

    (A) C4

    (B) C8

    (C) T8

    (D) L2

    (E) S1

157. Sural nerve

158. Ulnar nerve

159. Supraclavicular nerve

160. Lateral femoral cutaneous nerve

161. A 12-year-old boy is accidentally hit in the head by a baseball bat during a game at school. His parents are out of town and he needs to have stitches in his scalp. You can do all of the following EXCEPT

    (A) you must find his parents before you do anything.

    (B) you can accept the consent the parents signed transferring medical decision making to the school.

    (C) you can accept a letter the family's housekeeper has giving her authority to agree to medical treatment in the parents' absence.

    (D) you can accept the approval of the patient's aunt.

(E) you can proceed with a medically necessary emergency procedure even if you cannot obtain consent.

162. Which one of the following is NOT typically associated with child abuse?

(A) Scalded buttock burns

(B) Cigarette burns

(C) Epidural hematoma

(D) Subdural hematoma

(E) Femur fracture

163. A 16-year-old girl presents to the labor and delivery room at 37 weeks of pregnancy. She complains of severe headaches. Her blood pressure is 150/100 mm Hg. PE shows an edematous patient. Regarding this patient's condition, which one of the following statements is NOT true?

(A) It occurs in approximately one percent of pregnancies.

(B) A young primigravida with poor prenatal care is at highest risk for preeclampsia.

(C) It is associated with rapid uterine enlargement, such as occurs with hydatiform mole, diabetes, and multiple gestations.

(D) It predicts a 33% probability of recurrence with subsequent pregnancies.

(E) Magnesium sulfate is the first-line drug in the United States for the prevention of preeclampsia from degenerating into eclampsia.

164. Appropriate screening tests in a sexually active 29-year-old woman would be

(A) a baseline mammogram and repeat mammograms yearly thereafter.

(B) a flexible sigmoidoscopy now and repeat studies every five years thereafter.

(C) a pelvic examination and a Pap smear now and every three years thereafter.

(D) administration of pneumococcal immunization.

(E) a complete blood count.

Questions 165-168 refer to the following:

A 45-year-old alcoholic male presents to the clinic with a 22-lb. weight loss over two months, and bulky, greasy, and malodorous stools associated with diarrhea and malnutrition. The physician ordered a 72-hour stool collection while the patient was on a high-fat diet. The result showed numerous fat globules and fat content greater than 15 gm/day.

165. All of the following disorders are associated with the malabsorption syndrome EXCEPT

(A) chronic pancreatic insufficiency.

(B) Crohn's disease.

(C) Mallory-Weiss tear.

(D) bacterial overgrowth syndrome.

(E) nontropical sprue.

166. All of the following tests are useful to make the diagnosis of malabsorption EXCEPT

(A) small intestinal biopsy.

(B) serum carotene.

(C) bentiromide test.

(D) urinary D-xylose test.

(E) barium enema.

167. All of the following medications have been implicated in causing malabsorption EXCEPT

(A) colchicine.

(B) neomycin.

(C) irritant laxative.

(D) prednisone.

(E) cholestyramine.

168. Which one of the following tests is most useful in making the diagnosis of malabsorption secondary to bacterial overgrowth syndrome?

    (A) Serum folate

    (B) Qualitative stool fat

    (C) Serum cobalamin

    (D) Urine 5-hydroxyindolacetic acid

    (E) C14-xylose breath test

169. A 45-year-old man comes to the clinic for a routine employment check-up. He was found to have a reactive (10 mm) PPD skin test. He is otherwise asymptomatic. His chest X-ray is normal. His physical exam was normal. What would be the next step in management of this patient?

    (A) Isoniazid and B12 prophylaxis

    (B) Sputum for acid-fast bacilli smears and cultures

    (C) CT scan of the chest

    (D) Repeat the chest X-ray in one year if symptoms occur

    (E) Repeat the PPD skin test in six months

For Questions 170-173, match the test required to make the correct diagnosis with each numbered case question.

    (A) Doppler ultrasound

    (B) Plain X-rays

    (C) MRI

    (D) Bone scan

    (E) Nerve conduction studies

170. A 31-year-old math teacher presents to the clinic with symptoms of numbness of the right upper extremity, diplopia, lower extremity spasticity, and urinary incontinence. These symptoms have been waxing and waning in severity and have progressed gradually over the course of several months.

171. A 56-year-old salesman is hospitalized for an elective laser surgery to his right eye for proliferative diabetic retinopathy. On routine questioning by the anesthesiologist, this patient complains of bilateral lower extremity tingling and pain. His fasting blood glucose level is 268 mg/dl.

172. The 46-year-old Vice-President of the United States was flown to Walter Reed Army Medical Center to evaluate his sudden pain and numbness on the left lower extremity. He has been on an airplane for an extensive period of time because of a lecture series across the country. He has no past medical history. Upon examination, the physicians found diminished pulses in the left dorsalis pedis artery. There was no calf pain, erythema, sensory loss, or motor weakness.

173. A 41-year-old architect is hospitalized because of evaluation of his severe anemia hematocrit of 23%. He has had no past medical history. This patient states he feels weak, tired, and excessively thirsty. His serum calcium level is 16 mEQ/L. On examination, he has skin pallor and reproducible tenderness on palpation of his anterior thorax.

174. An asymptomatic 60-year-old male returns for a routine check-up following pacemaker placement. Physical examination is unremarkable. Based on the oblique view chest X-ray (including image enlargement), shown on the following page, you recommend

Panel A

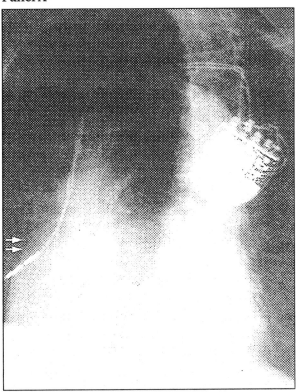

Panel B

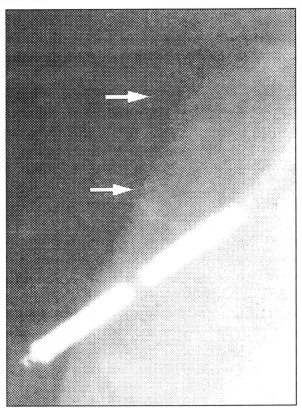

(A) consultation with a cardiotho-
racic surgeon.

(B) return visit in six months.

(C) penicillin, 500 mg po Q6H for 10
days.

(D) Sestamibi stress test.

(E) immediate replacement of the
pulse generator.

175. A 17-year-old woman presents to your office
wanting to be tested for HIV. She denies any
sexual contacts, and has never used intravenous drugs. She wants to be tested because
she says that "it's everywhere, and I just want
to make sure that I don't have it." You tell her
that

(A) you need to first discuss HIV
testing with her parents.

(B) you will test her for HIV but will
need to inform her parents if she
is positive.

(C) she does not need to be tested
because her pretest probability
for having the disease is so low.

(D) you will test her for HIV.

(E) None of the above.

176. An 82-year-old female was brought to the
emergency room after she collapsed during
a rehabilitation session. Past history was significant for hemiparesis resulting from a cerebral infarction. A past anterior wall myocardial infarction has recently been complicated by congestive heart failure. Several

days previously, a diagnostic vascular ultra-sonographic study could not confirm a suspected deep venous thrombosis of the right leg. The transesophageal study is shown in the figures below. You immediately begin treatment for

Panel A

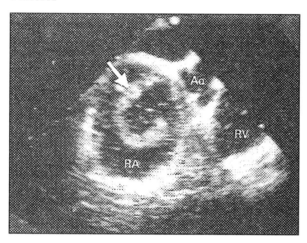

Panel B

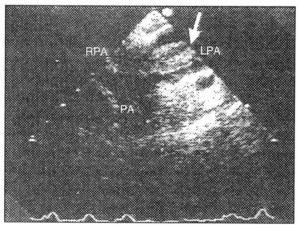

(A) ruptured aorta.

(B) ruptured ventricular free wall.

(C) massive pulmonary embolus.

(D) ruptured ventricular septum.

(E) Dressler's syndrome.

For Questions 177-180, match the correct disease with the first choice of the following antibiotics:

(A) Ampicillin

(B) First-generation cephalosporin

(C) Amphotericin B

(D) Acyclovir

(E) Erythromycin

177. A 30-year-old woman with sinusitis

178. A 48-year-old woman diagnosed yesterday with shingles

179. A 43-year-old HIV-positive patient with recurrent and refractory fungal infections

180. A 12-year-old student with an abscess of his leg recently drained in the emergency room

USMLE STEP 3
PRACTICE TEST 2

Day Two – Afternoon Session

(Answer sheets appear in the back of this book.)

TIME: 3 Hours
180 Questions

> **DIRECTIONS**: Each of the following numbered items or incomplete sentences is followed by an answer or a completion of the statement. Choose the **ONE** choice that **BEST** answers the question or completes the sentence.

1. Which one of the following pairs are measures of dispersion in Gaussian (normal) distribution?

   (A) Variance/mode

   (B) Range/mean

   (C) Standard deviation/median

   (D) Range/variance

   (E) Standard deviation/mode

2. A 68-year-old man comes to your office complaining of a hand tremor. The tremor becomes worse with voluntary movement. He notes that it improves with alcohol consumption. On physical exam, the tremor is coarse in nature. What is the most likely cause of this patient's tremor?

   (A) Parkinson's disease

   (B) Alcoholic neuropathy

   (C) Benign familial tremor

   (D) Intention tremor

   (E) Huntington's chorea

3. A 63-year-old previously healthy businessman is brought to your clinic by his wife because he got lost while driving home, a route he has been taking for over 20 years. Which one of the following diagnoses is most likely?

   (A) A stroke

   (B) Alcoholic blackout

   (C) Migraine

   (D) Early Alzheimer's

   (E) Pancreatic cancer

4. You are asked to evaluate a patient with a possible obturator hernia. All of the following are associated with the hernia EXCEPT

   (A) obstruction with medial thigh pain.

   (B) obstruction with lateral thigh pain.

   (C) herniation of small bowel.

   (D) augmented pain by thigh extension.

   (E) rectal palpation revealing a soft, tender mass.

Questions 5-12 refer to the following:

A 31-year-old man comes to see you in clinic. You have seen him a few times in the past for upper respiratory infections. He now comes in off-schedule with a hacking cough, fever, and a new lesion on his left leg. The lesion is non-tender, elevated, and is multi-lobulated. He has lost 20 pounds since he last came to see you four months ago.

5. An examination of his oral mucosa is likely to show

    (A) an edentulous palate.

    (B) thrush.

    (C) tonsillitis.

    (D) cleft palate.

    (E) enlarged uvula.

6. In association with the mouth lesions, which one of the following is the patient likely to have noted?

    (A) Conjunctivitis

    (B) Streptococcal pharyngitis

    (C) Herpangina

    (D) Dysphagia

    (E) Otitis

7. You review your chart on the patient. You are surprised to discover that you have failed to ask him about

    (A) childhood immunizations.

    (B) family history.

    (C) exposure to tuberculosis.

    (D) sexual history.

    (E) occupation.

8. The patient's chest radiograph is likely to show

    (A) a solitary nodule.

    (B) a cavity.

    (C) cardiomegaly.

    (D) enlarged pulmonary artery.

    (E) no abnormality.

9. You are fairly sure of the patient's underlying diagnosis. You ask him for

    (A) the name of his next of kin.

    (B) his permission to obtain an HIV test.

    (C) the names of all of his sexual partners.

    (D) the date of his last PPD.

    (E) the date of his last tetanus shot.

10. All of the following tests should be ordered at this point EXCEPT

    (A) complete blood count.

    (B) herpes serologies.

    (C) T-cell counts.

    (D) chemistry battery.

    (E) hemoccult.

11. Your disposition of this patient is

    (A) admission to the hospital.

    (B) discharge to home on trimethoprim-sulfamethoxazole.

    (C) outpatient bronchoscopy.

    (D) referral to the AIDS clinic.

    (E) referral to a dermatologist.

12. Before he leaves your office, you call the hospital to schedule

    (A) an abdominal CT scan.

    (B) a pulmonary arteriography.

    (C) a bronchoscopy.

    (D) a dermatology consult.

    (E) an MRI of the brain.

13. A 28-year-old patient with AIDS begins to demonstrate fever, weight loss, night sweats, and fatigue. He begins coughing and manifests hemoptysis. The attending physician suspects an infection. Laboratory diagnosis of sputum cultures demonstrates that pathogen produces niacin and cannot be grown on a blood agar plate. Which of the following is the most likely infectious agent responsible for these clinical findings?

    (A) Candida albicans

    (B) Cryptosporidium

    (C) Toxoplasma

    (D) Mycobacterium

    (E) Cytomegalovirus

14. A 65-year-old hypertensive male arrives at the "urgent care center" in his neighborhood with complaints of excruciating anterior chest pain, which radiates to the back, neck, and jaw. Physical examination reveals a diaphoretic male in acute distress with a blood pressure of 180/120, pulse of 110, respiration of 20, temperature of 98.4°F. Lungs are clear; there is a Cor grade II/VI high-pitched blowing decrescendo diastolic murmur best heard in the third left intercostal space; and the abdomen is benign. A two-dimensional transesophageal echocardiogram was performed. The horizontal imaging slices, shown in the figures below, were taken 3 centimeters above the aortic valve. The two images were taken at slightly different gray-scale gain settings. You diagnose

    (A) dissecting aortic aneurysm.

    (B) aortitis.

    (C) angiosarcoma of the aorta.

    (D) supravalvular aortic stenosis.

    (E) acute anterior wall myocardial infarction.

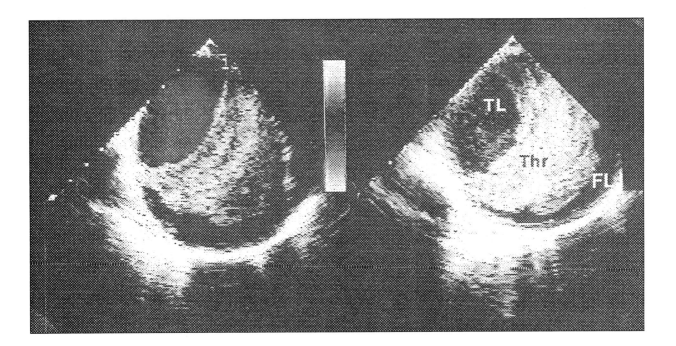

15. A 43-year-old female with chronic granulocytic leukemia was admitted to the hospital and given a course of chemotherapy. After treatment, neutropenia and fever developed. Soon after, grouped hemorrhagic pustules appeared on the patient's buttocks, which evolved into round ulcers with necrotic black eschars. Blood cultures grew *Pseudomonas aeruginosa*. What would be the next step in management of this patient?

    (A) Debridement of the ulcer

    (B) Chest X-ray

    (C) Gentamicin and pipracillin

    (D) Gentamicin and ampicillin

    (E) Radiation therapy

16. A 47-year-old schoolteacher whom you have followed for annual exams is brought in by her husband who says she has been getting progressively more confused and forgetful. She has never been like this before. He tells you her mother had Alzheimer's and her sister is schizophrenic. He does not know what to do and wants your help. You examine her, and she does not know you, cannot remember her husband's or children's names, and has a low-grade fever. You should

    (A) commit her to a psychiatric service.

    (B) admit her to a psychiatric service.

    (C) admit her for a medical workup.

    (D) refer her to a psychiatrist.

    (E) arrange for them to see a social worker who can tell them about Alzheimer's support groups.

17. The X-ray, shown in the figure in the next column, is illustrated in a medical journal with the heading: "What is your diagnosis?"

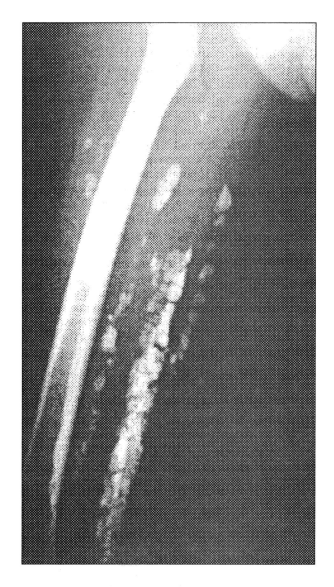

    (A) Atherosclerosis

    (B) Soft tissue calcifications

    (C) Extravasation of contrast material

    (D) Reaction to subcutaneously injected medications

    (E) Gout

Questions 18-20 refer to the following:

A 24-year-old graduate student was unable to attend classes because of severe nasal pruritus, rhinorrhea, nasal congestion, sneezing, and excessive tearing of the eyes. It is springtime and there is a high pollen count.

18. This patient visits the physician at the college health center for advice on how to alleviate his allergic symptoms. All of the following are the recommendations of the doctor EXCEPT

    (A) antihistamines.

    (B) topical nasal steroids.

    (C) immunotherapy.

    (D) nonsteroidal anti-inflammatory agents.

    (E) stay indoors with air-conditioning.

19. Upon further questioning of this patient, the doctor finds out that he has a strong family history of allergies. All of the following are associated with allergic rhinitis EXCEPT

    (A) allergic asthma.

    (B) sinusitis.

    (C) urticaria.

    (D) IgE-mediated systemic anaphylaxis.

    (E) contact dermatitis.

20. Several weeks later, this patient presents with bronchitis and is given erythromycin by another physician. He is still taking terfenidine—a nonsedating antihistamine—for his hay fever symptoms. Two days later he is hospitalized because of palpitations resulting in syncope. What would be the appropriate management of choice at this time?

    (A) Discontinue terfenidine (Seldane) and monitor the patient on telemetry

    (B) Start lidocaine

    (C) Cardiac catheterization

    (D) Echocardiogram

    (E) Perform a tilt-table test

21. A 65-year-old woman is brought in with acute bilobular pneumonia. She has fever, shaking chills, and acute confusion. She belongs to an HMO and your hospital is not one of the ones approved by it. The nearest HMO-approved hospital is 45 minutes away by ambulance. You

    (A) admit her emergently and call her HMO to tell them you will transfer her as soon as possible.

    (B) send her to the HMO hospital.

    (C) admit her and do not call the HMO at all.

    (D) call the hospital lawyer to complain.

    (E) tell her family you can do nothing.

22. A 35-year-old woman presents to your office after referral from a surgeon with a noted elevated TSH. Other laboratory testing confirms the diagnosis of primary hypothyroidism. Symptoms consistent with this would be all of the following EXCEPT

    (A) slow tendon reflex relaxation.

    (B) constipation.

    (C) cold intolerance.

    (D) urinary incontinence.

    (E) dry skin.

23. Which one of the following statements regarding the prevention of thromboembolism is INCORRECT?

    (A) Angina pectoris, advanced age, and mitral annular narrowing are risk factors for stroke.

    (B) Left atrial enlargement with no clinical symptoms is a risk factor for thromboembolic disease.

    (C) Warfarin decreases the incidence of stroke in patients with atrial fibrillation of non-rheumatic origin.

    (D) Patients with no cardiopulmonary disease have a very low risk of developing a thromboembolism.

    (E) Patients with lone atrial fibrillation are at increased risk for stroke.

24. Conchal hypertrophy is usually

    (A) located on the same side as septal deviation.

    (B) located on the opposite side of septal deviation.

    (C) unrelated to the deviation.

    (D) never seen with septal deviation.

    (E) located on both sides of the septum.

25. A 21-year-old female college student is brought in to you by her parents who complain that she has lost a significant amount of weight. You suspect that she has anorexia nervosa. True statements about this disorder include all EXCEPT

    (A) anorexic patients often exhibit obsessive-compulsive behaviors.

    (B) amenorrhea is an uncommon finding in females with anorexia nervosa.

    (C) patients with anorexia nervosa have a disturbed perception of their own weight and shape.

    (D) bulimic episodes may occur when a patient is not able to exert complete control over food.

    (E) anorexics frequently deny the severity of their illness, which makes therapy difficult.

26. A 58-year-old male smoker presents to the clinic suddenly with complaints of blood-tinged productive sputum on coughing and weight loss. He was found to have a temperature of 100.0°F and significant weight loss. There is no family history of cancer. What would be the next step in establishing the diagnosis?

    (A) PPD skin test

    (B) Culture of the sputum for acid-fast bacteria

    (C) Chest X-ray

    (D) Bronchoscopy

    (E) Starting therapy for bronchitis and waiting to see if the patient's symptoms are alleviated

27. HIV serology testing is routinely performed in all of the following groups at risk EXCEPT

    (A) patients presenting with STDs.

    (B) homosexual and bisexual men.

    (C) bisexual women.

    (D) individuals having multiple sexual partners.

    (E) individuals who frequently receive blood transfusions.

28. Your patient is a 17-year-old high school dropout. His parents tell you that recently he has been involved in a gang and suggest checking their son for alcohol intoxication. The young man is otherwise healthy, cooperative, and answers all of your questions. Regarding measurement of biochemical markers for alcohol in this patient, which one of the following statements is in accord with the U.S. Preventive Services Task Force recommendations?

    (A) Given the risk for alcoholism and drug abuse, urinary testing for drugs is appropriate.

    (B) Given the parents' concern about their son's gang involvement, testing for biochemical markers is appropriate.

    (C) This young man has two serious risk factors: being a high school dropout and being involved in a gang.

    (D) All of the above statements are correct.

    (E) None of the above statements are correct.

29. A 38-year-old man presents to your office with a sore throat. He says that for the last two days, he has had a sore throat and chills and a fever to 101.3°F. His sore throat has made it painful for him to swallow, but he doesn't have any difficulty swallowing. He denies cough or sputum. Physical examination reveals that he has a temperature of 101.8°F and his oropharynx has erythematous tonsils with whitish-grey exudates. He has tender cervical lymphadenopathy and his neck is supple. His lungs are clear to aus-

cultation. The most appropriate intervention would be to

- (A) begin treatment for bacterial pharyngitis immediately.
- (B) assure the patient that it is probably a viral illness and that he should go home and drink plenty of fluids.
- (C) send off pharyngeal swab for culture.
- (D) order a monospot test to rule out mononucleosis.
- (E) admit him to the hospital for 24-hour observation.

Questions 30-33 refer to the following:

Your 25-year-old patient has been losing platelets and is in need of a transfusion prior to going to surgery for an exploratory laparotomy.

30. To what level should he be transfused prior to surgery?
- (A) 20,000
- (B) 50,000
- (C) 100,000
- (D) 200,000
- (E) 500,000

31. Every unit of platelet transfusion should raise the platelet level by approximately how much?
- (A) 2,000
- (B) 5,000
- (C) 7,500
- (D) 10,000
- (E) 15,000

32. Twelve hours after surgery, your patient develops a temperature of 103.3°F and erythema and tenderness along the wound. You

suspect a wound infection. The most likely cause is

- (A) *Neisseria.*
- (B) *Legionella.*
- (C) *Enterobacter.*
- (D) *Streptococcus.*
- (E) *Mycoplasma.*

33. The most appropriate antibiotic to treat this is
- (A) isoniazid.
- (B) tobramycin.
- (C) penicillin.
- (D) amikacin.
- (E) acyclovir.

34. Your patient is a 32-year-old gravida 4 para 3 at 18 weeks gestational age who is found to have a UTI. However, sensitivities are not yet back to the offending organism, *E. coli.* Which one of the following is a safe empiric treatment for this UTI?
- (A) Ciprofloxin
- (B) Tetracycline
- (C) Bactrim
- (D) Ampicillin
- (E) Gentamicin

35. A 21-year-old sexually active female is seen for vaginal bleeding during intercourse. If colposcopy and Pap smear were unrevealing, the proper mode of action at this time would be to reassure the patient of the importance of a Pap smear and inform her that
- (A) all sexually active women should undergo annual screening for three consecutive years.
- (B) hysterectomy would protect against cervical cancer.

(C) if two consecutive smears have been normal, the next appointment for a Pap smear should be scheduled after three years.

(D) the patient is at risk of developing cervical cancer.

(E) use of condoms may protect against pregnancy, but not against cervical cancer.

For Questions 36-39, match the appropriate antidote for overdosage of each toxin.

(A) Ethanol

(B) Acetylcysteine

(C) Fab fragments

(D) Naloxone

(E) Deferoxamine mesylate

36. A 30-year-old alcoholic man presents after ingestion of methanol.

37. A 25-year-old woman presents after ingesting 40-500 milligram tablets of acetaminophen.

38. A 76-year-old man presents after accidentally taking too many of his pills of digoxin. His EKG is notable for third-degree AV block.

39. A 30-year-old man presents after a suicide attempt with ingestion of one full bottle of iron supplements.

40. Your patient is four days post-op exploratory laparotomy for lysis of adhesions and has an ileus. The next appropriate step is

(A) advancement of diet.

(B) keep NPO.

(C) passage of a nasogastric tube.

(D) take back to the operating room for a "second look" laparotomy.

(E) give an enema.

Questions 41-48 refer to the following:

A 33-year-old male is seen for a six-month history of dry, nonproductive cough. He also states that he has had intermittent fevers and has felt tired for the past two months. On physical examination you detect enlarged cervical, axillary, and inguinal lymph nodes. Respiratory tract examination reveals bilateral rales on auscultation of the lungs and bilateral infiltrates on chest X-ray. Your clinical suspicion is confirmed by a positive HIV test.

41. What is the drug of first choice for the prevention of this patient's respiratory tract condition?

(A) IV ampicillin

(B) IV tetracycline

(C) Aerosolized pentamidine

(D) Trimethoprim-sulfamethoxazole

(E) Pyrimethamine plus sulfamethoxazole

42. What is the drug of second choice for the prevention of this patient's respiratory tract condition?

(A) IV ampicillin

(B) IV tetracycline

(C) Aerosolized pentamidine

(D) IV trimethoprim-sulfamethoxazole

(E) Pyrimethamine plus sulfamethoxazole

43. Screening high-risk groups for HIV infection is performed by

(A) Western blot test.

(B) Eastern blot test.

(C) ELISA test.

(D) CD-4+ count.

(E) CD-8+ count.

44. The next step in testing for HIV in this patient requires

    (A) Western blot test.

    (B) Eastern blot test.

    (C) ELISA test.

    (D) CD-4+ count.

    (E) CD-8+ count.

45. Prophylaxis against *Pneumocystis carinii* pneumonia is initiated when the CD4+ lymphocyte count decreases to a level of

    (A) 100 cells/mm^3.

    (B) 200 cells/mm^3.

    (C) 300 cells/mm^3.

    (D) 500 cells/mm^3.

    (E) 1,000-1,500 cells/mm^3.

46. Prophylaxis against toxoplasmosis should be initiated when the CD4+ lymphocyte count is reduced to

    (A) 100 cells/mm^3.

    (B) 200 cells/mm^3.

    (C) 300 cells/mm^3.

    (D) 500 cells/mm^3.

    (E) 1,000-1,500 cells/mm^3.

47. To prevent a further deterioration of this patient's condition and development of mycobacterium avium intracellular infection, you should initiate prophylaxis when the CD4+ count reaches

    (A) 100 cells/mm^3.

    (B) 200 cells/mm^3.

    (C) 300 cells/mm^3.

    (D) 500 cells/mm^3.

    (E) 1,000-1,500 cells/mm^3.

48. If HIV serology tested negative, the CD4+ count in this patient would have been

    (A) 100 cells/mm^3.

    (B) 200 cells/mm^3.

    (C) 300 cells/mm^3.

    (D) 500 cells/mm^3.

    (E) 1,000-1,500 cells/mm^3.

For Questions 49-52, match the correct answer for each question.

    (A) Ask patient's permission to do HIV test

    (B) Report to Board of Health

    (C) Culture appropriately

    (D) Reassure

49. Patient with syphilis

50. Patient with CMV retinitis

51. Patient with suspected tuberculosis

52. Patient with pelvic inflammatory disease

Questions 53-60 refer to the following:

A 35-year-old woman comes into the emergency room with a fractured radius and ulna and multiple ecchymoses. She says she fell down a flight of stairs. The nurses tell you they have seen her in the ER many times before and that they think her husband beats her up. In fact, one of the nurses knows her husband and tells you he has a history of assault.

53. After you examine the patient, one of the first things you should do is

    (A) confront her about her husband's behavior.

    (B) accuse her of trying to kill herself.

    (C) obtain appropriate radiographs.

    (D) call the police.

    (E) call the social worker.

54. The radiographs of her arm demonstrate a compound fracture of both the radius and ulna. Radiographs of the other arm show old irregularly healed fractures of the radius and humerus and a metal pin near the humeral

head. The patient's abdomen on exam was tender in the right upper quadrant and an ultrasound shows a fluid-filled lesion under the liver. You suspect a hepatic hematoma. You should

- (A) tell the patient of your findings and inquire as to their etiology.
- (B) call the police.
- (C) tell her you know her husband beats her and he should be locked up.
- (D) call a home for battered women and arrange for her to go there.
- (E) call hospital security.

55. The patient sticks to her story of falling. You

- (A) gently tell her that all of her injuries are not likely due to falling down the stairs and tell her that domestic abuse is unfortunately fairly common and that there are ways to deal with it and protect her and her children.
- (B) call the police.
- (C) send the police to arrest her husband.
- (D) refuse to treat her if she does not tell you the truth.
- (E) call her family.

56. The patient still will not change her story. The nurse who knows her husband volunteers to talk to her. The nurse gently tells the patient that she knows about her husband. The patient breaks down and starts to cry. You offer to

- (A) call the police.
- (B) arrange admission to the home for battered women.
- (C) call her family.
- (D) call the hospital social worker.
- (E) talk to the husband.

57. The patient agrees and the social worker comes and tells her about her options regarding local homes for battered women. She has one child and the social worker assures her that the home will take her child in, too, and will not divulge her location to the husband. She thinks about this while the orthopedist sets her fracture, and then she decides she had better go home or her husband will hurt her child before she can get her out of the house. You, the nurse, and the social worker try to get her to change her mind, but she is adamant. You

- (A) send her out after she signs a release against medical advice.
- (B) refuse to ever see her again.
- (C) call the police.
- (D) call her family.
- (E) give her the ER phone number, the police emergency number, your pager, and the number for the home for battered women and urge her to change her mind.

58. She is brought to the ER one week later, with head trauma, by an ambulance called by her sister. The sister tells you the husband got angry at her for burning his dinner and beat her with a broom. She is unconscious, but her pupils respond to light. You should

- (A) refuse to take care of her.
- (B) inform the police of your suspicions.
- (C) call the husband.
- (D) do nothing.
- (E) accuse her sister of not watching her closely enough.

59. The patient eventually recovers from her injuries. You discuss her situation with her, telling her she is risking her life by returning to her husband. She thinks you are right but wants to discuss the issue with her sister and pastor. You recommend that

- (A) she goes to the home for battered women while she is making up her mind.
- (B) she goes home to her husband.

(C)   she spends time in protective custody.

(D)   she stays in the hospital until she decides what to do.

(E)   she seeks sanctuary in a church.

60. You are very worried about the patient because she decides to go home with her sister while she makes up her mind. The nurse in the ER who knows the husband is sure he will find her and hurt her again. You can

(A)   commit the patient.

(B)   commit the husband.

(C)   try to talk the patient into going to the home for battered women.

(D)   keep her in the hospital.

(E)   get her into the federal witness protection program.

61. A 23-year-old man presents to your office with diffuse pruritus for three weeks. He denies any other symptoms or past medical illnesses. On physical examination, you note numerous eczematous areas over his body with excoriations. He notes that he recently bought a new down comforter for his bed. The most likely diagnosis is

(A)   acne vulgaris.

(B)   contact dermatitis.

(C)   psoriasis.

(D)   urticaria.

(E)   lichens simplex chronicums.

62. Which one of the following screening procedures should take place routinely at 36 weeks of gestation?

(A)   Gestational diabetes

(B)   Group B streptococcal culture

(C)   HBV culture

(D)   Ultrasound

(E)   Rh factor

63. A 46-year-old black female, who was hospitalized on the oncology ward secondary to multiple myeloma, presents with nausea, vomiting, polyuria, constipation, and abdominal pain over the course of several days. Her oncologist found out that her serum calcium was 16 mg/dl. Her electrocardiogram revealed shortening of the Q-T interval. Soon her mental status began to deteriorate. What would be the immediate treatment in this situation?

(A)   Subcutaneous salmon-calcitonin

(B)   Laxatives for the constipation

(C)   Biphosphonates

(D)   Inorganic phosphate

(E)   Intravenous normal saline

Questions 64-66 refer to the following:

64. Histiocytosis X is known as all of the following EXCEPT

(A)   Hand-Schuller-Christian syndrome.

(B)   Letterer-Siwe disease.

(C)   eosinophilic granuloma.

(D)   pulmonary alveolar proteinosis.

(E)   histiocytosis X.

65. The treatment of histiocytosis X is by

(A)   antibiotics.

(B)   steroids.

(C)   surgery.

(D)   chemotherapy.

(E)   radiation.

66. The lesions of histiocytosis occur most often in the

(A)   kidneys and liver.

(B)   lungs and bones.

(C)   heart.

(D)   colon and bladder.

(E)   head and neck.

67. A 54-year-old black male with chronic hypertension presents to the emergency room with symptoms of malaise and weakness. His BUN was elevated to 56 mg/dl, and his creatinine level was elevated to 5.0 mg/dl. His blood pressure was 190/110 mm/hg and he was non-compliant with medication at home. This patient had no difficulty voiding. All of the following options can be undertaken in the management of this patient EXCEPT

 (A) hemodialysis.

 (B) diuretics.

 (C) kidney ultrasound.

 (D) urine analysis with microscopy.

 (E) low-protein diet.

68. A 47-year-old female visits her doctor during a routine check-up. She had symptoms of fatigue, sleep disturbances, poor appetite, anhedonia, and poor concentration for two to four weeks. Her physical examination and lab data were within normal limits. She has not had any mood elevations or flight of ideas. She has occasional feelings of hopelessness. What would be the initial management of choice?

 (A) Admit to a psychiatric institution

 (B) Group counseling

 (C) Lithium

 (D) Selective serotonin reuptake inhibitor

 (E) Electroconvulsive therapy

69. A 66-year-old black male was brought by ambulance to the emergency room complaining of severe substernal chest pain associated with nausea, diaphoresis, and shortness of breath. His electrocardiogram reveals ST segment elevations in leads II, III, and AVF. The rate was 52 beats per minute. Which one of the following cardiac events is associated with the above findings?

 (A) Inferior myocardial infarction

 (B) Pericardial effusion

 (C) Anterior myocardial infarction

 (D) Aortic stenosis

 (E) Dilated cardiomyopathy

70. A 40-year-old woman presents to your office with two weeks of clear rhinorrhea and pruritus in the eyes. She says that she has these symptoms usually during the autumn. She denies any fevers, chills or purulent discharge. Appropriate initial medications would be

 (A) antibiotics.

 (B) antihistamine.

 (C) oral steroids.

 (D) ocean spray.

 (E) None of the above.

Questions 71-78 refer to the following:

71. A 45-year-old alcoholic is admitted to your service with what appears to be an attack of acute pancreatitis. Classically, this patient will present with

 (A) mild LUQ pain.

 (B) excruciating LUQ pain.

 (C) fluid epigastric pain.

 (D) excruciating epigastric pain.

 (E) no complaints.

72. This pain may spread to the

 (A) left shoulder.

 (B) right shoulder.

 (C) LLQ.

 (D) LUQ.

 (E) neck.

73. The pain is aggravated when the patient is

 (A) supine.

 (B) prone.

 (C) left lateral decubitus.

 (D) right lateral decubitus.

 (E) sitting.

74. Besides the patient being an alcoholic, other reasons for this acute attack, to be gained from the history-taking, include all of the following EXCEPT

    (A) biliary tract disease.

    (B) hypolipidemia.

    (C) pancreatic ductal obstruction.

    (D) vascular compromise.

    (E) mumps.

75. You are now making rounds two days after you admitted the patient. He has a nasogastric tube placed and is feeling somewhat better. You do notice, however, that the patient now has

    (A) mild jaundice.

    (B) moderate hypotension.

    (C) severe fatigue.

    (D) a left shift of his white blood cells.

    (E) a high temperature.

76. An accumulation of blood and fluid in the lesser peritoneal sac may form a(n)

    (A) hematoma.

    (B) pseudocyst.

    (C) thrombus.

    (D) embolus.

    (E) ascitic collection.

77. Other diseases that could have presented in a similar severity include all of the following EXCEPT

    (A) acute appendicitis.

    (B) peptic ulcer perforation.

    (C) leaking duodenal ulcer.

    (D) splenic rupture.

    (E) megacolon.

78. Another disease presenting in the same location could be

    (A) diverticulitis of the colon.

    (B) acute pyelonephritis.

    (C) transverse colon obstruction.

    (D) early appendicitis.

    (E) colon cancer.

79. A healthy 28-year-old man calls you with concerns of being exposed to another person who was subsequently diagnosed with meningococcal meningitis. He asks you if he should do anything because he has heard that meningitis can be contagious. You prescribe him

    (A) two weeks of dapsone.

    (B) two days of rifampin.

    (C) two weeks of an intravenous third-generation cephalosporin.

    (D) a screening lumbar puncture.

    (E) None of the above, and reassure the patient that he has nothing to worry about.

80. You are the physician in charge of the care of an 81-year-old female patient with multiple medical problems. Her main concern is the recurrent bouts of pneumonia. A single dose of pneumococcal vaccine is believed to confer a lifetime immunity against pneumococcal pneumonia. It is recommended for all of the following conditions EXCEPT

    (A) COPD.

    (B) congestive heart failure (CHF).

    (C) chronic glomerulonephritis.

    (D) pregnancy in a glaucomic patient.

    (E) cirrhosis.

81. All of the following are indicated in the treatment of postoperative congestive heart failure EXCEPT

    (A) furosemide.

    (B) morphine.

(C) oxygen.

(D) phenylephrine.

(E) nitroglycerin.

82. A 45-year-old woman comes to your clinic with a two-month history of weight loss, increased thirst, and nocturia. Which one of the following tests is likely to be most useful as an initial evaluation step?

(A) CBC

(B) Brain MRI

(C) Blood glucose

(D) Chest radiograph

(E) ACTH stimulation test

83. A 63-year-old woman is brought in by her family because she has become withdrawn, does not appear to be interested in her surroundings, sweats a lot, and sleeps a lot. She is tachycardiac and hypertensive, which is new for her. As part of your initial evaluation you order

(A) thyroid function tests.

(B) ACTH stimulation test.

(C) aldosterone level.

(D) glucose tolerance test.

(E) fasting lipids.

For Questions 84-87, match each of the following prenatal diagnostic procedures with its clinical indication during pregnancy.

(A) Ultrasound

(B) Amniocentesis

(C) Chorionic villus sampling

(D) Blood sampling from the cord or chorionic plate

(E) Any two of the above.

84. Spina bifida

85. Family history of neural tube defect

86. Trisomy 21 (Down's syndrome)

87. Fetal sex

Questions 88-92 refer to the following:

Examination of the oropharynx reveals an erythematous cobblestone-appearing mucosa, and the patient has a temperature of 103.4°F.

88. All of the following may be an associated physical finding EXCEPT

(A) nasal discharge.

(B) cervical lymphadenitis.

(C) watery eyes.

(D) a systolic ejection murmur.

(E) mild splenomegaly.

89. This patient most likely has

(A) carcinoma of the pharynx.

(B) Vincent's angina.

(C) acute pharyngitis.

(D) mumps.

(E) AIDS.

90. Adequate treatment would include all of the following EXCEPT

(A) antibiotics.

(B) analgesics.

(C) increased fluid intake.

(D) increased physical exercise and work.

(E) antipyretics.

91. After two days of following your instructions, the patient returns with a mild rash and itching over his chest. Your next step should include

(A) discontinuance of all the medications.

(B) continuance of all the medications.

(C) prescription of an antihistamine.

(D) discontinuance of the antibiotic and replacing it with another antibiotic from a different class.

(E) biopsy of the rash.

92. When the patient returns in two weeks, he is cured but brings in his girlfriend, who is also your patient, with similar complaints. On examination you make a similar diagnosis. You should

(A) treat her.

(B) treat him.

(C) treat both of them.

(D) treat neither of them.

93. Complications from a chronic peptic ulcer include all of the following EXCEPT

(A) hemorrhage.

(B) pyloric obstruction.

(C) perforation.

(D) carcinoma.

(E) intestinal adhesions.

94. Pain in the perineum may come from all of the following EXCEPT

(A) fissure in ano.

(B) anal ulcer.

(C) folliculitis.

(D) carcinoma.

(E) perianal hematoma.

95. A 19-year-old man presents to your office wanting to be tested for syphilis. He tells you that his recent sexual partner was diagnosed with syphilis. No chancres are noted on examination. Lab results come back with a positive VDRL and a negative FTA. You tell him that the results indicate that

(A) he was once infected with syphilis, but was treated for it.

(B) he is now infected with syphilis and needs treatment for it.

(C) he has tertiary syphilis.

(D) he may be infected with syphilis, but will need to be rechecked in six months.

(E) he does not have syphilis.

Questions 96-99 refer to the following:

A right-hand-dominant worker presents to your office with right wrist pain. The Finkelstein test is positive.

96. This patient suffers from

(A) carpal tunnel syndrome.

(B) cubital tunnel syndrome.

(C) de Quervain's disease.

(D) Dupuytren's contracture.

(E) trigger finger.

97. The disease in Question 96 is classified as a

(A) compression syndrome.

(B) tenosynovitis.

(C) flexor tenosynovitis.

(D) extensor tenosynovitis.

(E) disease of palmar fascia.

98. The nerve closely associated with the above disease that must be observed during surgery is the

(A) ulnar nerve.

(B) radial nerve.

(C) median nerve.

(D) palmar cutaneous nerve.

(E) musculocutaneous nerve

99. The Finkelstein test is performed with

(A) the thumb flexed into the palm and ulnarly deviating the wrist.

(B) the thumb flexed into the palm and radially deviating the wrist.

(C) tapping the nerve in question.

(D)   passive flexion of both wrists.

(E)   alternate compressing of the radial and ulnar.

Questions 100-107 refer to the following:

A previously healthy 56-year-old man is admitted to the intensive care unit because of acute loss of consciousness while driving. Fortunately, he did not sustain significant injuries as a result of the ensuing accident. By the time you see him, he is alert, but aphasic, and cannot move his right hand or leg. He has no gag reflex. He seems to follow simple commands. He has no history of hypertension, heart disease, or blood clots. His father died of a stroke.

100.   After stabilizing him, you order

(A)   a bone scan.

(B)   a craniotomy.

(C)   a brain MRI.

(D)   a skull film.

(E)   a serum calcium.

101.   Testing demonstrates that the patient has findings consistent with a hemispheral infarct. There is no bleeding. You begin anticoagulation and pursue the possibility of

(A)   tuberculosis.

(B)   a thrombus in the heart.

(C)   a brain tumor.

(D)   cavernous sinus thrombosis.

(E)   sinusitis.

102.   You find no evidence of an obvious source for this stroke. The patient spikes a fever of 39°C the next morning. Your major concern at the moment is

(A)   atelectasis.

(B)   aspiration pneumonia.

(C)   sinusitis.

(D)   meningitis.

(E)   encephalitis.

103.   You find no obvious source of the fever and it resolves spontaneously. The patient begins rehabilitation and makes some progress in using his left hand to write. His gag reflex improves so that he can swallow and eat. As part of your evaluation of the patient's status and in an effort to determine the cause of his illness, you order all of the following EXCEPT

(A)   a sedimentation rate.

(B)   antinuclear antibodies.

(C)   a repeat MRI.

(D)   a bone scan.

(E)   speech therapy.

104.   The patient continues to be stable. The sedimentation rate comes back at 55 (normal, 0-10). The antinuclear antibody test is negative. MRI shows no extension of the lesion. Before you transfer him to the rehabilitation unit, you order

(A)   a chest CT.

(B)   skull films.

(C)   sinus films.

(D)   rheumatoid factor.

(E)   brain angiography.

105.   The angiogram shows beading of the vessels in the area of the infarct. You now suspect

(A)   a brain tumor.

(B)   cerebral vasculitis.

(C)   encephalitis.

(D)   meningitis.

(E)   pseudotumor cerebri.

106.   You transfer the patient to the rehabilitation unit and decide to further evaluate this new diagnosis. You order all of the following EXCEPT

(A)   C3 complement level.

(B)   temporal artery biopsy.

(C)   C4 complement level.

(D) liver-spleen scan.

(E) sural nerve biopsy.

107. You immediately add which one of the following measures to the patient's management regimen?

(A) High-dose prednisone

(B) Methotrexate

(C) Penicillamine

(D) Hemodialysis

(E) Coumadin

For Questions 108-111, match the likeliest diagnosis with the symptoms.

(A) Vitamin B12 deficiency

(B) Diabetic peripheral neuropathy

(C) Alcohol withdrawal

(D) Carpal tunnel syndrome

(E) Peripheral vascular disease

108. A 45-year-old woman with macrocytic anemia and paresthesias of her hands and feet

109. A 53-year-old man with asterixis and confusion

110. A 66-year-old man with a black toe

111. A 35-year-old woman with nocturnal paresthesias in her hands

112. A 54-year-old male is hospitalized with a urinary tract infection and is on intravenous antibiotics. On the fifth hospital day, he has a change of mental status and his fever is elevated to 103°F. His chest X-ray shows diffuse bilateral alveolar infiltrates consistent with adult respiratory distress syndrome. Arterial blood gas reveals Ph of 7.29, pCO$_2$ of 30, and pO$_2$ of 50. Blood cultures are positive for *E. coli*. This patient's blood pressure is 70/40 mm/hg. All of the following should be included in the management plan for this patient EXCEPT

(A) intubation and central line placement.

(B) intravenous hydration.

(C) intravenous corticosteroids.

(D) aminoglycosides.

(E) positive end expiratory pressure (PEEP) on the ventilator.

113. A 60-year-old female has recently begun treatment with alendronate for osteoporosis. She now presents to the emergency department complaining of severe odynophagia. The lesion, defined by the black arrows in the figure below is obtained as part of the diagnostic evaluation. Other causes of this lesion include all of the following EXCEPT

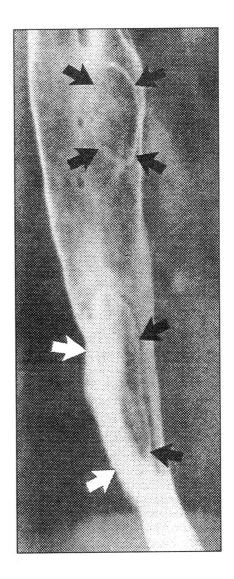

(A) cytomegalovirus.

(B) herpes virus.

(C) ingestion of KC1 tablets.

(D) malignancy.

(E) ingestion of omeprazole tablets.

114. An 81-year-old male patient with known prostate cancer presents to the ER with severe low back pain. A technetium 99 bone scan confirms your suspicion of metastatic bone disease. At this time, you should administer

    (A) chemotherapy to prevent further metastases.

    (B) high-dose radiotherapy to the low back to relieve pain.

    (C) high-dose morphine.

    (D) high-dose fentanyl.

    (E) high-dose hydromorphone.

Questions 115-118 refer to the following:

A 49-year-old man with a history of type II diabetes mellitus requiring insulin presents to your office with a foot ulcer. He says that he has noticed it for the past several weeks, but it has not caused him any pain or discomfort, and so he decided not to have it seen right away. Physical examination reveals that he is afebrile. The great toe on the right foot has a 2 centimeter ulceration with a small amount of purulent drainage.

115. The best explanation for the patient not feeling the ulcer is

    (A) diabetic neuropathy has caused him to lose sensation in his feet.

    (B) diabetic microvascular disease has caused his foot to necrose.

    (C) diabetic vascular disease has lead to lacunar infarct, which has caused him to lose sensation in his feet.

    (D) he wasn't paying attention.

    (E) None of the above.

116. The most likely pathogens involved are

    (A) *Staphylococcus aureus.*

    (B) beta-hemolytic *Streptococcus.*

    (C) *Bacteroides fragilis.*

    (D) *Haemophilus influenzae.*

    (E) All of the above.

117. Which one of the following historical factors would make *Pseudomonas aeruginosa* more likely?

    (A) Stepping on a sharp object while wearing shoes

    (B) Walking barefoot in the grass

    (C) Stepping on a piece of glass with barefeet

    (D) Stepping on a rusty nail

    (E) None of the above.

118. Of the following, the most appropriate treatment for diabetic foot ulcers includes

    (A) surgical debridement and broad-spectrum antibiotics.

    (B) surgical debridement and antibiotics for Gram-positive organisms.

    (C) surgical debridement and antibiotics for Gram-negative organisms.

    (D) no surgical debridement and broad-spectrum antibiotics.

    (E) no surgical debridement and antibiotics for Gram-positive organisms.

119. A 64-year-old man was transferred to your service earlier in the day from the CCU after a myocardial infarction was ruled out. He was mentally clear when you last saw him. He is afebrile and has no localizing signs. The likeliest cause of his altered mental status is

    (A) encephalitis.

    (B) a cerebrovascular accident.

    (C) septic emboli.

(D)   brain tumor.

(E)   confusion due to new surroundings.

120.   A 45-year-old woman is hospitalized for a flare-up of her lupus. She is being treated with high doses of prednisone. You are called to see her because she has developed a low-grade fever and is somnolent. On physical examination she seems to recoil slightly when you palpate her abdomen. All of the following diagnoses need to be considered EXCEPT

(A)   peritonitis.

(B)   ruptured viscus.

(C)   mesenteric infarction.

(D)   leiomyomata.

(E)   pancreatitis.

Questions 121-124 refer to the following:

A 72-year-old female whom you have seen once for an episode of low back pain comes in now with severe pain in her thoracic and lumbar spine.

121.   All of the following historical questions are important EXCEPT

(A)   age of menopause.

(B)   history of hormonal therapy.

(C)   history of transfusions.

(D)   trauma.

(E)   family history.

122.   Which one of the following tests will probably be most useful to order first in this patient?

(A)   MRI of the spine

(B)   Radiograph of the spine

(C)   Bone scan

(D)   CBC

(E)   ACTH stimulation test

123.   The patient has compression fractures of T8, T11, L1, and L2. You suspect

(A)   elder abuse.

(B)   tuberculosis.

(C)   osteoarthritis.

(D)   osteoporosis.

(E)   osteomyelitis.

124.   Which one of the following tests will be useful for long-term follow-up after initiation of treatment?

(A)   Radiographs

(B)   Bone scans

(C)   Bone densitometry

(D)   CT scans

(E)   MRIs

For Questions 125-128, select the most likely pathogen in these patients with diarrhea.

(A)   *Cryptosporidium*

(B)   *Shigella*

(C)   *Giardia lamblia*

(D)   *Clostridium difficile*

(E)   *Rotavirus*

125.   A 24-year-old female with a urinary tract infection

126.   A 50-year-old female returning from a hiking trip in the Rocky Mountains

127.   A 30-year-old intravenous drug user with thrombocytopenia

128.   A 50-year-old banker with dysentery

129.   A 59-year-old man is followed for the management of essential hypertension. All of the following are sequelae of essential hypertension EXCEPT

(A)   left ventricular hypertrophy.

(B)   retinal hemorrhage.

(C)   chronic glomerulonephritis.

(D)   atheromatous plaque formation in coronary arteries.

(E)   cerebrovascular disease.

Questions 130 and 131 refer to the following:

A 56-year-old patient who you have been treating for 15 years comes to your office with fear of oral cancer. He notes a row of smooth, small bumps at the posterior dorsum of his tongue.

130. You

(A)   tell him you will perform a biopsy.

(B)   tell him it is cancer.

(C)   reassure him that these bumps are normal.

(D)   refer him to a head and neck oncologist.

(E)   prescribe an antibiotic.

131. If the above patient were to have a right unilateral paralysis of his tongue, his tongue would

(A)   deviate to the right.

(B)   deviate to the left.

(C)   protrude normally.

(D)   retrude slightly to the right.

(E)   retrude slightly to the left.

For Questions 132-135 you are interpreting urine studies for a nephrologist who is out of the hospital. Based on the following results, what is the diagnosis?

(A)   Acidic pH

(B)   Increased specific gravity

(C)   Presence of blood

(D)   Presence of ketones

(E)   Presence of protein

132. A 46-year-old woman with nephrotic syndrome

133. A 33-year-old male on a fast for political reasons

134. A 79-year-old male with a recurrence of a kidney stone

135. A 33-year-old male with a cranial injury and with SIADH

136. Your patient has just had a breast biopsy and you are about to send her home. Which one of the following discharge criteria is LEAST important?

(A)   Taking in fluids

(B)   Being afebrile

(C)   Ability to void

(D)   Ability to have a bowel movement

(E)   Ability to ambulate

137. Which one of the following statements regarding elder abuse in the United States is NOT true?

(A)   The American Medical Association (AMA) recommends that physicians incorporate questions in routine history-taking to screen for elder abuse.

(B)   The physical or emotional dependence on the caregiver can be a risk factor.

(C)   Financial dependence on the caregiver can be a risk factor.

(D)   The prevalence of elder abuse is much lower in institutionalized patients compared to elders in the community setting.

(E)   Deterioration in health of the perpetrator can be a risk factor.

138. Of the following organisms, the one that has been possibly linked with gastric carcinoma is

(A)   *Neisseria gonorrhea.*

(B)   *Helicobacter pylori.*

(C) *Escherichia coli.*

(D) Epstein-Barr virus.

(E) None of the above.

139. A 40-year-old man presents to his primary care physician for a routine check-up. He was found to have a subperiosteal xanthoma over the upper tibia, orange-yellow tuberous xanthomas on the lower third of the forearm, elbows and knee, and bilateral arcus senilis. He has a strong family history of premature coronary artery disease. His serum cholesterol level was 304 mg/dl. This patient was otherwise asymptomatic and with no other physical findings. What would be the initial management plan for this patient?

   (A) Step I diet therapy

   (B) Biopsy of the xanthomas

   (C) Allopurinol

   (D) HMG-CoA reductase inhibitor

   (E) Gemfibrozil and niacin combination

140. A 78-year-old white male nursing-home resident presents with severe epigastric pain and coffee-ground emesis. He was transferred to the nearby university hospital, and an upper endoscopy was performed after the patient was stabilized with hydration and blood transfusions. The endoscopy results revealed chronic active gastritis, and the culture was positive for *H. pylori*. What is the next step in managing this patient?

   (A) H2 receptor blockers

   (B) Discontinuing all nonsteroidal anti-inflammatory agents

   (C) Proton-pump inhibitor

   (D) Triple antibiotics plus a proton-pump inhibitor

   (E) Advising the patient to discontinue alcohol intake and watchful waiting

For Questions 141-144, match the acid-base values with the appropriate clinical conditions.

You are evaluating a young woman following an overdose with salicylates. As part of your discussion of acid-base disorders, you ask the third-year medical student to match the following acid-base values with the appropriate clinical condition

	pH	pCO$_2$	HCl$_3$-
(A)	7.6	45	38
(B)	7.2	23	10
(C)	7.1	95	30
(D)	7.6	15	14

141. Vomiting

142. Diabetic ketoacidosis

143. Sedative overdose

144. Meningitis

145. A 40-year-old man comes to the emergency room because of weight loss. You have seen him before, and he looks worse than ever. He is cachectic and weak, and has disseminated candidiasis as well as a dry hacking cough. His chest radiograph shows a diffuse multilobe infiltrate. You are certain he has HIV/AIDS, but he refuses to be tested. You

   (A) send off his blood for HIV testing because you believe it is medically necessary.

   (B) report him to the Board of Health.

   (C) call his family.

   (D) refuse to take care of him.

   (E) admit him.

146. Sarcoid is characterized by all of the following EXCEPT

   (A) organ dysfunction results from distortion of tissue architecture.

(B) clinical manifestations occur only when a sufficient number of structures vital to tissue function are involved.

(C) following the initial inflammatory reaction, granulomas are formed.

(D) initially, there is an accumulation of mononuclear inflammatory cells in affected organs.

(E) an exaggerated humoral response heralds recovery.

147. A 68-year-old male with a history of hypertensive cardiac disease was admitted for evaluation of increasing congestive heart failure. The electrocardiogram shows low voltage QRS complexes and ventricular premature contractions. The echocardiogram shows increased thickness of the ventricular wall and septum. A percutaneous transvenous cardiac biopsy, stained with Congo red and viewed under polarized light, is shown in the figure below. You diagnose

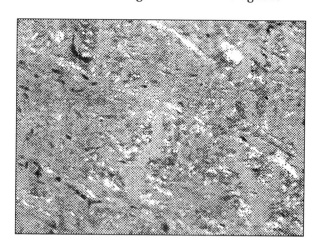

(A) hemochromatosis.

(B) sarcoidosis.

(C) endomyocardial fibrosis.

(D) amyloidosis.

(E) eosinophilic endomyocardial disease.

148. Which one of the following is correct with respect to a hand examination?

(A) Finger extension of 45°

(B) Finger extension of 90°

(C) Metacarpal phalangeal flexion of 45°

(D) Metacarpal phalangeal flexion of 60°

(E) Finger abduction of 90°

Questions 149-156 refer to the following:

You have diagnosed metastatic breast cancer in a 55-year-old woman who has failed chemotherapy in conjunction with autologous bone marrow transplantation. She knows her diagnosis and does not want to go through any more chemotherapy.

149. You discuss the patient's condition and decision with her family and tell them that she will probably die soon. Her son wants you to do everything that can be done to keep her alive. Your obligation is

(A) to do what your patient wants, within reason, as long as she is mentally competent.

(B) do what her family wants.

(C) try to change her mind.

(D) tell her you will do what she wants and then do what you think is best.

(E) take a family vote.

150. The patient's husband wants her "to not suffer," though she is not in pain at the moment. He wants her to receive large doses of morphine at home. You

(A) do as he wishes.

(B) discuss this with the patient.

(C) explain that this is not consistent with good medical practice or with the patient's best interests.

(D) volunteer to come to their home to administer the drugs.

(E)   teach the husband how to give injections.

151. The husband tells you that he will get drugs whether you prescribe them or not. You

(A)   call the police.

(B)   try to commit him.

(C)   try to get a restraining order on him so he cannot go near the patient.

(D)   discuss this in the presence of the patient and the entire family.

(E)   tell the family to find another doctor.

152. You are legally allowed to

(A)   help the patient commit suicide if this is what she wants.

(B)   prescribe narcotics in reasonable doses if the patient has pain.

(C)   help the family aid the patient in committing suicide.

(D)   give the patient a large supply of multiple narcotics.

(E)   teach the patient how to inject air intravenously.

153. The issue of a physician helping a patient to commit suicide is

(A)   a religious one.

(B)   being discussed before the Supreme Court of the United States.

(C)   legal.

(D)   between the patient and physician.

(E)   subject to patient-physician confidentiality.

154. The patient's family tells you they will call someone to help them "put the patient out of her misery." You should

(A)   call the police.

(B)   refuse to care for the patient.

(C)   obtain a restraining order against the family.

(D)   tell the patient about this and give her your opinion.

(E)   call the newspapers.

155. The patient herself inquires about the possibility of going to a hospice. You tell her

(A)   she does not qualify because it might take her a long time to die.

(B)   she is too old.

(C)   it is a good idea and you will have the social worker get her more information.

(D)   she is too healthy.

(E)   she does not have the right disease.

156. The patient's family wants her to stay in the hospital until she dies. You tell them

(A)   hospitalization is not medically necessary for her at present.

(B)   that you will admit her to the hospital.

(C)   that she should go to a different doctor.

(D)   that you would admit her, but the insurance company will not let you.

(E)   that this is a ridiculous idea.

157. Partial complex seizures most commonly manifest abnormalities in which one of the following areas of the brain on electroencephalography?

(A)   Temporal lobe-limbic region

(B)   Cerebellum

(C)   Midbrain-pons region

(D)   Frontal lobe

(E)   Medulla

Questions 158-165 refer to the following:

An 18-year-old female patient comes to the college outpatient clinic with a complaint of a sore throat and a temperature of 103°F. She states she is in good health, takes no medicines, and has no medical allergies.

158. All of the following areas should be examined EXCEPT

   (A) her oropharynx.

   (B) her heart.

   (C) her lungs.

   (D) her abdomen.

   (E) her peripheral pulses.

159. Upon examination of her neck you would expect to find

   (A) a normal neck.

   (B) tender lymphadenopathy.

   (C) non-tender lymphadenopathy.

   (D) a bruit.

   (E) a deviated trachea.

160. On inspection of the oropharynx, you notice a cobblestone-appearing and erythematous mucosal pharynx. Your most likely diagnosis is

   (A) squamous cell carcinoma.

   (B) acute pharyngitis.

   (C) Strep throat.

   (D) bronchitis.

   (E) epiglottitis.

161. A rapid Strep antigen test is positive. The antibiotic of choice here would be

   (A) penicillin.

   (B) vancomycin.

   (C) erythromycin.

   (D) clindamycin.

   (E) Flagyl.

162. This disease should be treated for

   (A) one day.

   (B) three to five days.

   (C) seven to ten days.

   (D) three to four weeks.

   (E) six to eight weeks.

163. Other treatment modalities include all of the following EXCEPT

   (A) rest.

   (B) fluids.

   (C) antipyretics.

   (D) exercise.

   (E) analgesics.

164. The patient comes back to your office two weeks after the initial visit stating she is much improved. She has no soreness in her throat or in her neck. You would now suggest which one of the following?

   (A) A chest X-ray

   (B) An arterial blood gas

   (C) A throat culture

   (D) Continuance of the antibiotic for two more weeks

   (E) Follow-up on an as-needed basis

165. She tells you before leaving that her boyfriend has been feeling ill lately with the symptoms that she initially had. You suggest which one of the following?

   (A) A course of antibiotics

   (B) Reassurance

   (C) Have him come to the office as soon as possible

   (D) Have him return only if it worsens

   (E) Tell him to take two aspirins and schedule an appointment

166. A 20-year-old black female with a history of sickle cell disease presents with a sickle cell crisis. She has noted gastroenteritis for the last three days and now notes back and rib pain. She is afebrile and the rest of her vital signs are stable. Her room air oxygen saturation is 98%. Appropriate initial interventions include all of the following EXCEPT

    (A) vigorous hydration.

    (B) complete blood count.

    (C) serum electrolytes.

    (D) analgesics.

    (E) supplemental oxygen.

167. A 32-year-old woman calls after taking penicillin for a sore throat. She has a mild rash over her back. You advise her to

    (A) finish the course of the antibiotic to cure the infection.

    (B) decrease the dose by one-half.

    (C) stop taking the drug totally.

    (D) stop taking the drug and come to the clinic for a change in antibiotic.

    (E) double the dose of the antibiotic.

168. The FTA-ABS (Fluorescent Treponemal Antibody Absorbed) is a test for

    (A) herpes.

    (B) HIV.

    (C) *Gonococcus.*

    (D) syphilis.

    (E) *Streptococcus.*

169. Your head nurse brings a "friend" today for an evaluation. He has been treated by an alternative care therapist with tryptophan for insomnia. He now complains of difficulty climbing stairs and a tingling sensation of his feet. Examination is remarkable for a proximal myopathy and peripheral neuropathy. The most likely findings on peripheral smear are

    (A) lymphopenia.

    (B) eosinophilia.

    (C) leukopenia.

    (D) basophilia.

    (E) lymphocytosis.

170. An 80-year-old woman presents with right upper quadrant pain and fever to 103°F increasing for four days. Her past medical history includes diabetes and chronic renal insufficiency. Physical examination reveals that she has a temperature of 102.8°F, a heart rate of 110, a blood pressure of 90/60, and a respiratory rate of 22. She has right upper quadrant tenderness to palpation and no rebound tenderness. Bowel sounds are normal. She is also noted to be slightly jaundiced. Rectal examination is guaiac-negative. The most likely diagnosis is

    (A) acute cholecystitis.

    (B) acute cholangitis.

    (C) acute pancreatitis.

    (D) acute cholelithiasis.

    (E) acute gastritis.

171. Your 62-year-old hypertensive patient has been on a diuretic and, by herself, she increased the dose. Her serum potassium is low. You order a stat EKG and see

    (A) elevated T-waves.

    (B) depressed T-waves.

    (C) normal sinus rhythm.

    (D) shortened Q-T interval.

    (E) bradycardia.

172. A 21-year-old HIV-positive male presents to the emergency room with progressive dyspnea. His CXR appears normal and his blood gas reveals a $PaO_2 = 55$. His treatment should include

    (A) steroids and Ciprofloxin.

    (B) steroids and trimethoprim/ sulfamethoxazole.

(C) azathioprine.

(D) Ganciclovir.

(E) None of the above.

173. Which one of the following criteria is NOT included in a current definition of death?

    (A) The total cessation of all vital functions

    (B) No reflex activity

    (C) The absence of hypothermia or CNS drug depression

    (D) No response to deep, painful stimuli

    (E) No EEG activity

174. A 58-year-old man came in to the physician's office for a routine physical exam. His history and exam were unremarkable except for an unusual bluish-black pigmentation over his face and fingers. Adding sodium hydroxide to his urine sample turned the specimen black. Spinal films revealed intervertebral disk spaces showing greater radiodensity than the adjacent vertebrae. What is the diagnosis?

    (A) Ochronosis

    (B) Porphyria cutanea tarda

    (C) Systemic lupus erythematosus

    (D) Pellagra

    (E) Sturge-Weber syndrome

Questions 175-178 refer to the following:

A 31-year-old nurse comes to see you because of a chronic cough that is occasionally streaked with blood. She only comes in because her supervisor has insisted that she be evaluated. She is sure her cough is due to a virus. She smokes a pack of cigarettes a day. She says she has been dieting "forever" but has finally started to lose some weight. She has been feeling tired lately but attributes this to working extra overtime. She works on a general medicine ward at the county hospital. She says her PPD was negative when she came to work at the hospital three years ago, but has not been repeated since. She has never had a chest radiograph. You order a radiograph which shows a faint lesion in the right upper lobe.

175. Your leading working diagnosis in this patient is

    (A) tuberculosis.

    (B) lung cancer.

    (C) histoplasmosis.

    (D) *Mycoplasma* pneumonia.

    (E) viral pneumonia.

176. You next order

    (A) serum serologic tests.

    (B) a PPD and positive control skin tests.

    (C) a chest CT.

    (D) sputum samples for cytology.

    (E) a chest tomography.

177. You would not place a PPD on this patient if

    (A) she were not a nurse.

    (B) she had a fever.

    (C) she had received a BCG vaccination in the past.

    (D) she had a history of pneumonia.

    (E) she worked on an AIDS ward.

178. You advise the patient

    (A) that you are going to begin treatment right away.

    (B) that she needs oxygen.

    (C) that she has nothing to worry about.

    (D) that she can go back to work tomorrow.

    (E) that she must go home and await the results of her tests.

179. A 25-year-old male medical student is brought to the emergency room by his fiancee who explained that over the past three weeks the patient has become increasingly irritable and suspicious. He has not slept in the past three nights and has become preoccupied with the belief that the ideas for his thesis are being stolen by government agents. The fiancee also states that about three months out of the past year the patient had felt too tired to go to class and spent most of the time sleeping. She recalled that the patient had an aunt who was "quite moody" and has been hospitalized twice in a psychiatric institution. After further interviewing and examination of the patient, a diagnosis of bipolar disorder is made. Which one of the following statements is NOT true of bipolar disorder?

   (A) The lifetime risk of bipolar disorder is .01%.

   (B) There is evidence of genetic transmission of the disease.

   (C) The treatment of choice for the acute manic state is lithium.

   (D) Electroconvulsive therapy (ECT) is useful in some situations of bipolar disorder.

180. A thoracic deformity seen with active rickets is

   (A) pectus-carinatum.

   (B) Harrison's groove.

   (C) pectus excavatum.

   (D) barrel chest.

   (E) localized bulges and depressions.

USMLE STEP 3 – PRACTICE TEST 2

Day One – Morning Session

ANSWER KEY

1. (D)	31. (A)	61. (B)	91. (C)
2. (D)	32. (E)	62. (C)	92. (D)
3. (A)	33. (A)	63. (E)	93. (B)
4. (C)	34. (E)	64. (D)	94. (D)
5. (B)	35. (D)	65. (A)	95. (B)
6. (C)	36. (D)	66. (A)	96. (D)
7. (A)	37. (C)	67. (A)	97. (C)
8. (D)	38. (B)	68. (A)	98. (A)
9. (E)	39. (A)	69. (B)	99. (D)
10. (E)	40. (B)	70. (E)	100. (B)
11. (A)	41. (B)	71. (D)	101. (A)
12. (E)	42. (C)	72. (C)	102. (D)
13. (B)	43. (D)	73. (D)	103. (E)
14. (A)	44. (A)	74. (B)	104. (A)
15. (D)	45. (C)	75. (C)	105. (A)
16. (B)	46. (B)	76. (D)	106. (C)
17. (A)	47. (E)	77. (E)	107. (C)
18. (E)	48. (C)	78. (A)	108. (D)
19. (D)	49. (B)	79. (C)	109. (B)
20. (A)	50. (B)	80. (A)	110. (D)
21. (D)	51. (D)	81. (C)	111. (E)
22. (D)	52. (D)	82. (B)	112. (A)
23. (B)	53. (C)	83. (E)	113. (C)
24. (E)	54. (B)	84. (B)	114. (A)
25. (C)	55. (C)	85. (D)	115. (D)
26. (D)	56. (D)	86. (E)	116. (C)
27. (B)	57. (B)	87. (B)	117. (A)
28. (C)	58. (E)	88. (A)	118. (B)
29. (A)	59. (D)	89. (B)	119. (A)
30. (E)	60. (C)	90. (E)	120. (A)

121.	(A)	136.	(A)	151.	(A)	166.	(B)
122.	(A)	137.	(D)	152.	(A)	167.	(B)
123.	(B)	138.	(B)	153.	(C)	168.	(B)
124.	(C)	139.	(D)	154.	(C)	169.	(A)
125.	(E)	140.	(D)	155.	(E)	170.	(C)
126.	(A)	141.	(D)	156.	(A)	171.	(D)
127.	(D)	142.	(D)	157.	(C)	172.	(B)
128.	(B)	143.	(C)	158.	(E)	173.	(D)
129.	(D)	144.	(C)	159.	(A)	174.	(A)
130.	(D)	145.	(B)	160.	(B)	175.	(B)
131.	(B)	146.	(C)	161.	(B)	176.	(B)
132.	(D)	147.	(E)	162.	(C)	177.	(B)
133.	(D)	148.	(E)	163.	(C)	178.	(C)
134.	(A)	149.	(B)	164.	(A)	179.	(C)
135.	(C)	150.	(B)	165.	(A)	180.	(C)

USMLE STEP 3 – PRACTICE TEST 2

Day One – Afternoon Session

ANSWER KEY

1. (E)	31. (E)	61. (C)	91. (D)
2. (E)	32. (E)	62. (D)	92. (B)
3. (A)	33. (D)	63. (E)	93. (D)
4. (E)	34. (B)	64. (E)	94. (D)
5. (A)	35. (A)	65. (C)	95. (B)
6. (D)	36. (B)	66. (C)	96. (B)
7. (C)	37. (B)	67. (C)	97. (D)
8. (D)	38. (C)	68. (D)	98. (E)
9. (E)	39. (A)	69. (E)	99. (C)
10. (C)	40. (C)	70. (A)	100. (C)
11. (E)	41. (C)	71. (E)	101. (C)
12. (C)	42. (D)	72. (D)	102. (C)
13. (E)	43. (D)	73. (A)	103. (B)
14. (B)	44. (A)	74. (C)	104. (B)
15. (D)	45. (C)	75. (A)	105. (D)
16. (A)	46. (D)	76. (D)	106. (D)
17. (C)	47. (E)	77. (C)	107. (E)
18. (D)	48. (B)	78. (D)	108. (A)
19. (B)	49. (D)	79. (B)	109. (C)
20. (C)	50. (D)	80. (E)	110. (A)
21. (D)	51. (E)	81. (C)	111. (A)
22. (A)	52. (C)	82. (C)	112. (A)
23. (D)	53. (C)	83. (D)	113. (B)
24. (A)	54. (B)	84. (B)	114. (E)
25. (D)	55. (C)	85. (A)	115. (B)
26. (D)	56. (D)	86. (E)	116. (A)
27. (A)	57. (E)	87. (E)	117. (B)
28. (C)	58. (C)	88. (A)	118. (E)
29. (B)	59. (B)	89. (B)	119. (A)
30. (B)	60. (D)	90. (C)	120. (B)

121. (E)	136. (A)	151. (B)	166. (A)
122. (E)	137. (D)	152. (C)	167. (C)
123. (D)	138. (D)	153. (D)	168. (D)
124. (C)	139. (E)	154. (E)	169. (C)
125. (A)	140. (D)	155. (D)	170. (A)
126. (E)	141. (D)	156. (A)	171. (E)
127. (B)	142. (B)	157. (E)	172. (D)
128. (B)	143. (B)	158. (D)	173. (A)
129. (E)	144. (A)	159. (E)	174. (B)
130. (B)	145. (D)	160. (C)	175. (B)
131. (A)	146. (B)	161. (B)	176. (B)
132. (B)	147. (C)	162. (B)	177. (A)
133. (A)	148. (A)	163. (E)	178. (D)
134. (E)	149. (E)	164. (C)	179. (C)
135. (B)	150. (A)	165. (D)	180. (A)

USMLE STEP 3 – PRACTICE TEST 2

Day Two – Morning Session

ANSWER KEY

1. (C)	31. (D)	61. (C)	91. (E)
2. (B)	32. (E)	62. (C)	92. (A)
3. (B)	33. (E)	63. (B)	93. (E)
4. (D)	34. (D)	64. (E)	94. (E)
5. (D)	35. (C)	65. (A)	95. (B)
6. (A)	36. (A)	66. (B)	96. (D)
7. (D)	37. (B)	67. (A)	97. (D)
8. (E)	38. (C)	68. (C)	98. (B)
9. (D)	39. (B)	69. (E)	99. (E)
10. (D)	40. (D)	70. (D)	100. (C)
11. (E)	41. (E)	71. (D)	101. (B)
12. (D)	42. (B)	72. (C)	102. (E)
13. (A)	43. (D)	73. (B)	103. (B)
14. (B)	44. (B)	74. (D)	104. (D)
15. (C)	45. (C)	75. (D)	105. (C)
16. (A)	46. (B)	76. (B)	106. (D)
17. (D)	47. (D)	77. (D)	107. (A)
18. (A)	48. (A)	78. (D)	108. (C)
19. (D)	49. (B)	79. (A)	109. (A)
20. (C)	50. (A)	80. (E)	110. (A)
21. (D)	51. (B)	81. (A)	111. (D)
22. (C)	52. (B)	82. (D)	112. (B)
23. (A)	53. (A)	83. (B)	113. (C)
24. (B)	54. (A)	84. (B)	114. (A)
25. (B)	55. (B)	85. (C)	115. (D)
26. (D)	56. (C)	86. (C)	116. (C)
27. (C)	57. (A)	87. (A)	117. (B)
28. (A)	58. (C)	88. (D)	118. (A)
29. (A)	59. (E)	89. (C)	119. (C)
30. (C)	60. (B)	90. (B)	120. (A)

121.	(D)	136.	(A)	151.	(D)	166.	(E)
122.	(A)	137.	(D)	152.	(C)	167.	(D)
123.	(C)	138.	(D)	153.	(B)	168.	(E)
124.	(D)	139.	(C)	154.	(B)	169.	(D)
125.	(B)	140.	(B)	155.	(A)	170.	(C)
126.	(D)	141.	(B)	156.	(D)	171.	(E)
127.	(B)	142.	(D)	157.	(E)	172.	(A)
128.	(C)	143.	(B)	158.	(B)	173.	(B)
129.	(B)	144.	(B)	159.	(A)	174.	(A)
130.	(C)	145.	(A)	160.	(D)	175.	(C)
131.	(D)	146.	(E)	161.	(A)	176.	(C)
132.	(A)	147.	(A)	162.	(C)	177.	(A)
133.	(B)	148.	(B)	163.	(A)	178.	(D)
134.	(E)	149.	(D)	164.	(C)	179.	(C)
135.	(D)	150.	(D)	165.	(C)	180.	(B)

USMLE STEP 3 – PRACTICE TEST 2

Day Two – Afternoon Session

ANSWER KEY

1.	(D)	31.	(B)	61.	(B)	91.	(D)
2.	(C)	32.	(D)	62.	(B)	92.	(C)
3.	(D)	33.	(C)	63.	(E)	93.	(D)
4.	(B)	34.	(D)	64.	(D)	94.	(E)
5.	(B)	35.	(C)	65.	(B)	95.	(E)
6.	(D)	36.	(A)	66.	(B)	96.	(C)
7.	(D)	37.	(B)	67.	(A)	97.	(D)
8.	(E)	38.	(C)	68.	(D)	98.	(B)
9.	(B)	39.	(E)	69.	(A)	99.	(A)
10.	(B)	40.	(C)	70.	(B)	100.	(C)
11.	(A)	41.	(D)	71.	(D)	101.	(B)
12.	(C)	42.	(C)	72.	(A)	102.	(B)
13.	(D)	43.	(C)	73.	(A)	103.	(D)
14.	(A)	44.	(A)	74.	(B)	104.	(E)
15.	(C)	45.	(B)	75.	(A)	105.	(B)
16.	(C)	46.	(A)	76.	(B)	106.	(B)
17.	(B)	47.	(A)	77.	(E)	107.	(A)
18.	(D)	48.	(E)	78.	(D)	108.	(A)
19.	(E)	49.	(B)	79.	(B)	109.	(C)
20.	(A)	50.	(A)	80.	(D)	110.	(E)
21.	(A)	51.	(C)	81.	(D)	111.	(D)
22.	(D)	52.	(C)	82.	(C)	112.	(C)
23.	(E)	53.	(C)	83.	(A)	113.	(E)
24.	(B)	54.	(A)	84.	(E)	114.	(B)
25.	(B)	55.	(A)	85.	(B)	115.	(A)
26.	(C)	56.	(D)	86.	(B)	116.	(E)
27.	(C)	57.	(E)	87.	(E)	117.	(A)
28.	(E)	58.	(B)	88.	(D)	118.	(A)
29.	(A)	59.	(A)	89.	(C)	119.	(E)
30.	(B)	60.	(C)	90.	(D)	120.	(D)

121. (C)	136. (D)	151. (D)	166. (E)
122. (B)	137. (D)	152. (B)	167. (D)
123. (D)	138. (B)	153. (B)	168. (D)
124. (C)	139. (D)	154. (D)	169. (B)
125. (D)	140. (D)	155. (C)	170. (B)
126. (C)	141. (A)	156. (A)	171. (B)
127. (A)	142. (B)	157. (A)	172. (B)
128. (B)	143. (C)	158. (E)	173. (A)
129. (C)	144. (D)	159. (B)	174. (A)
130. (C)	145. (E)	160. (B)	175. (A)
131. (A)	146. (E)	161. (A)	176. (B)
132. (E)	147. (D)	162. (C)	177. (C)
133. (D)	148. (A)	163. (D)	178. (E)
134. (C)	149. (A)	164. (E)	179. (A)
135. (B)	150. (C)	165. (C)	180. (B)

DETAILED EXPLANATIONS
OF ANSWERS

USMLE Step 3 – Practice Test 2
Day One – Morning Session

1. **(D)** Influenza outbreaks of varying severity occur annually. The virus is transmitted primarily via small particle aerosol resulting from coughing or sneezing (A). Following initial respiratory tract infection, the virus replicates, destroying ciliated epithelium (B). The quantity of virus in respiratory tract specimens correlates with the severity of illness (C). Viremia is a rare immunity disorder that appears to be subtype-specific and long lasting (E).

2. **(D)** Hemoglobin F levels are usually elevated in newborns compared with older individuals.

3. **(A)** While Hepatitis A (A), B (B), and E (E) can be transmitted through the fecal-oral modes of transmission, hepatitis A has a very short incubation period and therefore, represents the most likely viral cause of this patient's enteric hepatitis.

4. **(C)** *Streptococcus bovis* endocarditis is often associated with the onset of bowel cancers, as well as other lesions in the alimentary tract. None of the other answer choices have an association with the development of neoplastic lesions.

5. **(B)** This patient has toxoplasmosis encephalitis infection in the brain, which is the most common brain infection in the AIDS patient. Since this patient has positive titers for toxoplasmosis and also a CT scan, which suggests toxoplasmosis gondii infection by the ring-enhancing lesions, empiric treatment with sulfadiazine and pyrimethamine or sulfadiazine and clindamycin should be initiated. A stereotactic brain biopsy (A) is reserved for patients who do not respond to the initial three to five days of treatment for toxoplasmosis. Whole-brain radiation (C) treatment is for patients who have a malignancy, or more commonly a lymphoma, of the brain which is also common in AIDS patients. Amphotericin B (D) treatment is for patients who have cryptococcal meningitis. This patient does not exhibit any meningeal signs. This patient did not have a stroke. His blood pressure is normal and he does not require antihypertensive medication (E).

6. **(C)** Liver dysfunction is more commonly associated with the anticonvulsant valproic acid and much less commonly with phenytoin. Nystagmus on lateral gaze (A) is universally seen in patients with a therapeutic level of phenytoin and is a good clinical sign that the patient is taking the medication. A morbilliform rash (B) occurs in four percent of patients on phenytoin, and an alternative anticonvulsant should be chosen if this occurs. Gingival hypertrophy (D) is a common side effect of phenytoin. Other side effects are hirsutism, megaloblastic anemia, osteomalacia, lymphadenopathy, and a lupus-like syndrome. Phenytoin is also teratogenic.

7. **(A)** The patient in this case suffers from anorexia nervosa. This condition is a common cause of amenorrhea in the teenage group. Refeeding patients (B) who have been starving should be through a gradual means to avoid refeeding syndrome, a condition that may result

in dangerous electrolyte abnormalities. Depression (C) and isolation are common associated features of anorexia. Death (D) from this condition may result from effects of malnutrition as well as from suicide.

8. **(D)** Electroencephalography is a useful test to diagnose the presence and etiology of seizure disorders; however, it is not useful in the acute management of this condition. Airway and venous access (A) should be obtained immediately in patients presenting in status epilepticus to maintain oxygenation and to administer medications intravenously. Intravenous diazepam (B) should be the first drug administered to attempt to stop the seizure, as other epileptic medications will require more time prior to the onset of action. Patients in whom the etiology of the seizure is unknown should be administered dextrose (C). Oxygen (E) should be administered to improve the cyanosis commonly present in status epilepticus.

9. **(E)** In patients with grand-mal seizure, the postictal phase may last for several hours and is characterized by somnolence and fatigue. A common characteristic of grand-mal seizures is a loss of sphincter tone and incontinence (A). Seizures with minimal motor activity characterized by a blank stare (B) are characteristic of petite-mal seizures and are common in children. Prodromal symptoms (C) are common in patients with grand-mal seizures and can include a change in mood or a sense of apprehension. Febrile seizures (D) are common in children, but uncommon in adults.

10. **(E)** Seizures are often difficult to distinguish from syncope; however, these entities can be distinguished by certain clinical features and tests. A loss of awareness is not one of these, as this is present in many types of seizures, as well as in syncope. Electroencephalography (A) allows for the determination of a seizure focus. It is normal in patients with vasovagal syncope. Pulse rate during a seizure (B) is increased, while it is commonly reduced during a vasovagal syncopal episode. Motor activity (C) is absent during a syncopal episode and is increased during most seizure episodes. Warning symptoms (D) commonly occur prior to seizure episodes, as well as syncopal episodes, before which patients may feel diaphoretic and dizzy.

11. **(A)** Of the electrolyte abnormalities given, hypocalcemia most commonly induces seizures. Hypokalemia (B) more commonly manifests as muscular weakness and cardiac arrhythmia. Hypercalcemia (C) more commonly manifests with numerous symptoms, chiefly involving the heart, neuromuscular system, central nervous system, and GI tract. Hyperkalemia (D) manifests as cardiac dysrhythmias. Hypophosphatemia (E) may present with muscle weakness and hematological abnormalities.

12. **(E)** With a patient spiking a temperature to 104.1°F, especially a nursing home patient, a cause for the fever should be sought. By performing blood cultures (A), a chest X-ray (B), a sputum culture (C), and a complete blood count (D) you can evaluate the most common reasons for a temperature, as well as look for an elevation in the white blood cell count. There is no need currently to obtain an electrocardiogram (E).

13. **(B)** Lead poisoning occurs with excess exposure to lead. The symptoms are abdominal pain, anorexia, weakness, headache, nausea, vomiting, and constipation. Physical examination reveals a "lead line" in the gingiva, papilledema, ocular palsies, wrist drop, convulsions, delirium, and even coma.

14. **(A)** Hyperglycemia is the most likely cause of the mild reduction in sodium in this patient and occurs as a compensatory mechanism to main serum osmolarity in conditions of hyperglycemia, which are common in diabetics with infection. Nephrogenic diabetes insipidus (B) is a cause of hyperglycemia, not hypoglycemia. SIADH (C) does cause hypoglycemia, but is unlikely to present in this manner. Psychogenic polydypsia (D) is another cause of hyponatremia, but generally occurs in psychiatrically unstable patients.

15. **(D)** The vagus nerve, cranial nerve X, is tested by asking to raise his uvula. Laryngeal muscles can also be tested for the vagus. Testing gag reflex evaluates CN IX, glossopharyngeal nerve, and recurrent laryngeal branch of the CN X enervating laryngeal muscle.

16. **(B)** The facial nerve, cranial nerve VII, is tested partly by having the patient show you his

lower teeth. This tests the marginal mandibular branch. The other four branches may also be tested separately. These are the temporal, zygomatic, buccal, and cervical.

17. **(A)** The trigeminal nerve, cranial nerve V, is tested by the motor strength of the temporalis masseter muscles. The sensory branches (ophthalmic, maxillary, and mandibular) may also be tested individually over each anatomic area.

18. **(E)** The accessory nerve, cranial nerve XI, also known as the spinal accessory nerve, is tested by having the patient raise his shoulders or turn his head against resistance, testing the trapezius and sternocleidomastoid. The acoustic nerve (C), cranial nerve VIII, is divided into a cochlear and vestibular portion, which can be individually tested by tests of hearing and nystagmus, respectively.

19. **(D)** The mainstay treatments for symptomatic rheumatoid arthritis remains NSAIDs and glucocorticoids. The other medications are used in an attempt to slow down the progression of the disease.

20. **(A)** Young women who have heavy menses, and especially those with decreased intake of meat, can easily become iron deficient, which can be treated by oral supplementation. Blood transfusion (D) isn't necessary unless someone exhibits hemodynamic or cardiac compromise. Erythropoietin injection (E) won't help until the iron stores are refilled. B12 injections (B), as well, won't help unless the patient has pernicious anemia.

21. **(D)** The X-ray in panel B demonstrates marked dilatation of the central pulmonary arteries and right ventricular enlargement, which were not present on the X-ray taken three years earlier. The X-ray in panel B is consistent with pulmonary hypertension. Conditions that must be excluded include primary pulmonary hypertension, congenital heart disease, such as mitral stenosis, pulmonary thromboembolic disease, and pulmonary venoocclusive disease [(A), (B), (C), and (E)]. Persons with left-to-right shunts may develop progressive pulmonary vascular disease with its associated pulmonary hypertension. With disease progression, the worsening pulmonary hypertension results in a decline of the left-to-right shunt (D).

22. **(D)** An intoxicated patient is not competent to make decisions such as this.

23. **(B)** All of the other tests may be necessary but none can be performed on an agitated, combative patient. DTs is the likeliest explanation for this patient's acute decompensation.

24. **(E)** A bone scan would not be helpful at this time, but all of the other tests would be. The major differential diagnoses to be considered in this setting are gout, precipitated by surgery and presumably cessation of antihyperuricosemic agents, and septic arthritis, after what may have been a "dirty" operation.

25. **(C)** Chronic glomerulonephritis is a cause of secondary hypertension rather than a sequela of essential hypertension. Left ventricular hypertrophy is a common sequela of long-standing hypertension (A). Hypertension affects the retinal artery and its branches, the sequelae of which can be visualized on fundoscopic exam as retinal hemorrhages (B). Atheromatous plaques form in small- and medium-sized vessels in numerous vascular beds secondary to essential hypertension. These beds include the coronary and cerebrovascular circulation [(D) and (E)].

26. **(D)** Oral allopurinol does not play a role in the acute management of gouty arthritis, but can be useful after the acute attack subsides to reduce serum uric acid levels. Oral colchicine (A) at a maximum dose of 6 mg is often effective. Intravenous colchicine (E) may also be effective in cases where the oral dose is not. Oral indomethacin (B) and other NSAIDs can be effective for acute management. Intra-articular triamcinolone (C) should be reserved for uniarticular cases that do not respond to oral therapy.

27. **(B)** Waldenstrom's macroglobulinemia (primary macroglobulinemia) is associated with uncontrolled proliferation of lymphocytes and plasma cells, of which a large number of high molecular-weight monoclonal IgM proteins is produced. Retinal hemorrhages, exudates, and venous congestion with vascular segmentation may occur. All patients have anemia. Males are more commonly affected. Multiple myeloma (A) can present similarly, but plasma cells and immunoglobulins other than IgM are the predominant

cells in the marrow and lytic lesions, renal failure, and unexplained skeletal pain, and recurrent bacterial infections are common. Plasmacytoma of bone (C) consists of a tumor containing monoclonal plasma cells and no evidence of M-protein. This disease is not generalized but confined to one section of the bone. It is also called solitary myeloma. Chronic lymphocytic leukemia (D) can also present with anemia, pallor, hepatosplenomegaly, and lymphadenopathy. Elevation of the serum IgM protein is not present. Hyperviscosity syndrome (E) presents as chronic nasal bleeding, oozing from the gums, and blurry vision. IgM protein is not found in this syndrome.

28.　**(C)**　Primary pulmonary hypertension occurs in a population of less than 40 years of age. It presents with progressive dyspnea and right heart failure, rather than acute shortness of breath as in this case. Pulmonary embolus, unstable angina, aortic dissection, and aortic stenosis can all present with chest pain in a more acute manner, as described in this case [(A), (B), (D), and (E)].

29.　**(A)**　An rsR' pattern in V1 is seen characteristically in right bundle branch block. The most common EKG finding with pulmonary embolus is sinus tachycardia (B). Right ventricular strain pattern (C) can be seen due to the elevation in pulmonary pressure. Nonspecific T-wave changes (E) and a small Q-wave in III (D) are also common.

30.　**(E)**　Ventilation-perfusion scan would be the appropriate next test to obtain. Although it is the gold standard, pulmonary angiogram (A) is invasive and is, therefore, reserved for cases that cannot be definitively diagnosed by ventilation-perfusion scan. Doppler studies (B), plethysmography (C), and venography (D) are all methods of diagnosing deep venous thrombosis (DVT). Although they are of utility in helping to make the diagnosis of pulmonary embolus if positive, a negative test for DVT does not rule out the possibility of pulmonary embolism.

31.　**(A)**　Treatment consists of the immediate initiation of IV heparin by bolus infusion and continuous drip, followed by the initiation of Coumadin therapy. Immediate initiation of Coumadin therapy without heparin (B) would require at least two days before adequate anticoagulation could be obtained and, additionally, could be dangerous because of the risk of "Coumadin necrosis" in pa-

tients with Protein C or Protein S deficiency. Subcutaneous heparin at the dose proposed (C) is useful only for prophylaxis of DVT, not treatment of PE. Fibrinolytic therapy (D) is reserved for very select cases of massive PE, and is not appropriate in this patient.

32.　**(E)**　Chronic liver disease is associated with coagulopathy and a tendency for bleeding rather than thrombosis of large vessels. Bed rest (A), hip surgery (C), and pregnancy (D) all predispose to PE due to the presence of venous stasis, a risk factor for DVT. Pancreatic cancer (B) creates a hypercoagulable state and thus predisposes toward the development of PE.

33.　**(A)**　The most common source of pulmonary thromboembolic material is the deep ileofemoral vein. The popliteal vein (B) is also a potential source, but less common than the ileofemoral vein. Superficial vein thrombophlebitis (C) does not predispose to PE. Aortic mural thrombus (D) can also develop into PE, but this is less common.

34.　**(E)**　Venogram with intravenous contrast is the gold standard for the diagnosis of DVT. Nuclide venogram (A) has a high incidence of false positives. Plethysmography (D) is useful for diagnosing DVT above the knee, while Doppler study is more sensitive for clots below the knee (C). Fibrinogen scan (B) is also sensitive, but not as specific as plethysmography studies.

35.　**(D)**　Inflammation of the pericardium is associated with pericarditis, but not commonly associated with PE. Although more commonly associated with right-heart failure, massive pulmonary embolus can result in left-heart failure as well (A). Pulmonary vasoconstriction develops secondary to mechanical factors as well as the release of humoral factors, and the increased right-heart afterload may result in right heart failure [(B) and (E)]. Infarction of lung segments abutting the pleura (C) result in pleural irritation and pleuritic chest pain.

36.　**(D)**　Hyperbilirubinemia can lead to blue-green or even orange urine.

37.　**(C)**　Tetracycline ingestion can lead to yellow urine.

38.　**(B)**　Urinary tract infection can lead to cloudy white urine.

39. **(A)** Excessive fluid intake will lead to colorless urine due to its low concentration. Hematuria of any cause will lead to red urine (E). It can come from trauma, neoplasm, or infection.

40. **(B)** Sutures that are placed on the face should be removed in three to five days. This will allow the skin to heal while eliminating the formation of suture marks on an esthetic part of the body. Adhesive strips should be applied after the removal of the sutures, because the wound has not acquired enough strength yet to resist the forces of facial animation.

41. **(B)** Certain disease complexes are positively associated with certain HLA antigens within the population. Systemic lupus erythematosus is not associated with an increased incidence of the HLA B27 antigen. Rather, it is associated with an increased incidence of HLA DR3 and DR4. All of the other choices are associated with HLA B27 with the relative risk greatest for ankylosing spondylitis.

42. **(C)** Except for hypernatremia, all the other factors, whether desirable or undesirable, are associated with cardiopulmonary bypass.

43. **(D)** A fourth-degree burn is a full thickness burn into the subcutaneous tissues down to muscle and bone. The treatment for this is usually amputation or surgical resection of the affected part.

44. **(A)** A first-degree burn is a partial thickness burn into the epidermis and is somewhat akin to a sunburn. It can be effectively treated with topical agents.

45. **(C)** A third-degree burn is a full thickness burn through the entire dermis. The skin is non-viable and will not reepithelialize. The burned skin needs to be excised. The resultant wound may be left to contract on its own, or a skin graft may be applied to hasten healing and decrease contraction.

46. **(B)** A second-degree burn goes further into the dermis. These may be able to reepithelialize, but often if they get secondarily infected, they will progress to a third-degree burn and, therefore, require excision.

47. **(E)** This patient has systemic lupus erythematosus, which is a multisystemic disease of unknown origin associated with tissues and organs damaged by deposition of pathogenic antibodies and immune complexes. Virtually any organ can be affected by inflammation. The antinuclear ribonucleoprotein antibody serologic test is usually positive and elevated in patients with mixed connective tissue disease, not lupus. The ANA are elevated in 95% of patients with lupus, but it is not very specific. Anti-double stranded DNA antibody titers (B) are extremely useful in determining if the patient has lupus-induced glomerulonephritis. It is a sensitive and specific assay. A false-positive VDRL level (C) is usually seen in SLE patients because of the autoimmune mechanisms involved. A true-positive VDRL test is suggestive of syphilis infection. The anti-sm antibody test (D) is also positive in lupus patients as well as the presence of the LE cell on the peripheral smear, which is virtually diagnostic for SLE.

48. **(C)** All suspicious pigmented lesions should be biopsied. The biopsy should be incisional or excisional, depending on the size. A shave should not be performed with a pigmented lesion because it could alter the staging. Reassurance is not advised until a pathologic diagnosis is back (A). The lesion is not infectious and, as such, a culture and sensitivity is not necessary (B). Unless bony involvement is suspected, an arm X-ray is not indicated (D). Steroids would not be appropriate until a diagnosis is made (E).

49. **(B)** With no axillary lymphadenopathy, a wide local resection is adequate treatment for this lesion. Follow-up alone is not appropriate (A). Lymph node resection (C), radiation therapy (D), and chemotherapy (E) are not indicated with this tumor as it presents.

50. **(B)** Patient education after a cancer cure is vitally important. This patient is still at risk for melanoma and must be precautioned. Risk factors, such as sun exposure, must be reduced. Wearing adequate clothing is sufficient; she does not need to avoid the sunlight totally (C). Steroids (D) are not warranted.

51. **(D)** The chest X-ray shows a diffuse reticulonodular pattern. Bronchoalveolar lavage is helpful in this case, showing small budding yeasts. The clinical history of travel to an endemic area

also suggests infection with histoplasma (D). Although also a yeast, *Candida albicans* (C) typically presents as thrush or esophagitis. Pneumonia by *Candida albicans*, which is extremely rare, occurs by hematogenous dissemination. Either wet mounts or Gram-stained smears of material from the affected lesions show budding yeast with characteristic pseudohyphae. *Streptococcus pneumoniae (E)*, another cause of pneumonia, appear as Gram-positive cocci in chains. The presence of intranuclear inclusions and multinucleated giant cells on Giemsa-, Wright-, or Papanicolaou-stained specimens is suggestive of *Herpes simplex* (B). In *Pneumocystis carinii* (A) infections, methenamine silver stains the cyst wall. Wright-Giemsa stains stain trophozoites, nuclei of cysts, and intermediate forms. Immunofluorescent and inmunoperoxidase staining are currently gaining in popularity.

52. **(D)** Tachycardia may be due to such factors as pain, fever, and hypovolemia, among others. It is not itself an indication for intubation. All the other factors represent profound physiologic derangements that are indicative of the need for ventilatory support.

53. **(C)** Breast self-examination is important in the early diagnosis of breast cancer. A breast mass that is felt should immediately be evaluated. It should not be ignored (A). A mammogram (B) or biopsy (E) should not be performed until the doctor confirms the presence of a mass. A mastectomy (D) should not be performed until the diagnosis is cancer, and only if that is to be the treatment.

54. **(B)** Stein-Leventhal syndrome is characterized by enlarged cystic ovaries, amenorrhea, and obesity. This syndrome is part of the broad spectrum of symptoms seen in women with polycystic ovarian disease, which also include mild hirsutism and chronic anovulation. An elevated LH level with a normal FSH level is associated with this syndrome. Prolactin-secreting tumors (A) of the pituitary gland are associated with galactorrhea and amenorrhea. An MRI scan of the brain can diagnose this disorder by detecting the micro- or macroadenoma. Infertility is common. Hirsutism is rare. Hypothalamic hypothyroidism (C) is a rare disorder associated with low thyroid-releasing hormone levels, and low or normal TSH levels. Gonadotropin levels are usually low.

Cushing's syndrome (D) is associated with obesity and hirsutism along with amenorrhea. The FSH and LH levels are usually normal. The ACTH level is elevated in Cushing's disease. Premature ovarian failure (E) is associated with low estrogen levels and elevated FSH and LH levels, via the negative feedback system. Premature loss of oocytes prior to the age of 40 characterizes hypergonadotropic amenorrhea. Amenorrhea and infertility are common.

55. **(C)** The decreased FEV1 makes this an obstructive disease. The fact that it completely reverses with bronchodilator treatment makes it a reactive airway disease, as opposed to a chronic obstructive pulmonary disease.

56. **(D)** Her symptoms of fever, cough productive of rusty sputum, and rigors is consistent with *Streptococcus pneumoniae* pneumonia.

57. **(B)** The findings of no chest pain, positive smoking history, and flattened diaphragms on chest radiograph are all consistent with chronic obstructive pulmonary disease.

58. **(E)** The absence of physical findings on auscultation, and the absence of chills and fever make pneumonia less likely. The yellow-green sputum implies some infectious etiology, such as acute bronchitis.

59. **(D)** Introducing normal saline drops to each nares will only aggravate the symptoms of allergic rhinitis and will not alleviate the inflammation. The newest and most effective treatment available now to relieve the symptoms of allergic rhinitis are inhaled nasal steroids (A) such as Beconase and Nasocort. This has been shown to decrease the inflammation and reduce the number of eosinophils in the nasal discharge. Oral antihistamines (H1 blockers), such as Terfenidine and Loratadine, have been shown to decrease the symptoms of allergic rhinitis (B) by blocking the receptor on the mast cells so that degranulation does not take place and the inflammatory cells are not released to cause symptoms. Staying in an air-conditioned room or car (C) helps to keep the patient from being exposed to pollen or ragweed, which is the offending allergen causing the symptoms. Alcohol intake, even in moderate amounts,

along with ingestion of antihistamines, would cause excessive sedation and drowsiness (E). The combination is not advised.

60. **(C)** Hepatitis A is a self-limited infection, which is almost always transmitted by the fecal-oral route, with an incubation period of two to six weeks. Fecal shedding of the virus occurs over a two to three week period, declining with the appearance of anti-HAV in the serum (A). This coincides with the peak level of serum transaminases (B). Serum antibodies are initially predominantly IgM in type (E). This IgM response is rapidly followed by an IgG antibody response. IgG anti-HAV persists in the serum for many years (D). No HAV carrier state has been described following acute infection with hepatitis A (C).

61. **(B)** Zollinger-Ellison syndrome is associated with multiple endocrine neoplasia syndrome type I in 20% of patients. Symptoms of abdominal pain and diarrhea are secondary to an elevated basal acid output and recurrence of disease. Serum gastrin, measured by radioimmunoassay, is the most reliable diagnostic test. A calcium or secretin stimulation test can confirm the diagnosis by helping to elevate the gastrin and basal acid output. The ulcers in this syndrome are located in unusual locations such as postbulbar jejunum or duodenum. Pancreatitis (A) would present with severe abdominal pain and nausea or vomiting. Serum amylase and lipase levels would be elevated, not gastrin levels. *H. pylori*-induced duodenal ulcer (C) would present with epigastric pain, but usually H2 blockers would temporarily relieve the pain. The serum gastrin level would not be elevated to such a degree. Multiple endocrine neoplasia type II (D) is associated with medullary thyroid carcinoma, pheochromocytoma, and parathyroid hyperplasia. Zollinger-Ellison syndrome is affiliated with MEN type I, which is more likely to be characterized by parathyroid and pituitary adenomas, and pancreatic islet cell tumor. Celiac sprue (E) would present with malabsorption symptoms secondary to dietary intake of wheat gluten. Serum gastrin levels are usually normal in this disorder.

62. **(C)** Current prevalence of spousal abuse is estimated as 10% of North American women. Domestic violence (e.g., spousal abuse) occurs in families of every racial and religious background and in all socioeconomic strata of society (A). The violence will recur, and when it does it will likely be more severe. Fear of escalation of violence and even murder are common reasons for women to stay in the abusive relationship (D). Group psychotherapy appears to work best for abusers (E). It facilitates the sharing of experiences with other persons who have had similar experience.

63. **(E)** In this young patient, with walk-in pneumonia and with fluffy infiltrates on chest radiograph, *Mycoplasma* is the most likely causative organism. *Strep. pneumoniae* and *H. influenzae* pneumonia usually present with more marked complaints and with a consolidated infiltrate on chest radiograph. *Legionella* is extremely rare in the young patient and classically affects older smokers. Tuberculosis is usually more indolent and classically presents with upper lobe infiltrates.

64. **(D)** Screening for gestational diabetes should be performed at 28 weeks. Other components of the 28-week screen are a repeat screen for Rh and a repeat CBC.

65. **(A)** This patient is likely to recover if he can be supported through this acute episode. Intubation is necessary at this point and is what you should recommend.

66. **(A)** The radiographic study of the small bowel demonstrates multiple jejunal diverticula. A malabsorption syndrome may result due to bacterial overgrowth within these diverticula in a manner analogous to a blind loop. The bacterial overgrowth syndrome usually responds to treatment with oral antibiotics. Usually, a 10-day course of an effective antimicrobial program is adequate to correct the malabsorption for months. Some persons may need repeat courses of treatment (A). Nutritional therapy, such as medium-chain triglyceride oil and vitamin supplementation, is recommended by some experts. Pancreatic enzyme supplements are recommended in cases of malabsorption due to pancreatic insufficiency (E). It has been speculated that diets low in fiber are an important etiological factor in the development of colonic diverticula. However, the role of dietary fiber in the treatment of small intestinal diverticular disease requires clinical studies (D). Surgical consultation is required only if the

diverticula bleed, perforate, or become acutely inflamed (B). There is no clinical indication to consult an oncologist (C).

67. **(A)** Bacterial meningitis generally presents with a more dramatic clinical presentation, including severe headache, high fever, and acute onset with more rapid progression. This is a classic presentation for Lyme disease (B). Leptospirosis (C) may have such nonspecific symptoms early in the course, although conjunctival suffusion is also common. This is also a classic presentation for influenza syndrome (D), although cough may also be present. Acute mononucleosis related to EBV may present in this manner, often accompanied by hepatosplenomegaly.

68. **(A)** A positive Lyme titer may be seen in any spirochete illness, including syphilis. It may also occur in certain autoimmune conditions associated with a positive rheumatoid factor or antinuclear antibody. Mycoplasma pneumonia (B) is not a spirochete infection. Psittacosis (C) is caused by a *Chlamydia* infection and may present in a similar fashion, but is not associated with a positive Lyme antibody. Herpes infection (D) is not associated with positive Lyme titers.

69. **(B)** Erythema chronicum migrans is the name of the annular erythematous rash, which develops at the site of the tick bite 3-30 days after exposure. Erythema nodosum (A) is a rash, which develops most commonly in the lower extremities, usually immune complex-mediated and associated with conditions such as inflammatory bowel disease or tuberculosis. Erythema multiforme (C) is a rash composed of "target lesions," which may blister and is associated with drug reactions, infections, or malignancy. Erythema marginatum (D) is the rash associated with rheumatic fever.

70. **(E)** The pathogenic organism in Lyme disease is the spirochete, *Borrelia burgdorferi*, a tick-transmitted organism. *Chlamydia trachomatis* (A) in its different strains can cause conjunctivitis and blindness, nonspecific urethritis, and lymphogranuloma venereum. *Ureaplasma urealyticum* (B) is a common cause of nonspecific urethritis. *Rickettsia prowazekii* (C) is the cause of typhus. *Blastomyces dermatitidis* (D) is a fungal pathogen causing pulmonary and skin involvement.

71. **(D)** Streptomycin is not of clinical utility in the treatment of Lyme disease. Amoxicillin (A) is the preferred treatment in pregnant or lactating women or children under the age of eight. Tetracycline (B), 250 mg QID, is effective treatment in adults. Erythromycin (C) is useful in patients with allergy to penicillin. Ceftriaxone (E) is effective for more advanced disease.

72. **(C)** Cranial neuritis or, in this case, Bell's palsy, is one of the most common neurologic manifestations of Lyme disease. Vasculitis stroke (A) is uncommon in Lyme disease and does not present with a facial nerve palsy as described in this patient. Encephalitis (B), transverse myelitis (D), and sensory radiculopathy (E) may occur in Lyme disease, but do not cause a facial nerve palsy.

73. **(D)** Although Lyme disease may occasionally cause a mild hepatitis, jaundice is rare. First-degree A-V block (A) is one of the most common cardiac manifestations of Lyme disease. Lymphadenopathy (B) is also common in Lyme disease. Oligoarthritis and joint effusion, including the knee (D), are common. Acrodermatitis (E) is a red violaceous skin lesion, which may develop in tertiary Lyme disease.

74. **(B)** Exposure to ticks should be avoided by covering exposed skin in the outdoors and using insect repellent. Prophylactic vaccination (A) against Lyme disease is not currently available. Prophylactic antibiotics (C) prior to camping trips is not advisable. Avoid skin contact with the patient (D). Avoiding close contact with house pets (E) is not necessary, as the vector is carried by the deer and the mouse.

75. **(C)** The normal glucose levels rule out diabetes mellitus [(A) and (B)]. When the patient is exposed to water deprivation, he still cannot concentrate his urine, as evidenced by his urine osmolality of 150. This rules out psychogenic polydipsia (D) and makes the diagnosis of diabetes insipidus. Diabetes insipidus can be caused by lithium.

76. **(D)** Although estrogen replacement therapy can decrease the incidence of myocardial infarction (A), stroke (B), osteoporosis (C), and death from any cause (E), the incidence of endometrial and breast cancer are slightly increased.

77. **(E)** His symptoms are classic for cluster headaches and can continue intermittently for days and recur years later. Migraine headaches (A) are classically described as throbbing, and tension headaches (B) are classically described as a tightening.

78. **(A)** Anuria is defined as an output of less than 100 cc per day in an adult. Oliguria is defined as a urine output of less than 500 cc per day in an adult. The reasons for anuria and oliguria are further divided into prerenal, renal, and postrenal.

79. **(C)** Vertigo is the sensation of a patient's surroundings whirling when his eyes are open. Syncope (A) is a fainting episode. Dizziness (B) is a light-headed feeling related to orthostasis. Presbycusis (D) is the loss of hearing due to aging. Entrapment (E) is the process of an extraocular muscle getting trapped in the orbit, limiting motion.

80. **(A)** Acute tubular necrosis results from severe hypoxia and ischemia to the distal and proximal renal tubules and from injury from toxins as well. Ischemia of the nephrons are present in septic shock and, subsequently, brown casts are found in the urinary sediment. Oliguria usually accompanies acute tubular necrosis.

81. **(C)** This patient has rhabdomyolysis, which is necrosis of the skeletal muscle tissue from either trauma or a viral infection. The muscle enzyme, creatinine phosphokinase, is released into the bloodstream and, thus, elevated. The urine dipstick would be positive for blood, but there would be no detectable red blood cells in the urine on microscopy. The pigment myoglobin is present in the urine.

82. **(B)** This young female patient has systemic lupus erythematosus, which is associated with glomerulonephritis and kidney damage secondary to autoimmune mechanisms. Immune complexes bind to the glomerular basement membrane. Steroids and cyclophosphamide are the treatments of choice. Red blood cell casts are associated with nephritis.

83. **(E)** This debilitated gentleman has pulmonary tuberculosis, which can also be disseminated and involve other organs such as the bone, heart, and kidneys. Interstitial nephritis from tu-

berculosis can appear as white blood cells in the urinary sediment without bacteria growing on the urine culture. This is called a sterile pyuria.

84. **(B)** There has been some evidence to support the use of HMG-CoA reductase inhibitors in the primary prevention of coronary artery disease. Also, tight control of hypertension can decrease the incidence of coronary artery disease. Although aspirin (C) has been shown to be effective in secondary prevention of coronary artery disease after a myocardial infarction, it has not been shown to be effective in primary prevention.

85. **(D)** Pulmonic regurgitation presents as a basal diastolic murmur.

86. **(E)** Mitral stenosis presents as an apical diastolic murmur.

87. **(B)** Ventricular septal defect presents as a midprecordial systolic murmur.

88. **(A)** Aortic stenosis presents as a basal systolic murmur.

89. **(B)** Hyporesonant lungs are not a sign of pulmonary emphysema. Pulmonary emphysema is the result of loss of interstial elasticity and interalveolar septa leading to air trapping. The volume of the lungs is increased. Signs include a barrel chest (A), hyperresonant lungs (C), rales (D), and decreased breath sounds (E).

90. **(E)** Knowledge of her childhood vaccination history would not be especially helpful at this stage.

91. **(C)** In a patient with an acutely swollen joint, the first thing that must be done is to determine whether the joint is infected. This can be accomplished only by joint aspiration.

92. **(D)** In a setting such as this, special handling of the fluid sample is necessary to maximize the chances of growing the suspected organism.

93. **(B)** These lesions are characteristic of DGI in a patient presenting in this manner.

94. **(D)** While the skin lesions can contain live organisms and be infective, it is very unusual to grow the gonococcus from them.

95. **(B)** Patients with DGI who have joint effusions must be presumed, at least initially, to have an infected joint and should be treated with intravenous antibiotics in the hospital at least until response is evident. If the joint proves not to be frankly infected, oral antibiotics can be substituted.

96. **(D)** The Board of Health or similar institution must be notified. They will then trace and treat contacts. The only individuals at risk are sexual contacts, not co-workers or other casual contacts.

97. **(C)** These lesions typically resolve spontaneously without scarring.

98. **(A)** When a young patient presents with gradually increasing shortness of breath and has bilateral interstitial infiltrates on chest radiograph, PCP pneumonia must be on the differential diagnosis and an HIV test should be considered.

99. **(D)** Hypercalcemia is a classic cause of shortened Q-T intervals.

100. **(B)** This lesion is unlikely to be related to the patient's metabolic disturbance, and its pursuit at this point is not necessary.

101. **(A)** A list of all the medications the patient has been ingesting is very important.

102. **(D)** Excess ingestion of vitamin D is a well-described cause of hypercalcemia.

103. **(E)** Spinal anesthesia can be utilized for any surgery below about the T7 to T8 dermatome. Above this, a block can have undesirable cardiac respiratory side effects. Surgery of the cervical region with spinal anesthesia would also lead to respiratory insufficiency and/or failure.

104. **(A)** A high oral glucose challenge test should be followed up with a three-hour oral glucose tolerance test. If two out of three of the hourly values are elevated, the patient has gestational diabetes. Before considering insulin therapy (B) or a strict ADA diet (D), one needs to confirm the suspected diagnosis, as mentioned above. Oral hypoglycemics (C) are contraindicated in pregnancy. Elevated blood sugar is not a normal finding in a low-risk pregnancy (E) and needs further evaluation.

105. **(A)** While all of the five choices are associated with diabetic pregnancies, congenital anomalies are the major cause of perinatal mortality for the infant of the diabetic mother.

106. **(C)** An IVP is not indicated at this point, but all of the other tests are useful and indicated in this patient.

107. **(C)** A family history of a connective tissue disease is an important piece of information in this patient.

108. **(D)** All of the findings can be explained by, or are consistent with, lupus.

109. **(B)** Nephrotic syndrome is often found in patients with lupus. The absence of a positive urine sediment makes glomerulonephritis (A), which can be found in lupus, unlikely. The other conditions are not consistent with the clinical presentation.

110. **(D)** Positive anti-DNA antibodies are often associated with active SLE. Low complement levels, high sedimentation rate, and other autoantibodies are often seen with active disease. Elevated CPK (C) would be unusual.

111. **(E)** Lupus cerebritis is often seen in patients with active disease and can present with new seizures.

112. **(A)** High-dose prednisone (60 mg. or above) is the first line of treatment for acute lupus. Cyclosporine (C), cyclophosphamide (E), or other immunosuppressive agents might be added to it. Nonsteroidals (B) are merely symptomatic in this condition. Low-dose prednisone (D) is not helpful in active lupus.

113. **(C)** A patient with lupus and a history of pleurisy and a negative chest physical examination often has a normal chest roentgenogram. However, one should obtain the radiograph because sometimes a pulmonary process can be seen before it is heard through the stethoscope.

114. **(A)** With the history of ascites, when someone presents with fever, the ascites should always be tapped to rule out spontaneous bacterial peritonitis, especially with the classic symptoms of nausea, vomiting, and sometimes increased

hepatic encephalopathy. The diagnosis is made on a cell count of greater than 500 cells or greater than 250 polymorphonuclear cells.

115. **(D)** Guillain-Barre syndrome is an acute immune polyneuropathy which mainly affects the motor nerves. It is associated with a prior upper respiratory infection or camplobacter jejuni. Death can occur because this neurologic disease can cause paralysis of the respiratory system. Myasthenia gravis (A) is an autoimmune disease caused by circulating antibodies against the acetylocholine receptors in the postsynaptic muscle membranes. It presents initially with extraocular muscle weakness causing ptosis and diplopia. Multiple sclerosis (B) can present initially with optic neuritis. Cerebral spinal-fluid analysis reveals oligoclonal bands, and the CT of the brain reveals white matter lesions. Steroids are the treatment of choice initially. Shy-Drager syndrome (C) is caused by degeneration of the central autonomic neurons. Amyotrophic lateral sclerosis (E) presents initially as upper extremity fasiculations. The cerebral spinal-fluid analysis is normal. It is a motor neuron disease with degeneration of the anterior horn cells of the spinal cord. Early on, deep tendon reflexes are preserved.

116. **(C)** The first teeth to erupt in a child are the central incisors, and they erupt at about six months of age. The next to erupt, in approximate order, are the lateral incisors (7-10 months), the first molars (12-16 months), the canines (16-20 months) and, finally, the second molars (20-30 months). There are only 20 deciduous teeth in the child.

117. **(A)** The mandibular central incisors will erupt first, and these are in the anterior mandible, or lower jaw.

118. **(B)** Chest pain that worsens on inspiration usually occurs from a rib problem that may be seen with a rib fracture (A) or costochondritis (C). Intercostal myositis (D) will also simulate this pain. Shingles (E) or recurrent zoster will give pain from its dermatologic sequelae. While a myocardial infarct (B) will give substernal chest pain, it will occur all the time and is not solely related to inspiration.

119. **(A)** Calcium oxalate and calcium phosphate comprise the majority of urinary stones. The other stones are less common. About 85% of urinary stones are radiopaque (as opposed to gallstones, where only 10-15% are seen on X-ray).

120. **(A)** The most common causative organism for pneumonia in cystic fibrosis patients is *Pseudomonas aeruginosa*, although other organisms can occur.

121. **(A)** In hemolytic anemias, the life span of the red cell is reduced from the normal 90-120 days (A). In hereditary spherocytosis, molecular abnormalities of the protein of the cytoskeleton are present. Ankyrin is a protein that links spectrin to protein 3. Deficiencies of both spectrin and ankyrin are present. The degree of spectrin/ankyrin deficiency correlates with the degree of spherocytosis, as measured by the osmotic fragility test; it also correlates with the severity of hemolysis and response to splenectomy (B). Defects in protein 3 present only in the dominant form of hereditary spherocytosis (C). As the red blood cells age, they gradually lose a portion of their lipid bilayer, thus becoming more spherocytic (D). The spheroidal contour and rigid structure of these red blood cells inhibit their passage through the spleen. In the toxic environment of the splenic cords, further loss of the cell membrane occurs. This "splenic conditioning" produces a subpopulation of hyperspheroidal cells (E).

122. **(A)** Discussing this step with the family is the appropriate course of action.

123. **(B)** Genu valgum (knock knee) is lateral deviation of the leg from midline and usually occurs bilaterally. Genu varum (bowleg) (A) is the condition when the legs deviate toward the midline. Genu recurvatum (C) occurs when the knees are fixed in hyperextension with decreased ability to flex. Genu medialis (D) and genu lateralis (E) are not medical terms.

124. **(C)** The most common cause of genu valgum is prominent development of the medial femoral condyles. Laxity of the knee ligaments may also be responsible. The amount of deviation is measured with the patient standing and the knees next to each other; the distance between the medial malleoli is measured.

125. **(E)** Tumors rarely cause fluid in the knee joint. Fluid may be synovial fluid, pus, or blood.

The most common reasons for fluid in the joint are gout (A), pseudogout (B), trauma (C), and arthritis (D).

126. **(A)** Anserine bursitis results from fluid in the bursa anserina, which is on the medial aspect of the knee. A Morrant-Baker's cyst (B), semimembraneous bursitis (C), and popliteal abscess (D) all occur in the popliteal area. Infrapatellar bursitis (E) occurs as an anterior knee cyst.

127. **(D)** Refusal of a mentally competent individual to follow your medical recommendation is neither illegal nor evidence of insanity. Documentation of your advice and the patient's refusal, with or without his signature, is important.

128. **(B)** Carpal tunnel syndrome is caused by compression of the median nerve. There will be a positive Tinel's sign, which is a tingling sensation over a nerve indicating a lesion or regeneration. There will also be a positive Phalen's sign, which is pain on flexion of the wrist indicating a compression similar to what is going on within the carpal tunnel. Cubital tunnel (A) is compression of the ulnar nerve. de Quervain's disease (C) is a stenosing tenosynovitis of the extensor compartment of the wrist. Dupuytren's disease (D) is a disease of the palmar fascia of the hand, leading to finger contractures. A wrist fracture (E) will present with point tenderness over the fracture, as well as a history of trauma.

129. **(D)** For a median nerve compression, treatment modalities include a cock-up wrist splint (A), steroid injections (B) into the carpal tunnel, surgery (C) to release the transverse carpel ligament, and rest (E). Observation is not indicated, as this is normally a disease of progression.

130. **(D)** Based on the clinical presentation alone, the most likely diagnosis is measles. This condition would have been prevented with an appropriate immunization series. Measles vaccine as a component of MMR should be given at 15 months of age and at four to six years. The other choices are not correct, since none confer lifelong immunity against measles.

131. **(B)** This patient has Marfan's syndrome, which is an autosomal dominant disorder. There is a mutation in the fibrillin gene on chromosome

15. Ectopia lentis, laxity of joints, and aortic root dilatation are common manifestations. Aortic dissection from aortic insufficiency and aortic root dilatation results from elongated chordae tendineae. This is usually the most common cause of mortality. Mitral valve prolapse (A) is present in 85% of the patients with Marfan's syndrome. This is usually asymptomatic. Spontaneous pneumothorax (C) would initially present with shortness of breath and chest pain. Pulmonary emboli (D) is not the most common manifestation in Marfan's syndrome. The patient would present initially with tachypnea. Ventricular arrhythmias (E) cause sudden collapse and death in patients with hypertrophic cardiomyopathy.

132. **(D)** In a young individual who is known to have converted from a negative to a positive PPD, a chest radiograph should be obtained to identify the presence of active pulmonary disease, which would affect the choice of therapy. Repeating the PPD (A) is not advised, since a false-positive would be unusual and repeating a positive test would likely cause the patient a great deal of discomfort at the site of antigen application. There is no reason to check her liver functions (B) at this point in time. Such testing would be beneficial on a regular basis once treatment is initiated to identify early adverse hepatic reactions to drugs. A sputum sample for culture (C) would not be helpful at this time, since it is unlikely to be positive and would take several weeks to grow. Such an individual would not be expected to have infection in her kidneys or bladder, so a urine culture (E) would not be indicated.

133. **(D)** Carcinoma of the prostate gland is the third most common cause of morbidity from cancer in men. It is not usually adenocarcinomas and does not cause gynecomastia unless hormone therapy is given. Cirrhosis of the liver (A) causes hyperestrogenemia due to decreased hepatic extraction of androstenedione, leading to increased conversion of estrone to estradiol, leading to gynecomastia. Spirinolactone (B), cimetidine, digitalis, and phenothiazines are just some of the drugs that cause gynecosmastia. Thyrotoixicosis (C) causes increased production of androstenedione, which is converted to estradiol, and leads to gynecomastia. Germ-cell testicular tumors (E) cause gynecomastia by secreting human chorionic gonadotropin, which in turn increases testicular secretion of estradiol.

134. **(A)** Chronic primary adrenocortical insufficiency is associated with hyperkalemia, hyperreninemia, and hypotension. The hyperpigmentation is secondary to excessive ACTH production from the pituitary gland. Hyporeninemic hypoaldosteronism (B) causes hyperchloremic metabolic acidosis. There is mineralocorticoid deficiency and low renin concentrations, as well as severe hyperkalemia. Cushing's disease (C) is secondary to excess cortisol levels. This can be from an elevation of ACTH from the pituitary gland. Conn's syndrome (D) is primary hyperaldosteronism. This disease causes hypertension, hypernatremia, and hypokalemia. Secondary adrenal insufficiency (E) is from inadequate stimulation of the adrenal cortex by ACTH. Clinically significant mineralocorticoid deficiency is rare. Hyperkalemia and hyperpigmentation are rare.

135. **(C)** Alcoholics may appear sober at blood levels that would produce clinical signs of intoxication in nonhabituated persons, a phenomenon known as tolerance. This occurs because, after repeated exposure to a drug (in this case, ethanol), the body compensates (C). Alcohol withdrawal is characterized by tremulousness, autonomic overactivity, and, in some cases, seizures, hallucinosis, and delirium (A). Wernicke's syndrome is characterized by ophthalmoplegia, ataxia, and mental clouding (B). The "acetaldehyde syndrome" occurs when an alcoholic consumes alcohol while taking disulfiram (D). Blackouts are amnestic episodes, which occur following excessive amounts of alcohol (E).

136. **(A)** Care must be exercised with rewarming to prevent cardiovascular complications. There is a significantly increased susceptibility to ventricular fibrillation between 28-30°C, which may be exacerbated by unnecessary jostling or manipulation (A). At temperatures below 18°C, asystole may supervene (B). There is no increased risk for pulmonary embolism. However, respiratory rate and tidal volume decrease progressively with decreasing temperature (C). Hyperkalemia often occurs and is independent of rewarming (D). Since rebound hypoglycemia may occur with rewarming, hyperglycemia should not be treated (E).

137. **(D)** Due to enzyme damage, renal concentrating ability is lost, producing a very dilute urine (D). Electrolyte abnormalities are common and include hyperkalemia, hyponatremia, and hyperphosphatemia (A). Disseminated intravascular coagulation, as well as thrombocytopenia and granulocytopenia, may also occur (B). Decreased tissue perfusion and hypoxemia produce lactic acidemia, which results in metabolic acidosis (C). Hyperamylasemia may reflect underlying pancreatitis (E).

138. **(B)** This transesophageal echocardiographic study demonstrates two echolucent spaces at the anterior and posterior wall of the aortic root, consistent with abscess cavities (B). Normal endothelium is nonthrombogenic, but when damaged or denuded, it is a potent inducer of coagulation. The sterile thrombus formed on the endothelial surface is known as nonbacterial thrombotic endocarditis (NBTE). Libman-Sacks endocarditis is an NBTE, which occurs in persons with systemic lupus erythematosus (A). Marantic endocarditis is an NBTE, which occurs in persons with chronic wasting illness (E). Septic pulmonary emboli result from endocarditis of the tricuspid valve (C). The Gram-negative fastidious, slow-growing HACEK organisms (*Haemophilus, Actinobacillus, Cardiobacterium, Eikenella, Kingella*) are part of the normal oropharyngeal flora. Subacute endocarditis with very large vegetations is typical of these organisms (D).

139. **(D)** The skin is the most frequent source of microorganisms responsible for endocarditis in injection drug abusers. *Staphylococcus aureus* accounts for over 50% of the cases of endocarditis [(D) and (E)]. *Streptococcus bovis* produces endocarditis in persons with underlying gastrointestinal lesions. Viridans streptococci cause approximately half of the cases of endocarditis in non-intravenous drug abusers and five percent of the case in intravenous drug abusers (A). Fungi, especially *Candida albicans*, account for approximately 5-10% of cases (B). Gram-negative bacilli, especially *Pseudomonas aeruginosa*, also account for approximately 10% of the cases (C).

140. **(D)** In endocarditis, the bacteremia is continuous and characterized by a constant number of organisms per milliliter of blood. It is not related to the height of the person's temperature nor the site of blood sampling [(D) and (A)]. Three

blood cultures should be obtained, at least one hour apart, to demonstrate a continuous bacteremia (B). Only one culture should be obtained from each venipuncture site (E). For fastidious organisms or fungi, the rate of culture positivity is increased if specimens are observed for more than three weeks, with periodic sampling for Gram stain and subculture, even in the absence of turbidity (C).

141. **(D)** This cross-section of a contrast-enhanced computed axial tomographic scan of the abdomen shows bilateral, wedge-shaped, low-density areas in both kidneys, consistent with embolic renal infarction (D). Acute interstitial nephritis secondary to drugs typically presents with oliguria. The urinary sediment usually contains red blood cells and numerous leukocytes. Diagnosis of this diffuse lesion is made by renal biopsy (A). Excessively high levels of drugs may produce acute tubular necrosis, which typically presents with decreased urine flow. Urine sediment contains casts of damaged tubular cells, red blood cells, and inflammatory cells (B). Papillary necrosis typically presents with hematuria and flank or abdominal pain. A "ring shadow" on pyelography is characteristic (C). There is no evidence of cystic disease on this study (E).

142. **(D)** ADH increases water reabsorption (i.e., decreases urine output) by acting on collecting tubules of the kidney. Anti-diuretic hormone antagonists such as demeclocycline inhibit the action of ADH by affecting the insertion of H2O channels into the kidney cell membrane, thereby inhibiting the reabsorption of water. The other answers all imply diuretics which affect salt concentration directly and water absorption indirectly. Carbonic anhydrase inhibitors (A) such as acetazolamide inhibit carbonic hydrase in the proximal convoluted tubule cells, which results in bicarbonate depletion and resultant increased water secretion into the lumen. This causes diuresis. Loop diuretics (B) also affect salt excretion, but by a different mechanism. Loop diuretics inhibit the cotransporter molecule of sodium, potassium, and chloride, thereby causing more salt ions to be in the lumen of the kidney tubule and by osmotic diffusion, more water to be excreted. Thiazides (C) inhibit sodium transport at the level of the distal convoluted tubule. Potassium-sparing diuretics

(E) affect sodium ion channels and Na+/K+ ATPase pumps in the collecting tubules and cause increased urine flow in this manner.

143. **(C)** Pediculosis is an infestation of the body with lice. *Pediculus humanus capitis* infestation involves the scalp; *Pediculus humanus corporis* primarily infests the body, especially if the clothing is not changed (C). Female lice cement their eggs (nits) firmly to hair or clothing seams. An intensely irritating maculopapular or urticarial rash may occur in sensitized persons. Head lice are most often transmitted directly from person to person, but may also be transmitted by shared headgear or grooming implements. Head infestation is most common in school-aged females with long hair. *Pulex irritans*, the human flea, generally does not infest the body. Rather, the flea sucks blood from the body for a few minutes or hours. Bites usually cause pruritus (A). *Dirofilaria immitis*, the dog heartworm, most typically presents as an asymptomatic isolated pulmonary nodule (B). The bedbug, *Cimex lectularius*, feeds for 3-15 minutes at night or in subdued light. Bites result in pruritic, irritating lesions in sensitized persons (D). *Latrodectus mactans*, the black widow spider, may bite if its web is disturbed. The bite, which may be swollen and erythematous, is often followed by chest tightness and abdominal cramping (E).

144. **(C)** Radiologic findings in psoriatic arthritis may be similar to findings in other rheumatologic diseases, such as rheumatoid arthritis or Reiter's syndrome. Radiologic findings shown include an asymmetric distribution (A), subchondral cysts (B), new periosteal bone formation (D), and marginal erosions (E). Soft tissue swelling is not confined to the joint distribution and accounts for the "sausage digits," which may be seen clinically (C).

145. **(B)** Some lifestyle choices are well-established risk factors that contribute to the development of coronary artery disease. Smoking is one of the most serious culprits. Pacemakers (A) and other advanced medical technology (D) are utilized in a tertiary prevention of the disease. Control of diet (C) and stress (E) is less contributory to declining morbidity and mortality rates in patients with coronary artery disease than quitting smoking.

146. **(C)** Although pleural and peritoneal mesotheliomas (D) are mostly asbestos-related tumors, bronchogenic carcinomas remain the principal cause of mortality in people exposed to asbestosis. Less commonly, laryngeal carcinoma (A) may also be associated with asbestosis. Smokers have a fifty- to one hundred-fold increased risk for developing bronchogenic cancer with asbestosis exposure. The presence of COPD (B) is highly possible in a heavy smoker, but clinical presentation is more compatible with a malignancy. The absence of relevant information in the patient's history eliminates tuberculosis (E).

147. ~~(E)~~ *D* The X-ray illustrates dextrocardia in situs inversus, which is a mirror image position of the internal organs. Typically, the heart is structurally normal (D). Longevity is normal (A). Due to the reversed position of the internal organs, pain due to acute appendicitis occurs in the left lower quadrant, while pain due to biliary colic presents with symptoms/signs in the left upper quadrant (B). There is no evidence of tuberculosis on this X-ray (E).

148. **(E)** The testes should be examined together using the thumb and forefinger of each hand. The shape (A), size (B), consistency (C), and sensitivity to pressure (D) should all be ascertained. There is no need to determine the weight (E) and, further, it would be difficult to clinically achieve this.

149. **(B)** Compression of the subclavian artery is usually from external compression or secondary to a peripheral neuritis in the upper extremity. Scalenus anterior syndrome (A) is a disturbance of the ulnar nerve, which can lead to subclavian compression. A cervical rib (C) and hyperelevation of the arm (E) can cause direct compression of the subclavian artery. The costoclavicular syndrome (D) produces a similar compression to that of the scalenus anterior muscle. The subclavian steal syndrome (B) is a subclavian artery stenosis in patients with atherosclerosis or narrowing secondary to catheterization.

150. **(B)** This patient probably has benign prostatic hypertrophy but may have prostate cancer. However, the initial intervention in evaluating this should be a digital rectal examination.

151. **(A)** Chronic liver disease generally results in thrombocytopenia secondary to hypersplenism, rather than thrombocytosis. Myeloproliferative disease (B), such as essential thrombocythemia or chronic myelocytic leukemia, may result in elevated platelet counts, often greater than one million. Postsplenectomy (C) results in a secondary thrombocytosis for several weeks. Inflammatory bowel disease (D) and other chronic inflammatory diseases can cause secondary thrombocytosis. Malignancy (E) may result in chronically elevated platelet counts.

152. **(A)** The symptoms of severe polydipsia with a normal osmolality is concerning for diabetes insipidus. Diabetes mellitus (B) was excluded by the serum glucose. Although psychogenic polydipsia (C) is a possibility, the urine osmolality should be expected to be lower.

153. **(C)** This patient has rhabdomyolysis, which involves necrosis of the muscle tissue and thus elevations in CPK levels and myoglobin in the urine. Immediate treatment involves judicious intravenous hydration with replenishment of electrolytes to prevent formation of myoglobin casts within the kidney tubules and worsening of the renal failure. Steroids (A) are not used to treat rhabdomyolysis. Viral infections account for only five percent of rhabdomyolysis cases, and antiviral treatment is not recommended (B). This patient most likely has rhabdomyolysis secondary to a viral syndrome, which had resolved on its own. *Legionella* pneumonia is the most common cause of bacterial lung infection associated with rhabdomyolysis. These patients may benefit from erythromycin and adjunct rifampin therapy (D). This patient has no evidence of a lung infection. Dialysis (E) may be necessary in certain patients who fail to respond to supportive therapy alone.

154. **(C)** A history of peptic ulcers is not associated with any particular etiology of dysphagia. The etiology of dysphagia can usually be determined by a careful history. Solid-food dysphagia is more common in structural lesions of the esophagus, while liquid-food dysphagia is more common with neuromuscular dysphagia (A). A prolonged duration of symptoms suggests non-malignant process, while new-onset dysphagia is more worrisome for malignancy (B). A history of

heartburn suggests the possibility of a reflux-associated peptic stricture (D). Associated weight loss is often seen with dysphagia related to esophageal carcinoma (E).

155. **(E)** The classic finding of achalasia on barium swallow includes the "bird's beak esophagus," a gradual tapering of a dilated esophagus to a narrowed gastroesophageal junction. Esophageal cancer usually appears as a stricture or asymmetrical narrowing in the esophagus on barium swallow (A). A Schatzki's ring appears immediately above the gastroesophageal junction as a fixed, symmetrical "shelf-like" irregularity (B). Barium swallow in patients with diffuse esophageal spasm shows aperistaltic contractions and is often described as a "cork-screw esophagus" (C). Peptic stricture is difficult to differentiate from other causes of structural dysphagia by barium swallow alone, but does not show an aperistaltic, dilated esophagus (D).

156. **(A)** Esophageal manometry is the gold standard for the diagnosis of achalasia. Twenty-four-hour pH probe is the gold standard for the diagnosis of gastroesophageal reflux disease (B). Proton pump inhibitors are useful in the treatment of peptic ulcer disease and gastroesophageal reflux disease, but are generally not useful in patients with achalasia (C). Full thickness esophageal biopsy cannot be performed through an endoscope and would not be useful in attempting to diagnose achalasia (D). Pneumatic balloon dilation is usually the treatment of choice for achalasia, however, due to the associated risk of esophageal perforation, this procedure is generally not performed unless the diagnosis of achalasia is confirmed (E).

157. **(C)** Esophageal cancers in the distal esophagus most commonly arise from Barrett's mucosa, a metaplastic transformation of the normal esophageal squamous mucosa into a specialized columnar epithelium (SCE). SCE can progress to dysplasia and subsequently into adenocarcinoma. Squamous cell cancers are also common in the esophagus (A), but occur more commonly in the proximal esophagus. Sarcomas are rare in the esophagus (B). Unfortunately, patients with esophageal cancer rarely develop symptoms until the tumor has progressed beyond the stage of carcinoma-in-situ (D). As discussed, Barrett's mu-

cosa is a metaplastic transformation of the esophagus, which is a preneoplastic lesion (E).

158. **(E)** All of these blood types are acceptable for transfusion, as the patient's blood type already contains A and B antigens and Rh antigen. However, transfusion reactions may still occur to other antigen types, such as Kell and Duffy. The frequency of A blood type is 40%, while the frequency of the B type is 10%; AB is 3%; and O type is 45%.

159. **(A)** Painless jaundice usually represents a chronic obstruction of the biliary tract from tumor or sclerosing cholangitis. Cholelithiasis can present with jaundice, but usually is associated with right upper quadrant pain because of the acuity of the obstruction.

160. **(B)** Color of stools (A) should be asked to rule out acholic stools in obstruction, melena in upper gastrointestinal bleed from cirrhosis, or steatorrhea in pancreatic duct obstruction. The color of urine (C) can darken with non-obstructive jaundice, as in hemolytic anemia.

161. **(B)** The elevation in total bilirubin with the elevation in alkaline phosphatase is most consistent with a cholestatic liver disease. Viral hepatitis (A) usually presents with elevated transaminases. Cirrhosis of the liver (D) and hepatocellular carcinoma (C) usually don't have an elevation in alkaline phosphatase unless the biliary tracts are involved. Hemolytic anemia (E) alone won't elevate the alkaline phosphatase.

162. **(C)** Elevation in alkaline phosphatase can be found in biliary obstruction or bone resorbing diseases. When there is a concomitant elevation in the gamma-glutamyl transpeptidase or 5'-nucleotidase, the elevation in alkaline phosphatase is most likely from the biliary tracts.

163. **(C)** Since the laboratory results show that the biliary tracts are likely involved, direct visualization under ERCP is probably the best test to assess the area. Right upper quadrant ultrasound (A) is a good test for patients with right upper quadrant pain, but in this patient with a possible cancer or primary sclerosing cholangiotism it will not be the best test. EGD (B) will not visualize the biliary tracts well. HIDA scan (D) is essentially

helpful only in ruling out cholecystitis. Open liver biopsy (E) may be needed later, but can probably come after ERCP, as open liver biopsy is more invasive.

164. (A) Unfortunately, there have been no medical therapies which have been shown to change mortality in patients with primary sclerosing cholangitis. The only treatment remains liver transplantation.

165. (A) Treatment of pruritus in patients with primary sclerosing cholangitis can be mitigated with cholestyramine.

166. (B) There is a high incidence of inflammatory bowel disease in patients with primary sclerosing cholangitis, and they should all undergo colonoscopy before undergoing liver transplant.

167. (B) With a variance of 25, the standard deviation is 5 mg/dL. In a normally distributed sample population, we know that 95% of the values fall within two standard deviations of the mean. Therefore, the range of values will be 198 minus or plus 10 = 188 to 208.

168. (B), **169. (A)**, **170. (C)**, **171. (D)** Factitious hypoglycemia is thought to be at least as common as hypoglycemia from insulinoma; several tests help to distinguish between these conditions. When insulin is cleaved from its precursor proinsulin molecule, C-peptide is released in a 1:1 ratio with insulin. Thus, in insulinoma (A), both insulin and C-peptide levels are increased. Administration of exogenous insulin (B), which lacks C-peptide, produces hypoglycemia in the face of high insulin levels, but normal or low C-peptide levels. Antibodies to insulin, if present, suggest chronic insulin injection. Neither exogenous insulin nor sulfonylureas elevate proinsulin. Sulfonylureas (C) do increase both insulin levels and C-peptide levels. Hypoglycemia secondary to solid extrapancreatic tumors (D), such as sarcomas, may result from massive utilization of glucose, which exceeds hepatic production. Plasma insulin levels are suppressed.

172. (B), **173. (D)**, **174. (A)**, **175. (B)** The patient in 172 is not a transplant candidate because he is still actively drinking and the new liver would be likely to be damaged like the old. The patient in 173 needs a renal transplant. The patient in 174 needs

a heart transplant. The patient in 175 is not a candidate because her renal function is virtually normal.

176. (B) The Wright's-stained peripheral blood smear shows two spirochetes (A). The typical history suggests relapsing fever, a condition caused by *Borrelia* (B). The louse-borne form is transported from person to person by the human body louse, while the tick-borne form is transmitted via ticks. The illness responds to antimicrobial therapy. Quarantine measures are not required (D). The FTA-ABS is one of two standard treponemal tests. Although treponemes appear as spirochetes on dark-field examination, the history is not consistent with a treponemal infection (C). Rocky Mountain spotted fever is caused by *Rickettsia*, which are small, obligate intracellular pathogens (E).

177. (B) The clinical suspicion for pulmonary embolism in this patient is very high because of the oral contraceptives, acuity of symptoms, and lab tests. Of all low probability VQ scans, 30% are false negatives. If the clinical suspicion is high, the gold standard test should be done, which is a pulmonary arteriogram.

178. (C) Regardless of a predisposing condition, presenting signs and symptoms include increasing testicular pain or discomfort, heaviness, and swelling of the testes. Periodic screening for seminoma by testicular examination is recommended for all men with a childhood history of cryptorchidism, orchiopexy, and testicular atrophy (D). There are inadequate grounds for using an occult blood test or sigmoidoscopy (A) as a screening means for colorectal cancer. These tests may be used for colorectal cancer in asymptomatic individuals. There is also insufficient evidence for digital rectal examination (B). Screening of patients with no signs or symptoms for oral cancer is not routinely recommended (E).

179. (C) The arteriogram demonstrates severe bilateral renal artery stenosis. This diagnosis should be considered when hypertension occurs in a previously normotensive person older than 55 years or when hypertension accelerates in a previously well-controlled patient. Symptoms of hypokalemia, such as muscle weakness, tetany, or polyuria, may occur. Metabolic alkalosis and deterioration of renal function may also be present.

Definitive treatment is with percutaneous transluminal angioplasty or surgery (C). A Captopril renal scintigram is an excellent screening procedure for renovascular hypertension, especially for persons thought to have unilateral disease. Sensitivity and specificity exceed 95% (A). Three-dimensional phase-contrast MRI is also an excellent noninvasive screening procedure, with sensitivities and specificities reported to be greater than 90% (B). Peripheral vein renin determinations are typically not useful in the diagnosis or therapy of persons with renal artery stenosis. A ratio of less than 1.5:1 does not exclude the diagnosis, particularly in persons with bilateral disease (D). Interventional therapy is superior to medical therapy if the patient is able to tolerate the procedure. The dosage of Captopril is excessive (E).

180. **(C)** With acute cholangitis or inflammation of the bile ducts, there is elevation of the liver function tests. The urine may have bilirubin present and will not be normal (D). The serum bilirubin will also be elevated.

USMLE Step 3 – Practice Test 2
Day One – Afternoon Session

1.   **(E)**   Tetanus toxoid plus diphtheria vaccine is mandatory for all patients with HIV. The same is true for yearly immunizations against influenza regardless of patient's age. Yearly screening for TB should be mandatory, not optional (B). Positive HIV seropositivity is not a contraindication for vaccinations (C). IPV (inactivated polio vaccine) is the recommended vaccination for HIV patients.

2.   **(E)**   Patients with acute GI bleeding should be maintained NPO in case of possible operative or endoscopic interventions. Blood should be typed and crossed (A) for possible transfusion. Normal saline should be infused (B) to correct hypovolemia. Vital signs should be monitored frequently (C) as this is a simple and useful indicator of volume status and bleeding. Immediate GI and surgical consultations (D) should be obtained in patients with significant GI bleeding.

3.   **(A)**   CAT scan is not generally a useful test in the initial diagnostic evaluation of GI bleeding. Flexible sigmoidoscopy (B) can be useful to evaluate for hemorrhoids or a distal source of bleeding. Tagged RBC scan (C) is a sensitive method of detecting the site of lower GI bleeding. Upper endoscopy (E) is a reasonable test to consider in this patient, as he is taking ibuprofen and can have a rapidly bleeding peptic ulcer.

4.   **(E)**   Hematocrit obtained very soon after the initiation of acute GI bleeding is unlikely to reveal anemia in patients without a prior history of anemia. A microcytic anemia (A) may be seen in patients with chronic GI bleeding. Normocytic and macrocytic anemia (B and C) are not generally associated with GI bleeding. A mixed microcytic and macrocytic anemia (D) is more commonly seen in malnourished and/or alcoholic patients with folate and iron-deficiency anemia.

5.   **(A)**   Diverticulosis commonly presents as painless, sudden, massive hematochezia. Diverticulitis (B) usually presents with abdominal pain, fever, and tenderness. Although esophagitis (C) can occur with ibuprofen use, esophagitis is rarely so severe as to cause massive lower GI bleeding. Inflammatory bowel disease (D) is more commonly associated with bloody stool and diarrhea rather than massive hematochezia. Small bowel lymphoma (E) may present with hematochezia, but is a rare diagnosis.

6.   **(D)**   NSAID medications, such as ibuprofen, cause platelet dysfunction, which is manifested by an increased bleeding time. PT and PTT (A and B) are not affected by NSAID medications. Although platelets become dysfunctional, the platelet count (C) is not affected. Factor VIII (E) is a vitamin K-dependent factor, which is dysfunctional in malnourished patients and patients with liver disease.

7.   **(C)**   Administration of packed platelets will reverse the coagulopathy related to NSAID medications. The administration of DDAVP would also be an alternative. The platelet effects of ibuprofen will last for several days; therefore, surgery cannot be delayed (A). FFP will not correct hematological abnormalities (B) related to platelet dysfunction. It would not be safe to proceed with surgery without reversing the effects of the ibuprofen, especially in a patient with GI bleeding (D). Hematological consultation (E) is not indicated in this situation.

8.   **(D)**   Endoscopic therapy can be effective for isolated angiodysplasias; however, multiple lesions generally respond better to angiographic or surgical therapy. Angiodysplasia is a very common cause of lower GI bleeding in elderly patients (A). Angiodysplastic lesions can be seen throughout the GI tract (B), especially in patients with chronic renal failure. There may be an association between angiodysplasia and aortic stenosis, but there is no association between this condition and mitral valve disease (C). Angiodysplasia (E) is associated with malignancy.

9. **(E)** Infectious gastroenteritis is not a cause of postoperative fever. Wound infection (A) is a common cause of postoperative fever. Pulmonary events related to anesthesia, such as atelectasis or pneumonia, may occur postoperatively and manifest as fever (B and C). Urinary tract infection (D) related to perioperative Foley catheterization is a common cause of postoperative fever.

10. **(C)** This patient's symptoms are most consistent with diabetes mellitus.

11. **(E)** The most important thing to do first is correct the patient's hypoglycemia before it causes neurological impairment.

12. **(C)** A common mistake is to continue insulin injections despite decreased or no oral intake and in the presence of nausea and vomiting.

13. **(E)** A ventilation-perfusion scan is not indicated for this patient.

14. **(B)** Continuous insulin infusion is contraindicated here.

15. **(D)** MRSA colonization or infection is not particularly associated with diabetes. All of the other conditions are associated with juvenile-onset diabetes mellitus.

16. **(A)** Diabetic ketoacidosis is most common among juvenile-onset or insulin-dependent diabetics.

17. **(C)** He should be admitted to a hospital, but a regular ward bed is sufficient.

18. **(D)** Non-hospitalized diabetics are most likely to develop pneumococcal pneumonia, as are otherwise healthy individuals.

19. **(B)** *Herpes simplex* lesions are typically vesicular.

20. **(C)** Gonococcal lesions often present as painless papules on the skin.

21. **(D)** Papillomavirus infections cause warts.

22. **(A)** Chancroid is characteristic of *Hemophilus ducreyi*.

23. **(D)** These symptoms are most consistent with genital herpes.

24. **(A)** This patient is likely to be "sundowning," a condition of confusion, usually nocturnal, that elderly people sometimes suffer from in the strange environment of a hospital. This condition usually responds to haloperidol.

25. **(D)** No intervention is indicated in a PPD-positive patient over age 35 who has a normal chest radiograph and no history of recent contact with a patient with tuberculosis.

26. **(D)** As long as she is not obviously septic, she can be discharged on appropriate empiric antibiotics and be followed closely as an outpatient.

27. **(A)** An HIV-positive patient who develops an opportunistic infection, such as thrush or Kaposi's sarcoma, is considered to have AIDS by convention.

28. **(C)** A CBC is necessary at this point because the patient's fatigue could easily be due to anemia, particularly iron-deficiency anemia in an individual who may still be menstruating. None of the other tests is indicated at this stage.

29. **(B)** This condition does not appear to be familial in nature.

30. **(B)** This condition is defined by its association with reproducible painful areas, usually over bursae and other periarticular structures, which are called trigger points. The other findings would not be expected in this patient.

31. **(E)** This condition is often associated with some degree of depression.

32. **(E)** This pattern is most common with the condition this patient has.

33. **(D)** This condition is a frequent cause of absenteeism.

34. **(B)** Relatively small bedtime doses of amitriptyline or related agents can be quite beneficial.

35. **(A)** Fibromyalgia is the best diagnosis for this patient.

36. **(B)** Temporal arteritis can produce a picture like this and is a medical emergency because it can lead to acute blindness if not promptly treated.

37. **(B)** Patients who are HIV-positive and have CD4 counts below 50 are at significant risk for CMV retinitis and should be regularly screened for it even if they are asymptomatic.

38. **(C)** The rash of psoriasis is usually scaling, pruritic, and erythematous, and commonly occurs on extensor surfaces, in and around the ears, and on the scalp. Other sites include the umbilicus.

39. **(A)** Pernicious anemia is likely in this patient, given her history, family history, and lab findings.

40. **(C)** The patient is likely to be choking on a piece of his dinner and the easiest first maneuver is the Heimlich procedure. If this does not dislodge the obstruction, an attempt at a tracheostomy (A) may then be necessary.

41. **(C)** Sinusitis has not been associated with RSV, but all of the other conditions have.

42. **(D)** This is the most likely etiology of this condition and should be covered by any antibiotics administered before culture confirmation is obtained.

43. **(D)** At this point, child abuse is not in your differential diagnosis and need not be brought up. The other findings would be consistent with ingestion of an exogenous toxin.

44. **(A)** Lead poisoning would explain all of this patient's findings.

45. **(C)** A high level is consistent with lead intoxication. A low level, though, does not categorically rule out the possibility, and further testing should be done if clinical suspicion is high.

46. **(D)** All of the other conditions are manifestations of severe plumbism.

47. **(E)** In this setting, an elevated sedimentation rate would strongly suggest polymyalgia rheumatica. Since the patient has such prominent headaches and some visual changes, temporal arteritis would also be suspected and must be treated, since it can rapidly result in blindness if untreated, even before the results of other diagnostic studies, such as a temporal artery biopsy, are available.

48. **(B)** The patient's CBC will show profound thrombocytopenia, leukopenia, and anemia, and the likeliest cause in someone with sickle cell anemia is an aplastic crisis.

49. **(D)** This patient should be considered to have meningitis until proven otherwise, and the only way to make this diagnosis is via a lumbar puncture.

50. **(D)** Isolated coin lesion with a pleural effusion on CXR is unlikely to be secondary to sarcoidosis, rather, a malignancy should be considered. Bilateral hilar adenopathy (A) is usually asymptomatic and reversible without therapy. Diffuse parenchymal changes (B) are known as a Type III X-ray and are usually chronic. "Eggshell calcifications" (C) are sometimes seen in chronic sarcoidosis. Bilateral hilar adenopathy and diffuse parenchymal changes (E), or Type II chest X-ray, may result in symptoms of cough and dyspnea.

51. **(E)** Swan-Ganz catheterization is not useful in helping to make the diagnosis of any sarcoidosis. Bronchoalveolar lavage (A) reveals an increased proportion of lymphocytes. Pulmonary function testing (B) typically reveals decreased lung volumes and diffusion capacity with hypoxemia. Gallium 67 lung scan (C) shows a pattern of diffuse uptake. Fiber-optic bronchoscopic biopsy (D) is most likely to give a definitive diagnosis, although the histologic findings of non-caseating granulomas are not specific for sarcoidosis.

52. **(C)** The rash described in this patient is classic for erythema nodosum, the most common skin lesion in patients with sarcoidosis. Lupus pernio (A) is also common, but more commonly presents as a dusky purple discoloration, often on the face. Erythema gangrenosum (B) and fungal rashes (D) are not commonly associated with sarcoidosis. Although the rash of cryoglobulinemia may present on the extensor lower extremity, it is not associated with sarcoidosis (E).

53. **(C)** Occular involvement occurs in approximately 25% of patients, usually manifesting

as uveitis. GI tract involvement (A) is uncommon and usually asymptomatic. Pancreas involvement (B) is unusual. Nervous system involvement (D) occurs in only five percent of patients and may involve the facial nerve. Heart involvement (E) also occurs in only about five percent of patients.

54. **(B)** In the United States, the majority of patients are black, although in Europe, the majority of patients are white. The majority of patients with sarcoidosis present between the ages of 20-40 (A). Sarcoidosis is not contagious (C). Males appear to be somewhat less susceptible to the disease than females (D).

55. **(C)** Antibody-mediated processes are not thought to be important in the immunopathogenesis of sarcoidosis, although a hyperglobulinemia is often seen clinically. Granuloma formation is common in affected sites (A) and is a result of mononuclear phagocytes and epithelioid cells. Large numbers of activated T-cells accumulate in affected organs (B) and T-cell responses are thought to be important in the pathogenesis of this condition. IL-2 is a T-cell stimulus for proliferation and appears to be important in sarcoidosis for maintaining T-cell activation (D). It is not known why some patients with sarcoidosis develop a fibrotic disease; however, the fibrotic response appears to be mediated through the release of growth factors such as fibroblast growth factor and platelet-derived growth factor (E).

56. **(D)** Eye involvement may lead to blindness and, thus, occular involvement is an indication for treatment. Death is attributable to sarcoidosis in only 10% of patients (A) with this condition. About 50% of patients with sarcoidosis will remit spontaneously (B), not 90%. Sarcoidosis is not known to be a risk factor for the development of lymphoma (C).

57. **(E)** Lymph node involvement rarely causes problems for patients and should only be an indication for treatment in cases of massive lymphadenopathy (A). Treatment for sarcoidosis is generally in the order of weeks to months (B), not life-long. Inhaled glucocorticoids (C) are not useful for pulmonary disease. Although levels of angiotensin-converting enzyme are elevated in the serum of two-thirds of patients, treatment is usually not based on this marker (D).

58. **(C)** Urgent urological consultation is indicated. The patient's fever suggests an obstructing stone. Ninety percent of renal stones are radiodense and will be detected on a plain X-ray (A); however, IVP (B) is still necessary to determine the exact location of the stone and to determine whether the kidney proximal to the stone is functioning. Most ureteral stones pass spontaneously (D). Only about 10% require interventional therapy.

59. **(B)** Uric acid stone formation is associated with acidic urine, not alkaline urine. Calcium stones are the most common stone type (A) and are most commonly due to idiopathic hypercalciuria. Cystine stones occur secondary to a defect in renal tubular absorption of cysteine (C and E). The disorder is inherited, and the stones are manifested early in life. This type of stone is formed only by patients with cystinuria. Urea-splitting organisms, such as proteus, may result in struvite stones, which can grow quite large (staghorn calculi) (D).

60. **(D)** Ceftriaxone is effective against Gram-negative organisms and obtains excellent penetration into the urine. The other agents are used primarily for the treatment of Gram-positive infections.

61. **(C)** Triamterene is a potassium-sparing diuretic, which is associated with the formation of urinary calculi. Hydrochlorothiazide (A) results in a fall in urinary calcium excretion. Sodium citrate therapy (B) makes the urine alkaline and increases urinary citrate levels; both factors reduce the risk of calcium stones. Inorganic phosphates (D) decrease calcium absorption, but should not be used unless other therapies are ineffective due to the risks associated with this therapy. Cellulose phosphate (E) is an ion-exchange resin, which binds to calcium, preventing its absorption, and is occasionally used in the treatment of stones related to absorptive hypercalciuria.

62. **(D)** Acarbose is an alpha-glucosidase inhibitor which interferes with intestinal absorption of complex carbohydrates and thus lowers the glucose load absorbed in the body. Metformin (A) is a biguanide which works by decreasing hepatic glucose production by 30% and increasing glucose utilization in skeletal muscle. In one large study,

metformin lowered the fasting blood glucose level by an average of 52 mg/dl. NPH insulin (B) is long-acting and remains in the body eight to twelve hours after injection. Type II diabetics who take NPH insulin simply relieve their pancreas of the need to produce that amount of insulin during the day. It can now cope with the extra glucose coming in. Sulfonylureas (C) work by binding to a sulfonylurea receptor on the pancreatic islet cell and thus facilitate insulin secretion. Regular insulin (E) works in half an hour to one hour, and lowers the blood glucose by increasing glucose uptake in cells.

63. **(E)** Clinical findings suggestive of a toxic infant or child include all of the following: poor or delayed capillary refill (A), tachycardia (B), nasal flaring, grunting, prolonged expiration, tachypnea, chest retractions, stridor (D), slow irregular or decreasing respiratory rate (C), and fever. Diarrhea is not a sign of toxicity in infants and children.

64. **(E)** All febrile infants less than 24 days of age warrant a sepsis evaluation and hospitalization for parenteral antibiotic therapy pending the results of cultures.

65. **(C)** You may treat him emergently while his parents are sought, since this is a potentially life-threatening condition.

66. **(C)** The history of prolonged mechanical ventilation is suggestive of a midtracheal stenosis. A known complication of prolonged endotracheal intubation, this lesion probably results from hyperinflation of the endotracheal tube (C). The lesion demonstrated here is in the trachea, not the esophagus (A). A foreign body, depending on its radiodensity, appears as a filling defect, rather than a stricture (B). A laryngeal carcinoma of sufficient size to produce obstructive symptoms would be readily observable by laryngoscopic examination. On CAT examination, a mass lesion would be observed in addition to a stricture. The haziness in the upper portion of this CAT study is artifact, rather than a significant lesion (E). A substernal goiter may produce tracheal compression and deviation. A mass effect is usually seen on a PA chest film. A CAT study, not required for diagnosis, would also demonstrate a mass effect (D).

67. **(C)** Corticosteroids have not shown to improve the outcome in patients with adult respiratory distress syndrome. In fact, steroids can make the patient more immunocompromised and, thus, the *E. coli* sepsis would be further propagated. This patient has *E. coli* sepsis, which needs immediate intervention because of the high mortality involved. He should be transferred to the intensive care unit and monitored with a Swan-Ganz catheter or central venous line to see the cardiac pressures and to give fluid accordingly. If hypotension is also involved, then this patient has septic shock. The hypoxia should be treated with intubation and ventilatory management (A). This patient also has adult respiratory distress syndrome (ARDS), which has a very high morbidity and intubation is required. Intravenous hydration (B) is required if this patient has hypotension. Aminoglycoside therapy (D), such as gentamicin, is used for Gram-negative bacteremia and should be given immediately. This antibiotic has nephrotoxicity and frequent levels should be checked. *E. coli* is a Gram-negative aerobic bacterial organism. The source of the sepsis is probably the urinary tract. PEEP (E), or positive end expiratory pressure, is usually required in any patient with adult respiratory distress syndrome to increase the oxygenation.

68. **(D)** This patient has a urinary tract infection most likely secondary to *E. coli* and an invasive foley placement. She has uncomfortable symptoms of dysuria and hesitancy and, therefore, she should be treated with trimethoprim-sulfamethoxazole empirically along with removing the foley catheter. An intravenous pyelography (A) is an invasive procedure, which should only be performed if there is a strong suspicion for a kidney stone or obstruction. This procedure should not be a first step in diagnosing a urinary tract infection. Intravenous normal saline (B) would indeed flush the kidneys and aid in alleviating the symptoms of a urinary tract infection, but along with this, one should remove the foley and give antibiotics. Penicillin (C) would not be a good drug of choice since it usually covers Gram-positive organisms and also because resistance is very high with penicillin. *E. coli* is a Gram-negative bacterial organism. Several days may pass before the results of the urine and blood cultures become available. If the patient is symptomatic, treatment should be initiated empirically first (E).

69. **(E)** By the end of the fourth week, the septum primum grows from the roof of the common atrium and extends toward the endocardial cushions. The endocardial cushion are rapidly growing intracardiac cell masses that assist in formation of the atrioventricular septum (A), atrioventricular canals, and the aortic and pulmonary channels. The ostium primum is the opening between the septum primum and the endocardial cushions. The ostium secundum is formed from perforations in the closing septum primum to allow blood to flow from the right to the left primitive atria. The septum secundum develops as the venous sinus horn is incorporated into the right atrium; this septum never forms a complete partition in the common atrium (C). The opening left by the septum secundum is the foramen ovale (D). The foramen ovale allows blood to flow from the right the left atrium during fetal blood circulation; at birth the increase in left atrial pressure closes the foramen ovale. In 20% of people, the septum primum and secundum do not completely fuse (E), and a probe patent foramen ovale exists; however, it does not allow intracardiac shunting of blood.

70. **(A)** The scabies mite, *Sarcoptes scabiei*, is illustrated in the figure. The mite burrows into the skin, particularly along the sides of the fingers, flexor surfaces of the wrists, and at the elbows (A). Head and body lice have three pairs of nearly equal sized legs bearing claws for gripping hairs or fibers (B). Fleas are wingless insects 2-4 mm long that feed on the blood of humans (C). Bedbugs are flat, mahogany-brown, 5-7 mm long wingless insects, which feed almost exclusively on humans (D). Myiasis refers to infestations by maggots, primarily due to the larvae of metallic-colored screw-worm flies or botflies (E).

71. **(E)**, 72. **(D)**, 73. **(A)**, and 74. **(C)** Specificity is defined as the proportion of people with no disease and with a negative test result. It is calculated as follows:

Specificity = true negatives/true negatives + false positives = 60/35 + 60 = 0.63 or 63%.

It is used to confirm a diagnosis. Positive predictive value is defined as a ratio of true positives to the sum of all positive tests.

Positive predictive value = True positives/true positives + false positives = 25/25 + 35 = 0.417 or 41.7%.

Odds ratio = True positives x true negatives/false positives x true negatives = 25 x 60/35 x 15 = 2.86 or 28.6%.

Attributable risk = True positives/true positives + false positives – true negatives/true negatives + false negatives = 25/25 + 35 – 15/15 + 60 = 41.7% – 36.8 % = 4.9%.

75. **(A)** Mechanisms that lead to these conditions [(B), (C), (D), and (E)] are multifactorial and not very well-understood.

76. **(D)** This lesion is suggestive of a melanoma because of its color and irregularity, and its size is such that surgical removal is warranted.

77. **(C)** The patient's elevated BUN with relatively normal creatinine suggests gastrointestinal blood loss rather than renal insufficiency (A). The fatigue and weakness is probably due to anemia from bleeding rather than from thyroid disease (E).

78. **(D)** In a patient with sharp abdominal pain and distention, you must consider an abdominal or peritoneal process. To look for free air under the diaphragm, a lateral decubitus film is very sensitive.

79. **(B)** A 66-year-old patient with acute left side jaw pain may be having an anginal attack or an infarction. Obtaining an EKG can assist you with the diagnosis. Cardiac pain often is referred to the jaw.

80. **(E)** All of the rhythms noted can be seen with digitalis toxicity. Any rhythm can be seen, but classically (and uncommonly), bidirectional ventricular tachycardia is noted, and, commonly, multifocal atrial tachycardia is noted.

81. **(C)** The anterior hypothalamus, not the posterior hypothalamus, contains the body's thermostat; it senses the temperature of the blood perfusing the brain and activates peripheral control mechanisms to bring core temperature to its preferred set-point. Disorders of heat dissipation (A) include dehydration, autonomic dysfunction, and the neuroleptic malignant syndrome. The elderly are at risk for "classic" heatstroke. Exertional heatstroke occurs in hot, humid weather. Other risk factors predisposing to heatstroke include alcohol,

encephalitis, thyrotoxicosis, and cocaine abuse. The typical victim of heatstroke is confined at home without benefit of air conditioning or fans during hot, humid weather (B). Other lab abnormalities in heatstroke include lactic acidosis, muscle enzyme abnormalities, hypocalcemia, hypophosphatemia, hyperkalemia, and thrombocytopenia (D). Disseminated intravascular coagulation is also present in severe cases of hyperthermia. Neuroleptics, such as haldoperidol, can result in neuroleptic malignant syndrome; alcohol and diuretics can cause dehydration; anticholinergic agents can interfere with sweating—all of which exacerbate symptoms of heatstroke (E).

82. **(C)** Tight control of diabetes does not cure neuropathy, but intensive therapy slows progression of diabetic neuropathy. There is no cure for diabetic neuropathy, only the symptoms can be treated. The more severe and long-standing the diabetes, the worse the neuropathy. Distal symmetrical diabetic polyneuropathy (A) is the most common because of its refractoriness to therapy. Diabetic third nerve palsy, proximal neuropathies compression neuropathy (carpal tunnel syndrome), and autonomic neuropathies can also occur in long-standing diabetes. Diabetic proximal motor neuropathy (B) is vascular in origin because the blood vessels that supply the motor nerves become damaged and result in progressive nerve ischemia. The Diabetes Control and Complications Trial Research Group showed that intensive treatment with insulin injections delays onset and slows progression of diabetic neuropathy, retinopathy, and nephropathy. Very little can be done to restore sensation (D), but foot ulcers, osteomyelitis, and Charcot joints can be prevented by having a physician check the foot every six months and by keeping the toenails clipped and cleaned. Symptoms of pain caused by neuropathy can sometimes be alleviated (E) by adjusting the doses of amitriptyline, phenytoin, desipramine, and topical capsaicin. Topical capsaicin works by inhibiting substance P in the superficial nerve fibers and diminishing the sensation of tenderness.

83. **(D)**, 84. **(B)**, 85. **(A)**, and 86. **(E)** Alcoholic liver disease (A) covers a spectrum of liver dysfunction, ranging from fatty liver to alcoholic hepatitis to alcoholic cirrhosis. Liver function tests commonly show an SGOT which is more than twice that of the SGPT. Total bilirubin is often elevated when al-

coholic liver disease has progressed to alcoholic hepatitis or alcoholic cirrhosis. Other findings in alcoholic cirrhosis include spider angiomata (tiny blanching cutaneous vessels) and muscle wasting. Viral hepatitis (B), due to hepatitis B and C, is often due to blood-borne transmission such as intravenous drug use. Constitutional symptoms are often associated with viral hepatitis, and liver function tests usually show an SGPT which is greater than the SGOT. Cholangiocarcinoma (C) is a tumor of the bile ducts. It commonly presents as progressive jaundice and weight loss in elderly patients or patients with a history of primary sclerosing cholangitis. Liver function tests show an elevated total bilirubin and alkaline phosphatase. Acute cholangitis (D) is an infection of the biliary tree, most commonly secondary to an impacted stone in the common bile duct. Patients present with pain, jaundice, and fever. Liver function tests show an elevated alkaline phosphatase and total bilirubin count, although transaminases are usually also elevated during the early period. Acute cholecystitis (E) usually occurs secondary to a stone impacted in the neck of the gall bladder. Liver function tests are often normal, as there is no obstruction of bile from the liver.

87. **(E)** Rheumatoid arthritis is a disease of unknown cause leading to proliferative inflammation of the articular synovium. Generalized joint pain and tingling and warm joints are classic. Unlike gout, there is no response to colchicine, and the uric acid level is normal.

88. **(A)** Acute gout classically awakens the patient at night with burning, tingling numbness, and warmth of a joint, particularly the great toe. When the metatarsophalangeal joint of the great toe is affected, it is termed *podagra*. Trauma, cold, infection, and certain drugs may precipitate the acute attack.

89. **(B)** Suppurative arthritis usually involves a joint distant from the original clinical infection. The patient will have a temperature and the joint will be warm, painful, and tender. Fluctuance is present and pus may often be aspirated.

90. **(C)** Pseudogout, or articular chrondro-calcinosis, is similar in presentation to acute gout because of its abrupt onset and painful swelling. The difference is that the symptoms are intense for just a couple of days and then subside.

91. **(D)** Gonococcal arthritis is an infectious arthritis and is the most common extragenital complication of gonorrhea. It must be considered in any individual who is sexually active, especially in someone who gives a history of recent urethritis. The pattern of arthritis is often migratory in nature.

92. **(B)** *H. influenzae* is the most likely cause of this patient's meningitis out of the choices given. *S. pneumoniae* (A) is a common cause of meningitis; however, it is a Gram-positive coccus. *L. monocytogenes* (C) is also a cause of meningitis in the elderly; however, it is also a Gram-positive organism. *S. aureus* (D) is an unusual cause of non-iatrogenic meningitis and also is not a Gram-negative organism. *E. coli* (E) is a Gram-negative rod; however, it is an extremely uncommon cause of bacterial meningitis.

93. **(D)** The deep layer of the closure should be of a resorbable material, because you will close over it and not remove it. Chromic gut is a resorbable material. Silk (A), nylon (B), steel (C), and cotton (E) are all non-resorbable and must be removed.

94. **(D)** With a peptic ulcer, there is moderate tenderness localized to an area 2-3 cm in diameter located just below the xiphoid. It may radiate to the back, but it does not start there. The pain rarely extends to beneath the costal margins laterally unless perforation occurs, leading to generalized abdominal pain.

95. **(B)** The most common symptom of esophageal carcinoma in the United States is progressive dysphagia over a period of several months. Advanced lesions are associated with weight loss and coughing after drinking fluids. In the presence of these classic symptoms, the irregularly narrowed esophageal lumen is most consistent with esophageal carcinoma (B). Esophageal dilatation, often with a distal beak, is characteristic of achalasia (A). Esophageal varices appear as multiple vertical filling defects of the esophagus (C). In diffuse esophageal spasm, the barium study shows segmental contractions. These appear as curling or multiple ripples in the wall, known as the "corkscrew esophagus" (D). Schatzki's ring appears as a symmetric thin web located in the terminal esopha-

gus (E). It also presents with intermittent, not progressive, dysphagia.

96. **(B)** If an individual has a weapon and threatens to kill someone in the physician's presence, it is the physician's "duty to warn" the potential victim.

97. **(D)** Giving patient records to a patient's employer would be unacceptable in terms of physician-patient confidentiality if the patient has not given his/her consent.

98. **(E)** If a physician charges for procedures, visits, etc. that he/she has not performed, this is considered fraud.

99. **(C)** A physician who helps a patient to die because the patient wants him/her to is participating in physician-assisted suicide, which is still not considered legal.

100. **(C)** You cannot refuse to take care of her or report her to anyone because she does not do what you recommend. The best course of action is to discuss her situation with her and her family and a counselor who might be able to help her.

101. **(C)** Otitis externa is an infection of the outer ear. It is also known as "swimmers ear" since it is seen often in swimmers and divers. There is very intense outer ear pain. Hearing losses, either conductive (A) or sensorineural (B), will usually not be painful. Otitis media (D) may present as an earache, but is not common in 33-year-olds; it is more often seen in an infant or toddler. Migraine headaches (E) usually do not present with an earache, but rather a headache with associated photophobia.

102. **(C)** The best treatment for an otitis externa is a combination topical antibiotic and steroid. It will work better than IV (A) and oral (B) antibiotics because of better penetration. Incision and drainage (D) will not work well because of the lack of a localized collection of pus. Tympanoplasty (E) will not resolve an infection of the outer ear.

103. **(B)** Gastric outlet obstruction is the likely diagnosis. In patients with peptic ulcer disease,

scarring can cause this phenomenon, and it presents in the patient noted in this question. On obstructive series, only the stomach is noted to be dilated, and not the small or large intestines (D and E).

104. **(B)** Cocaine use during pregnancy may result in premature labor and placental abruption. Fetuses exposed to cocaine are at increased risk for developing intrauterine and postnatal growth retardation, microcephaly, intracranial hemorrhage, and seizures. Cardiac septal defects (A) and cleft palate (D) are characteristic of fetal alcohol syndrome (A). Spina bifida occulta (C) results from maternal folate deficiency and can be prevented by prophylactic intake of folate during pregnancy. Gray baby syndrome (E) is associated with maternal use of chloramphenicol during pregnancy.

105. **(D)** This patient has a urinary tract infection most likely secondary to *E. coli* and an invasive foley placement. She has uncomfortable symptoms of dysuria and hesitancy and, therefore, she should be treated with trimethoprim-sulfamethoxazole empirically along with removing the foley catheter. An intravenous pyelography (A) is an invasive procedure, which should only be performed if there is a strong suspicion for a kidney stone or obstruction. This procedure should not be a first step in diagnosing a urinary tract infection. Intravenous normal saline (B) would indeed flush the kidneys and aid in alleviating the symptoms of a urinary tract infection, but along with this, one should remove the foley and give antibiotics. Penicillin (C) would not be a good drug of choice since it usually covers Gram-positive organisms and also because resistance is very high with penicillin. *E. coli* is a Gram-negative bacterial organism. Several days may pass before the results of the urine and blood cultures become available. If the patient is symptomatic, treatment should be initiated empirically first (E).

106. **(D)** Hematuria is the presence of blood in the urine. There are many reasons for it, which must be ascertained in the history. The presence of pain (A), the amount of blood (B), the time during voiding that it occurs (C), and medication history (E) are all important because they will help define the cause of hematuria as well as where in the urinary tract the blood may be entering. The

presence of any smell in the urine (D) will not be diagnostic.

107. **(E)** Hematuria may result for many reasons. These include: trauma (A), as in a blunt or penetrating injury; infection (B), as in urinary tract infection; neoplasm (C), as in renal cell carcinoma; and coagulopathy (D), as in advanced liver disease with elevated PT and PTT. Routine aspirin use (E) may prolong bleeding times, but will not usually lead to hematuria.

108. **(A)** A blood glucose will help you to diagnose glycosuria, but will not be helpful with hematuria. A urinalysis (B) will determine the presence of blood in the urine. An IVP or intravenous pyelogram (C) will study the urinary tract and allow you to visualize any abnormalities that may be the source of bleeding. A cystoscopy (D) will allow you to actually visualize the urinary tract to see any abnormalities. A PT/PTT (E) will tell you about the patient's bleeding times and coagulation profile and may give you insight into the reasons for the hematuria.

109. **(C)** Measurement of alpha-fetoprotein, human chorionic gonadotropin, and unconjugated estrogen in maternal serum ("triple screen") is recommended to prenatally detect affected fetuses with Down's syndrome or trisomy 110. An abnormal test requires definitive evaluation [(A) and (B)]. Due to the false-positive rate, more definitive testing is necessary if abnormalities are detected on the blood screening (D). Several options are available, including amniocentesis, chorionic villous sampling, ultrasonography, or periumbilical blood sampling, depending on which of the three tests is abnormal. The risks/benefits of each of these procedures must also be taken into consideration (C). Preconceptual folic acid supplementation, continued for the first three months of pregnancy, reduces the risk of neural tube defects (NTD). For women at increased risk of NTD, 0.4 mg is recommended (E)

110. **(A)** If a test were ideally specific, all persons with a positive test would manifest a predefined disease (A). A specific test is used to confirm the presence of a disease, not to exclude it (C, D, and E). Usually, some, or even many, persons with the disease will have a falsely negative test (B).

111. **(A)** If a test were ideally sensitive, all persons with a predefined disease would have a positive test result (A). The sensitivity of a test is used to exclude the presence of a disease (B, C, and E). Usually, some persons without the disease will have a false-positive test result (D).

112. **(A)** The karyotype of a normal female is illustrated in this figure. The chromosomes obtained from a single somatic cell during metaphase have been rearranged by size and varying arm length (A). The normal male pattern differs from the female by the presence of one Y chromosome in the place of one X chromosome (B). Down's syndrome is characterized by trisomy of chromosome 21 (C). Turner's syndrome (45, X) is characterized by the absence of one X chromosome in females with short stature and gonadal dysgenesis (D). Klinefelter's syndrome (47, XXY) occurs in approximately one of every 500 males and is the most common cause of male infertility (E).

113. **(B)** It is appropriate to draw these baseline tests: if the student is negative, they should be repeated in a few months to see if he has become infected.

114. **(E)** The constellation of symptoms that develop in far-advanced renal failure is termed uremia. Signs of uremia include hypertension, anorexia, vomiting (C), edema, a metallic taste in the mouth, and orthopnea. This patient probably had renal failure from long-standing hypertension. She developed encephalopathy secondary to retention of urea, sulphate, and phosphate and thus passage of these toxins across the blood-brain barrier cause a change in mental status and asterixis (A). Asterixis are myotonic twitches and "flaps" in the hands secondary to advanced uremia. Sensory abnormalities occur as well as peripheral neuropathy (B). Kussmaul's respirations (D) and dyspnea occur in a uremic patient secondary to respiratory compensation from metabolic acidosis in renal failure. Alopecia, or baldness, (E) is not a symptom of uremia.

115. **(B)** In this patient with acute renal decompensation and mental status changes, immediate hemodialysis should take place. If this does not occur soon, then hyperkalemia can occur and result in an arrhythmia and subsequent death. Plasmapheresis (A) is only useful to remove immune-complexes in autoimmune diseases such as TTP or myasthenia gravis. Peritoneal dialysis (C) is too slow in removing the toxins in the blood and thus should not be the immediate treatment modality of choice. This patient does not have urinary tract obstruction and a distended bladder, thus a foley catheter is not needed (E). Diuresis (D) would be useful if this patient had signs of fluid overload such as rales, dyspnea, and edema. Otherwise, it would only make the encephalopathy worse.

116. **(A)** A low-protein, not high-protein, diet is necessary in a renal patient to retard the progression of renal insufficiency and to prevent hyperfiltration. As renal insufficiency progresses, the capacity of the kidney to adjust to variations in sodium and water intake becomes limited. If excessive sodium intake is taken, then there is a risk of the renal patient developing congestive heart failure, edema, and worsening hypertension. Excessive potassium intake may result in potassium retention and cardiac problems (D). Milk of magnesia, certain magnesium containing antacids, and certain vitamin supplements that contain magnesium should be restricted in renal patients because these patients cannot excrete magnesium (B). All over-the-counter doses of medications should be discussed with the physician taking care of the patient because the dosages and frequency need to be adjusted in a renal patient (C). Erythropoietin can be supplemented in a chronic renal failure patient to maintain the hematocrit and to avoid blood transfusion (E).

117. **(B)** Proctalgia fugax, which presents with intense perineal pain (A), is more common in men than women. It is near the coccyx or within the rectum (C), usually subsides within five minutes (D), and is usually the reason for the pain of the levator ani muscles (E).

118. **(E)** A surgical consultation is the best course here.

119. **(A)** A chest tube to decompress the pneumothorax is the best treatment.

120. **(B)** This is a typical case of spontaneous pneumothorax, beginning at a young age.

121. **(E)** The cause of spontaneous pneumothorax is unknown.

122. **(E)** The aortic area is the right second interspace close to the sternum.

123. **(D)** The pulmonic area is the left second interspace close to the sternum.

124. **(C)** The tricuspid area is just lateral to the lower left edge of the sternum.

125. **(A)** The mitral area is at the left fifth interspace just medial to the midclavicular line.

126. **(E)** The patient's symptoms and physical examination are consistent with a dilated cardiomyopathy. Chronic alcoholism, Adriamycin usage, valvular disease, and viral diseases can all cause dilated cardiomyopathy.

127. **(B)** In a patient with a suspicious oral lesion, a cervical lymph node, and weight loss, one must be extremely suspicious for oropharyngeal cancer. Pharyngitis (A) will not give you this clinical picture. Oral candidiasis or thrush (C) will also not give you this picture of a very sick man. There is also no cervical lymphadenopathy. Lymphoma (D) will usually not have an ulcerated oral mass. Kaposi's sarcoma (E) seen with HIV-positive patients, will have weight loss and lymphadenopathy, but the lesion of Kaposi's is different from oral cancer. It tends to be more vascular and bluish-red.

128. **(B)** A head and neck surgeon (B) probably sees and treats the most cancer and is the best to render a second opinion. A dentist (A) may often make the diagnosis but may not be the best one for a second opinion. An internist (C) probably doesn't see enough oropharyngeal cancer to make the appropriate diagnosis and the same will hold true for a nutritionist (E). An oncologist (D) is an internist who treats cancer patients with chemotherapy, but may not see as much as a head and neck surgeon to offer the best second opinion.

129. **(E)** In working up the head and neck cancer patient, you are obligated to look for local, regional, and metastatic disease. By obtaining a biopsy (A) of the specimen and performing a panendoscopy (B) (which includes a nasopharyngoscopy, laryngoscopy, bronchoscopy, and esophagoscopy), you can adequately evaluate the local and regional tissues. A chest X-ray (C) and liver function tests (D) will help you assess possible metastatic disease. A colonoscopy (E) would not be indicated.

130. **(B)** This patient has lost weight and has no appetite. Increasing his oral diet (A) would probably not be effective. Initiation of total parenteral nutrition (TPN) (C) is not necessary because his GI tract is functional and should be used. TPN also has a lot of adverse side effects. Since you can use the GI tract, there is no need to place a gastrostomy tube (E) or jejunostomy tube (D). Just a simple nasogastric tube may be used to adequately supplement the diet.

131. **(A)** Squamous cell carcinoma of the oropharynx can be best treated with surgery if amenable or resectable. Radiation (B) or chemotherapy (C) are adjunctive and used (usually) either pre- or postoperatively.

132. **(B)** The most important risk factor for oropharyngeal carcinoma is the combination of tobacco and alcohol. Stopping these is the best advice you can give. Improved nutrition (A) and low cholesterol diet (E) are not as important. Hypertension control (C) and potassium supplementation (D) will not lower his chance of recurrence.

133. **(A)** During the first year of diagnosis and treatment of head and neck cancer, the follow-up should be every three months. After the first year, the visits may start to be slowly spaced apart, provided there is no clinical recurrence.

134. **(E)** This woman has had a syncopal episode with a possible hip fracture. The minimal tests that should be obtained are an EKG (A), a chest X-ray (B), hip films (C), and a head CT scan (D). There is no reason to obtain an MRI of the neck.

135. **(B)** In this woman with a murmur, she may very well have valve damage and may be showering emboli from the heart. Not only could these emboli go to the carotid arteries of the brain, they could go to the other vessels of the body as well, leading to occlusion. You would not obtain an echocardiogram for the presence of a murmur only (A) or a heart valve only (C). There are other ways to evaluate for an aneurysm (D) or to test the ejection fraction (E).

136. **(A)** A bruit of the carotid artery leads to a stenosis which will present as a bruit. When this is heard, it is wise to quantify the amount of occlusion. The best non-invasive way to do this is by performing an ultrasound examination of the neck. A CAT scan of the neck (B) or MRI of the neck is not warranted. An MRI, or magnetic resonance imaging, is non-invasive and can be used to study the arteries. Angiograms of the arteries (D) is invasive and is usually performed when contemplating surgery. Plain films (E) would not reveal soft tissue occlusions or plaques.

137. **(D)** Angiograms of the arteries are the best way to delineate the lesion and plan the surgery. An ultrasound (A) is not detailed enough. A CAT scan (B) or an MRI (C) will not give you the most accurate information. Plain films (E) will not show the arteries because they are soft tissue.

138. **(D)** A carotid endarterectomy (D) is the procedure that will remove the occlusion from the artery and lead to a hopefully successful result. Angioplasty (A) is not performed with carotid arteries because of the possible risk of embolization. Bypass (B) and ligation (C) are not performed either.

139. **(E)** This contrast-enhanced computed axial tomographic (CAT) scan of the head demonstrates more than 30 ring-enhancing lesions. In the late cerebritis and early capsule phases of brain abscess, the typical CAT scan shows a hypodense lesion surrounded by a uniformly enhancing thin-walled ring upon contrast administration. A variable hypodense area of edema extends beyond the ring (A). However, a similar CAT appearance may also be observed in metastatic cancer, resolving cerebral infarcts, and granulomas (B, C, and D). The most useful diagnostic tests in diagnosing herpes simplex encephalitis are MRI and EEG. MRI shows a virtually pathognomonic increased signal, particularly on T2 weighted sequences. When the CAT is positive, the lesion appears as an area of low absorption in the temporo-parietal area, which may be associated with a mass effect. The lesion enhances with contrast (E).

140. **(D)** The pretreatment contrast-enhanced scan of the brain demonstrates a ring-enhancing mass with irregular borders in the left basal ganglia (A). There is marked edema around this mass (C). The mass effect has produced compression of the left lateral ventricle, shifting the ventricle to the right (B and D). The falx cerebri is displaced to the right of midline, in a manner consistent with subfalcial herniation (E).

141. **(D)** Hydrocephalus refers to net accumulation of cerebrospinal fluid within the cerebral ventricles, resulting in their enlargement (A). Both communicating and noncommunicating hydrocephalus are obstructive (E). Noncommunicating hydrocephalus results from lesions that obstruct the intracerebral CSF circulation at or proximal to the foramina of Luschka and Magendie (B). Communicating hydrocephalus results from obstruction of the basal cisterns or convexity subarachnoid space so that the ventricular system communicates with the spinal subarachnoid space. However, the CSF is not able to drain through the arachnoid villi into the superior sagittal sinus (C). Both types of hydrocephalus are treated by shunting (D).

142. **(B)** This child's electroencephalogram (EEG) demonstrates complex repetitive discharges composed of spiky elements mixed with slower waveforms diffusely throughout the left hemisphere (B, A, and C). By contrast, the right hemisphere shows abnormally slow background activity (E). Normal background alpha activity of 11 to 12 Hz per second is demonstrated on the normal, awake EEG (D).

143. **(B)** This patient has onychomycosis, which is very prevalent in the general population over the age of 60. This cosmetic nail dystrophy is caused primarily by dermatophytes in 90% of the cases. Amphotericin B is given by intravenous route only and is a toxic anti-fungal agent for this non-threatening cosmetic condition. Thus, amphotericin B is not recommended for onychomycosis. Griseofulvin (A) is a fungistatic agent effective only against dermatophytes. It is water-soluble and works by incorporating itself into the newly minted nail plate. Thus, therapy with this agent is a long-term endeavor (around six to nine months) to eradicate onychomycosis. Itraconazole (C) is an oral azole anti-fungal agent, which is incorporated into the nail plate as it is formed and thus it binds tightly to its keratin components. This drug stays in the toenails for six to nine months, and once a week dosing may be used for maintenance. Terbinafine hydrochloride (D) is given in doses of 250 mg per day for 6-12 weeks. It is an expensive

medication. This drug has the advantage of entering the nail plate from the nail bed and remaining in the affected area for months after treatment is discontinued. Fluconazole (E) is also an oral azole drug approved for the treatment of fungal disease of the nails. This agent has the disadvantage of not having a very strong affinity for keratin.

144. **(A)** Tension headaches are most likely in a patient in this age group, with headaches described as a band-like pain and worse at the end of the day. Temporal arteritis (B) is less common in this age group and is often associated with visual symptoms and tenderness in the temporal region. Migraine headaches (C) often present in association with visual and/or GI symptoms and may include additional neurological symptoms. Cluster headaches (D) are generally unilateral, not bilateral, and often in association with ocular symptoms. Trigeminal neuralgia (E) is a condition more common in older women, which results in bouts of severe pain over the trigeminal nerve distribution, often triggered by touch, chewing, or cold.

145. **(D)** Angina is the likeliest diagnosis.

146. **(B)** Gastroesophageal reflux is the likeliest diagnosis.

147. **(C)** Costochondritis is the likeliest diagnosis.

148. **(A)** Sickle cell crisis is the likeliest diagnosis.

149. **(E)** Testing of asymptomatic patients for stroke is not routine and is only performed in the presence of very strong risk factors, one of which is the pre-existing cardiovascular or cerebrovascular disorder. Advanced age (A), smoking (B), or alcohol use (C) alone or in any combination do not warrant screening for cerebrovascular disease. Preventive measures at this time should only include counseling about smoking, alcohol use, exercise, and dietary fat consumption.

150. **(A)**, 151. **(B)**, 152. **(C)**, 153. **(D)** Random cortisol levels are not useful in screening for hypercortisolism because of the diurnal variation of the hormone. The overnight dexamethasone test is the most widely used screening test. If normal, Cushing's syndrome is virtually excluded. Typi-

cally, a low-dose dexamethasone suppression test, followed by a high-dose dexamethasone suppression test is performed to evaluate a patient with cortisol excess. The high-dose dexamethasone test helps to distinguish ACTH-independent and ACTH-dependent causes of Cushing's syndrome and to distinguish between pituitary and ectopic causes of ACTH-dependent Cushing's syndrome. Thus, in adrenal causes of cortisol excess, which are autonomous and independent of ACTH, plasma levels are not affected by even high-dose dexamethasone testing. Because the hypothalamic-pituitary axis is suppressed with adrenal lesions, plasma levels of ACTH are low. However, both pituitary and ectopic causes are ACTH-dependent. Pituitary adenomas have an altered set point for glucocorticoid inhibition, but retain a partial ability to respond to high-dose dexamethasone.

154. **(E)** Hydroxychloroquine is a treatment modality for SLE and is not associated with the development of a lupus-like syndrome. Hydralazine (A) and procainamide (C) are most strongly associated with a lupus-like syndrome, as is isoniazid (B). Phenothiazine (D) is also associated with this syndrome, though less commonly than the above-mentioned agents.

155. **(D)** The slide shows three large Negri bodies (eosinophilic viral inclusion bodies) in the cytoplasm of a cerebellar Purkinje cell. Such inclusions are pathologic hallmarks of rabies (D). Subacute sclerosing panencephalitis is characterized by intranuclear inclusions. Electron microscopy of virus-infected cells shows nucleocapsids, but no complete or budding viral particles (A). Progressive multifocal leukoencephalopathy is characterized by multiple foci of enlarging demyelinating "plaques." Astrocytes are tremendously enlarged and contain hyperchromatic, deformed, and bizarre nuclei, with frequent mitotic figures. Oligodendrocytes have enlarged, densely staining nuclei, containing viral inclusions formed by crystalline arrays of JC virus particles (B). Creutzfeldt-Jakob disease is characterized by small round vacuoles (spongiform changes) within the neuropil, cortical neuronal depletion, hypertrophy, and proliferation of glial cells, and absence of inflammation. Amyloid fibrils and plaques composed of CJD protein can be detected immunochemically. The presence of protease-resistant protein (PrP), either *in situ* or after extraction, permits rapid

confirmation of the diagnosis (C). Cerebral edema, with swelling of astrocytic foot processes, and anoxic changes in neurons are seen in Reye's syndrome. Ultrastructural changes in the mitochondria paralleling those observed in the liver also occur (E).

156. **(A)** A perforated duodenal ulcer will present as acute right lower quadrant pain. Pain, tenderness, and rigidity will be pronounced where the contents of the perforation drain down the right pericolic gutter.

157. **(E)** The patient presentation is suggestive of lumbosacral strain. Colchicine (E) is a useful therapy for patients with gout, not lumbosacral strain. Bed rest, warm compresses, and NSAID therapy (A, B, and C), are useful for the acute management of lumbosacral strain. Physical exertion should be avoided during the acute episode; however, a back and abdomen strengthening program can be helpful to prevent the recurrence of lumbosacral strain (D).

158. **(D)** Although the patient requests additional testing, she should be counseled regarding the lack of need for additional testing at this time. Aggressive or defensive comments are not prudent in this situation. CT scan (B) is unlikely to be of any yield in this situation. Referral to an orthopedic surgeon (C) is not indicated in this situation.

159. **(E)** None of the proposed tests is likely to reveal abnormalities in patients with lumbosacral strain. The diagnosis is mostly a clinical one. Back X-rays (A) are useful to evaluate for bone spurs or fractures. EMG/nerve conduction studies (B) are not indicated in this patient. CT scan and myelograms (C and D) are useful to evaluate a herniated disk, but this is not a likely concern at this time in this patient.

160. **(C)** Patients with ulcerative colitis may develop rheumatoid factor-negative spondyloarthropathy; however, they are not predisposed to develop lumbosacral strain. Leg-length discrepancy (A) is thought to predispose toward the occurrence of chronic low back pain secondary to lumbosacral strain. Frequent lifting and obesity (B and E) also predispose toward episodes of lumbosacral strain and can be improved by proper lifting techniques and conditioning of abdominal and lower back muscles. An abnormal forward pelvic tilt or accentuated lordosis (D) also predisposes toward the development of low-back pain.

161. **(B)** This patient has chronic myelogenous leukemia, which is characterized by splenomegaly and an extreme elevation of the granulocyte count. This is a myeloproliferative disorder, which can result in blast crises and leukostasis. The leukocyte alkaline phosphatase level would be depressed in chronic myelogenous leukemia and elevated in a leukemoid reaction secondary to an infection. Alpha-fetoprotein (A) is a tumor marker, which is elevated in hepatomas and certain testicular carcinomas. The angiotensin-converting enzyme level (C) would be elevated in sarcoidosis. It is a non-specific test. The ceruloplasmin level (D) is a plasma protein, which is a screening tool to diagnose Wilson's disease. It would be less than 200 in a patient with excess copper accumulation in the liver and brain, which is diagnostic for Wilson's disease. CA-125 (E) is a tumor marker which is elevated in ovarian carcinoma.

162. **(B)** The X-ray shows marked expansion of bone and a bowing deformity of the right tibia, with the mixed lytic and sclerotic changes characteristic of Paget's disease. The remodeling of the Pagetic bone typically follows the lines of stress produced by muscle pull or gravity, accounting for the characteristic lateral bowing of the femur or the anterior bowing of the tibia (B). The disease may also present with lytic lesions that cause expansion of the cortex, exhibiting features suggestive of malignancy (C). In the skull, the early phase of osteolytic activity may present as osteoporosis circumscripta, with sharply demarcated radiolucency in the frontal, parietal, and occipital bones (E). Fissure fractures, which may herald complete fractures, occur more frequently in persons with bowing. Complete fractures of the long bones occur most often in the femur, but are not evident here (A). Rickets results from defective bone and cartilage mineralization. Radiologic manifestations, most evident at the epiphyseal growth plate, include widening, increased thickness, and cupping. The metaphyseal border is hazy due to decreased calcification of the hypertrophic zone and inadequate mineralization (D).

163. **(E)** Whipple's disease is an infectious systematic disease affecting many organs, but most severely the small intestine. PAS-positive macrophages in the mucosa are diagnostic; CNS signs

(memory loss, nystagmus, confusion, etc.) are often present. The macrophages are filled with rod-shaped bacilli which disappear after antibiotic therapy and reappear on cessation of antibiotics. Biopsy of the small intestine also shows blunting of villi and dilated jejunal lymphatics. This is a protein-losing enteropathy which causes steatorrhea and neurological abnormalities. Lymphoma of the small intestine (A) would also present with abdominal pain, fever, and diarrhea, but biopsy would show malignant lymphoid cells in the mucosa or submucosa, not PAS-filled macrophages. Celiac sprue (B) can cause malabsorption because of intolerance to wheat, barley, and oats. Biopsy of the small intestine would show villous atrophy. Isospora belli infection (C) causes diarrhea and fever in AIDS patients. Neurological signs are not usually present. Lymphangiectasia (D) is characterized by diarrhea, mild steatorrhea, and edema. It is a protein-losing enteropathy with abnormal dilated lymphatic channels found on a biopsy of the small intestine.

164. **(C)** Carpel tunnel syndrome or median nerve compression is not associated with painful, palmar swelling. Thenar space infection (A), palmar abscess (B), ulnar bursa abscess (D), and acute tenosynovitis (E) are all infectious, inflammatory processes, which are associated with painful, palmar swelling.

165. **(D)**, 166. **(A)**, 167. **(C)**, 168. **(D)** Immunologically mediated inflammatory reactions have been classified into four separate groups. IgE mediated allergic reactions (Type I) are the result of antigens IgE interacting with IgE antibodies, which are bound to mast cells and basophils, which subsequently release reactive mediators. Anaphylactic and allergic diseases occur through this mechanism. Cytotoxic (Type II) reactions (B) occur through compliment-mediated damage, resulting in cell lysis or tissue damage. Immune complex formations (Type III) are a mechanism of combating antigens (C); however, these complexes may deposit and damage tissues or blood vessels, accounting for diseases such as systemic lupus erythematosus or serum sickness. Delayed-type hypersensitivity reactions (Type IV) (D) account for diseases related to granuloma formation, such as tuberculosis and fungal infection. In these conditions, T-cell mediated responses result in the recruitment of macrophages, which undergo giant cell transformation, accounting for the development of granulomas.

169. **(C)** Shortness of breath can be due to respiratory or metabolic reasons. In this patient, a metabolic acidosis can lead to tachypnea and a feeling of shortness of breath. The oxalate crystals in the urine are classically associated with ethylene glycol poisoning.

170. **(A)** Symptoms of digoxin toxicity include nausea, vomiting, palpitations, visual changes with colors, haloes noted around lights, and nearly any type of arrhythmia.

171. **(E)** Flumazenil is a benzodiazepine inhibitor and can be used acutely to reverse benzodiazepine overdose. However, with longer-acting benzodiazepines, flumazenil may need to be repeated.

172. **(D)** Pupillary constriction with decreased respiratory effort are classic for opioid toxicity.

173. **(A)** In this child you would expect to see the signs of dehydration and hypovolemia, since intake is decreased and output is increased. You would not see a decreased pulse. You would see an increased pulse (B) and decreased blood pressure (C) as a result of the hypovolemia. The mucous membranes (D) would be dry because of decreased body fluid, and urine would be concentrated (E) in an attempt to conserve fluid.

174. **(B)** The family history (B) would not be as useful as the other choices. Gestational age (A) of the baby is important in assessing the ability to thrive. Immunization status (C) is important to know, to rule out any disease that could be present that could have been prevented normally. The diet (D) is important in assessing nutrition, and recent travel (E) may indicate the acquisition of a disease not usually found in the native land.

175. **(B)** Pyloric stenosis is obstruction of the pyloric lumen due to pyloric muscular hypertrophy. There is a discrete 2-cm firm mass, or "olive," deep in the epigastrium which can be palpated. A duodenal obstruction (A), which is caused by stenosis or atresia of the duodenum, a large bowel

obstruction (C), or esophageal atresia (D) will not have an associated palpable mass. In a diaphragmatic hernia (E), the abdominal contents are in the thorax, giving the child great breathing difficulties.

176. **(B)** This child needs intravenous fluid administration. He should not be sent home (A). Increasing his oral intake (C) will not work because he is vomiting. Anti-emetics (D) and anti-diarrheals (E) will only treat the symptom and not the problem. They should also be used with caution in the newborn.

177. **(A)** SBP can present without a fever, and can additionally present without abdominal pain, nausea, or vomiting. It is a common cause of hepatic encephalopathy and is more common in patients with a large amount of ascites.

178. **(D)** Ascites fluid cell count greater than 250 polymorphonuclear leukocytes/microliter is diagnostic for SBP. Patients should be treated regardless of Gram-stain (B and C) or culture (A), which can both be negative.

179. **(C)** The most common cause of SBP is *E. coli.*

180. **(A)** Aminoglycosides (gentamicin) should be avoided in the treatment of SBP because they can induce renal failure, especially in patients with liver failure, and they penetrate the peritoneal fluid poorly.

USMLE Step 3 – Practice Test 2
Day Two – Morning Session

1. **(C)**, 2. **(B)**, 3. **(B)**, 4. **(D)** Disorders caused by the transmission of a single mutant gene are inherited through either autosomal dominant, recessive, or X-linked patterns. Color blindness is X-linked and therefore cannot be passed on from male to male vertically. Sickle cell anemia is a common autosomal recessive disorder which requires two copies of the mutant allele for full phenotypic presentation, although carriers may also display milder abnormalities. Cystic fibrosis is also transmitted as an autosomal recessive trait. The disease occurs in 1 in 2,000 Caucasian births, and 4-5% of Caucasians are heterozygous carriers for the disease. Nonalcoholic steatohepatitis is not known to be genetically linked at this time. It is associated with diabetes, hyperlipidemia, and certain medications.

5. **(D)** Acute promyelocytic leukemia is a subtype (M3) of acute myelogenous leukemia. It is often associated with disseminated intravascular coagulation triggered by elevated fibrin degradation products and schistocytes in the peripheral blood. Acute lymphocytic leukemia (A) is more common in children and associated with hepatosplenomegaly and lymphadenopathy, neither of which appear in this patient. Disseminated intravascular coagulation is uncommon unless there is an underlying sepsis. Chronic myelogenous leukemia (B) is characterized by an elevated WBC count or left upper quadrant pain, both of which are associated with splenomegaly and neither of which are present in this patient. Multiple myeloma (C) is characterized by a proliferation of plasma cells. Most patients develop anemia and, like the patient described, may present with lethargy, fatigue, and pallor. Various organs are involved, the spleen being a notable exception. Susceptibility to infection and clotting disorders is increased. However, DIC is unlikely to develop, except in the presence of a significant infection. Chronic lymphocytic leukemia (E) is characterized by accumulation of B lymphocytes. Males are affected more than females, and the spleen is often involved.

6. **(A)** The pleural fluid analysis suggests an exudative effusion. Nephrotic syndrome results in a transudative effusion, not an exudative effusion. Systemic lupus erythematosus (B) and other connective-tissue diseases can result in an exudative effusion. Bronchogenic carcinoma (C), lymphoma, and metastatic cancer (E) may cause exudative pleural effusions. Parapneumonic effusion (D) is a non-empyemic effusion, which occurs secondary to the inflammation of a bacterial pneumonia and is generally exudative.

7. **(D)** The computed axial tomographic scans of the abdomen show polycystic disease, affecting both the liver and kidneys. Both hepatic and renal cysts increase in size and/or number over time (D). At least two genes have been associated with this syndrome. In the most commonly manifested clinical disease, the genetic defect is localized to the short arm of chromosome 16 (B). Intracranial aneurysms occur in approximately 10% of affected persons (A). Approximately one-third of affected persons will show microscopic hematuria on a random urinalysis. Forty percent will have at least one episode of gross hematuria (C). Hypertension develops in at least 60% of affected persons (E).

8. **(E)** This patient appears to be manipulating the system to obtain codeine. It is possible he is addicted to codeine, is selling it, or is providing it for someone else. In any case, the pharmacist has done the correct thing in calling you. You should calmly but firmly confront the patient with this situation and explain that you cannot give him prescriptions for narcotics that he is getting from other physicians. Pharmacists will often set up a system whereby only one designated physician can write such a prescription for the patient.

9. **(D)** The working diagnosis of this patient is basal cell carcinoma, which accounts for most cases of skin malignancies in the United States. The easy way to identify a form of skin cancer is memorizing that cancers above the upper lip are

more likely to be basal cell carcinoma (BCC), whereas those below the upper lip are more likely to be squamous cell carcinoma (SCC). Epidemiological studies show that light-skinned populations are approximately 50 times more likely to develop this condition at some point in their lives (A). In fact, it is the most common form of cancer in light-skinned populations (B) and is responsible for 40% of all cancer in the United States. Sensitivity and prolonged exposure to UV radiation are among the factors contributing to skin cancer. However, genetic predisposition is the major risk factor (C).

10. **(D)** Intertrigo is a superficial dermatitis in the skin folds as a result of warm, moist skin, and secondary infection with bacteria. It is, therefore, seen in the skin and not the hair roots (A), cornea (B), retina (C), or the tympanic membrane (E).

11. **(E)** It is vitally important to review old records whether it be charts, X-rays, or lab results. You will save time and expense as well as avoiding mistakes or repetitive procedures. To give pain medication (A), order X-rays (B), or perform procedures such as passage of an NG tube (C) or rectal examination (D) may be premature and/or unnecessary.

12. **(D)** Lymphedema usually begins gradually. Initially, the enlarged limb is soft and pitting. As the condition becomes chronic, the skin takes on a woody texture. The tissues become indurated and fibrotic. The edema is no longer pitting. In this case of massive obesity, the lymphangiogram shows normal lymphatic vessels and regional lymph nodes (A). The radionuclide promptly migrates cephalad (B). The magnetic resonance imaging study demonstrates massive subcutaneous deposition of fat, without evidence of fluid accumulation (C and D). The irregular high-intensity subcutaneous signals on the coronal section represent venous varicosities (E).

13. **(A)** The history and physical exam are most consistent with pseudomembranous colitis from antibiotic usage. A flat plate (B) should be done to exclude toxic megacolon, which can complicate this disease. Complete blood count (C) should be done to rule out severe anemia. Stool samples should be sent off for both *C. difficile* toxin to rule in pseudomembranous colitis and for culture to rule out other kinds of bacterial colitis

(D and E). A flexible sigmoidoscopy is not necessary in the initial workup for this disease.

14. **(B)** An uncommon complication of *C. dif.* colitis is toxic megacolon, which can lead to bowel perforation. If a patient has a dilated colon, he should be admitted for observation and decompression if necessary.

15. **(C)** The symptoms are classic for *C. dif.* colitis, and it almost always follows long-term antibiotic usage. It classically presents after usage with clindamycin or amoxicillin, but can present after almost any antibiotic usage, except for metronidazole.

16. **(A)** Initial treatment for *C. dif.* colitis is metronidazole. If that doesn't work, then oral vancomycin is another possibility.

17. **(D)** AZT given during pregnancy as recommended has been found to decrease the rate of transmission by two-thirds. HIV transmission has been found to occur in utero; therefore, caesarean section does not prevent transmission (A). Breast feeding has been implicated in the transmission of the virus to infants and, therefore, is not recommended to women in the United States (B). Not all babies born to HIV-infected women will be infected with the virus (C). Perinatal transmission is estimated to occur in 33-50% of affected pregnancies if no antiretroviral therapy is used. HIV disease has not been shown to cause chromosomal abnormalities (E).

18. **(A)** If you suspect an overdose of sleeping pills, gastric lavage is a relatively easy way to remove any undissolved or partially dissolved medication.

19. **(D)** The likeliest diagnosis is acute bronchitis, which should respond to an oral antibiotic.

20. **(C)** Diabetics frequently have peripheral neuropathy and subsequently injure their extremities and do not even know it. They often have difficulty healing their wounds as well, due to vascular disease. It is important to educate these patients on the importance of wound care. A biopsy (A) would not be needed on this ulcer, and the patient would probably have trouble healing it. A culture (B) would only show polymicrobial disease

and not be of too much significance initially. To obtain a primary closure (D) would be fraught with difficulty and not be indicated, especially if the wound is infected. An angiogram (E) should be ordered if revascularization is planned, and this wound initially should be treated conservatively.

21. **(D)** The characteristic pattern illustrated here is known as the Brockenbrough-Braunwald sign (E). In this simultaneous arterial and left ventricular pressure tracing of a person with hypertrophic obstructive cardiomyopathy, the first three beats show a peak systolic gradient of 25 mm Hg (A). On the first sinus beat after the premature ventricular contraction (PVC), the peak systolic gradient increases to over 100 mm Hg (B). The pulse pressure (arterial systolic pressure minus diastolic pressure) decreases (C). The decrease in pulse pressure following a PVC results from a reduced stroke volume caused by increased dynamic obstruction (D).

22. **(C)** Risk factors for the development of placenta previa include multiparity, advanced maternal age, previous C-section, large placenta, and cigarette smoking.

23. **(A)** and 24. **(B)** Diagnosis is reliably confirmed by ultrasonography in 95% of cases. For the remaining instances, diagnosis can be substantiated by direct vaginal examination of the cervix. If ultrasound is unavailable, the diagnosis of placenta previa can be made by radioisotope scanning (rarely used).

25. **(B)** A double setup is a vaginal examination performed with the immediate capability of converting to caesarean section. It is instituted when the exact location of a suspected placenta previa cannot be delineated by ultrasonography. The double setup is an elective procedure for hemodynamically stable patients. It should be performed in the operative room with the mother prepared for an emergent operative delivery, under general anesthesia.

26. **(D)** Early decelerations are characterized by slowing of the fetal heart rate beginning with the onset of uterine contractions. Early decelerations are believed to occur from vagal stimulation, as the fetal head is compressed, and are benign. Late decelerations are identified by a decrease in fetal heart rate that occurs after the onset of uter-

ine contractions and ends after the contractions are completed. Variable decelerations are unrelated to time of onset, duration, or magnitude of uterine contractions. Variable decelerations occur consequent to umbilical cord compression. Some authorities consider beat-to-beat variability to be the most sensitive indicator of fetal well-being obtainable from fetal heart beat patterns.

27. **(C)** Fetal scalp blood sampling should be performed when the heart rate pattern appears ominous. Normal fetal scalp pH ranges from 7.28 to 7.30. A fetal scalp pH less than 7.20 is a menacing sign and indicates immediate delivery of the fetus. A pH between 7.20 and 7.25 is equivocal and requires repeating 15 minutes later to determine fetal well-being.

28. **(A)** Abruptio placenta indicates premature separation of the placenta from the uterus, before delivering the fetus. It occurs in 0.2-2.4% of all deliveries. It is associated with gestational hypertension, preeclampsia, multiparity, cigarette smoking, and cocaine abuse. Congenital hypofibrinogenemia does not protect from, but predisposes to, the placental abruption. In women with a history of one abruption, the recurrence rate is 10 times that of the normal population.

29. **(A)** Because rupture of an old scar is rare and the morbidity and mortality of such a rupture is low, the American College of Obstetricians and Gynecologists states that the parturient who has had a previous C-section with a lower uterine segment transverse incision can be permitted a trial of labor. A high incidence of rupture is associated with closure uterine incision scars.

30. **(C)** None of the responses, with the exception of ectopic pregnancy, can have such potentially life-threatening consequences if missed. In ectopic pregnancy, the fertilized ovum implants at any site other than the endometrial cavity. The fallopian tube is the most likely site. The growing trophoblast can erode into the tubal muscularis and maternal blood supply, causing hemorrhage and shock. A threatened abortion (A) is considered when any bloody discharge appears to come from the pregnant uterus. A missed abortion (B) occurs when the embryo is no longer viable but is retained in utero, usually for at least six weeks. Fibroids (D) can cause significant uterine bleeding, but are uncommon in this age group. Salpingitis

(E) is an infection of the fallopian tubes, usually caused by chlamydia or gonorrhea.

31. **(D)** Dysuria, or difficult or painful urination, may result in hesitancy or straining. The most common cause is a partial obstruction of the urethra. A vaginal wall carcinoma (A), intrauterine pregnancy (B), uterine fibroid (C), and bladder paralysis (E) may also lead to dysuria, but are less common. In adults, infection often occurs secondary to lower urinary tract obstruction associated with pregnancy, STDs, or instrumentation.

32. **(E)** This Genta-stained biopsy specimen demonstrates *Helicobacter pylori* filling a gastric pit. Clinical trials have demonstrated that eradication of this organism with triple therapy decreases the rate of duodenal ulcer recurrence following ulcer healing. Several treatment regimens have been proposed, including one combining tetracycline, metronidazole, and bismuth (E). Famotidine, a more potent H-2 receptor antagonist than cimetidine, is administered at bedtime, initially at a dose of 40 mg (D). There is no evidence of a malignancy in this biopsy specimen (B). Although both psychotherapy and decreasing cigarette consumption can be suggested, neither measure will eradicate the organism and are not the preferred strategy (A and C).

33. **(E)** All of the other tests are emergently needed.

34. **(D)** This is a typical presentation for a woman with preeclampsia.

35. **(C)** Pancreatitis is not a feature or association of preeclampsia, while all of the others are.

36. **(A)** Diuretics can exacerbate preeclampsia and should be avoided.

37. **(B)** A consumptive coagulopathy can be a manifestation of preeclampsia.

38. **(C)** Delivery cures preeclampsia in nearly all patients without underlying renal disease.

39. **(B)** Fortunately, the prognosis of preeclampsia is quite good after delivery.

40. **(D)** In an emergency room, pain and apprehension is a major reason for hypertension.

While his hypertension may be under poor control (A), it is not as likely a cause as his pain. A pheochromocytoma (B) is also a possibility, but not likely. Factitial readings (C) are again a possibility, but not as likely as his pain and apprehension. Hypovolemia (E) will lead to hypotension, not hypertension, as with someone in shock. The heart rate will also increase.

41. **(E)** When performing a history of the hand, various questions are important. The dominance of the hand (B) is important because the physical examination may be subtly different between hands, and your treatment may vary based on hand dominance. Occupation (C) of the patient is important for similar reasons. Previous hand trauma (D) is essential because you want to discriminate new trauma from old trauma in your exam. Tetanus status (A) is important with any trauma because of needed prophylaxis. While family history (E) is important for a general review of systems, it takes on smaller importance when examining the hand.

42. **(B)** The flexor digitorum profundus of the ring finger flexes the DIP joint of the ring finger. The flexor digitorum superficialis (A) flexes the PIP joint. The extensor digiti communis of the finger extends the finger (C). The flexor carpi ulnaris (D) and flexor carpi radialis (E) flex the wrist and deviate it to the ulnar and radial sides, respectively.

43. **(D)** There is no indication to repair a flexor tendon in the emergency room. This usually requires an operating room. The administration of tetanus toxoid (A), irrigation and exploration of the wound (B), closure of the skin (C), and hand splinting (E) are all appropriate at this time.

44. **(B)** The Allen's test is used to ascertain arterial supply to the hand by alternately compressing the radial and ulnar arteries and assessing inflow. The Trendelenburg test (A) is used for testing lower extremity venous competence. The McMurray test (C) is used for testing the medial meniscus of the knee. Kocher's test or sign (D) is used to examine the thyroid gland in which pressure on the lateral lobe produces stridor. Kernig's sign (E) is used for testing the presence of meningitis.

45. **(C)** The ulnar nerve provides sensation to the small finger and the ulnar half of the ring finger. The radial nerve (A) provides sensation to the

dorsal radial three-and-one-half fingers. The median nerve (B) provides sensation to the volar radial three-and-one-half fingers. The musculocutaneous nerve (D) provides sensation to the radial half of the anterior surface of the forearm. The hypothenar (E) is not a nerve in the hand.

46. **(B)** A neuropraxia occurs when there is a pressure injury of the nerve and no signs of obvious trauma, as in this case. A neurotmesis (C) occurs when there is complete division of the nerve. An axontmesis (D) occurs when there is interruption of the axons of the nerve, but not the supporting structure of the nerve. An inexperienced examiner (A) is always a possibility, but not as likely. A laceration around the field of exploration (E) is a possibility, but not as likely.

47. **(D)** This patient has hepatitis C infection along with early cirrhosis. He is at risk of chronic, persistent hepatitis C and hepatoma. A hepatitis C vaccine is not yet available. When someone is stuck with a needle from a hepatitis C virus-positive patient, the options are to watch and wait or to administer immune serum globulin. The hepatitis B vaccine is available to all persons at risk for obtaining hepatitis B and, therefore, they should be vaccinated prior to an incident occurring. All individuals found to be anti-HCV-positive need to be considered potentially infectious and should be counselled concerning infectivity (A). An HCV-positive patient has a 0-3% chance of transmitting the virus to a sex partner. Neonatal transmission occurs in about six percent of infants born to HCV-positive mothers. Household articles should not be shared (B), and cuts or skin lesions should be covered to prevent the spread of infectious secretions or blood. Interferon alpha-2b (C) at a dosage of three million units three times a week, subcutaneously, has been shown to normalize alanine aminotransferase and reduce fever degeneration and necrosis. The response rate to interferon therapy for hepatitis C is about 50%, but the majority of patients relapse when therapy is discontinued. Liver biopsy (E) is indicated in patients with confirmed hepatitis C viremia and sustained elevations of aminotransferases over a period of six months.

48. **(A)** The most drastic complications that can occur after a myocardial infarction are papillary muscle rupture and free wall rupture. With a new enlarged cardiac silhouette on chest radiograph and decreased voltage on EKG with hypotension, the myocardial rupture needs to be ruled out and can be confirmed by an emergent echocardiogram.

49. **(B)** Aseptic meningitis is the most likely diagnosis based on the presence of predominantly lymphocytic cells, and normal protein and sugar levels. Common causes of aseptic meningitis include viral infections and medications. Bacterial meningitis (A) generally results in a CSF examination with predominantly polymorphonuclear cells and a reduced glucose and elevated protein. Migraine headache (C) generally results in a normal CSF exam, which this patient does not have. Subarachnoid hemorrhage (D) results in a bloody CSF appearance with elevated protein.

50. **(A)** The spleen lies obliquely with its long axis along the tenth rib, and the area of splenic dullness is in the left posterior axilla, not exceeding a vertical distance of more than 9 cm. The area of splenic dullness can usually be determined by palpation and percussion.

51. **(B)** The bone marrow aspirate, showing an increased number of plasma cells, confirms the clinical diagnosis of multiple myeloma. The marrow must contain at least 10% plasma cells. In chronic lymphocytic leukemia, there is a proliferation of lymphocytes, which are indistinguishable on light or electron microscopy from normal small B-lymphocytes (C). No metastatic cells are present in this specimen (A and E). Myeloid metaplasia is characterized by bone marrow fibrosis and extramedullary hematopoiesis (D).

52. **(B)** The bone lesions of myeloma are caused by the proliferation of tumor cells and the activation of osteoclasts, which destroy the bone. The bone lesions are lytic in nature (B) and are rarely associated with osteoblastic new bone formation (A). The observed bony abnormalities, which include punched-out lytic lesions, osteoporosis, and/or fractures, are observed in approximately 80% of myeloma patients (C). The biconcave or "fishmouth" vertebral deformity, which is classic for sickle cell anemia, results from bony infarcts (D). The "bamboo spine," seen in ankylosing spondylitis, results from marginal bridging

of the syndesmophytes, interapophyseal joint fusion, and "squaring" of the lumbar and thoracic vertebrae (E).

53.　**(A)**　The classic triad of multiple myeloma is bone marrow containing more than 10% plasma cells, lytic bone lesions, and an M-component in the urine or serum (A). These constitute the minimal criteria for the diagnosis of myeloma, although a plasmacytoma may be substituted for the marrow plasmacytosis. These abnormalities must not be explained by other diseases, such as metastatic carcinoma, chronic infection, and connective tissue diseases. Although they do not constitute criteria, anemia, hypercalcemia and Bence-Jones proteinuria are common findings in persons with myeloma (E).

54.　**(A)**　Normally, light chains are filtered, reabsorbed in the tubules, and catabolized. The excessive amount of light chains presented to the renal tubule causes protein overload, resulting in tubular damage. The protein presents as large, waxy, laminated casts, composed primarily of monoclonal light chains (B), in both the distal tubules and collecting ducts (A). Hyperuricemia, glomerular deposition of amyloid, and recurrent infections also cause renal failure in persons with myeloma (C and E). Deposition of monoclonal heavy chains in the renal glomerulus, known as heavy chain deposition disease, can result in nephrotic syndrome and renal failure (D).

55.　**(B)**　As with many diagnoses in medicine, it is always best to compare with the old when faced with something new. In the case of this chest X-ray, the lesion may have been stable or unchanged over the years and, as such, there would be less to do or to be concerned about.

56.　**(C)**　A soft palate carcinoma will have no effect on the status of the gums. Dilantin (A) will cause an overgrowth or hyperplasia of the gums. Gingivitis (B) is a local inflammation of the gums which causes swelling. Scurvy (D) causes the gums to become deep red and purple as well as swollen and tender. An odontogenic or tooth abscess (E) will cause a swelling under the gums, causing them to swell over the involved tooth.

57.　**(A)**　Subacute bacterial endocarditis is the correct diagnosis.

58.　**(C)**　Pericarditis is the correct diagnosis.

59.　**(E)**　Hypocalcemia is the correct diagnosis.

60.　**(B)**　Atrial fibrillation is the correct diagnosis.

61.　**(C)**　Rickets is infantile osteomalacia, and results from vitamin D deficiency. A lab value seen with this is decreased serum calcium. The serum phosphorus is decreased as well. Serum alkaline phosphatase is increased, not decreased (D).

62.　**(C)**　In infants and children, the primary form of tuberculosis may not be contagious, since they may not cough. In addition, a childhood primary TB has a brief, self-limited, and often asymptomatic course.

63.　**(B)**　Her symptoms are consistent with temporal arteritis. To ensure the diagnosis and to start treatment with steroids, an urgent temporal artery biopsy should be done.

64.　**(E)**　The physician should initiate a careful search for possible carcinogens at the work site. Physicians involved in occupational medicine should act in accord with the code of ethical conduct. Therefore, confidentiality of whatever is learned about patients served is recommended. It is broken only when *required* by law (B) or because of overriding public health considerations (C). Since the occurrence of two similar cases in a year could have been by chance alone, releasing information to management or other workers (D) is not only unethical, but also not justified at this time. Likewise, expressing an opinion based solely on suspicions (A) is not a professional approach.

65.　**(A)**　This patient has scurvy, which is caused by vitamin C deficiency. The elderly and urban poor are at an increased risk for dietary deficiency of ascorbic acid. Wounds heal poorly and joints, muscle, and subcutaneous tissues may become sites of hemorrhage. Vitamin B12 deficiency (B) can result from intestinal malabsorption disorders and leads to pernicious anemia. Symptoms include parasthesias, numbness and tingling of the hands, and stiffness of the legs with unsteadiness. Neurological symptoms are secondary to subacute degeneration of white matter in the dorsal and lateral columns of the spinal cord. Niacin deficiency (C) causes glossitis, anorexia, weight loss, and abdominal discomfort. Niacin deficiency is called pellagra. Vitamin B1 deficiency, or thiamine (D) deficiency, causes cardiovascular compromise— "beriberi" and Wernicke-Korsakoff syndrome. Vitamin A deficiency (E) causes night blindness.

66. **(B)** This patient has meningitis. The best procedure to test if the infection is from a viral or bacterial source is to perform a lumbar puncture, examine the cerebral spinal fluid for white blood cells, and do a Gram stain to look for bacterial organisms. If this patient has meningococci meningitis, it is a medical emergency and penicillin should be instituted even before the cultures are back. A lumbar puncture is crucial to the diagnosis. If this patient has no focal neurological signs, then performing a head CT (A) prior to performing a lumbar would be a waste of time and resources and would not yield much information. A skin biopsy would take too long, and this patient could expire in the meantime from wide-spread dissemination. Thus, this invasive procedure is useless. Cerebral spinal fluid cultures should be sent to the microbiology lab for bacterial and fungal cultures prior to blood culture (D), since the patient's symptoms are referred in the brain. Intravenous hydration (E) is important because of volume depletion and fever, but a lumbar puncture should still be performed first.

67. **(A)** Morphine is generally regarded as the narcotic against which all others are compared in terms of analgesic potency. Of the agents listed, Sufentanil (E) is the next most potent, being 70-100% as potent as morphine.

68. **(C)** Isolated mild hypertension on one check should be confirmed on another visit before treatment is started for hypertension.

69. **(E)** The polymerase chain reaction (PCR) is a molecular technique that can be used to generate banding patterns that can be tracked through a family. It is a DNA amplification technique, which is based on knowing the nucleic acid sequence for a particular gene region. Diagnostic testing, using PCR, allows amplification of very specific pieces of DNA from extremely small samples. The technique is so sensitive that one can amplify and analyze DNA from a single hu-

man sperm, which contains one duplex target DNA molecule (A). Using this technique, tests can occasionally be performed on archival samples (B). Due to its extreme sensitivity, testing performed by the PCR technique is vulnerable to minute contamination by any DNA, including skin cells from laboratory personnel, cross-contamination from a previous sample, or other amplified DNA present in the laboratory (C). PCR is also vulnerable to infidelity during replication, which may cause artifactual mutations (D).

70. **(D)** Her blood pressure elevation may be a transient reaction to the headaches or her stress, and her headaches may be stress-related. The prudent course is to see her again soon and reassess her, both for her blood pressure and her headaches.

71. **(D)** Time is an important factor in considering the type of surgery for retinal detachment. Peripheral or macular detachments exceeding 24 hours can be treated electively (A and B). Urgent surgical intervention is required for a recent or impending macular detachment (C).

72. **(C)** The blood smear shows Gram-negative diplococci (C). *Staphylococcus aureus*, one of the most important human pathogens of the staphylococci, is a Gram-positive nonmotile, catalase-positive coccus. The name, *Staphylococcus*, means "bunch of grapes," which describes the appearance of the clusters and clumps of Gram-positive cocci seen on Gram-stained specimens (A). *Streptococci* are Gram-positive bacteria with a spherical-to-ovoid shape, typically forming chains when grown in liquid media. The chief nonenterococcal group D streptococcal species that causes human infection is *Streptococcus bovis* (B). *Streptococcus pneumoniae* are encapsulated, Gram-positive cocci, which occur in chains or pairs. When in pairs, they are typically lancet-shaped. The capsule, not evident on Gram's stain, requires special negative stains, such as an India ink preparation, for visualization. Confusion arises because the organism sometimes stains negatively on Gram-stain preparations of purulent or exudative material (D). This clinical picture would be atypical for *Escherichia coli*, a small, Gram-negative bacillus (E).

73. **(B)** Weber's test involves the placement of a tuning fork on the midline of the skull and

asking the patient to compare intensities. Lateralization of sound to one ear indicates a conductive loss on the same side. There is a perceptive loss on the other side.

74. **(D)** This patient has *Mycoplasma* pneumonia, which is prevalent in young adults in college or in the military. This pneumonia is associated with a hacking cough and bullous myringitis. It is also associated with cold agglutinin. The X-ray findings are usually worse than the physical exam. Oral erythromycin is the correct treatment of choice. A CT of the chest (A) is not necessary in this patient, and it would not give us any additional information. Steroids (B) are contraindicated in this infectious pneumonia. Steroids will only exacerbate the pneumonia. Steroids are useful in pneumonitis disorders of the lung. Hospitalization (C) is not required in this situation because this patient is young and healthy with no other underlying disorders, and cephalosporins are not the treatment of choice. This patient does not have asthma symptoms or wheezing on exam. Her X-ray is suggestive of pneumonia. Thus, beta-adrenergic agonists (E) are not needed.

75. **(D)** The specificity is defined as: of all patients who don't have the disease, how many test negative (92/100). The sensitivity is defined as: of all patients who do have the disease, how many test positive (98/100 = 98%).

76. **(B)** Tympany replaces resonance with a pneumothorax. Emphysema (A) leads to hyper-resonance replacing resonance. Dullness replaces resonance in the lower lung with pleural effusion (C). Dullness replaces resonance in the upper lung with neoplasm (D) or atelectasis (E).

77. **(D)** In renal failure, the serum creatinine does not represent a steady-state measurement of renal function; therefore, any calculations of creatinine clearance based on serum creatinine are not accurate. Twenty-four-hour urine studies (A) pose the same problem, as the creatinine clearance can change significantly in 24 hours. The dosing of aminoglycosides needs to be changed as they are renally excreted, and the best way to dose them is to follow levels until they reach their trough and then redose (D). Considerations to stopping the aminoglycoside should be made, however, if the patient is remaining septic, aminoglycoside therapy should probably be contin-

ued. Toxicity is minimized by achieving a predose trough of 2 ug/mL and a peak under 10 ug/mL. Furthermore, the maintenance dose will decrease as creatinine clearance slows.

78. **(D)** Introducing normal saline drops to each nares will only aggravate the symptoms of allergic rhinitis and will not alleviate the inflammation. The newest and most effective treatment available now to relieve the symptoms of allergic rhinitis are inhaled nasal steroids (A), such as Beconase and Nasocort. This has been shown to decrease the inflammation and reduce the number of eosinophils in the nasal discharge. Oral antihistamines (H1 blockers), such as Terfenidine and Loratadine, have been shown to decrease the symptoms of allergic rhinitis (B) by blocking the receptor on the mast cells so that degranulation does not take place and the inflammatory cells are not released to cause symptoms. Staying in an air-conditioned room or car (C) helps to keep the patient from being exposed to pollen or ragweed, which is the offending allergen causing the symptoms. Alcohol intake, even in moderate amounts, along with ingestion of antihistamines would cause excessive sedation and drowsiness (E). The combination is not advised.

79. **(A)** Anemia in a 65-year-old male requires that other sources of gastrointestinal bleeding be excluded prior to definitive therapy of hemorrhoids. Most hemorrhoids respond to conservative therapy, including sitz baths, rectal suppositories, and stool softeners. Internal hemorrhoids usually respond to high-fiber diets (E) and avoidance of prolonged sitting at stool. Complications of hemorrhoids, such as prolapse and thrombosis, sometimes require more definitive therapy. These procedures should not be undertaken until proctosigmoidoscopy or colonoscopy is performed (B, C, and D).

80. **(E)** In the screening for colorectal cancer, the test most widely used for the detection of blood in the stool is a guaiac-based test for peroxidase activity. Heme in red meat and peroxidase activity in turnips and horseradish may cause false-positive tests (A and B). Ingestion of salicylates, which may produce occult gastrointestinal bleeding, can cause false-positive results for colon cancer (C). Vitamin C, which is an antioxidant, may interfere with the reaction, producing a false-negative test (D). Oral supplements do not directly

interfere with this test. However, the black-colored stool may cause difficulty in the interpretation of a positive test (E).

81. **(A)** The barium enema shows several filling defects, which have a benign appearance. Colonoscopy (A), with excisional biopsy (B), is recommended. Results of chemistry screening have not been reported. In the absence of elevations of liver-function tests, liver-spleen scanning is not recommended (D). The lesions have not yet been identified as malignant. At this point, it is premature to obtain a chest X-ray in an otherwise healthy male (E). Because carcinoembryonic antigen (CEA) lacks both sensitivity and specificity, it should not be used as a screening marker for colorectal cancer (C).

82. **(D)** The high-power photomicrograph demonstrates a well-differentiated glandular adenoma. Although themselves benign, they are associated with the development of colonic adenocarcinoma. These adenomatous polyps are thought to require a minimum of five years to become clinically significant. Since all of the observed lesions were excised, a repeat colonoscopy is not recommended for a minimum of three years (D). There is no evidence of carcinoma in this specimen (B). Therefore, any other diagnostic investigations are inappropriate (A, C, and E).

83. **(B)** As iron deficiency develops, the MCV decreases. As the anemia becomes more severe, the MCHC also decreases. An extremely low serum ferritin is definitive evidence in predicting absent marrow iron stores. Treatment in this setting can be initiated with ferrous sulfate (B) and does not require further confirmation with a bone marrow aspiration/biopsy (A). Iron-containing vitamin cocktails are expensive and lacking in the appropriate iron concentrations (D). With this mild degree of anemia and the absence of symptoms, the risks associated with a blood transfusion make this therapy inappropriate (E). With clear evidence of iron deficiency, even though the underlying causes of it have been eliminated in this case, treatment should still be initiated promptly (C).

84. **(B)** The lesion demonstrates a transition zone between normal colonic epithelium and the anaplastic glands of an adenocarcinoma. Ninety-five percent of all colon carcinomas are adenocarcinomas (B), the majority of which secrete mucin

(A). Villous adenomas are characterized by long, slender papillary projections with scant lamina propria (C). There is no evidence of angiodysplasia or arteriovenous malformation in this specimen (D). Colonic hamartomas are non-neoplastic tumors composed of an abnormal mixture of normal tissues (E).

85. **(C)** Serum carcinoembryonic antigen (CEA) is a broad spectrum tumor marker, which is elevated in a variety of adenocarcinomas, including colon, lung, pancreas, and breast. It may be increased in a number of nonmalignant conditions, including bronchitis, diverticulitis, and liver disease (C). It may also be increased by smoking (A). The lack of sensitivity and specificity makes CEA an inappropriate screening test for carcinoma of the colon (B). A decline in CEA during chemotherapy of metastatic disease usually suggests a favorable response to treatment (D). Even though CEA elevations may precede other evidence of colon cancer recurrence, routine monitoring with CEA does not distinguish curable from incurable colon cancer patients (E).

86. **(C)** Furosemide is often held prior to surgery because volume depletion can exacerbate hypotension with the induction of general anesthesia. As a general guideline, with a few specific exceptions, patients should continue taking their usual medications prior to surgery.

87. **(A)** Persons with paranoid reaction will have persecutory or grandiose delusions.

88. **(D)** Persons with depression will have insomnia, despondency, and indecisiveness.

89. **(C)** Persons with hysterical personality will have emotional immaturity.

90. **(B)** Persons with anxiety will have tachycardia, sweating episodes, fatigue, and muscle tenseness.

91. **(E)** Thyroid storm is a severe exacerbation of hyperthyroidism brought on by the stresses of illness or surgical operation. Preoperative evaluation of thyroid function helps to determine the right intraoperative dose of an antithyroid agent to prevent the crisis from happening. Measurements of total serum T4 and T3 (A), TSH (D), radioactive iodine uptake (C), and thyroid resin

uptake (B) are all indicated tests in the evaluation of hyperthyroid patients preparing for a surgical procedure.

92. **(A)** In a patient newly diagnosed with mild type II diabetes mellitus, the first treatment should be attempts at dietary control with a goal of 1,800 calories/day.

93. **(E)** Diabetes presenting in a young patient with high glucose levels is most likely type I diabetes mellitus, and oral hypoglycemics will be ineffective.

94. **(E)** Although the patient likely has type II diabetes mellitus, the fact that she recently had an episode of non-ketotic hyperosmolar coma makes it unlikely that treatment with oral hypoglycemics or metformin will be effective.

95. **(B)** When dietary control fails for Type II diabetes mellitus, oral hypoglycemics can be tried, and then metformin, if necessary, before insulin needs to be considered.

96. **(D)** This patient has thrombocytopenia secondary to antiplatelet antibodies from drug-induced quinidine. The lesions on the lower extremities constitutes purpura, and this patient must now be considered allergic to quinine or quinidine. Scurvy from severe vitamin C deficiency (A) produces large ecchymosis and bleeding gums. It is unusual for vitamin C deficiency to happen overnight and to occur within a hospital setting where the patient is usually well fed. Prednisone (B) is a steroid used to treat palpable purpura secondary to hypersensitivity vasculitis, such as in systemic lupus erythematosus. Intravenous penicillin (C) is the immediate treatment of choice in meningococcemia, which also presents as purpura. However, this patient is not toxic or febrile. She has no signs of meningitis. Chemotherapy (E) is the treatment of choice if this patient has Kaposi's sarcoma, which would resemble ecchymoses rather than purpura.

97. **(D)** Glomerulonephritis is not a manifestation of acute rheumatic fever, although it can be a manifestation of prior streptococcal infection. Erythema marginatum (A) is the name of the rash associated with rheumatic fever. Subcutaneous nodules (B) and chorea (C) are also major criteria for the diagnosis of rheumatic fever. Carditis (E) can be a pancarditis, but most commonly affects the mitral valve.

98. **(B)** This patient has symptoms of benign prostatic hypertrophy and he is also hypertensive. The best medication for this patient is an alpha-adrenergic blocker such as terazosin. This drug will relax the smooth muscle wall lining the blood vessels as well as relax the smooth muscles lining the prostate gland, resulting in fewer symptoms of urgency and frequent micturition. Verapamil (A) is a calcium-channel blocker which is used in hypertension. It also causes constipation. This drug should not be used in patients with systolic dysfunction of the heart because it has a negative inotropic effect. Clonidine (C) is a centrally acting alpha-2 blocker which is used in hypertension. It can cause dry mouth and dizziness. It should be avoided in stroke patients because its effects occur centrally. Nifedipine (D) is also a calcium channel blocker, which acts through vasodilation of the blood vessels by relaxing the smooth muscle of the vasculature. It does not alleviate symptoms of benign prostatic hypertrophy. Hydrochlorothiazide (E) is a diuretic, which acts by increasing salt-loss and, thus, plasma volume. This in turn decreases blood pressure in certain patients with high plasma volume hypertension and salt-retainers. This drug would make the symptoms of increased urinary frequency worse in this patient.

99. **(E)** Prostate specific antigen is secreted by prostate cells. Levels normally increase with age (A). Use of age-adjusted PSA levels increases the accuracy of the test (B). PSA levels may be increased in benign clinical conditions, including benign prostatic hyperplasia, prostatitis, and prostatic infarction (D). In persons with benign prostatic hypertrophy, who are treated with finasteride, the age-adjusted PSA range should be decreased by 50% (C). Early detection by PSA has not affected disease mortality to any significant extent (E).

100. **(C)** Rubella vaccine should be given again at age 12.

101. **(B)** Galactorrhea can be caused by medicines that block dopamine (which acts in the pituitary as a prolactin-inhibiting factor), thereby causing increased release of prolactin. Phenothiazines act by blocking dopamine and classically can cause galactorrhea, as can metoclopramide,

methyldopa, verapamil, and some antidepressants.

102. **(E)** Although placing a PPD (A), obtaining a chest radiograph (B), and beginning treatment are all appropriate (C and D), these all need to be done within the hospital. Although the patient may not be ill enough to be admitted, for a public-health concern, she should begin treatment for her TB before she returns to the community.

103. **(B)** This is the treatment of choice. The patient most likely has thrombophlebitis with a pulmonary embolus. Oral Coumadin (C) will ultimately be substituted for heparin before she is discharged, but its onset is too slow for acute treatment.

104. **(D)** This is a typical presentation for pleurisy. Other possible findings are a rub on physical examination and ST-T segment elevations on electrocardiogram.

105. **(C)** The patient is essentially bedridden with her hemiplegia and is at risk for aspiration.

106. **(D)** This scenario is most consistent with alcohol withdrawal after two days.

107. **(A)** A chronic alcoholic is at risk for subacute bacterial peritonitis, which can be a life-threatening illness with minimal initial symptoms. The other conditions would be associated with worsening symptoms.

108. **(C)** Hematemesis is unusual in this condition, but all of the other conditions can be associated with hematemesis and cirrhosis.

109. **(A)** It is not unusual for bedrest to precipitate a gouty attack in a susceptible patient.

110. **(A)** In this setting, particularly in a patient already receiving antibiotics, you should treat empirically for a fungal infection while awaiting cultures. Symptomatic treatment of the fever is appropriate after amphotericin has been added.

111. **(D)** A fundoscopic exam would be least revealing because it focuses on the eye and retina and would rarely be involved with a preoperative physical exam or with a patient complaining of hemoptysis and dyspnea.

112. **(B)** A chest X-ray is the next appropriate test to order. It is inexpensive, easy to obtain, and reveals a lot of information. An EKG (A) would be ordered with cardiac concerns. A CT of the chest with contrast (C) or without contrast (D) is expensive and not ordered early in a work-up. Incentive spirometry (E) is an exercise to help expand the lungs and prevent atelectasis; it is not a test.

113. **(C)** Laryngitis will not lead to hemoptysis or coughing up of blood. Hemoptysis may, however, be seen with carcinoma of the lung (A), mitral stenosis (B), pulmonary infarct (D), and chronic bronchitis (E).

114. **(A)** Wheezing is produced by the rapid passage of air through a bronchus that is narrowed, not dilated (B). Crackles (C) are caused by a series of tiny explosions produced when previously deflated airways are reinflated. Friction along pleural surfaces (D) produces pleural rubs. Alveoli filled with fluid (E) may sound muffled or decreased.

115. **(D)** You should not proceed with the orthopedic surgery. In this patient with lung carcinoma and a torn ligament, the emergency lies with the carcinoma. You should proceed with a thoracic surgery consultation (A), a CT of the chest (B), a metastatic survey of the body (C), and pulmonary function tests (E). This will allow you to get the advice of an expert as well as stage the disease and see how well the lungs are prior to surgery.

116. **(C)** Oat-cell carcinomas may secrete ectopic ACTH or ADH and are associated with carcinoid syndrome. Flushing, wheezing, diarrhea, and cardiac valve lesions may develop.

117. **(B)** For most lung carcinomas, cigarette smoking is the number-one risk factor, and smoking cessation greatly prolongs life. Avoiding tendon injury (A) will not prolong life. Visiting a doctor (C) should prolong life, but not if smoking continues. Eating healthily (D) and lowering cholesterol (E) are important, but in these patients, smoking cessation is more important.

118. **(A)** Cigarette smoking affects wound healing and the skin or integument, but this effect does not pose a danger or shorten life expectancy as it does when it affects the other organ systems.

119. **(C)** This India ink smear of fresh centrifuged cerebrospinal fluid shows the mucinous capsule of cryptococcus as a translucent halo surrounding the budding yeast (C). The latex agglutination test to detect cryptococcal polysaccharide antigen in the CSF is an important adjunct to diagnosis. *Toxoplasma gondii* is an intracellular protozoan, which exists in three forms: the tachyzoite, the tissue cyst containing bradyzoites, and the oocyst, which contains sporozoites. In central nervous system infection, cysts containing bradyzoites are frequently found contiguous with the necrotic tissue border (A). *Neisseria meningitides* is a Gram-negative diplococcus (B). *Treponema pallidum* is a thin helical cell, with 6-14 spirals, tapered on either end. It is too thin to be seen by routine Gram stain, but can be visualized in wet mounts by darkfield microscopy, by silver stains, or by fluorescent antibodies (D). *Streptococcus pneumoniae* is an encapsulated Gram-positive diplococcus (E).

120. **(A)** An acute anxiety attack results in tachypnea, driving the CO_2 down, thus creating an acute respiratory alkalosis. Compensatory mechanism is a metabolic acidosis. Given the patient's overall good pulmonary health, her oxygenation will be excellent, of course, until the arterial oxygenation is low despite a near normal saturation; this could be an acute pulmonary embolism. Choice (C) is a primary respiratory alkalosis with a compensatory metabolic acidosis with severe hypoxemia. This could be ARDS. Choice (D) represents a person with stable COPD who is retaining CO_2.

121. **(D)** *S. aureus* is the most commonly isolated microbial agent. Since the disease process is endotoxin-mediated, antibiotics are not useful in eradicating this condition or even relieving signs and symptoms. The mainstay of therapy is massive fluid replacement, as in any other forms of circulatory shock with cardiovascular compromise.

122. **(A)**, 123. **(C)**, 124. **(D)**, 125. **(B)** Monocular visual loss results from a lesion of one eye or its retina or optic nerve. Binocular visual loss results from lesions anywhere in the visual pathways from the retina to the occipital pole and is best understood by referring to a diagram of the visual fiber pathways in any standard medical textbook. Lesions of the optic chiasm (A) produce bitemporal hemian-opsia. Lesions involving only upper or lower fibers of the radiations cause a lower or upper quadrant defect in the opposite half-field. Temporal lobe radiation lesions (B) cause "pie in the sky" visual field defects. Parietal lobe radiation lesions (C) cause "pie in the floor" visual field defects. Incomplete damage to the visual cortex (D) results in congruous homonymous scotomas.

126. **(D)** The intraoperative transesophageal echocardiogram demonstrates a large right atrial mass, which obstructs the right ventricular inflow. In adults, myxomas are the most common benign tumors. In children, rhabdomyomas are the most common. In adults, most myxomas are located in the left atrium. Right atrial myxomas produce symptoms of low cardiac output and systemic venous hypertension. Hepatomegaly, edema, ascites, and cyanosis are common (A, B, C, and E). Pulmonary emboli have been reported. However, systemic emboli, especially cerebral, are uncommon with right atrial tumors but are reported to occur in two-thirds of persons with left ventricular myxomas (D).

127. **(B)** "Antiphospholipid antibodies" (aPL) refers to a group of antibodies, including lupus anticoagulant antibodies (LAC) and anticardiolipin antibodies (aCL), which bind to negatively charged phospholipids. The antiphospholipid syndrome describes the association of aPL in several clinical settings. Unfortunately, there is high interlaboratory variability in quantitative aCL levels. Despite this, screening for these antibodies has become standard practice in many clinical settings. Screening women with fewer than three early pregnancy losses is not recommended because fetal outcome usually is favorable without intervention (B). Both arterial and venous pregnancy-related thromboses are indications for screening (A). Recurrent strokes and ischemic encephalopathy, particularly occurring in persons younger than age 50, have been epidemiologically associated with antiphospholipid antibodies (C). Antiphospholipid antibodies are commonly associated with collagen vascular disorders, particularly systemic lupus erythematosus (D). Thrombocytopenia and hemolytic anemia are also indications for performing the test (E).

128. **(C)** Hypercalcemia results from excessive vitamin D, hyperparathyroidism, multiple myeloma, carcinoma, or nephritis. The symptoms

include headaches, diarrhea, anorexia, fatigue, and weakness. Hydronephrosis (A) is dilation of the pelvis and calices of one or both kidneys resulting from obstruction to the flow of urine. Hypocalcemia (B) is decreased body calcium resulting from inadequate intake, hypoparathyroidism, or poor intestinal absorption. Hypotension (D) is decreased blood pressure and results from myriad causes, as does hypertension (E) which is elevated blood pressure.

129. **(B)** With a worsening blood gas characterized by increasing CO_2 and shortness of breath, the patient is getting tired. There is a problem with ventilation. The patient needs to be placed on a ventilator with an endotracheal tube. Diuresis (A) will help somewhat, but probably will not be entirely sufficient in this patient with a weak heart. A tracheotomy (C) is not needed because an airway may be established with an endotracheal tube. Cardioversion (D) and a pacemaker (E) would be needed if there were conductive problems, with the heart, which don't exist here.

130. **(C)** When a patient has, in sound mind, explained that he does not want any form of life-sustaining measures, your responsibility is to respect that under all circumstances.

131. **(D)** Alternating current (AC), the more common cause of electrical injury, is more dangerous than direct current (DC) because it can produce tonic muscle contractions, preventing the victim from releasing the source of electricity. This may also result in tetanic muscle spasms, leading to asphyxia. Cardiac arrest and coma are also more likely to occur at current frequencies of 50-60 cycles per second, which are associated with this type of injury (D). Electrical burns result from the conversion of electrical energy into heat (A). The extent of injury is directly proportional to voltage. Low-voltage contact does not result in the magnitude of tissue necrosis seen with high-voltage injury (B). Tissue resistance is important in determining both the initiation of current flow and its subsequent path. If skin resistance is high, there will be considerable local tissue destruction (C). Nervous tissue is highly susceptible to injury due to its low resistance (E).

132. **(A)** Given the patient's background of "physician-shopping" and her concerns about her health, you should consider a complete physical examination for several reasons. Some of these reasons include establishing a trusting physician-patient relationship, fulfilling patient expectations, providing the therapeutic benefit of touch, and, finally, establishing her baseline health status.

133. **(B)** The organisms involved in human bites are typically polymicrobial. Human bites, therefore, are much worse than most animal bites, and should be treated with broad-spectrum antibiotics. Leptospirosis (C) is a concern with rat bites, not human bites.

134. **(E)** Mefloquine is the drug of choice for individuals planning trips to Africa. It should be administered one week prior to the trip and continued for at least four weeks after return.

135. **(D)** Elevated MSAFP is associated with open neural tube defects. In addition, increased MS-AFP is also associated with ventral abdominal wall defects, fetal demise, and multiple gestations.

136. **(A)** The patient's clinical history indicates subarachnoid hemorrhage. The CT scan is only about 80% sensitive in ruling out subarachnoid hemorrhage, and if your index of suspicion is high, the gold standard lumbar puncture should be done, which would show xanthochromia.

137. **(D)** Usually, viral gastroenterites such as rotavirus (A) and norwalk virus (B) will not cause a bloody diarrhea. *Vibrio cholerae* (E) classically causes a secretory diarrhea that appears like "rice water." The non-toxigenic forms of *Escherichia coli* (C) are normal gut flora and normally don't cause disease. *Yersinia enterolitica* is a microorganism that causes diarrhea with blood and abdominal complaints.

138. **(D)** Silicosis is an occupational disorder characterized by inhalation of crystalline silicon dioxide particles from working in rock mining, sand blasting, or glass blowing. The main symptom is shortness of breath. Silica crystals are present in the lung nodules and pulmonary fibrosis can result from long-term, chronic exposure.

The classic radiological sign is "eggshell hilar calcifications." Antinuclear antibodies are present in up to 40% of patients with silicosis. Tuberculosis (A) usually presents with fever and weight loss. The nodules also may cavitate on the chest X-ray. Histoplasmosis (B) can also present with hilar adenopathy, but weight loss and fever are common as well as a history of exposure to pigeons prevalent in a geographic location (Ohio's Mississippi Valley). MAI infection (C) is common in end-stage AIDS. High fevers and weight loss are prevalent. Byssinosis (E) is an occupational airway disorder that occurs in workers exposed to cotton, hemp, or flax. The symptoms of chest tightness and dyspnea are most prominent during the initial working shift following a weekend, and tend to diminish over the course of each work-week. Long-term exposure to cotton dust can result in interstitial fibrosis.

139. **(C)** Except with rare metaplasia, a peptic ulcer will not progress to adenocarcinoma. Because of the erosion and bleeding, an obstruction (A) and hemorrhage (B) may occur. If it progresses, erosion through the wall may occur, leading to a perforation—often with devastating consequences if not detected.

140. **(B)** The most likely cause of his acute renal failure is post-contrast acute tubular necrosis. The treatment is to ensure that the patient is not hypovolemic and to follow the serum creatinine. This usually occurs three to four days after iodine contrast is given.

141. **(B)** Indomethacin and all NSAID medications can exacerbate asthma symptoms. Hydrochlorothiazide (A), a thiazide-type diuretic, and diltiazem (C), a calcium channel blocker, have no major pulmonary side effects. Although methotrexate (D) can cause a pneumonitis, it does not commonly exacerbate asthma. Vitamin E (E) also has no major pulmonary side effects.

142. **(D)** This patient will be receiving cumulative doses of daunorubicin, the chemotherapeutic agent that is an antitumor antibiotic. This anthracycline has been associated with lethal cardiomyopathy in patients given cumulative doses in excess of 550 mg/sq. m. A baseline resting left ventricular ejection fraction should be performed prior to chemotherapy in order to assess cardiac toxicity along the multiple courses of chemo-

therapy with daunorubicin. Bleomycin is a chemotherapeutic agent that should be limited to a total cumulative dosage of 400 units to avoid severe pulmonary fibrosis. A baseline pulmonary function test (A) should be performed before treatment. The antimetabolite methotrexate and the alkylating agent cyclophosphamide are both chemotherapeutic agents that cause renal toxicity. Thus, a baseline serum BUN and creatinine level (B) should be acquired prior to starting chemotherapy. The patient should also be very well hydrated in order to prevent hemorrhagic cystitis and intratubular crystallization. All antineoplastic agents cause myelosuppression but some are more toxic than others. Mitomycin-C and nitrosureas cause a delayed myelosuppression. A baseline bone marrow aspiration (C) should not be performed prior to using any chemotherapeutic agent unless a diagnosis is specifically required. Vincristine and vinblastine are plant alkaloids which cause dose-limiting neurotoxicity. A baseline nerve conduction study (E) is not recommended in an asymptomatic patient prior to receiving the vinca alkaloids as chemotherapy.

143. **(B)** The definitive diagnosis of *Herpes simplex* virus requires isolation of the virus (D). Cytologic examination of cells scraped from clinical lesions may be useful for making a presumptive diagnosis, but does not distinguish HSV from other viral infections, such as *Varicella zoster* (A). The sensitivity of viral isolation is higher in vesicular than in ulcerative lesions and during the initial attack (C). Immunofluorescence and ELISA approach sensitivity of viral isolation techniques for detecting HSV from genital or oral-labial lesions, but are only half as sensitive as viral isolation in detecting the virus from cervical or salivary secretions of asymptomatic carriers (B). Acute and convalescent serum can be useful in documenting seroconversion during primary HSV-2 infection (E).

144. **(B)** The ex-husband has no rights regarding your patient's medical care.

145. **(A)** This patient has subacute thyroiditis secondary to a viral infection. This benign disorder is more common in women and is associated with an elevated free T4 and low TSH. The thyroid gland is usually enlarged and tender. This disorder subsides on its own without treatment, but the pain and fever can be alleviated rapidly by steroids

or aspirin. The 24-hour uptake scan is decreased because the preformed thyroid hormones are released from the thyroid gland during the acute flare up. Steroids decrease the inflammation. Propylthiouracil (B) and Tapazole are both used in Grave's disease to decrease the production of thyroid hormones within the thyroid gland. This patient does not have Grave's disease because there is no evidence of exophthalmos or pretibial myxedema. The scan would show increased uptake in Grave's disease. Radioactive iodine treatment (C) to the thyroid gland would decrease excess production of thyroid hormones and is used to treat Grave's disease. This treatment would permanently affect the thyroid gland. In subacute viral thyroiditis, the symptoms are temporary and radiation would be harmful. Antibiotics (D) are useful only if the thyroid gland showed suppuration and the fever was high-grade. In this case, the thyroiditis was secondary to a viral infection. Fine needle aspiration of the thyroid nodule (E) would be useful only to obtain cytology fluid from a thyroid cyst or look for a tumor from a solid thyroid nodule.

146. **(E)**   Discoid lupus is associated with a 30-year-old woman with alopecia and a scarring rash on her face.

147. **(A)**   Kaposi's sarcoma is associated with a 42-year-old male with a nontender, purplish, elevated lesion on his forearm.

148. **(B)**   Poison ivy is associated with a nine-year-old boy who has been hunting insects in the woods.

149. **(D)**   Psoriasis is associated with a 67-year-old male with scaling erythematous lesions on his scalp and arms.

150. **(D)**   Ask the patient to come directly to the emergency room. The patient's symptoms are very concerning for ongoing myocardial ischemia or infarction. If so, this would require an admission into the hospital. However, a direct admission probably wouldn't be prudent, as some assessment should be done emergently in the emergency room.

151. **(D)**   Ask the patient to come directly to the emergency room. The patient's symptoms are very concerning for an ectopic pregnancy. Although

you might be able to do some of the workup in the office, the ultrasound, the obstetrician, and the laboratories would all be easier to work with in the emergency room.

152. **(C)**   Ask the patient to come to the office the same day. Although amoxicillin can have a side effect of a rash, you need to see the rash yourself and make sure that it's not hives preceding an anaphylactic response.

153. **(B)**   Ask the patient to schedule an appointment in two to three days. Erythromycin is commonly associated with gastrointestinal disturbances. The treatment for it is the use of antiemetics and reassurance.

154. **(B)**   This patient most likely has pneumocystis pneumoniae carinii infection because he is immunocompromised, and thus the treatment of choice would be intravenous trimethoprim-sulfamethoxazole and oxygen. An elevation of the A-a gradient, an elevation of the LDH, and bilateral interstitial infiltrates on an X-ray suggest PCP. Intravenous penicillin (A) is used to treat penicillin-sensitive Strep, pneumoniae, or severe Strep throat infection. Penicillin is not a good antibiotic of choice because of the emergence of penicillin-resistant organisms. A bronchial lavage and transbronchial biopsy (C) would be a diagnostic tool to identify the organism responsible for the pneumonia, but it is not useful for treatment. Intravenous Ganciclovir (D) would be useful to treat cytomegalovirus pneumonia, but the initial presumptive diagnosis in an immunocompromised individual should be PCP first. CMV pneumonia should first be diagnosed by a transbronchial biopsy before treatment is initiated. Steroids (E) are given in conjunction with intravenous trimethoprim-sulfamethoxazole if the patient is severely hypoxic with PCP.

155. **(A)**   In a high clinical suspicion of acute arterial occlusion, the first therapeutic option needs to be consideration of intravenous heparin.

156. **(D)**   A 5-cm abdominal aortic aneurysm is an asymptomatic pulsatile mass and is an incidental finding on abdominal radiograph. The presumptive diagnosis should be confirmed by ultrasonography, computed tomography, or angiography. At 5 cm, the risk of rupture approximates 10%. The mortality associated with elective

surgery is five percent (D), whereas the mortality of repairing a ruptured aneurysm is much higher and approximates 20% (E).

157. **(E)** The sural nerve is derived from S1 and S2.

158. **(B)** The ulnar nerve is derived from C8 and T1.

159. **(A)** The supraclavicular nerve is derived from C3 and C4.

160. **(D)** The lateral femoral cutaneous nerve is derived from L2 and L3.

161. **(A)** You do not have to wait until the parents are contacted.

162. **(C)** Epidural hematomas are not typically associated with child abuse. However, such factors as scalded buttock burns (A), cigarette burns (B), subdural hematomas (D), retinal hemorrhage (seen in shaken baby syndrome), and fracture of the femur (E) are common presentations of child abuse.

163. **(A)** Preeclampsia occurs in approximately six to seven percent of pregnancies of which .02-.07 degenerate into eclampsia. The hallmark of preeclampsia is vasospasm, which is secondary to increased serum levels of renin, aldosterone, angiotensin, and catecholamines. Magnesium sulfate is used to prevent eclamptic convulsions (E). Its main action is at the myoneural junction, where it inhibits the release of acetylcholine and the excitability of the muscle membrane.

164. **(C)** These should be started with women at age 18 or when first sexually active. Mammograms and screening flexible sigmoidoscopies should be done later in life. Since the patient is not immunocompromised, a pneumococcal immunization is probably unnecessary and a complete blood count is probably not necessary.

165. **(C)** Mallory-Weiss tear of the distal esophagus results from protracted vomiting and can result in an upper GI bleed. This does not cause malabsorption because the lesion is not even close to the small intestine. Chronic pancreatitis can lead to pancreatic insufficiency (A), resulting in loss of pancreatic digestive enzymes and, thus,

malabsorption. This is very common in alcoholics. Crohn's disease (B) can cause malabsorption secondary to a decrease in the absorptive surface from active inflammation and also from bile salt depletion from ileal disease. Bacterial overgrowth syndrome (D) can result from multiple causes such as dilation of the bowel, blind loop of bowel, and stasis secondary to diabetes. Nontropical sprue (E) results in malabsorption due to damage to the differentiated villus epithelial cells of the small intestine. Gluten in the diet results in impaired transport of nutrients through damaged villi in the jejunum.

166. **(E)** A barium enema test would only give information on the colon and not on the small intestine where most of the nutrients are absorbed. Plain abdominal X rays may be useful if one wishes to make the diagnosis of chronic pancreatitis and calcification of the pancreas is visualized. An upper GI series can also be useful. The gold standard in making the diagnosis of most causes of malabsorption is the small intestinal biopsy (A). Cultures and histology can also be taken on a biopsy and many rare causes of malabsorption such as lymphangiectasia, mastocytosis, giardias, and amyloidosis can be diagnosed. A serum carotene level less than 0.06 mg/dl is a good indicator for malabsorption secondary to decreased absorption of major nutrients needed for the body. The bentiromide test (C) is an excellent noninvasive test to diagnose malabsorption secondary to pancreatic insufficiency. The enzyme arylamine excretion malabsorption is secondary to pancreatic insufficiency. The enzyme arylamine excretion would be less than 50% in six hours. The most cost-effective and least invasive test is the urinary D-xylose test (D). This test distinguishes between malabsorption due to small intestinal disease and that due to pancreatic exocrine insufficiency. After administering 25 grams of D-xylose orally, a five-hour urinary excretion of less than 5 grams of D-xylose is virtually diagnostic of small intestinal malabsorption.

167. **(D)** Prednisone is an oral steroid, which can actually relieve the symptoms of malabsorption if the cause of malabsorption is adrenal insufficiency or Crohn's disease. Prednisone can decrease the inflammation in the small intestinal brush border. Colchicine (A) is toxic to the kidneys and to the GI tract if given in large doses for a long

period of time. This drug is used for gout, and it can result in malabsorption in certain instances. Neomycin (B) is an antibiotic, which can result in malabsorption in the small intestine from bacterial overgrowth. Irritant laxatives (C) can result in small intestinal malabsorption by causing caustic metabolites in the brush border. Cholestyramine (E) is used for hypercholesterolemia and for a high-fiber diet. It can also cause malabsorption of important medications that the patient is taking for other reasons. This drug causes bloating and excessive flatulence.

168. **(E)** The C14-xylose breath test is a sensitive and specific test for bacterial overgrowth. Following administration of oral xylose, breath radioactively labeled CO2 is measured at 30 and 60 minutes, respectively. The presence of increased numbers of bacteria within the lumen of the proximal small intestine correlates with an elevation in CO14 released in a breath. Serum folate (A) may actually be increased in bacterial overgrowth syndrome, but it is increased in all other causes of proximal small intestinal diseases. A qualitative stool fat (B) is a basic screening test for any cause of malabsorption; thus, it is sensitive, but not specific. Numerous fat globules are seen under the high-powered microscope. Serum cobalamin (C) is decreased from malabsorption in the distal small bowel. This can be secondary to pernicious anemia, chronic pancreatitis, and bacterial overgrowth syndrome. Urine 5-hydroxyindolacetic acid (D) is markedly elevated in carcinoid syndrome and minimally elevated in any other type of malabsorption. It is not useful to diagnose bacterial overgrowth syndrome.

169. **(D)** This patient has been exposed to tuberculosis but does not have active pulmonary infection. Thus, watchful waiting is the prudent thing to do and a follow-up chest X-ray is indicated if symptoms of weight loss, sweating, fever, and anorexia occur suggestive of active tuberculosis. Isoniazid and B12 prophylaxis (A) are indicated if the patient is younger than 35 years old and has a positive PPD status. If the patient is older than 35 years old, then the American Thoracic Society recommends no prophylaxis against TB because of the higher risk of liver toxicity. Obtaining sputum for acid-fast bacilli is not needed because this patient has no symptoms of cough and has a normal chest X-ray (B). Thus, the yield

would be negligible. A CT of the chest (C) would most likely be normal if the chest X-ray is normal and the patient is asymptomatic. This test would be useless and certainly not indicated in the management of this patient. A repeat PPD test is indicated only if the initial testing is negative (E). In this case, the PPD skin test was positive to 10 mm induration and, thus, another skin test is not necessary, not even in the future.

170. **(C)** This patient has multiple sclerosis, which is a demyelinating disease of unknown etiology. It is more common in young females and presents with different neurological symptoms. Oligoclonal bands are seen in the cerebral spinal fluid. Patients can present with optic neuritis, diplopia, monocular visual loss, sensory deficits of one limb, progressive motor weakness, and gait disturbances. The MRI scan of the brain makes the diagnosis. It would reveal hyperdense white matter changes, and lesions in the cerebellum, as well. Treatment of multiple sclerosis is with beta-interferon and steroids.

171. **(E)** This patient has diabetic peripheral neuropathy, which is caused by long-standing uncontrolled diabetes. Uncontrolled diabetes can cause end-organ damage to the eyes, kidneys, nerves, and autonomic nervous system. Diabetic peripheral neuropathy usually presents as distal symmetrical lower extremity numbness, tingling, and pain. The etiology is thought to be secondary to axonal degeneration and neuron ischemia. Deep-tendon reflexes are also diminished. Nerve conduction studies are the gold standard test in establishing the diagnosis of peripheral neuropathy.

172. **(A)** This patient has deep vein thrombosis of the left lower extremity. This can possibly lead to pulmonary embolism. Deep venous thrombosis is thought to be caused by venous stasis, a hypercoagulable state, and venous trauma. This patient has been in an immobile condition secondary to extensive traveling in the airplane for a long time and this can predispose to venous stasis. A noninvasive imaging study to establish the diagnosis of deep venous thrombosis is a duplex, Doppler sonogram of the lower extremities. Calf, popliteal, and thigh thrombosis can be asymptomatic and, thus, an ultrasound is necessary.

173. **(B)** This man has multiple myeloma, which is a neoplastic malignancy caused by proliferation of plasma cells. These plasma cells secrete immunoglobulins, which can be detected by serum protein electrophoresis. Twenty-five percent of patients with multiple myeloma have hypercalcemia. Forty percent of patients with multiple myeloma have a normochromic, normocytic anemia, which causes the pallor and fatigue. A plain X-ray of the thoracic bones can detect the lytic lesions, which are characteristic of multiple myeloma. Vertebral compression fractures, pelvic fracture, and skull fractures are also common. A bone scan is not useful because it would only detect osteoblastic, not lytic lesions. An MRI scan would not be useful because it detects lesions that are painful on movement. This patient has pain on palpation. The treatment for multiple myeloma is chemotherapy and prednisone. Radiation is for palliation only.

174. **(A)** The chest X-ray shows a fracture of the retention wire in the atrial J pacemaker lead. This wire, which normally maintains the J shape of the lead, has migrated from the body of the lead. Retention wires protruding from the lead body or those that protrude and migrate require removal (A) because of the high risk for laceration and cardiac tamponade (B). There is no indication for replacing the pulse generator in an asymptomatic patient, particularly one in whom the problem is with the lead, not the generator (E). There is no clinical indication for antibiotics or stress testing (C and D).

175. **(C)** The accuracy of any diagnostic test depends on the pre-test clinical probability. In this case, the chance that this patient is HIV positive is so low that the likelihood of her having a false positive on the HIV antibody test is likely higher than or equal to the chance that she will test positive for HIV. The specificity of various commercial tests varies from 95% to 99%. Since the predictive value of the ELISA is dependent upon the prevalence, a positive test should be confirmed by a Western blot or PCR technique.

176. **(C)** In panel A, this transesophageal echocardiogram shows a large, free floating, echodense mass in the right atrium. In panel B, there is a large mass in the left pulmonary artery (C). The aorta appears intact (A). Myocardial rupture, typically occurring in the first week following myocardial infarction, causes cardiac tamponade (B). Rupture of the ventricular septum is established by the demonstration of a left-to-right shunt (D). Dressler's syndrome, characterized by fever and pleuropericardial chest pain, may produce a pericardial effusion (E).

177. **(A)** Ampicillin works well against Gram-negative bacteria such as *H. influenza* that are often present and the cause of sinusitis.

178. **(D)** Shingles or herpes zoster is treated well by the antiviral drug acyclovir.

179. **(C)** Refractory fungal infections and opportunistic fungal infections, which are frequently seen in HIV-positive patients, are treated well with the antifungal medication amphotericin B.

180. **(B)** First-generation cephalosporins work well against Gram-positive cocci, such as staphylococcus, that are frequently seen with infections of the skin.

USMLE Step 3 – Practice Test 2
Day Two – Afternoon Session

1.   **(D)**   Range, variance, and standard deviation are the three measures of dispersion or variability, whereas mean, median, and mode represent central tendency of Gaussian distribution. The Gaussian, or normal, distribution is characterized by a bell-shaped, curved line. Its special properties are due to a population mean equal to zero, population standard deviation equal to one, and the area under the curved line equal to one.

2.   **(C)**   Benign familial tremor or senile tremor is a coarse tremor that worsens with movement or posture of the affected limb. It is improved with anxiolytics or alcohol. Parkinson's disease (A) is associated with a "pill rolling tremor" and with other symptoms of Parkinson's disease. Alcoholic neuropathy (B) is not commonly associated with a tremor. Intention tremor (D) is a result of cerebellar injury and results in a tremor, which increases with voluntary attempts to reach a target. Choreiform movements (E) are involuntary, rapid twitching movements, which in the case of Huntington's disease, occur with a genetic predisposition.

3.   **(D)**   An individual with early Alzheimer's disease can suddenly forget some routine activity in his life.

4.   **(B)**   An obturator hernia is a herniation of a segment of small bowel (C) through the obturator foramen. It is associated with obstruction and medial thigh pain (A), not lateral thigh pain. It is augmented by thigh extension (D), and a tender mass will be palpated on rectal exam (E).

5.   **(B)**   This patient is quite likely to have oral candidiasis.

6.   **(D)**   Thrush often involves the esophagus and causes painful swallowing.

7.   **(D)**   The patient's sexual history might well be critical to his diagnosis.

8.   **(E)**   The pulmonary disease most likely to be associated with this patient's underlying process often presents with a negative chest radiograph.

9.   **(B)**   You should suspect that this patient is likely to have HIV/AIDS and a serum test should be obtained.

10.   **(B)**   Herpes serologies would not be helpful. All of the other tests are important.

11.   **(A)**   This patient needs to be hospitalized for appropriate evaluation and treatment of his multiple infectious diseases.

12.   **(C)**   This patient needs a bronchoscopic examination to identify the cause of his pulmonary disease, which you suspect to be *Pneumocystis carinii* pneumonia. He will need a dermatology consult later (D) to evaluate the lesion on his left leg, which is likely to be Kaposi's sarcoma, but this is not as emergent as the bronchoscopy.

13.   **(D)**   This question can be answered merely on the clinical symptoms alone. Owing to the fact that this patient has AIDS and coughs, he could be infected with mycobacterium tuberculosis, mycobacterium intracellulare, or mycobacterium avium. All three of these infectious agents can cause pulmonary tuberculosis and are difficult to differentiate. Candida albicans (A) in immunosuppressed, or AIDS patients will produce thrush, or white patches in the mouth. Infection by Cryptosporidium (B) in immunosuppressed patients results in watery diarrhea. Identification comes from fecal rather than sputum smears. Toxoplasma (C) is an infectious agent that utilizes the domestic cat as its host. Infection primarily occurs only in immunosuppressed patients who subsequently experience fever, jaundice, and intracranial calcifications. Laboratory diagnosis is aimed at identification of increased levels or IgM surface antibody. Cytomegalovirus (E) infection, also known as mononucleosis, is characterized by fever, fatigue, and histologic demonstration of abnormal lymphocytes. Laboratory diagnosis involves histologic examination of blood smears

and subsequent identification of CMV by immunofluorescence.

14. **(A)** Dissection of the aorta begins most frequently in an intimal tear in the ascending aorta, a short distance above the aortic valve. Risk factors for dissection are arterial hypertension and medial degeneration of the aorta. Aortic angiography was formerly the definitive diagnostic procedure. The development of accurate noninvasive tests, such as MRI, CAT, and transesophageal echocardiography, has altered the diagnostic approach. Due to its speed, safety, and accuracy, transesophageal echocardiogram has become a first-line diagnostic test, especially for proximal dissections. This study shows a separation of the true lumen and the false lumen of the dissecting aneurysm. The color-coded flow signal in blue identifies flow away from the aortic valve in the true lumen. The echogenic crescent-shaped thrombus almost completely fills the false lumen, leaving only a narrow unobstructed mural rim (A). Aortitis, resulting from several causes, produces inflammation of the aorta. This may result in an obstruction of the aorta or its major arteries (B). The majority of primary malignant cardiac tumors are angiosarcomas. They usually originate in the right atrium or pericardium. Primary tumors of the aorta are rare. Presentation may mimic aortic dissection (C). There is no evidence of either a localized or diffuse narrowing of the aorta on this study (D). In myocardial infarction, two-dimensional and color flow Doppler echocardiography are useful in assessing regional wall motion and overall ventricular performance (E).

15. **(C)** This patient has ecthyma gangrenosum, which is frequently pathognomonic of *Pseudomonas septicemia*. It is associated with a very poor prognosis with a mortality rate of 80%. Immediate treatment with antipseudomonal antibiotic drugs need to be instituted right away. This gangrenous, black, eschar ulcer is usually associated with patients who are immunocompromised, such as this leukemia patient. Debridement of the ulcer (A) should only be done after antibiotics to cover this Gram-negative organism have been started. A chest X-ray (B) can be performed to rule out a pneumonia, but the source of the bacteremia is most probably the ulcer. Gentamicin and ampicillin (D) are used in combination for *Enterobacter* infections, not *Pseudomonas* infections. Radiation therapy (E) would only

immunocompromise the patient further by reducing the white blood cell counts and exacerbating the pseudomonal sepsis.

16. **(C)** Before you can attribute this patient's condition to psychiatric or other potentially irreversible diseases, you must look for treatable causes of altered mental states.

17. **(B)** The X-ray demonstrates extensive soft tissue calcifications of the thigh (B). In atherosclerosis, deposition of calcium should follow the course of the blood vessels (A). The deposition is too extensive to be extravasation contrast material or a reaction to subcutaneously injected medications (C and D). In tophaceous gout, deposition of monosodium urate most commonly occurs in the skin in and around the joints, especially those of the hands and feet. Subcutaneous deposition may also occur, but muscle involvement has not been reported (E).

18. **(D)** This patient has signs and symptoms of allergic rhinitis secondary to pollen exposure. Clinical features include nasal pruritus, postnasal discharge, pale nasal mucous membranes, edematous turbinates coated with thin, clear secretions, and eye tearing. These symptoms are secondary to IgE-mediated inflammatory release of histamines and basophils from the mast cells. Nonsteroidal anti-inflammatory agents are not the treatment of choice for allergic rhinitis. Antihistamines (A) block the H1 receptor on the mast cell and, thus, prevent release of the inflammatory mediators that cause these symptoms. Topical nasal steroids (B) reduce the inflammation upon direct contact with the nasal mucous membranes. Immunotherapy (C) is useful to desensitize the patient from the offending allergen. Turning the air-conditioning on (D) during peak outdoor pollen counts can reduce the amount of pollen one is exposed to, if one stays indoors.

19. **(E)** Contact dermatitis is a type of eczema that develops as a consequence of exposure to an external, noninfectious agent. It is not immunologically mediated; it is a T-cell-mediated allergy. Examples of contact dermatitis include poison ivy exposure, hair dye scalp irritation, and dermatitis from certain lotions. Contact dermatitis differs from IgE-mediated allergies. Allergic asthma (A) refers to bronchoconstriction triggered by inhalant allergens, and it is IgE mediated. At least 40%

of patients with allergic rhinitis manifest asthma symptoms at some point in time. Maxillofrontal headaches, postnasal discharge, and persistent nasal stuffiness, resulting from allergic rhinitis, can lead to sinusitis (B). Urticaria (C) or hives are also IgE mediated and can cause wheals and flares on the skin. Systemic anaphylaxis from allergenic substances can cause angioedema, wheezing, hypotension, chest tightness, and even a sense of impending doom. This is the most serious and potentially catastrophic IgE-mediated reaction (E).

20.　**(A)**　This patient took a combination of terfenidine and erythromycin, which has been shown in certain cases to cause prolonged Q-T intervals and subsequent arrhythmias resulting in syncope or even death. Terfenidine has since been taken off the market by the FDA. The treatment of choice would be to monitor the patient for a few days and discontinue the H1 antihistamine. Lidocaine (B) is only useful for ventricular arrhythmias that cause hemodynamic instability. A cardiac catheterization and echocardiogram (D) are useful to evaluate the patient with suspected organic heart disease. This patient is too young to have any cardiac ischemia, and the cause for the palpitations is known by history. A tilt-table test (E) is useful in patients who experience syncope to rule out orthostatic and vasovagal causes of syncope.

21.　**(A)**　This is a medical emergency and it is appropriate for her to be admitted to the nearest hospital. The HMOs usually reimburse for this as long as they are informed at the outset.

22.　**(D)**　Elevation in TSH is relatively sensitive for hypothyroidism. Symptoms of hypothyroidism include dry hair, dry skin (E), cold intolerance (C), constipation (B), weight gain, slow tendon reflex relaxation (A), periorbital edema, pretibial edema, and generalized lethargy.

23.　**(E)**　Lone atrial fibrillation is a very low risk for developing thromboembolic complications, including stroke. Epidemiological analysis has found several risk factors that increase the incidence of stroke. Among these are mitral annular calcification, angina pectoris, advanced age (A), and left atrial enlargement, with or without clinical symptoms of thromboembolism (B). Conversely, warfarin use in patients at risk of developing atrial fibrillation (C) and the absence of cardiopulmonary diseases are associated with low incidence of thromboembolism.

24.　**(B)**　Conchal hypertrophy of the nose is usually located on the side opposite a deviated septum. The airway is larger on the side away from the deviation, and there is a compensatory overgrowth of the concha.

25.　**(B)**　Starvation places the body in a high-stress state, which increases cortisol levels. This in turn decreases the pulsatile release of gonadotropin-releasing hormone, which leads to decreased secretion of FSH and LH, thus leading to amenorrhea. Obsessive-compulsive behavior (A) involving highly ritualized behavior can involve almost every aspect of an anorexic's life. Patients with anorexia have a disturbed perception of their body (C), feeling that they are overweight when in reality they are emaciated. Bulimic episodes, where the patient engages in bingeing/purging episodes, can occur (D). The difference between bulimia and anorexia is that bulimics do not drop below 85% of normal body weight. Anorexics often believe that they are the only ones who have a true understanding of reality and that everyone else is dysfunctional (E).

26.　**(C)**　This patient could have pneumonia, pulmonary tuberculosis, or lung cancer. To initially work this patient up, a chest X-ray has to be performed to see if there are infiltrates, effusions, mass lesions, or bronchiectasis. If the chest X-ray suggests lung cancer, then a CT scan of the lungs and bronchoscopy can be performed. If the chest X-ray shows bilateral upper lobe of tuberculosis, then sputum for acid-fast bacilli can be sent. A PPD skin test (A) should be performed on all individuals suspected of having been exposed to tuberculosis. This test does not inform us if active tuberculosis is present even if the test is positive. A chest X-ray has to be performed first. A smear and culture of sputum for acid-fast bacilli (B) can be sent three times on three consecutive days if the chest X-ray is suspicious for pulmonary tuberculosis. Bronchoscopy (D) with biopsy or culture is the gold standard for obtaining tissue samples in the lung to make the diagnosis of cancer, tuberculosis, or pneumonia. This test can be performed only after an initial chest X ray is done to guide the bronchoscopist to the tissue sample site. Empiric treatment (E) for presumed bronchitis is not satisfactory since a more serious disease such as cancer or tuberculosis can be missed.

27. **(C)** Bisexual women are not at increased risk of acquiring HIV infection. An increased risk has been associated with STDs (A), same-sex practices by men (B), multiple sexual partners of either sex (D), and individuals receiving multiple blood transfusions (E).

28. **(E)** Routine screening for biochemical markers of alcohol and other drugs is not recommended in the absence of symptoms. The presence of risk factors in this patient do not themselves warrant the screening; the boy does not have past or present history of drug use.

29. **(A)** The clinical suspicion for bacterial pharyngitis is very high with the triad of the fever, the exudates, and the tender lymphadenopathy. A pharyngeal swab (C) is probably not necessary due to the extremely high clinical suspicion of bacterial pharyngitis.

30. **(B)** Any patient being prepped for surgery should have a platelet count of greater than 50,000. This is suitable enough to allow for coagulation during surgery. Spontaneous bleeding may occur if the count is less than 20,000.

31. **(B)** A unit of transfused platelets should raise the platelet count by approximately 5,000. Consumptive coagulopathies may decrease this number.

32. **(D)** *Streptococcus* and *Clostridium* are the most likely agents for an early postoperative wound infection. Since penicillin is a good antibiotic for both, empiric treatment may be indicated. *Staphylococcus* wound infections will occur a few days later, if at all.

33. **(C)** Penicillin is the antibiotic treatment of choice for *Streptococcus*.

34. **(D)** Ampicillin is considered a Class B drug. Animal reproductive studies have not demonstrated a fetal risk, or animal studies have shown a fetal risk that has not been observed in women in their first trimester. It is safe to use in pregnancy. Ciprofloxin (A), Bactrim (C) and gentamicin (D) are considered Class C drugs—either

animal studies have shown adverse effects on the fetus, or there are no controlled studies in animals or women. Tetracycline (B) is a Class D drug—evidence of human risk exists but the benefits may be acceptable despite the risks.

35. **(C)** The American Cancer Society recommends that Pap smears be taken three years after two negative smears taken one year apart. The American College of Obstetrics and Gynecology recommends annual screening for all women (A) who have been sexually active or have reached the age of 18. Hysterectomy has no association with cervical cancer (B). There is no histologic evidence at this time to put the patient at increased risk of developing cervical malignancy (D). Due to the association of cervical dysplasia with human papilloma virus (HPV), condoms (E) may also protect against developing cervical malignancy.

36. **(A)** The treatment for methanol intoxication is supportive care and intravenous ethanol.

37. **(B)** Treatment for acetaminophen overdose is acetylcysteine, and dosages depend on acetylcysteine levels.

38. **(C)** In digoxin overdose exhibiting with conduction disturbances, antidigoxin Fab fragments is the treatment.

39. **(E)** Deferoxamine mesylate is the appropriate treatment for iron overdose.

40. **(C)** In a patient with an ileus, bowel function either slows down or stops. If left untreated and allowed to worsen, it can lead to serious complications. It is important to decompress the bowel by placement of an NG tube. Keeping the patient NPO (B) may not be enough because the bowel and abdomen may still distend. Advancing the diet (A) will only worsen things and an enema (E) will not cure the problem. Although the patient may require exploratory surgery (D), it may not be immediately required.

41. **(D)**, 42. **(C)**, 43. **(C)**, 44. **(A)**, 45. **(B)**, 46. **(A)**, 47. **(A)**, and 48. **(E)** The agent of first choice in the prophylaxis and treatment of PCP is trimethoprim-sulfamethoxazole. A favorable risk:benefit ratio for prophylaxis against PCP, toxoplasmosis, and mycobacterium avium intercellular is obtained when the CD4+ count is no less than 200 cells/mm^3. Prophylaxis against toxoplasmosis

should be initiated when the CD4+ count is reduced to 100 cells/mm³. CD4+ count should be in a range of 1,000-1,500 cells/mm³ in individuals who are free from HIV infection.

49. **(B)** Documented syphilis is a condition that must be reported to the local Board of Health.

50. **(A)** CMV retinitis is usually found only in association with HIV/AIDS. However, to perform the HIV blood test in a competent patient, you must obtain his/her permission.

51. **(C)** The patient should have appropriate cultures performed for tuberculosis.

52. **(C)** This condition can be due to any number of organisms, and baseline cultures should be collected before treatment.

53. **(C)** You should proceed with your medical evaluation first.

54. **(A)** You should give her a chance to explain the etiology of your physical findings.

55. **(A)** You can only advise this patient. If she is competent, you cannot force her to stay away from her husband or to press charges.

56. **(D)** The hospital social worker can make arrangements for appropriate and expeditious placement for the patient and her children. You should not attempt to confront the husband alone.

57. **(E)** She is a competent adult and you cannot force her to do something against her will, even if it is in her own best interest.

58. **(B)** In this instance, the patient is not competent and there is a witness to the husband's abuse. It is appropriate to tell the police what you think is happening.

59. **(A)** The home for battered women is the safest place for her, since she will be in a protected environment, the location of which is usually confidential.

60. **(C)** Again, since she is competent, you can only advise her at this point; you cannot force her to do anything.

61. **(B)** Contact dermatitis presents with pruritus and notable areas of eczematous areas. To make the diagnosis, a careful social and dietary history needs to be done.

62. **(B)** Although not included in the protocol of the American College of Obstetricians and Gynecologists, screening for group B *Streptococcus* is recommended by most obstetricians.

63. **(E)** This patient has severe, life-threatening hypercalcemia, which can result in a fatal arrhythmia or comatose situation if not treated promptly. Rapid promotion of renal calcium excretion by saline infusion is very effective and promotes calciuresis. Rehydration followed by diuresis by furosemide is the immediate management of choice in severe hypercalcemia. Synthetic salmon-calcitonin (A) temporarily lowers the serum calcium concentration by 1-3 mg/dl over the course of six to eight hours. This is not fast enough for this patient. Laxatives (B) will not decrease the calcium level. It will only alleviate the symptom of constipation, which is one of the signs of hypercalcemia. Patients with severe hypercalcemia have decreased deep-tendon reflexes. Biphosphonates (C) such as etidronate or alendronate work by decreasing the function of the osteoclasts in the bone and thus diminishing bone resorption. This, in turn, decreases the serum calcium. This process takes several days. Biphosphonates are used in chronic hypercalcemia; not acute hypercalcemia. Inorganic phosphate (D) alters extracellular calcium-phosphate equilibrium to promote calcium deposition into bone and soft tissue. This treatment should be reserved as a final therapeutic option because of the high risk of metastatic calcification.

64. **(D)** Histiocyosis X is a group of diseases typified by proliferation of histiocytes. The disorders it includes are: Hand-Schuller-Christian syndrome (A), which involves the lungs and bones and usually begins in early childhood. Letterer-Siwe disease (B) involves the bone, liver, spleen, skin, and lymph nodes and usually occurs before age three. Eosinophilic granuloma (C), involving the bones and lungs, occurs in patients between 20 and 40. It does not include pulmonary alveolar proteinosis.

65. **(B)** Steroids are the most effective treatment of Histiocytosis X, especially when there is lung involvement. Antibiotics (A), surgery (C), chemotherapy (D), and radiation (E) do not offer effective treatment.

66. **(B)** The areas of involvement of histiocytosis X are most often the lungs and bones. It does, however, effect other organs.

67. **(A)** This patient has renal failure, probably secondary to long-term chronic hypertensive nephropathy with sclerosis. The indications for immediate hemodialysis would be oliguria, anuria, BUN greater than 100 mg/dl, severe hyperkalemia, large pericardial effusion with impending tamponade, and uremic "frost" on the skin. This patient has none of the above signs and, thus, immediate hemodialysis is not necessary at this time. Diuretics (B) such as furosemide would lower the blood pressure by decreasing the total plasma fluid volume in the body. Bilateral kidney ultrasound (C) would give us information if the kidney failure is chronic (small, fibrosed kidneys) or acute (normal size kidneys). It would also tell us if amyloid (large kidneys) is involved or obstructive nephropathy is the cause of the renal failure. Urine analysis with microscopy (D) would give us information about protein content and white or red blood cell casts in the urine. This would rule out glomerulonephritis or nephrotic syndrome. A low-protein diet (E) with avoidance of excess dairy products and meats will prevent further decline of the glomerular filtration rate by decreasing the protein load on the kidneys. This, along with better blood pressure control, would prevent further decline in the renal function and possibly postpone dialysis for a long time.

68. **(D)** This patient has symptoms and signs of major depression and thus she should be treated before her symptoms get worse and she begins to think about suicide. The initial treatment of choice would be a selective serotonin reuptake inhibitor such as Prozac, Zoloft, or Paxil. These second-generation antidepressants have very few side effects. This class of medication works in two to three weeks, and the dose can be adjusted accordingly. This patient does not have to be institutionalized (A) because there is no evidence of suicidal ideations and she is not an immediate threat to herself or others at the present time. Group counseling (B) is effective if the patient has major depression from outside stress factors such as a death in the family, sexual abuse, or post-traumatic stress disorder. This patient has no precipitating cause for her depression. Lithium (C) is a drug used for patients with manic-depression. This patient has no evidence for a component of mania. Electroconvulsive therapy (E) should be used if the patient has been refractory to antidepressants and has not responded to a maximum dose of antidepressants. ECT is effective and rapid 90% of the time. Usually 6-12 treatments are given per week.

69. **(A)** Inferior wall myocardial infarctions usually are associated with bradyarrhythmias, nausea, and relatively mild damage to the myocardium compared to anterior wall myocardial infarctions. Q waves are seen in leads II, III, and AVF after the damage has been completed. Vagal nerve stimulation during the infarction causes nausea and vomiting. Usually the right coronary artery is involved. Patients with a large pericardial effusion (B) have diffuse ST elevations in all leads if pericarditis is present. However, nausea and vomiting are not typically present. Also, pericardial pain differs from ischemic pain, in that ischemic pain is not exacerbated by chest movement or lying down. Patients who have an anterior wall myocardial infarction (C) have ST elevations and Q waves in the anterior lateral leads, such as V1, V2, and V3. The thrombus would involve the left anterior coronary artery or the left main artery. Aortic stenosis (D) is associated with a harsh, systolic murmur in the early stages and there is usually no obvious change on the electrocardiogram, but the echocardiogram may show hypertrophic cardiomyopathy. Dilated cardiomyopathy (E) can lead to arrhythmias and decompensation of congestive heart failure, leading to possible myocardial infarction.

70. **(B)** Her symptoms are consistent with allergic rhinitis. The treatment can be nasal inhaler steroids or antihistamines. Oral steroids (C) are associated with too many side effects to be safe to use for this harmless, but annoying, medical problem. Antibiotics (A) aren't helpful in allergic rhinitis. Ocean spray (D) is helpful only in patients with dry mucous membranes.

71. **(D)** Acute pancreatitis will classically present with excruciating epigastric pain. The patient may even collapse from the pain. The pain is derived from the stimulation of the adjacent celiac plexus.

72. **(A)** Later on in the attack, the pain will radiate to one or both lumbar regions. If there is irritation of the phrenic nerve, there will be pain in the left shoulder. Occasionally, the pain may spread over the entire abdomen, especially the right lower quadrant.

73. **(A)** The pain is aggravated when the patient is supine. Therefore, the patient will assume a sitting (E) and leaning forward position in an attempt to lessen the pain.

74. **(B)** Hyperlipidemia, not hypolipidemia, is a cause of pancreatitis. The two most common causes are excessive alcohol intake and biliary tract disease (A). Pancreatic ductal obstruction (C), vascular compromise (D), and mumps (E) are other causes.

75. **(A)** Slight jaundice is usually evident one to two days after the onset of the pancreatitis from the hemolysis of blood. Two to three days after the attack there may be blue or green ecchymosis appearing in the flank (Grey-Turner's sign), resulting from hemolyzed blood. Or there may be a bluish discoloration of the umbilicus (Cullen's sign) from the same reason.

76. **(B)** A pseudocyst may form from an accumulation of blood and fluid in the lesser peritoneal sac. A hematoma (A) is clotted blood. A thrombus (C) is a blood clot within a vessel. An embolus (D) is a mass occluding a blood vessel which could be a clot, fat, or even air. Ascites (E) is an accumulation of serous fluid in the peritoneal cavity.

77. **(E)** Megacolon, or colonic dilation, results from lack of ganglionic cells to innervate the colon or from chronic contraction of the anal sphincter. It does not have the severity in presentation that acute pancreatitis would have or acute appendicitis (A), peptic ulcer perforation (B), leaking duodenal ulcer (C), or splenic rupture (D).

78. **(D)** Early appendicitis and acute pancreatitis usually present in the epigastrium. Diverti-culitis of the colon (A), obstruction of the transverse colon (C), and colon cancer (E) present in the infra-epigastrium. Acute pyelonephritis (B) presents in the lower quadrants.

79. **(B)** Meningococcal meningitis is contagious, and all close contacts should be treated prophylactically with rifampin for two days.

80. **(D)** Neither pregnancy nor glaucoma is an indication for the administration of pneumococcal vaccine. Once-only immunization appears to be effective protection in patients with chronic heart, lung, kidney, and liver disorders (A, B, C, and E). Other indications for the vaccine include functional or organic hypo- and asplenia chronic alcoholism, Hodgkin's disease, and HIV seropositivity. Additionally, since elderly patients are at increased risk for developing a disseminated pneumococcal infection, they also should be considered as candidates for prophylaxis with the pneumococcal vaccine.

81. **(D)** Although hypotension can accompany congestive heart failure, administering phenylephrine, an alpha-agonist, would only serve to increase the afterload against which an already failing heart would have to pump. This may worsen the condition. Furosemide (A) is given to reduce pre-load and treat associated pulmonary edema. Morphine (B) is given to reduce pre-load and treat pain. Nitroglycerin (E) will reduce pre-load and protect against myocardial ischemia. Oxygen (C) is also used to protect against ischemia.

82. **(C)** The patient's symptoms are consistent with new-onset diabetes mellitus, and one would expect her to have an elevated blood glucose, even in a non-fasting sample.

83. **(A)** Elderly individuals who have hyperthyroidism can present with so-called "apathetic hyperthyroidism," in which some of the symptoms are more like those one would expect from a hypothyroid younger person.

84. **(E)** Ultrasound is regarded as a noninvasive procedure that can be used at any time during the pregnancy. Its most common obstetrical indications include pregnancy dating, determination of fetal sex, assessment of fetal growth, assessment of placental implantation, fetal presentation, position, and lie. Multiple pregnancy,

intrauterine growth retardation, and many congenital disorders (e.g., spina bifida) can also be diagnosed by ultrasound examination.

85. **(B)** Amniocentesis, usually ultrasound-guided, is a transabdominal, fine-needle aspiration of amniotic fluid. The fluid is cultured and assessed for chromosomal abnormalities. Amniocentesis can be performed starting the second trimester (12 weeks of gestation), when ample fluid containing fetal cells is present. Some of the indications for amniocentesis are women over 35 years of age, a history of a previous child with chromosomal anomaly, and a family history of neural tube defect. In spina bifida, amniocentesis shows high levels of alfa-fetoprotein in amniotic fluid secondary to leakage from the open neural tube. Although levels of this glycoprotein are high in maternal and fetal serum, they are highest in the amniotic fluid which is in direct contact with the herniated fetal spine. Screening for neural tube defects begins with measurement of maternal serum AFP (MSAFP) levels.

86. **(B)** Lower than normal amniotic AFP levels may be diagnostic of Down's syndrome.

87. **(E)** Chorionic villus sampling (CVS) can be performed as early as 6-11 weeks of gestation to extract DNA. Determination of fetal sex, more reliable than with ultrasonography, and diagnosis of hemoglobinopathies are the major indications for CVS. Ultrasound-guided percutaneous umbilical blood sampling is performed to sample fetal blood directly so that intravascular transfusion of blood into the fetus is possible.

88. **(D)** A systolic ejection murmur (D) would not be heard with pharyngitis. It is associated with diseases such as mitral valve prolapse. Nasal discharge (A) is common with pharyngitis, as it is with all upper respiratory tract infections. Cervical lymphadenitis (B) is common and is usually tender on exam. Watery eyes (C) may also be seen, and mild splenomegaly (E) may be palpated with pharyngitis, especially if the etiology is viral.

89. **(C)** The presentation of the patient, as well as the examination, is very typical for acute pharyngitis. The patient is young and the appearance is not that of carcinoma (A). Vincent's angina (B) is an odontogenic infection associated with poor dentition and bad infection. Signs of this infection

are commonly unilateral. Mumps (D) presents with parotid swelling, and AIDS (E) may present with cervical lymphadenopathy, but the other signs do not fit.

90. **(D)** Rest is one of the recommended treatments, not increased physical exercise and work. Antibiotics (A) would be indicated, especially if the case were bacterial. Analgesics (B) provide symptomatic relief. Increased fluid intake (C) is important to prevent further dehydration, and antipyretics (E) are needed to counter the high fevers and chills.

91. **(D)** This patient most likely has developed an allergy to a medication and, of the ones given, the most likely one is the antibiotic. It is appropriate to discontinue the antibiotic and replace it with one from a different class. Discontinuance of all medications (A) is really not necessary. You should never continue all medications (B) if you feel that one of them is giving the patient an allergy. Prescription of an antihistamine (C) would cure the symptoms, but do nothing for the problem. Biopsy of the rash (E) would be inappropriate for an allergic rash.

92. **(C)** Since the patient and his girlfriend both have it, they have inoculated each other. This is known as a so-called "ping-pong" infection where you treat one partner only to have it come back. This is seen with venereal diseases, as well. The appropriate treatment is to treat both parties. Some practitioners would have treated both parties from the initial visit.

93. **(D)** Carcinoma is not a complication from a peptic ulcer. With acid production from the ulcer, you may have erosion which will lead to a perforation (C) and, with time, a pyloric obstruction (B). Hemorrhage (A) will occur if the erosion occurs around a vessel. If there is an abdominal process occurring, there will be some eventual scarring and a high likelihood of intestinal adhesions (E).

94. **(E)** While a perianal hematoma will cause a swelling in the perineum, it will rarely cause pain. A fissure in ano (A) and an anal ulcer (B) will cause pain from the erosion and breakdown of the skin and mucosa. Folliculitis (C) is inflammatory in nature and is often painful. Carcinoma (D) is painful when inflammation and erosion have occurred.

95. **(E)** The VDRL is very sensitive for syphilis, but is not very specific; it has a high false-positive rate. The utility of the FTA is to confirm a positive VDRL, and if the FTA is negative, the patient does not have syphilis and has a false-positive VDRL.

96. **(C)** The Finkelstein test is performed with the thumb flexed into the palm of the fist and actively or passively deviating the wrist ulnarward with the wrist in neutral. Stenosing tenosynovitis of the first dorsal compartment of the wrist (de Quervain's disease) will cause pain. The first dorsal wrist compartment contains the APL and EPB.

97. **(D)** de Quervain's disease is a stenosing tenosynovitis of the extensor tendons. Carpel tunnel syndrome is a compression syndrome (A). Trigger finger is a tenosynovitis (B) of a finger tendon pulley. Dupuytren's disease is a disease of the palmar fascia (E).

98. **(B)** The cutaneous branch of the radial nerve lies next to and by the incision used to treat the disease. It must be watched for closely, or a painful neuroma may develop if severed during surgery.

99. **(A)** The Finkelstein test is performed with the thumb flexed into the palm and ulnarly—not radially (B)—deviating the wrist. The test is positive when it causes pain. Tapping of a nerve is the Tinel's sign (C). Passive flexion of both wrists is Phalen's sign (D). Both Tinel's sign and Phalen's sign are usually positive in carpel tunnel syndrome. Alternately compressing the radial and ulnar arteries and accessing blood flow is the Allen's test (E).

100. **(C)** MRI of the brain would be the best immediate test to determine the cause of this patient's symptoms.

101. **(B)** A thrombus in the heart, either in a chamber or on a valve, could break off and lodge in the brain, causing a stroke-like event. Tuberculosis (A) or sinusitis (E) would not cause symptoms and signs such as this. You would have seen a brain tumor (C) or cavernous sinus thrombosis (D) on the diagnostic imaging test.

102. **(B)** The absence of a gag reflex places this patient at greater risk for aspiration pneumonia.

103. **(D)** A bone scan would not be helpful. A sedimentation rate (A) and antinuclear antibodies (B) would help elucidate the possibility of an inflammatory process. A repeat MRI (C) would allow you to assess the size of the lesion and determine whether the anticoagulation has caused any bleeding. Speech therapy (E) is mandatory in this aphasic patient.

104. **(E)** This test will give you more detailed information regarding the vasculature in the brain. You want to do this before transfer because of the possibility of a dye reaction or dehydration after the study.

105. **(B)** Vascular beading is most consistent with vasculitis, which fits in with the elevated sedimentation rate, too.

106. **(B)** This picture is not consistent with temporal arteritis, which is what you would be evaluating with a temporal artery biopsy. You are interested in pursuing evidence of a systemic vasculitis. C3 (A) and C4 (C) levels might be low if significant amounts of complement are being consumed in an autoimmune process. A liver-spleen scan (D) might show infarcts due to vasculitis. The sural nerve (E) is often asymptomatically involved in systemic vasculitis.

107. **(A)** High-dose prednisone is the first-line treatment of choice in cerebral vasculitis. You might add an immunosuppressive agent, such as cyclosporine, azathioprine, or cyclophosphamide to this.

108. **(A)** Vitamin B12 deficiency is the likeliest diagnosis.

109. **(C)** Alcohol withdrawal is the likeliest diagnosis.

110. **(E)** Peripheral vascular disease is the likeliest diagnosis.

111. **(D)** Carpal tunnel syndrome is the likeliest diagnosis.

112. **(C)** Corticosteroids have not been shown to improve the outcome in patients with adult respiratory distress syndrome. In fact, steroids can make the patient more immunocompromised

and, thus, the *E. coli* sepsis would be further propagated. This patient has *E. coli* sepsis, which needs immediate intervention because of the high mortality involved. He should be transferred to the intensive care unit and monitored with a Swan-Ganz catheter or central venous line to see the cardiac pressures and to give fluid accordingly. If hypotension is also involved, then this patient has septic shock. The hypoxia should be treated with intubation and ventilatory management (A). This patient also has adult respiratory distress syndrome (ARDS), which has a very high morbidity and intubation is required. Intravenous hydration (B) is required if this patient has hypotension. Aminoglycoside therapy (D), such as gentamicin, is used for Gram-negative bacteremia and should be given immediately. This antibiotic has nephrotoxicity and frequent levels should be checked. *E. coli* is a Gram-negative aerobic bacterial organism. The source of the sepsis is probably the urinary tract. PEEP (E), or positive end expiratory pressure, is usually required in any patient with adult respiratory distress syndrome to increase the oxygenation.

113. **(E)** The double contrast esophagram illustrates a giant esophageal ulcer, demarcated by the black arrows. Pill-induced esophageal injury includes both esophagitis and esophageal ulcers. Ulcers may result from a variety of medications, including alendronate and potassium (C). Esophageal damage may be prevented by washing the medication down with copious amounts of water and avoiding recumbency following pill ingestion. Viral infections, including cytomegalovirus and herpes virus, can also result in esophageal ulcers or severe esophagitis (A and B). Malignancy may present as an esophageal ulcer (D). Esophageal ulcers are often a therapeutic problem and may require treatment with high-dose H2-receptor antagonists or proton pump inhibitors (E).

114. **(B)** The local palliative treatment for the local pain is preferred over systemic administration of narcotics. Since the pain from metastases is limited to the lower spine, local therapy should be the treatment of first choice at this time. Low-dose narcotic analgesics (C, D, and E), may be an appropriate first choice in diffuse pain. Chemotherapeutic agents are not known to control metastatic cancer pain (A).

115. **(A)** Classically, diabetics with neuropathy will have a stocking/glove distribution of loss of sensation, initially just affecting their hands and feet and slow progression proximally.

116. **(E)** Classically, diabetic ulcers are often infected with multiple organisms, including anaerobes.

117. **(A)** Although it is described commonly, diabetics do not often get ulcers infected with *Pseudomonas aeruginosa*. The times that you need to be concerned about it particularly are when diabetic patients step on a sharp object that punctures through a shoe. Shoes, for some reason, have a higher count of *Pseudomonas aeruginosa* than other places.

118. **(A)** These often need to be debrided because diabetics have such poor wound healing. Broad-spectrum antibiotics need to be used because of the commonly polymicrobial nature of these ulcers.

119. **(E)** This is commonly known as "sundowning," and is not unusual for older individuals in hospital environments when evening comes and they are not familiar with their surroundings.

120. **(D)** Fibroids would not cause symptoms and findings like these. All of the other conditions could produce such a picture with only minimal pain and physical findings in a patient immunosuppressed with high doses of steroids.

121. **(C)** Transfusion history is unlikely to be relevant to the patient's current symptoms.

122. **(B)** Spine films will be the most helpful in directing you to a diagnosis.

123. **(D)** These are typical findings for osteoporosis.

124. **(C)** Bone densitometry is the best and most accurate way to follow response to therapy of osteoporosis.

125. **(D)**, 126. **(C)**, 127. **(A)**, 128. **(B)** *Cryptosporidium* is an organism which can cause severe diarrhea in patients with AIDS (A). *Shigella* and *G. lamblia* are common in homosexual AIDS patients, but less likely in an individual contracting the disease

through intravenous drug use. *Shigella* is an enterinvasive pathogen which causes bloody diarrhea (B). *G. lamblia* is commonly acquired by drinking water from streams (C). *C. difficile* is usually a superinfection related to antibiotic administration with subsequent changes in the colonic bacterial flora (D). *Rotavirus* is a common pathogen in children (E).

129. **(C)** Chronic glomerulonephritis is a cause of secondary hypertension rather than a sequela of essential hypertension. Left ventricular hypertrophy is a common sequela of long-standing hypertension (A). Hypertension affects the retinal artery and its branches, the sequelae of which can be visualized on fundoscopic exam as retinal hemorrhages (B). Atheromatous plaques form in small- and medium-sized vessels in numerous vascular beds secondary to essential hypertension. These beds include the coronary and cerebrovascular circulation (D and E).

130. **(C)** The bumps that the patient is worried about are the circumvallate papillae. They are located at the posterior dorsum of the tongue and are normal. There is no need to perform a biopsy (A), or tell him it is cancer (B). There is no need to refer him to an oncologist (D), since they are benign. Since they are non-infectious, there is no need for an antibiotic (E).

131. **(A)** With a unilateral paralysis of the tongue, the tongue deviates toward the deviated side. So with a right unilateral paralysis, the tongue would deviate to the right.

132. **(E)** Protein will be present in a patient with nephrotic syndrome because of the disease. If the proteinuria is persistent, a 24-hour urine study should be performed to quantify it.

133. **(D)** Ketones will be present in anyone who is fasting. Acetoacetic acid will be present.

134. **(C)** Blood will be present with the presence of a kidney stone because of the localized trauma resulting from the stone.

135. **(B)** Specific gravity, which usually corresponds to osmolarity except with osmotic diuresis, is increased with the syndrome of inappropriate ADH.

136. **(D)** With any postoperative ambulatory surgery patient, certain criteria must be met prior to discharge. These include taking in fluids (A) while not vomiting, being afebrile (B), having stable vital signs, being able to void (C) on one's own and not with catheterization, and having the ability to ambulate (E). Not having a bowel movement occurs with many patients due to either the anesthesia or decreased GI motility. Whereas it may be a problem if not occurring for several days, it is usually not a problem for several hours or a day.

137. **(D)** The prevalence of elder abuse is about four percent. It is much higher in institutionalized elderly patients compared to those who live in the community. Risk factors include age over 75 years, isolation, physical, emotional, or financial dependence (B and C) on the caregiver, history of family violation, and deterioration in health of the victim or the perpetrator (E).

138. **(B)** In addition to being linked with peptic ulcer disease, there is now some evidence that *Helicobacter pylori* infection is linked with gastric carcinoma.

139. **(D)** This patient has hypercholesterolemia and a strong family history of coronary artery disease. He also manifests signs of hypercholesterolemia, such as tuberous xanthomas and arcus senilis. This patient should immediately be started on a lipid-lowering regimen, which includes the statin drugs such as pravastatin and lovastatin (HMG-CoA reductase inhibitors). These drugs work by inhibiting the rate-limiting step in the production of cholesterol in the liver. Pravastatin sodium has been shown to reduce the risk of a first myocardial infarction by 31%. Keeping the patient on a low-cholesterol diet (A) is helpful also, but it cannot be the only choice of treatment in the initial management of this patient because of his high risk profile of coronary disease. Biopsy (B) of the xanthoma would only reveal cholesterol plaques, and this would not give us any other information that can aid in the management of this patient. Allopurinol (C) is the treatment of choice for hyperuricemia and tophaceous gout, which can mimic xanthomas. Gemfibrozil and niacin (E) can both lower the serum triglyceride levels, but they are not ideal to lower the serum LDL and serum cholesterol levels. These two drugs combined can, in rare instances, cause myopathy.

140. **(D)** This patient has had an upper GI bleed secondary to *H. pylori*-related gastritis. The treatment of choice is tetracycline, metronidazole, and ampicillin, along with the proton-pump inhibitor, to eradicate the infectious organism. This will prevent recurrence of the gastritis in 90% of cases. H2 blockers alone (A) will only alleviate symptoms of epigastric pain and decrease the acid load in the stomach, but it will not prevent the gastritis from recurring if the organism is not eradicated first. Nonsteroidal anti-inflammatory agents alone can cause gastritis if there is evidence of long-term, chronic use. But in this case, we have evidence that the gastritis is caused by *H. pylori* and not by anti-inflammatory agents (B). Omeprazole is a proton-pump inhibitor (C), which plays an important role in decreasing the acid load in the stomach. This will alleviate symptoms of epigastric pain. Along with the proton-pump inhibitor, antibiotics are needed for two to three weeks to eradicate the infectious etiology of the inflammation. Since this patient resides in a nursing home, it would be unusual for the cause of the upper GI bleed to be alcohol intake. Watching and waiting would only result in recurrence of the gastritis and upper GI bleed (E).

141. **(A)**, 142. **(B)**, 143. **(C)**, 144. **(D)** All of these examples represent uncompensated acid-base abnormalities.

Metabolic alkalosis (A) typically begins with increased loss of acid from either the stomach or the kidney. Hyperadrenocorticism, severe potassium depletion, excessive intake of alkali, and volume depletion, such as occurs with vomiting, may all result in metabolic alkalosis.

Metabolic acidosis (B) may occur if there are abnormally high net bicarbonate losses. Renal disease, diarrheal disease, and consumption of acidifying salts may produce a normal anion gap metabolic acidosis. Increased anion gap acidosis results when the kidneys fail to excrete inorganic acids or if there is a net accumulation of organic acids, such as occurs in diabetic ketoacidosis.

Respiratory acidosis (C) occurs if there is a failure to ventilate properly. Most commonly, this is seen in conditions associated with primary failure in the central nervous system ventilatory drive controls, conditions associated with failure in transport of carbon dioxide from the alveolar space, and conditions associated with primary failure in the transport of carbon dioxide from tissues to alveoli.

Respiratory alkalosis (D) may result when hyperventilation decreases the carbon dioxide tension. This occurs in conditions which result in increased stimulation of the central nervous system respiratory center, such as occurs in infections or brain tumors. This may also occur in conditions associated with tissue hypoxia.

145. **(E)** As long as the patient is mentally competent, you cannot obtain an HIV test without his permission.

146. **(E)** It is currently thought that sarcoid results from an exaggerated cellular immune response to a variety of antigens or self-antigens. Hyperglobulinemia is thought to result from a nonspecific polyclonal stimulation of B-cells by activated T-cells. Antibodies are not thought to play any significant role in the pathogenesis of the disease (E). The initial manifestation of the disease is an accumulation of mononuclear inflammatory cells, especially T-helper lymphocytes and mononuclear cells, in affected organs (D). Granuloma formation follows this initial inflammatory response (C). Organ dysfunction results primarily from distortion of the architecture of the affected tissue by the accumulated inflammatory cells and granulomas (A). The disease becomes clinically manifest when a sufficient number of structures vital to tissue function are involved (B).

147. **(D)** The cardiac biopsy specimen shows amyloid protein, which produces an apple-green birefringence under polarized light. Congestive heart failure and a variety of arrhythmias are the primary manifestations of cardiac disease. The heart is affected commonly in primary amyloid, but very rarely in secondary forms (D). In hemochromatosis, an excessive amount of iron is deposited in parenchymal tissues. Cardiac involvement is characterized by congestive heart failure and a variety of arrhythmias (A). Sarcoidosis is characterized by noncaseating granulomas, which may be surrounded by lymphocytic infiltrates or by patchy fibrosis. Arrhythmias, including complete heart block, are common (B). Endomyocardial fibrosis, usually occurring in children or young adults residing in tropical and subtropical Africa, is characterized by fibrous endocardial lesions of the inflow portion of either or both ventricles (C). Eosinophilic endomyocardial disease, also known as Löffler's endocarditis, or

fibroplastic endocarditis, may represent a part of the spectrum of hypereosinophilic syndrome, with cardiac damage resulting from the toxic effects of eosinophilic proteins (E).

148. **(A)** Finger extension is from 0 to 45°. Metacarpal phalangeal flexion is from 0 to 90°.

149. **(A)** As long as the patient is mentally competent or has made a "living will" directing her care should she become incompetent, you must honor her wishes above anyone else's.

150. **(C)** You tell him that it is proper to give the patient what she needs for pain control, but not more.

151. **(D)** The husband is probably just expressing his frustration with the entire situation and discussing it in everyone's presence may be the best way to deal with it. As long as he has not broken any law, you have no legal recourse against him.

152. **(B)** You can treat the patient's pain as completely as possible. However, at this time, physician-assisted suicide is not condoned as a legal procedure. Cases are currently in the court system dealing with this issue.

153. **(B)** As indicated, this issue has been brought to court and is now being considered at the level of the Supreme Court.

154. **(D)** Your obligation is to your patient; thus, you must discuss this with her and you can give her your opinion. Until the family actually does something, the police and courts should not be involved.

155. **(C)** A hospice is a very good place for terminally ill individuals, since it provides a more peaceful environment than a hospital and also causes less strain to the family than taking care of a dying patient at home.

156. **(A)** A patient should not be kept in the hospital just because the family desires it. Insurance companies will not pay for medically unnecessary hospitalizations, and the family would be charged. A hospice or nursing home is a good alternative to sending the patient home.

157. **(A)** Temporal lobe spikes or slow foci are most commonly seen in the temporal lobe in patients with partial complex seizure disorders. The cerebellum, midbrain, and medulla are generally not involved in patients with partial complex seizures (B, C, and E). Although partial complex seizures may involve the frontal lobe (D), EEG abnormalities are not usually seen in this region.

158. **(E)** A healthy 18-year-old female is presenting with signs and symptoms of a pharyngitis. The least that should be examined is the oropharynx (A) and lungs (C). The heart (B) should be auscultated for any murmurs or abnormalities that may have arisen. The abdomen (D) should be examined for the presence of organomegaly. Peripheral pulses (E) will not play a diagnostic role here.

159. **(B)** With an acute pharyngitis there is usually tender lymphadenopathy. It is usually not non-tender (C). A bruit (D) would be heard with narrowed carotids, which is unlikely here, and a deviated trachea (E) would be seen with a tension pneumothorax, also unlikely. It would also, therefore, not be a normal neck (A).

160. **(B)** This is the classic description of an acute pharyngitis. Squamous cell carcinoma (A) is usually ulcerated, erythematous, or leukoplakic. Strep throat (C) is likely, but you need a culture to know for sure. Bronchitis (D) and epiglottitis (E) will usually have a normal-appearing pharynx.

161. **(A)** Penicillin is the antibiotic of choice where the etiologic agent is *Streptococcus*. The other antibiotics do not work as well against *Streptococcus*.

162. **(C)** Acute pharyngitis should be treated for 7–10 days. Most people will start to have clinical resolve after about 48 hours, but the full course must be taken to adequately cure.

163. **(D)** When treating an acute pharyngitis, or most viral and bacterial infections, the mainstay of treatment is rest (A), fluids (B), antipyretics (C), and analgesics (E). Exercise (D) should not be performed.

164. **(E)** This patient is now cured and no scheduled follow-up is necessary. She need only

be seen on an as-needed basis. A chest X-ray (A), arterial blood gas (B), and throat culture (C) are unnecessary tests, which are not indicated here, but only if the clinical picture worsened. Continuance of the antibiotics (D) is not warranted, since you have a cured patient.

165. **(C)** Her boyfriend ought to be treated, but he should be seen first. You should not blindly give antibiotics (A) without seeing the patient, nor should you reassure him. (B). To return only if it worsens (D) or to take two aspirin (E) is not correctly treating him, since a patient ought to be examined and a diagnosis made prior to instituting therapy.

166. **(E)** Treatment for sickle cell crisis includes hydration (A), analgesics (D), and transfusions if the patient is severely anemic. Serum electrolytes (C) should be measured in this patient because of the gastroenteritis. Supplemental oxygen (E) has not been shown to shorten the course of a sickle cell crisis.

167. **(D)** This patient has an allergic reaction to the penicillin. She should stop taking the drug and have the antibiotic changed. She should not finish the course (A) or decrease it by half (B) or double the dose (E). To stop taking the drug totally (C) would solve the allergy problem, but not adequately treat the infection.

168. **(D)** The FTA-ABS is a test for syphilis. It will not test for herpes (A), HIV (B), *Gonococcus* (C), or *Streptococcus* (E).

169. **(B)** The most likely cause of this clinical picture is the eosinophilia myalgia syndrome, a multisystem disease that is occasionally fatal. The disease has been associated with ingestion of products that contain L-tryptophan. The disease is characterized by blood eosinophilia, with greater than 109 eosinophils per liter.

170. **(B)** The classic triad of jaundice, right upper quadrant pain, and fevers is often found with cholangitis and is called Charcot's triad. These patients often appear to be very ill and toxic.

171. **(B)** With hypokalemia or decreased serum potassium, the T-waves on the EKG will be low or flat (B). When there is hyperkalemia, or increased serum potassium, the T-waves will be peaked or elevated (A). The rhythm may or may not be sinus and the rate may be bradycardic (E) or tachycardiac. The Q-T interval (D) may not be affected.

172. **(B)** This patient has *Pneumocystis carinii* pneumonia. It occurs in about 85% of HIV-infected patients when the CD4 count is less than 200/uL. The chest film may be normal, show cysts, pneumothoraces, nodular lesions, or diffuse infiltrates. In patients with PaO_2 of less than 70 mm Hg or A-a gradient greater than 35 mm Hg, steroids are indicated as additional therapy. Ciprofloxin (A) is not indicated for PCP. Azathioprine (C) is an immunomodulator, but is not a treatment for PCP. Ganciclovir (D) is a common therapy for another HIV-related disease: cytomegalovirus.

173. **(A)** The total cessation of all vital functions was included in the traditional definition of death. With the advent of highly sophisticated technology, the definition of death was equated to brain death. Since artificial pulmonary ventilation can be maintained indefinitely and blood circulation can be supported with pacemakers or extracorporeal circulation, the current definition emphasizes the cessation of brain-regulated functions. Therefore, irreversible and complete cessation of cortical and subcortical activity must be documented before declaring a person dead.

174. **(A)** Ochronosis (also known as alkaptonuria) is an autosomal recessive trait characterized by deficiency in homogentisic acid oxidase, an enzyme necessary in the production of the acid produced by the metabolism of phenylalanine and tyrosine. Ochronosis can produce ankylosis of joints and other cartilaginous structures. Darkening of the skin is present which represents deposits of homogentisic acid in cartilage and the dermis. Porphyria cutanea tarda (B) also causes skin discoloration. In contrast to ochronosis, either hyper- or hypopigmentation may develop. Patients also develop vesicular and bullous lesions, which were not seen in this patient. Lupus patients (C) can present with a photosensitive rash on the trunk and face along with arthralgias, malaise, and an elevation of antinuclear antibody titers. A "malar" rash is common. Pellagra (D) is secondary to niacin deficiency. The characteristic rash found in this nutritional deficiency is a dark, scaling, blistering lesion which is sharply demar-

cated. This dermatitis is usually preceded by diarrhea. Pellagra is associated with dementia, diarrhea, and dermatitis. Sturge-Weber syndrome (E) is associated with seizures and a hemangiomatous lesion on the face. Visual loss can occur because of involvement of the ophthalmic division of the trigeminal nerve.

175. **(A)** The patient is a health care worker with symptoms consistent with tuberculosis who has not had proper screening for this disease over the years.

176. **(B)** The positive control tests are necessary to determine whether a negative PPD is due to lack of exposure or anergy. Patients with tumors or active tuberculosis can be anergic.

177. **(C)** BCG vaccination is used in some parts of the world to protect against tuberculosis. People who have received BCG will be PPD-positive and may have a significant skin reaction to a PPD.

178. **(E)** Once you make a definitive diagnosis, you will begin treatment, but empiric treatment is not necessary (A). She should not return to work until it is clear what her diagnosis is and it is under adequate treatment (D). If she has tuberculosis, she should have negative sputum tests before patients are exposed to her again.

179. **(A)** Bipolar disorder is a mood disorder that is characterized by recurrent episodes of mania and major depression. The lifetime risk of bipolar disorder is one to two percent. The treatment of choice is lithium carbonate for the acute manic state, and 10-14 days may be required before the full effect is reached. A favorable response to lithium (C) is reported in 65-75% of bipolar manic patients. Family studies indicate there is evidence of familial transmission in this disease (B). Relatives of patients are two to three times more likely to incur a mood disorder. Electroconvulsive therapy (D) is usually reserved for severely depressed or manic patients who have not responded to pharmacotherapy, for whom medication is contraindicated, or for whom immediate effective intervention is needed (e.g., suicidal patients).

180. **(B)** Harrison's grooves are transverse grooves in the lower thorax that occur during active rickets from the pull of the diaphragm. A pectus carinatum (A) occurs when softened upper ribs bend inward, increasing the AP dimension of the chest. A pectus excavatum (C) occurs when the lower sternum sinks, causing a caving-in of the chest. Barrel chest (D) often results from emphysema. Localized bulges and depressions (E) usually occur in early life, such as from an enlarged precordium.

USMLE STEP 3

Practice Test 3

USMLE STEP 3
PRACTICE TEST 3

Day One – Morning Session

(Answer sheets appear in the back of this book.)

TIME: 3 Hours
180 Questions

DIRECTIONS: Each of the following numbered items or incomplete sentences is followed by an answer or a completion of the statement. Choose the **ONE** choice that **BEST** answers the question or completes the sentence.

---

1. Drug resistance to chemotherapeutic agents is a major reason for treatment failure. All of the following are true regarding drug resistance EXCEPT

    (A) multidrug resistance (due to P-glycoprotein overexpression) to one class of chemotherapeutic agents generally implies cross-resistance to other classes of chemotherapeutic classes, even those which are functionally and structurally disparate.

    (B) overexpression of P-glycoprotein decreases intracellular concentrations of antineoplastic agents by actively extruding them across the cell membrane.

    (C) inherent multidrug resistance occurs in tumors developing from normal tissues that express the mdr1 gene, which codes for P-glycoprotein.

    (D) apoptosis, an active form of cellular suicide, may be important in the development of multidrug resistance.

    (E) multidrug resistance involving topoisomerase II can be observed with all classes of antineoplastics.

2. Surface components and extracellular products produced by Group A streptococci include all of the following EXCEPT

    (A) M protein.

    (B) hyaluronidase.

    (C) pyrogenic exotoxins.

    (D) streptolysins.

    (E) CAMP factor.

3. A 50-year-old woman has been diagnosed with primary biliary cirrhosis. She has portal hypertension and ascites. Her physician placed her on a waiting list for liver transplantation. All of the following are absolute contraindications for liver transplantation EXCEPT

(A)   HIV seropositivity.

(B)   extrahepatic malignancy.

(C)   advanced cardiac disease.

(D)   fulminant liver failure.

(E)   severe emphysema.

4.   A 60-year-old woman has been noted by her family to be withdrawn and has lost interest in her environment. She has lost her appetite and her weight has fallen. She is having some difficulty sleeping. Which one of the following tests would be among the first to be obtained to evaluate her condition?

(A)   Antinuclear antibody titers

(B)   Urinalysis

(C)   CT scan of the abdomen

(D)   Thyroid-function tests

(E)   Antimitochondrial antibodies

For Questions 5-8, match the following presenting symptoms with the likely diagnosis.

(A)   CVA tenderness

(B)   Calf tenderness and swelling

(C)   Hemoptysis

(D)   Otorrhea

(E)   Projectile vomiting

5.   A six-week-old infant with pyloric stenosis

6.   A 44-year-old woman with a urinary tract infection

7.   A 55-year-old woman status postmastectomy with a deep-vein thrombosis

8.   An 18-year-old in a motorcycle accident with a basilar skull fracture

9.   A 72-year-old white male, with no past medical history and in good physical condition, visited his primary care physician for a routine check-up. Upon questioning the patient in detail, it was revealed that he had mild urinary hesitancy and frequency, and was getting up at night to void several times. On

examination, the only abnormality was a mildly enlarged, nontender prostate gland. All of the following are options in management of this patient EXCEPT

(A)   transrectal prostate biopsy.

(B)   serum prostate-specific antigen.

(C)   terazosin.

(D)   finasteride.

(E)   transurethral ultrasound of the prostate gland.

10.   An obese 49-year-old female comes to the clinic for advice on weight loss. Which one of the following is true regarding weight reduction?

(A)   An aggressive exercise regimen negates the need for a reduction in caloric intake.

(B)   A proper weight reduction regimen should result in a reduction of five to ten lb. per week.

(C)   Judicious use of diuretics is a useful supplement to dietary modifications.

(D)   Gastric stapling procedure is contraindicated in patients with morbid obesity.

(E)   None of the above.

11.   A 43-year-old man comes to your clinic with an unstable knee and a history of an old football injury. He is otherwise healthy. You arrange for him to undergo arthroscopy of his knee. All of the following are appropriate presurgical tests EXCEPT

(A)   blood count.

(B)   chemistries.

(C)   prothrombin time.

(D)   platelet count.

(E)   HIV test.

12.   A 29-year-old man presents to the emergency room with urethral discharge. He denies any other significant past medical

problems and denies any previous sexually transmitted diseases. Urethral swab results show gonorrhea. The patient receives treatment for gonorrhea. Which one of the following is also appropriate empiric treatment?

- (A) Treatment for *Herpes simplex virus*

- (B) Treatment for *Chlamydia trachomatis*

- (C) Treatment for syphilis

- (D) Treatment for HIV

- (E) Treatment for trichomonas

13. Which one of the following humoral factors plays the most important role in the febrile response?

- (A) Nitric oxide

- (B) Interleukin-1

- (C) Fibroblast growth factor

- (D) Vascular endothelial growth factor

- (E) Atrial natriuretic peptide

14. A 23-year-old male with HIV disease presents with symptoms of severe watery diarrhea, crampy abdominal pain, weight loss, and flatulence. There were no leukocytes or blood in the fecal matter. Cryptosporidial oocysts and mucus were seen in the fecal matter. His physician suspects cryptosporidiosis. All of the following are likely to be part of the patient's diagnostic picture EXCEPT

- (A) cryptosporidium oocysts are found in the patient's water supply.

- (B) a histological study of infected epithelium would reveal small, spherical, basophilic structures along the brush border.

- (C) symptomatic cryptosporidiosis rules out the possibility of any condition other than immuno-suppression.

- (D) paramomycin decreases the severity of symptoms in cryptosporidiosis.

- (E) oocystoda, a coccidian protozoan parasite found in feces of infected individuals with cryptosporidiosis.

15. A 40-year-old female patient is seen in the clinic for complaints of fatiguability and anorexia. Physical examination is unremarkable. Blood tests reveal a WBC of 10.5 with 15% eosinophils. All of the following conditions are associated with eosinophilia EXCEPT

- (A) allergic reaction to sulfa compounds.

- (B) Loffler's syndrome.

- (C) Hodgkin's disease.

- (D) chronic hepatitis B infection.

- (E) *Strongyloides* infection.

Questions 16-19 refer to the following:

A 58-year-old man, with a history of smoking and drinking, comes to your office diagnosed with an ulcer and cervical adenopathy. You are worried about carcinoma.

16. The best way to get an accurate diagnosis would be to do which of the following?

- (A) CT scan of the head and neck

- (B) Panendoscopy

- (C) Biopsy of the lesion

- (D) Barium swallow

- (E) Liver-function tests

17. The most important risk factor for this man developing head and neck cancer is which one of the following?

- (A) His family history

- (B) His social history

- (C) His weight loss

- (D) His high cholesterol level

- (E) His hypertension

18. All of the following may be important in the evaluation of metastasis EXCEPT

    (A) chest X-ray.

    (B) liver-function tests.

    (C) BUN and creatinine.

    (D) bone scan.

    (E) brain scan.

19. The most appropriate next step for this patient is

    (A) immediate surgery.

    (B) admission to the hospital for performance of tests.

    (C) encourage smoking and drinking cessation and have patient return in one month.

    (D) follow-up in three months.

    (E) follow-up in six months.

20. A 76-year-old obese man with prostatic carcinoma is evaluated for prostatectomy. He had a documented myocardial infarction. The patient gives no further history relating to his heart. The patient does not report recent heart attacks or palpitations. Chest X-ray confirms your findings on physical examination and shows flattening of the lumbar lordosis. His ability to flex or extend the vertebral column is significantly reduced. You consider a subarachnoid block with a patient in a sitting position for anesthesia. Which of the following statements would NOT justify your choice?

    (A) Sitting position would aggravate the pain.

    (B) In the sitting position, patients find it easier to flex the spine.

    (C) Sitting helps to prevent rotation of the vertebral bodies.

    (D) Sitting helps to prevent distortion of the vertebral bodies.

    (E) The midline of the lumbar spinal column is not obscured by fat pads rolling over it and is easily accessible.

Questions 21-28 refer to the following:

A 53-year-old man followed in your clinic is brought to the emergency room by his wife. He has developed acute pain and swelling in his right knee. The patient is in a great deal of pain. He is noted to be febrile, with an oral temperature of 102°F, and he is hypertensive, with a blood pressure of 164/104 in his right arm.

21. The most important test to order first is

    (A) a sedimentation rate.

    (B) a synovial fluid analysis of the fluid you have aspirated from his knee.

    (C) electrolytes.

    (D) blood cultures.

    (E) urinalysis.

22. All of the following are important questions to ask early in your assessment of this patient EXCEPT

    (A) has he ever had a similar episode?

    (B) has he had any recent invasive procedures or trauma?

    (C) is he taking any medications and, if so, which ones?

    (D) is his father still alive?

    (E) does anyone in his family have similar joint problems?

23. The patient tells you that he has had one or two similar episodes in his knees in the past. He takes a diuretic for his hypertension, and the dose was recently increased. He has not had any invasive procedures recently. He is unaware of any other family members with similar problems. You begin to consider the possibility that he has

    (A) pseudogout.

    (B) gout.

    (C) osteoarthritis.

    (D) rheumatoid arthritis.

    (E) Reiter's syndrome.

24. While waiting for the results of the synovial fluid analysis, the patient's CBC returns, revealing a HGB of 14 and a white count of 18,000, with a left shift. You decide to get an X-ray of the knee while waiting for the results of his

    (A) urine uric acid.

    (B) serum uric acid.

    (C) rheumatoid factor.

    (D) antinuclear antibody.

    (E) Lyme titer.

25. The reason you have ordered an X-ray is

    (A) to identify osteomyelitis.

    (B) to identify loose bodies.

    (C) to identify a fracture.

    (D) to look for erosions.

    (E) to look for vascular calcification.

26. You call the laboratory to find out the results of the synovial fluid analysis. You are told that the Gram stain is negative, the white count is over 100,000, and no crystals are seen. Your initial assessment is

    (A) the lab has made a mistake.

    (B) the patient has rheumatoid arthritis.

    (C) the patient has pseudogout.

    (D) the patient has a joint infection.

    (E) the patient does not have gout.

27. You are very worried about the high white count in the synovial fluid. Because of this, you decide to treat the patient with

    (A) antibiotics.

    (B) intra-articular steroids.

    (C) intravenous steroids.

    (D) indomethacin.

    (E) allopurinol.

28. The next day, the preliminary synovial fluid and blood cultures are negative. The patient's joint is still hot and swollen and his pain is only minimally decreased by the analgesics he is receiving. You decide to administer

    (A) intravenous colchicine.

    (B) different antibiotics.

    (C) intravenous prednisone.

    (D) allopurinol.

    (E) probenecid.

29. You are reviewing the buffy coat blood smear, shown in the figure, of a 28-year-old female, who was admitted with hepatosplenomegaly, thrombocytopenia, anemia, and bone pain. You now recommend

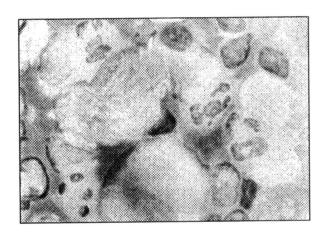

    (A) hexosaminidase A, 1000 U subcutaneous.

    (B) Alglucerase, 30 IU/kg intravenous.

    (C) renal transplantation.

    (D) orthotopic liver transplantation.

    (E) bone marrow transplantation.

30. A 67-year-old male with known hypertension comes in to his physician's office presenting with symptoms of urgency, urinary hesitancy, and frequent micturition at night. On examination, he has an enlarged prostate gland. Which one of the following antihypertensive medications is best suited for this particular patient?

    (A) Verapamil

    (B) Terazosin

    (C) Clonidine

    (D) Nifedipine

    (E) Hydrochlorothiazide

31. You are transfusing a patient for anemia. All of the following are possible reactions to the transfusion EXCEPT

    (A) fever.

    (B) hypotension.

    (C) hypertension.

    (D) tachycardia.

    (E) diaphoresis.

32. A 57-year-old white male presents to his physician's office complaining of severe heartburn and a "sour" taste in his mouth after eating a meal. He was diagnosed with mild reflux and given antacids. After three weeks the patient returned to the office, having tried the antacids, and stated that he did not get relief of his heartburn symptoms. He was referred to a gastroenterologist who performed an upper endoscopy and found Barrett's esophagus. What is the newest and most effective management of Barrett's esophagus in the 1990s?

    (A) Laser ablation plus proton-pump inhibition

    (B) H-2 blockers

    (C) Proton-pump inhibition alone

    (D) Repeat upper endoscopy with biopsy in three years

    (E) Endoscopic retrograde cholangiopancreatography (ERCP)

33. A 78-year-old white male nursing home resident is visited by his geriatrician. The patient is found to be mildly demented with a masked facial expression, seen with "pill-rolling" tremors, and a shuffling, slow gait. This patient denies any symptoms and is not incontinent. What would be the next best intervention?

    (A) Brain biopsy

    (B) Lumbar puncture

    (C) Thyroid function tests

    (D) Spinal cord MRI scan

    (E) Watchful waiting

34. You see a patient in the emergency room with a deep burn into the skin that is insensate. It is classified as

    (A) superficial.

    (B) first degree.

    (C) second degree.

    (D) third degree.

    (E) fourth degree.

35. You are monitoring the urine output of a 44-year-old male you have just admitted to the intensive care unit. Normal urine output per hour for this 80 kg male is closest to

    (A) 30 cc.

    (B) 60 cc.

    (C) 100 cc.

    (D) 120 cc.

    (E) 150 cc.

36. A 30-year-old male with known HIV disease presents to the infectious disease clinic complaining of symptoms of diarrhea, weakness, fatigue, weight loss, loss of appetite, and high fevers. He was found on examination to have diffuse lymphadenopathy and a hematocrit of 17%. His T-cell count was 20. Chest X-ray showed bilateral hilar adenopathy. Blood cultures grew *Mycobacterium avium intracellulare*. What would be the treatment?

    (A) Sulfadiazine and pyrimethamine

    (B) Clarithromycin, rifampin, and clofazimine

(C) Azithromycin alone

(D) Clarithromycin alone

(E) Isoniazid, pyrazinamide, ethambutol, and rifampin

37. A 42-year-old white male presents to the ER with a severe headache, transient visual disturbances, and diplopia. A CT scan of the head shows a focal frontal lobe mass with surrounding edema. What intervention is NOT used in the acute control of increased intracranial pressure in this situation?

(A) Hyperventilation

(B) Benzodiazepines

(C) Steroids

(D) Mannitol

Questions 38-41 refer to the following:

You are asked to manage a patient who takes Coumadin for a mechanical heart valve and who is about to undergo a tooth extraction and other oral surgery. He takes 5 mg of Coumadin every day. His PT is around 16 seconds.

38. The most appropriate way to manage this patient is

(A) allow the dentist to remove the teeth and perform surgery.

(B) stop the Coumadin the day before surgery.

(C) stop the Coumadin two days before surgery.

(D) stop the Coumadin two days before surgery and initiate heparin to keep the patient properly anticoagulated.

(E) stop the Coumadin and switch to aspirin.

39. When should the heparin be stopped prior to surgery?

(A) 2 hours

(B) 4 hours

(C) 8 hours

(D) 12 hours

(E) 24 hours

40. When should the Coumadin be restarted?

(A) The day before surgery

(B) The day of surgery

(C) The day after surgery

(D) Two days after surgery

(E) Three days after surgery

41. When should the heparin be turned off?

(A) One day before initiation of Coumadin

(B) On the day of Coumadin initiation

(C) One day after initiation of Coumadin

(D) When the PTT decreases

(E) When the PT returns to 16 seconds.

42. A 28-year-old healthy female, who failed to keep her last two prenatal appointments, walks in today, requesting an evaluation. Laboratory reports are unremarkable, except for a negative rubella serology. She does not recall her vaccination history. She thinks that she had "measles" as a child. You discuss all of the following EXCEPT

(A) primary infection confers lifetime immunity in immunocompetent hosts.

(B) vaccination with live attenuated virus confers immunity in more than 95% of immunocompetent persons for at least 16 years.

(C) immediate vaccination is recommended.

(D) congenital rubella usually results from maternal infection during the first trimester.

(E) in congenital rubella infection, the initial antibody response is IgG.

43. You examine a 49-year-old multigravida patient with redundant walls of the vagina protruding through the vaginal orifice. You diagnose a(n)

    (A) cystocele.

    (B) colpocele.

    (C) rectocele.

    (D) uterine prolapse.

    (E) enlarged introitus.

44. A 48-year-old man comes in with crushing substernal chest pain. You think he is having a myocardial infarction and send him to the CCU. The nurse reminds you that his insurance company has a 24-hour precertification clause for emergency admissions. This means that

    (A) you do not have to do anything.

    (B) you cannot admit him without talking to them first.

    (C) you have 24 hours to inform the insurance company of the admission.

    (D) you have to fill out special forms before the patient can go to the CCU.

    (E) you have to call the State Insurance Commission.

45. Long-term treatment for patients with sickle cell disease includes all of the following EXCEPT

    (A) hydroxyurea.

    (B) folic acid.

    (C) immunization.

    (D) suppression antibiotics.

    (E) avoidance of intense exercise.

Questions 46-49 refer to the following:

A 40-year-old man presents to your emergency room with four episodes of bright bloody emesis over one day. This has never happened previously. He denies any diarrhea, constipation, melena, or bright red blood per rectum, but states that he's had epigastric abdominal pain for several weeks. The only medication he is taking is several ibuprofen each day for chronic lower back pain. He smokes one pack of cigarettes per day and drinks five to six drinks per week. His blood pressure is 110/70, heart rate is 105, temperature is 99°F, respiratory rate is 15, and he is orthostatic. Abdominal exam reveals epigastric discomfort with palpation, but no rebound. Normoactive bowel sounds are noted. Rectal examination reveals guaiac-positive brown stool.

46. Of the following, all would be appropriate EXCEPT

    (A) type and cross for packed red blood cells.

    (B) stat gastrointestinal consult for esophagoduodenoscopy.

    (C) insertion of a nasogastric tube with normal saline flush.

    (D) abdominal CT.

    (E) initiation of treatment with intravenous H-2 blocker.

47. If this patient is 70 kilograms, an estimation of the blood loss based on physical examination would appropriately be

    (A) 0-900 cc of blood.

    (B) 900-1,500 cc of blood.

    (C) 1,500-2,100 cc of blood.

    (D) 1,500-2,700 cc of blood.

    (E) greater than 2,700 cc of blood.

48. The diagnosis of an acutely bleeding gastric ulcer is made by esophagoduodenoscopy. Of the following, the most appropriate intervention to do at this time would be

    (A) do not biopsy the ulcer nor sclerose the ulcer, but treat medically with H-2 blockers.

    (B) do not biopsy the ulcer, but sclerose the ulcer and treat medically with H-2 blockers.

(C) biopsy the ulcer and treat medically with H-2 blockers but do not sclerose the ulcer.

(D) biopsy the ulcer and sclerose the ulcer and treat medically with H-2 blockers.

(E) None of the above.

49. Of the following, all are known risk factors for peptic ulcer disease EXCEPT

(A) alcohol ingestion.

(B) smoking.

(C) pickled foods.

(D) *Helicobacter pylori* infection.

(E) chronic NSAID use.

50. A 65-year-old man who suffered a massive myocardial infarction cannot breathe without a respirator and has no electroencephalographic activity. He

(A) has coma vigile.

(B) has a reversible condition.

(C) is brain-dead.

(D) has rehabilitative potential.

(E) should not receive morphine.

51. At a routine physical examination, the blood pressure of a 70-year-old patient is recorded as 180/120 mm Hg. A complete history and complete physical examination reveal no other cardiovascular risk factors and no evidence of end organ damage or secondary causes of hypertension. As part of the management of this patient's condition, you, a primary care physician, decide to educate the patient on his condition. Which one of the following statements should be including in your counseling?

(A) Systolic hypertension in the elderly is not as significant as diastolic hypertension.

(B) Treating hypertension in the elderly usually is frustrating and often has no benefit for the patient.

(C) This patient is at increased risk for developing stroke and therefore should be placed on a combination of antihypertensive medications.

(D) You should leave the patient with a prescription for a single anti-hypertensive medication and reassurance.

(E) None of the above.

Questions 52-59 refer to the following:

A 30-year-old alcoholic female, found lying on the street, was brought in by the emergency medical service. Physical examination reveals a temperature of 99°F, blood pressure 110/70, pulse of 70, and respiration of 18. She is comatose, has alcohol odor on her breath, greenish-brown ecchymoses on the legs, and hepatomegaly.

52. While awaiting the results of laboratory tests, you administer all of the following EXCEPT

(A) thiamin, 100 mg IV push.

(B) dextrose, 1 g/kg IV bolus.

(C) naloxone, 0.01 mg/kg IV push.

(D) flumazenil, 0.2 mg IV push.

(E) diphenylhydantoin, 1 gm IV push.

53. The following laboratory results are reported by the laboratory

Sodium: 115 mEq/L
Potassium: 3.2 mEq/L
Chloride: 85 mEq/L
Bicarbonate: 22 mEq/L
Glucose: 70 mg/dL
BUN: 4 mg/dL
Creatinine: 0.5 mg/dL
Alcohol: 200 mg%

You now order

(A) plasma and urine osmolalities and urine sodium concentration.

(B) serum cortisol.

(C) thyroid-stimulating hormone.

(D)   repeat serum electrolytes.

(E)   plasma lipids.

54.   Regarding the alcohol level, which one of the following is true?

(A)   The blood alcohol will continue to decrease over the next several hours.

(B)   Coma is common in alcoholics at this blood alcohol level.

(C)   Coma is common in non-alcoholics at this blood alcohol level.

(D)   If this is the peak alcohol level, it can be expected to decrease at a rate of 10-25 mg% per hour.

(E)   This alcohol level explains the hyponatremia.

55.   The following results are now reported by the laboratory

Serum osmolality: 250 mOsmol/kg
Urine osmolality: 150 mOsmol/kg
Urine sodium: 35 mEq/L
Serum uric acid: 2.1 mg/dL

Just as you are about to begin treating the hyponatremia, the patient has a seizure. No focal neurologic signs are evident on your examination. While you are evaluating the seizures, you begin treatment of the hyponatremia with

(A)   water restriction, monitoring serum sodium.

(B)   demeclocycline, 300 mg/day.

(C)   isotonic saline (250 mM/L), to raise the serum sodium 0.5 mEq per hour.

(D)   hypertonic saline (514 mM/L), to raise the serum sodium 4-5 mM/L per hour.

(E)   hydrochlorothiazide, 25 mg daily.

56.   The patient is responding to your treatment of the hyponatremia. A repeat blood alcohol is reported as 176 mg%. In considering alcohol withdrawal as a potential cause of seizures in this patient, you reason that alcohol withdrawal seizures

(A)   do not occur at blood levels exceeding "legal intoxication."

(B)   typically occur more than 72 hours after cessation of alcohol.

(C)   may occur at this alcohol level, particularly if there are other medical stressors.

(D)   typically occur in clusters of six or more.

(E)   are almost always associated with focal neurologic findings.

57.   The laboratory reports a creatine kinase value of 200 U/L. All of the following are true regarding elevations of creatine kinase (CK) activity EXCEPT

(A)   in myocardial infarction, plasma MB-CK activity reaches a peak in 12-20 hours after the onset of chest pain.

(B)   intracerebral hemorrhage may produce an elevation of BB-CK.

(C)   bowel infarction may produce an elevation of BB-CK.

(D)   with rhabdomyolysis, the percentage of MB-CK to total CK exceeds 90%.

(E)   there is an increased percentage of MB-CK to total CK in muscular dystrophy.

58.   With your expert management, the patient had been gradually improving over the past several days, with normalization of her serum electrolytes. Today, she was found unresponsive to verbal commands and painful stimuli. A magnetic resonance imaging study, done as part of her evaluation, is shown in the figure on the next page. From this Tl-weighted image on the following page, you diagnose

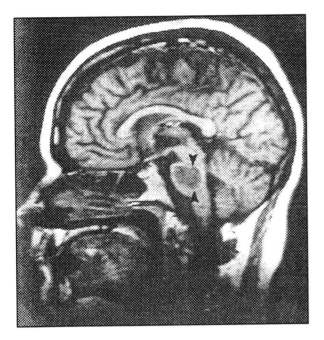

(A) pontine hemorrhage.

(B) central pontine myelinolysis.

(C) putaminal hemorrhage.

(D) cerebellar hemorrhage.

(E) Marchiafava-Bignami disease.

59. All of the following are true of central pontine myelinolysis EXCEPT

    (A) it is always fatal.

    (B) it may result from too rapid correction of hyponatremia.

    (C) it occurs more frequently in someone who develops hyponatremia chronically.

    (D) it results from osmotic demyelination.

    (E) neurons and axial cylinders are spared.

60. A 28-year-old male presents with symptoms of severe unilateral pain behind the right eye that lasts around one hour each day. These headaches are not associated with nausea or vomiting and occur once every three to four months. They occur mainly at night and are associated with right-sided nasal congestion and rhinorrhea. What is the most likely diagnosis?

(A) Migraines

(B) Cluster headaches

(C) Cerebral emboli

(D) Temporal arteritis

(E) Trigeminal neuralgia

61. A 79-year-old man with Alzheimer's has been admitted to your service from a nursing home because of pneumonia. He is breathing on his own, but is not responsive to commands. He has a low-grade fever and tachycardia. His wife has accompanied him and is his guardian. On previous recent hospitalizations, he has had "do not resuscitate" orders written in his chart. You should

    (A) assume the DNR orders remain in effect and write them.

    (B) discuss the situation with the wife to ascertain that she still agrees with these orders.

    (C) tell the house staff he will be a full code.

    (D) ignore him because he is probably going to die soon.

    (E) intubate him.

62. A seven-month-old female whom you follow in the well-baby clinic is brought to the walk-in pediatric clinic by his parents. They state that, since they came home from work the day before and picked her up at the baby-sitter's house, she has been lethargic, warm, and occasionally fussy. They have noticed that she has been rubbing the right side of her head. You suspect that the child has

    (A) meningococcal meningitis.

    (B) otitis media on the right.

    (C) pansinusitis.

    (D) pneumonia.

    (E) rubella.

63. A 23-year-old black male comes to the clinic for a follow-up visit. He recently moved to town and still has no medical records available. He tells you he has a history of severe episodic abdominal pain and pleurisy,

sometimes causing him to go to the emergency room. His old records will likely show that he has

    (A) diabetes mellitus with recurrent ketoacidosis.

    (B) sickle cell anemia.

    (C) Munchausen's disease.

    (D) pneumonia.

    (E) pancreatitis.

64. A cardiac thrill may be detected with

    (A) mitral regurgitation.

    (B) mitral stenosis.

    (C) myocardial infarction.

    (D) pulmonary hypertension.

Questions 65-68 refer to the following:

A 24-year-old woman with a history of insulin-dependent diabetes mellitus presents with two days of nausea and vomiting. She notes that two days previously, she had flu symptoms and did not eat and, therefore, did not take her insulin. Since then, she has felt weak with a sense of generalized malaise. Her nausea has been continuous and she has been vomiting up undigested food without blood or coffee-ground emesis. On physical examination, she is afebrile and has a respiratory rate of 26, a blood pressure of 130/80, and a heart rate of 110. The rest of the physical examination is essentially within normal limits. Laboratory tests reveal a sodium of 144, potassium of 3.8, chloride of 108, bicarbonate of 18, creatinine of 1.1, a glucose of 539, a white count of 11,000, and a hematocrit of 42%. This patient is appropriately diagnosed with diabetic ketoacidosis.

65. All of the following would be appropriate interventions EXCEPT

    (A) begin an IV insulin infusion.

    (B) begin crystalloid resuscitation.

    (C) begin a potassium IV infusion.

    (D) begin broad spectrum antibiotics.

    (E) begin oral phosphate.

66. Of the following, all can commonly initiate diabetic ketoacidosis EXCEPT

    (A) myocardial infarction.

    (B) sepsis.

    (C) noncompliance with insulin.

    (D) cystitis.

    (E) dehydration.

67. Of the following, which cannot occur with the treatment of diabetic ketoacidosis?

    (A) Hypokalemia

    (B) Hyperphosphatemia

    (C) Hypoglycemia

    (D) Fluid overload

    (E) Recurrent diabetic ketoacidosis

68. The proper time to stop IV insulin and change to subcutaneous insulin is determined by

    (A) accuchecks below 300.

    (B) correction of the anion gap.

    (C) physical examination signs of euvolemia.

    (D) absence of serum ketones.

    (E) absence of ketonuria.

69. A 54-year-old woman with a history of chronic renal insufficiency secondary to diabetes mellitus and hypertension presents to your clinic for routine follow-up. Her last creatinine clearance was 60 mg/24 hours. She is currently on enalapril and metoprolol for her blood pressure, and is on insulin for her diabetes mellitus. Her serum creatinine is stable at 2.5. Which one of the following therapeutic interventions is most important in slowing down the progression of her renal disease?

    (A) Close control of her diabetes mellitus

(B) Close control of her hypertension

(C) Close control of her hypercholesterolemia

(D) Stopping the ACE inhibitor

(E) Institution of dialysis

70. A medical student on your service turns in a history and physical he has written on a new patient for you to evaluate. In the course of this, you notice that his write-up is almost identical to that of the intern, which is already in the patient's chart. You

(A) decide this is a coincidence.

(B) fail the student for copying the intern's note.

(C) tell the chief resident that the intern is copying his notes from the medical student.

(D) discuss the problem with the student and the intern separately.

(E) tell the resident to settle the issue and report to you.

71. A 64-year-old vegetarian male, who has a past medical history of recurrent TIAs secondary to chronic atrial fibrillation with embolization into the area of the left middle cerebral artery, presents to his physician's office for a routine follow-up appointment. He is taking 12.5 mg per day of warfarin, but his INR and PT levels are still not in the therapeutic range. What would be the next step in management of this patient to prevent future transient ischemic attacks?

(A) Consume less green leafy vegetables

(B) Cardioversion

(C) Continue to increase the dose of warfarin

(D) Carotid endarterectomy

(E) Aspirin

Questions 72-75 refer to the following:

You are dictating a discharge summary for a 34-year-old healthy female, following an uncomplicated labor and delivery. A nurse arrives to inform you that the woman's previously healthy full-term male son has just developed respiratory distress.

72. The next day, a blood culture done as part of the evaluation of the distressed infant is positive. The most likely organism is

(A) group A streptococcus (*Streptococcus pyogenes*).

(B) *Candida albicans*.

(C) *Mycobacterium avium intracellulare*.

(D) group B streptococcus (*Streptococcus agalactiae*).

(E) *Corynebacterium diphtheriae*.

73. You request permission to perform a lumbar puncture. You indicate to the mother that, in early onset disease, the likelihood of meningitis is

(A) 80-90%.

(B) 30-40%.

(C) 100%.

(D) 10%.

(E) 60-70%.

74. Upon first seeing her infant with an arterial line, an endotracheal tube, and a venous catheter, the mother inquires as to the etiology of this infection. You indicate that all of the following increase the risk of infection EXCEPT

(A) prematurity.

(B) prolonged labor.

(C) rupture of the membranes six hours previously.

(D) maternal fever.

(E) chorioamnionitis.

75. Regarding future pregnancies, you advise the mother of which one of the following?

    (A) Ampicillin should be administered prophylactically during any future delivery.

    (B) She should have a tubal ligation immediately.

    (C) Ampicillin should be administered prophylactically throughout the next pregnancy.

    (D) Due to emerging drug resistance, vancomycin should be administered prophylactically during any future delivery.

    (E) You indicate that no special precautions are necessary.

76. A 35-year-old known alcoholic male presents to his primary care physician for a routine check-up. Routine lab data revealed an elevation of hepatic transaminases. The patient is asymptomatic. Physical exam reveals evidence of mild cirrhosis. All of the following should be done in this patient for health maintenance EXCEPT

    (A) PPD and anergy skin test.

    (B) hepatitis B and C profile screening.

    (C) advise the patient not to overuse acetaminophen.

    (D) liver biopsy.

    (E) advise the patient to join Alcoholics Anonymous.

77. In a newborn with intrauterine CMV infection, you expect to find which one of the following signs at birth?

    (A) Hepatitis

    (B) Thrombocytopenia

    (C) Cerebral calcifications

    (D) Hepatosplenomegaly

    (E) No signs

Questions 78-81 refer to the following:

A 69-year-old male, under your care for hypertension and cholelithiasis, was evaluated for abdominal pain during his recent vacation in Europe. He refused treatment and now requests your opinion of the diagnostic studies, which were performed in Europe.

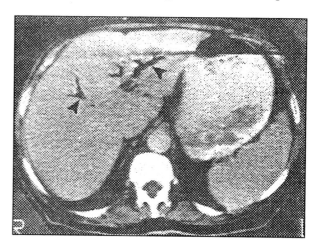

78. You indicate that the computed axial tomographic study of the abdomen, shown in the figure above, illustrates

    (A) hepatic granulomas.

    (B) metastatic lesions in the liver.

    (C) air in the biliary tree.

    (D) hepatic varices.

    (E) polycystic liver disease.

79. You indicate that the upper gastrointestinal series, illustrated in the figures on the following page, shows

    (A) gastric ulcer.

    (B) duodenal ulcer.

    (C) cholecystoduodenal fistula.

    (D) duodenal diverticula.

    (E) constricting gastric carcinoma.

Panel A

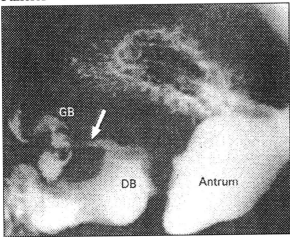

Panel B

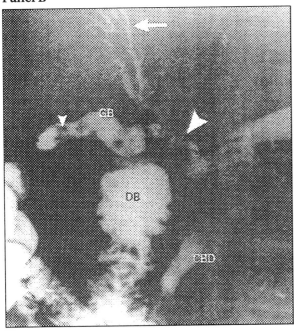

80. Based on the diagnostic studies, you recommend

    (A) surgery.

    (B) ursodeoxycholic acid, 10 mg/kg daily.

    (C) extracorporeal shock wave lithotripsy.

    (D) ranitidine, 300 mg HS.

    (E) amoxicillin, 750 mg plus metronidazole 500 mg TID for two weeks.

81. All of the following findings on plain abdominal radiographs suggest underlying disease of the gallbladder or biliary tract EXCEPT

    (A) deposition of calcium in a fibrotic gallbladder wall gives an eggshell appearance known as "porcelain gallbladder."

    (B) air in the biliary tree suggests choledochoduodenal fistula.

    (C) limey bile produces a hazy opacification of the gallbladder.

    (D) a large calcified gallstone may appear in the ileum in association with small bowel obstruction.

    (E) edema of the gallbladder wall is visible in acute cholecystitis.

82. You are the attending physician in the emergency room. A third-year medical student presents the case of an 80-year old obtundent female brought in by the EMS two hours ago. Physical examination reveals temperature of 99°F, pulse of 110, blood pressure 120/80, respiration of 20, with decreased skin turgor, and dry mucous membranes. Lungs are clear. Neurologic examination is nonfocal. The admission chemistry profile is

Glucose, mmol/L: 60
Sodium, mmol/L: 144
Potassium, mmol/L: 5
Chloride, mmol/L: 98
Bicarbonate, mmol/L: 20
BUN, mmol/L: 27
Creatinine, mmol/L: 490
Osmolarity, mOsmol/L: 380

You begin treatment for

    (A) diabetic ketoacidosis.

    (B) lactic acidosis.

    (C) nonketotic hyperosmolar coma.

    (D) dehydration.

    (E) drug overdose.

83. A 40-year-old man presents with epigastric burning radiating to his neck. He notes that these symptoms are worse at night before sleeping and after meals. He denies any association with exertion. Appropriate suggestions to him would include all of the following EXCEPT

   (A) decrease alcohol usage.

   (B) eat smaller meals.

   (C) use antacids.

   (D) treat with antibiotics.

   (E) keep his head higher when he sleeps.

Questions 84-86 refer to the following:

You are asked to see a 32-year-old male in a motorcycle accident complaining of neck pain.

84. In the emergency room you should

   (A) allow the patient to move the neck.

   (B) immobilize the neck totally.

   (C) take the patient to the operating room for a neck fusion.

   (D) place tongs on the patient in the emergency room.

   (E) perform a cervical block to decrease pain.

85. The lateral C-spine X-ray shows normal alignment and no fracture. Your next step is to

   (A) remove the cervical collar.

   (B) allow the patient to move his neck fully.

   (C) perform a complete C-spine series including an open-mouth odontoid.

   (D) send the patient home with a soft collar.

   (E) send the patient home with a steroid dose pack.

86. The radiologist tells you no fracture is seen at all. You should not feel comfortable in removing the collar until

   (A) there is absence of clinical symptoms.

   (B) follow-up X-rays show no fracture.

   (C) the neurosurgeon tells you to do so.

   (D) all four extremities are moving.

   (E) the patient asks you to do so.

87. A 72-year-old male with hypertension was admitted to the hospital with acute renal failure. He also complained of sudden visual impairment of the left eye and pain in the left foot. During the hospitalization, although distal pulses were palpable, two toes turned purple, with one of them requiring

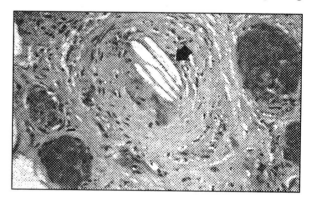

amputation. Based on the pathology section of the amputated digit, shown here, your diagnosis is

   (A) vasculitis.

   (B) Gram-negative sepsis.

   (C) cholesterol embolization.

   (D) bacterial endocarditis.

   (E) syphilis.

88. A 42-year-old man whom you treat periodically for vague musculoskeletal pains comes

in complaining of a backache. It is not severe, does not radiate, does not wake him up, and is relieved by acetaminophen. It occurs every few months after he works on his car. His physical examination is completely negative. The patient heard about a new kind of magnetic resonance imaging machine on television and insists he needs to have this test. You

(A) agree and send him.

(B) explain to him that this procedure is not necessary for him at this time.

(C) call his insurance company for preapproval.

(D) tell him he does not know what he is talking about.

(E) tell him you will send him to another physician for a second opinion.

89. A 65-year-old postmenopausal white female presents to the emergency room after having fallen in her apartment and injuring her right hip. X-rays revealed a right trochanter fracture, and the orthopedic surgeons performed an open reduction and internal fixation of the hip. Dual-photon imaging studies revealed that the patient had a very low bone-mineral density, suggestive of osteoporosis. To prevent future fractures, her primary physician can suggest all of the following EXCEPT

(A) alendronate.

(B) adequate lighting at home.

(C) plain sodium fluoride.

(D) transdermal estrogen patch.

(E) salmon calcitonin nasal spray.

Questions 90-93 refer to the following:

You are having lunch in a small restaurant across the street from the hospital, before going to make your afternoon rounds. You have a salad and coffee. A few tables away you see one of your surgical colleagues, to whom you refer most of your patients who need abdominal procedures, dining with a young woman who you know is not his wife. You try to keep from being seen by him, but you cannot help noticing that he is drinking multiple martinis throughout lunch. You manage to leave the restaurant without him seeing you, but you meet him shortly thereafter on one of the wards. He is in his scrubs and is looking over the chart of a patient who is scheduled to have surgery that afternoon. He greets you and you can smell alcohol on his breath.

90. You should

(A) tell him you saw him with another woman and you plan to speak to his wife.

(B) ask him the name of the woman with whom he was dining.

(C) ask him if he plans to go ahead and operate.

(D) tell him he is drunk and should go home.

(E) pretend you did not see him at lunch.

91. He tells you he saw you in the restaurant but thought you were avoiding him. He also says he plans to go ahead and operate and seems surprised that you should question it. You

(A) tell him you saw him consuming quite a few drinks, you can smell alcohol on his breath, and you think it would be better if he did not operate on anyone today.

(B) tell him you will call the police.

(C) tell him you will call his wife if he operates.

(D) say nothing.

(E) tell all the patients he is drunk.

92. He gets angry with you because of your advice and begins yelling at you in the hallway. You should

(A) yell back.

(B) leave him and go talk to the Chief of Surgery.

(C) call the police.

(D) listen.

(E) walk away.

93. This physician should be considered

(A) stupid.

(B) incompetent.

(C) stubborn.

(D) impaired.

(E) violent.

94. A 45-year-old black male presents to the emergency room with complaints of severe, excruciating right flank pain associated with nausea. He has no significant past medical history and does not drink alcohol. On examination, he has right costovertebral angle tenderness and a temperature of 100°F. Urine microscopy shows calcium oxalate crystals. Urine analysis reveals no white blood cells and negative leukocyte esterase. All of the following are appropriate management choices for this patient EXCEPT

(A) intravenous hydration.

(B) intravenous pyelogram.

(C) renal ultrasound.

(D) measuring serum BUN and creatinine.

(E) intravenous antibiotics.

95. Epidemiological control of meningococcal disease in the U.S. has been mostly achieved by virtue of

(A) frequent use of immunologic manipulations.

(B) improved life conditions of low socioeconomic strata.

(C) increased patient compliance.

(D) decreased number of patients per primary care physician.

(E) lowering the cost of routine vaccinations.

96. A 50-year-old woman presents to your office with symptoms of dysuria and urinary fre-quency for three days. She denies any flank pain, fevers, or chills. Her past medical history is only significant for glucose-6-phos-phate-dehydrogenase deficiency. Urinalysis reveals positive nitrites and leukocyte es-terase, with 15 white blood cells per high-power field and 4+ bacteria. All of the follow-ing antibiotic choices would be appropriate EXCEPT

(A) cephalexin.

(B) sulfamethoxazole-trimethoprim.

(C) Ciprofloxin.

(D) doxycycline.

(E) All of the above are appropriate for this patient.

Questions 97 and 98 refer to the following:

You have admitted an 80-year-old woman to the ICU in respiratory distress. Her blood gas on room air reveals retention of CO_2.

97. This is primarily a problem of

(A) oxygenation.

(B) ventilation.

(C) both oxygenation and ventila-tion.

(D) neither oxygenation nor ventila-tion.

(E) anemia.

98. To improve this woman's respiratory status, you would consider

(A) sedation.

(B) mechanical ventilation.

(C) increased inspired oxygen.

(D) decreased inspired oxygen.

(E) incentive spirometry.

Questions 99-102 refer to the following:

A 65-year-old man is brought to the emer-gency room by a family member with com-plaints of cough and fever. Sputum appears rust-colored. Vital signs are

Temperature: 102°F
Pulse: 110
Blood Pressure: 90/60
Respirations: 30

99. Physical examination is most likely to reveal

   (A) rales in the right base.

   (B) bilateral wheezing.

   (C) crepitus over the anterior clavicle.

   (D) absent breath sounds and hyperresonance in the left upper lung.

   (E) normal breath sounds.

100. Sputum Gram stain is most likely to reveal

   (A) Gram-positive cocci in pairs and chains.

   (B) Gram-positive cocci in clusters.

   (C) intracellular Gram-positive bacilli.

   (D) Gram-negative bacilli and cocci.

   (E) acid-fast bacilli.

101. If the pathologic organism was found to be *S. aureus*, this patient should be treated with

   (A) intravenous oxacillin.

   (B) intravenous penicillin.

   (C) intravenous vancomycin.

   (D) oral vancomycin.

   (E) oral first-generation cephalosporin.

102. After three days of therapy, the X-ray is unchanged from admission.

   (A) Sputum should be obtained for cytology.

   (B) The spectrum of antibiotic coverage should be broadened.

   (C) Chest X-ray should be followed on a daily basis for the next three days.

   (D) Consultation should be obtained for open lung biopsy.

   (E) Current management should be continued.

103. A 35-year-old female presents to your clinic with acute onset of severe anterior chest pain that is worsened by inspiration. She had a recent upper respiratory illness which seemed to resolve itself. The likeliest cause of her symptoms is

   (A) a myocardial infarction.

   (B) costochondritis.

   (C) lupus.

   (D) tuberculosis.

   (E) coxsackievirus infection.

104. Men in their 20s and 30s should be taught self-examination of which one of the following organs because of the increased chance of cancer?

   (A) Tongue

   (B) Breast

   (C) Penis

   (D) Testes

   (E) Scrotum

Questions 105-108 refer to the following:

A 65-year-old woman is brought to the ER because of a spiking fever and cough. She was brought by ambulance from a nursing home where she has been rehabilitating after a mild stroke . Chest radiograph shows acute lobar pneumonia. Her sputum stain reveals Gram-positive cocci. She seems somewhat depressed. The nurse's aide who has accompanied her tells you that she was widowed just before her stroke and her children do not live nearby.

105. You tell the patient she has bacterial pneumonia and needs to be admitted for a few days of antibiotics. She tells you she does not want to live and thus does not want to be treated. You

   (A) tell her you will send her home.

(B) tell her she does not know what she is talking about and is not competent to make a decision.

(C) talk to her about her depression and call the psychiatrist to see her, too.

(D) commit her.

(E) treat her in the ER.

106. The patient finally agrees to be admitted and receive treatment. She tells you that she is "low" because of her husband's death and her inability to take care of herself due to the stroke. The psychiatrist has prescribed an antidepressant. He says he is not worried about any suicidal tendencies. You

(A) call her family to inform them of her condition.

(B) commit her.

(C) insist she be hospitalized on a psychiatric ward.

(D) decide not to give her the antidepressant.

(E) tell her she is overreacting.

107. The next day one of the nurses tells you the patient is talking to her about her plans to kill herself. You

(A) tell the nurse not to worry because the psychiatrist said she was not suicidal.

(B) put her in protective isolation.

(C) change her antidepressant.

(D) call the psychiatrist back.

(E) commit her.

108. The psychiatrist tells you on the phone that he does not need to see her again because he is sure the patient is not suicidal. You argue that she has plans, but he claims that this is not important. You

(A) accuse him of malpractice.

(B) go to his office and call him incompetent in the presence of his colleagues.

(C) get another psychiatrist to render an opinion.

(D) commit the patient.

(E) tell the nurse not to worry.

109. A 63-year-old female patient with a history of MEN II is seen in the ER for mild pain in her arms and thighs. Your diagnostic work-up reveals metastases of previously unidentified chromaffin tissue cancer. The drug of first choice for the management of this patient's cancer pain at this time is

(A) fentanyl.

(B) NSAIDs.

(C) levorphanol.

(D) leritine.

(E) hydrocodone.

110. A 45-year-old woman with lupus comes to the clinic because of fatigue and malaise. She has just returned from a week-long vacation in the Caribbean where she spent most of her time lying on the beach. She is quite tanned. Her white count is 1,200 and her HGB is 10, both of which are much lower than her usual values. You suspect

(A) viral infection.

(B) leukemia.

(C) photosensitive reaction.

(D) aplastic anemia.

(E) pernicious anemia.

111. A 63-year-old man with a history of peptic ulcer disease is brought in by his wife because of recent onset of confusion. His wife says he takes a lot of liquid antacids every day and drinks three glasses of milk a day. His laboratory examination reveals an elevated serum calcium. You suspect

(A) an occult malignancy.

(B) hyperparathyroidism.

(C) milk-alkali syndrome.

(D) vitamin D intoxication.

(E) vitamin A intoxication.

112. A 62-year-old female recently had myco-plasma pneumonia. During treatment, she was found to have anemia with a positive Coomb's test. All of the following indicate hemolysis EXCEPT

    (A) low haptoglobin level.

    (B) elevated lactate dehydrogenase level.

    (C) elevated potassium.

    (D) low reticulocyte count.

    (E) elevated uric acid level.

Questions 113-115 refer to the following:

A 75-year-old man presents to your clinic with a hoarse voice and a 15-pound weight loss over the past six months without trying to diet. He admits to smoking two to three packs per day for 50 years and drinks three to four nights a week. His wife died one year ago from an unknown cancer.

113. You are worried about this patient having oral cancer. The most ominous aspect of his history and physical is

    (A) his voice.

    (B) his age.

    (C) his weight loss.

    (D) his smoking and drinking history.

    (E) his wife's death from cancer.

114. On examination of his oropharynx, you notice a 2 x 3 cm leukoplakic lesion on the base of his tongue by his right vocal cord. All of the following are other significant physical findings EXCEPT

    (A) an erythroplakic 5 x 5 mm lesion on the soft palate.

    (B) cervical lymphadenopathy.

    (C) a II/VI systolic ejection murmur.

    (D) decreased breath sounds.

    (E) hepatomegaly.

115. Causes of oropharyngeal leukoplakia include all of the following EXCEPT

    (A) trauma.

    (B) lingual thyroid.

    (C) aphthous ulcer.

    (D) lichen planus.

    (E) hyperkeratosis.

116. You are attending a postmortem conference to discuss an unusual presentation of echinococcus. A 56-year-old male from Saudi Arabia presented with dyspnea. A chest X-ray, a slice from a cross-sectional

Panel A

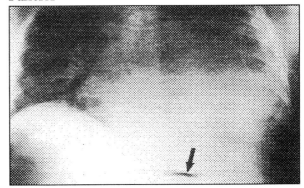

Panel B

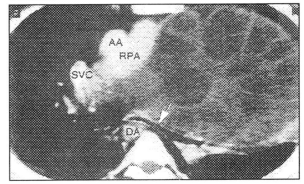

Panel C

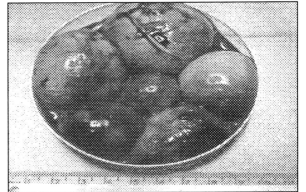

preoperative computed tomographic chest scan, and unruptured daughter cysts are shown in Panels A-C, on the previous page, respectively. All of the following management issues are addressed at the conference EXCEPT

(A) stable, calcified cysts do not require intervention.

(B) if surgical intervention is required, cysts should be isolated and killed prior to excision.

(C) hyponatremia may complicate surgical therapy.

(D) ethanol intoxication occurs as a complication of surgical therapy.

(E) leakage of cyst fluid may result in anaphylaxis.

Questions 117-120 refer to the following:

A 61-year-old woman with a history of squamous cell carcinoma of the lung presents to the emergency room with cough and shortness of breath while eating.

117. The most likely diagnosis is

(A) gastroesophageal reflux disease.

(B) congestive heart failure.

(C) pneumocystis pneumonia.

(D) tracheoesophageal fistula.

118. The best test to confirm this diagnosis is

(A) bronchoscopy.

(B) esophagoscopy.

(C) barium esophagram.

(D) chest X-ray.

119. Risk factor(s) for this condition include

(A) prolonged endotracheal intubation.

(B) AIDS.

(C) DVT.

(D) Zollinger-Ellison syndrome.

(E) All of the above.

120. All of the following can be used for palliation EXCEPT

(A) esophageal stenting.

(B) gastrostomy tube and NPO.

(C) airway stenting.

(D) esophagectomy.

(E) cervical esophagostomy and feeding gastrostomy.

121. A 12-year-old female is admitted to the emergency room for attempted suicide in which she ingested "two bottles of Tylenol" 12 hours ago. What medication should be given to the patient immediately?

(A) Digoxin

(B) Epinephrine

(C) N-acetylcysteine

(D) Verapamil

122. A 24-year-old woman presents to your office with a complaint of a foul-smelling vaginal discharge for two weeks. Her last menstrual period was three weeks ago and normal, and she is sexually active. On pelvic examination, you note a thin watery discharge and no other abnormalities. On wet mount, you note numerous trichomonads. All of the following would be appropriate EXCEPT

(A) discuss barrier protection and the reasons for using latex condoms.

(B) begin treatment with metronidazole.

(C) begin treatment with Lotrimin cream.

(D) discuss considerations of testing for HIV.

(E) send cervical swab for GC/chlamydia.

123. A 74-year-old female, who was walking her dog in the snow, slipped and fell on the ice. She had severe left hip pain and she was unable to get up. An ambulance brought her to the hospital where a hip fracture was diagnosed by X-ray. All of the following are true regarding falls in the elderly EXCEPT

(A) each year approximately 30% of community-dwelling people over 65 years old sustain a fall.

(B) prevention of hip fractures and falls in the elderly needs to be addressed through public health awareness programs.

(C) over 90% of hip fractures occur in women over the age of 70.

(D) more than 5% of falls result in a hip fracture.

(E) estrogen, alendronate, calcium, vitamin D, and nasal calcitonin are all used to treat osteoporosis.

Questions 124-131 refer to the following:

An 18-month-old infant is seen in the ER for fever. The fever has been intermittently present for three days. Her complete physical examination detects no gastrointestinal, cardiovascular, pulmonary, neurological, or musculoskeletal abnormalities. She is not on medications. You diagnose fever of unknown origin.

124. Your diagnosis is

   (A) supported by normal PE.

   (B) suggested by history.

   (C) based on normal findings.

   (D) very tentative.

   (E) wrong.

125. What is the most likely cause of the infant's condition?

   (A) Viral infection

   (B) Infected congenital abnormality

   (C) Atypical pneumonia

   (D) Occult bacteremia

   (E) Occult viremia

126. What is the most common organism for this condition?

   (A) RSV

(B) Parainfluenza virus

(C) *Streptococcus pneumoniae*

(D) *Haemophilus influenzae* type b

(E) *Neisseria meningitidis*

127. Which of the following would support the presence of fever without a focus?

   (A) WBCs < 15,000/mm^3

   (B) WBCs < 5,000/mm^3

   (C) Fever > 38.5°C

   (D) Positive exposure history

   (E) All of the above.

128. You should consider doing all of the following EXCEPT

   (A) repeat examination.

   (B) keep in touch with parents.

   (C) obtain blood cultures every time she is having fever.

   (D) use acetaminophen if you have to use an antipyretic.

   (E) be cautious with antibiotic treatment.

129. Regardless of origin, temperatures above 39°C may lead to convulsions in a child. Which of the following statements is true about febrile seizures?

   (A) The convulsion takes a few seconds.

   (B) The convulsion is focal with lateralizing features.

   (C) Most children with febrile convulsions go on to develop epilepsy in later life.

   (D) Seizures do not manifest neurologic deficits.

   (E) The onset is usually between age two months and age three years.

130. To diagnose fever of unknown origin in a child, which one of the following criteria should be met?

(A) Presence of fever for more than a week

(B) Fever in a hospitalized child

(C) Fever despite investigations performed during the week the child has been hospitalized

(D) All of the above.

(E) None of the above.

131. Concerning antipyretic treatment in a child with fever, which one of the following statements is true?

(A) All children with a high fever should be treated with an antipyretic.

(B) Children with a history of febrile convulsions should receive antipyretics.

(C) Children with chronic respiratory disease should receive antipyretics.

(D) Both (B) and (C).

(E) None of the above.

132. A 45-year-old female presents with severe bilateral wrist pain, low-grade fever, and swelling of the metacarpophalangeal joints. On exam, she has decreased range of motion of the wrist joints and swan-neck deformities are seen on both hands along with ulnar deviation. Her rheumatoid factor was positive. All of the following are complications of rheumatoid arthritis EXCEPT

(A) arthritis of the cricoarytenoid joints

(B) splenomegaly and leukopenia.

(C) pancreatitis

(D) cervical spine disease

(E) cardiovascular disease

133. Which of the following conditions is an indication for hemodialysis in children?

(A) Ingestion of tricyclic antidepressants

(B) Ingestion of digitalis

(C) Ingestion of opiates

(D) Severe salicylate intoxication unresponsive to other management

(E) Methemoglobinemia

Questions 134-136 refer to the following:

A 32-year-old Peace Corps worker is stationed to work in a remote agricultural village in India and is concerned about exposure to mosquitoes and acquiring malaria. She is in excellent physical condition and has no past medical history. She has no known allergies. She visits her family physician for routine travelers advice.

134. All of the following are recommended for malaria prevention EXCEPT

(A) use of mosquito netting at night.

(B) use of mosquito repellent such as 25% DEET.

(C) mefloquine.

(D) chloroquine.

(E) wearing long-sleeve pants and shirts at night.

135. Upon completing her mission in India, she returns to the United States and subsequently has a high fever of 103.5°F, anorexia, malaise, and lethargy. She denies symptoms of cough and pleurisy. She is brought into the emergency room by her sister. Her physical exam is normal except for dry, oral mucous membranes. All of the following should be done in the management of this case EXCEPT

(A) blood cultures.

(B) stool cultures.

(C) a look at the peripheral smear.

(D) intravenous hydration.

(E) chest X-ray.

136. All of the following preventive measures should be undertaken in this patient prior to traveling to endemic, third world countries such as India EXCEPT

(A)   hepatitis B vaccine.

(B)   typhoid vaccine.

(C)   hepatitis A vaccine.

(D)   rabies vaccine.

(E)   water and food precautions.

Questions 137-140 refer to the following:

A 69-year-old man with a history of mild hypertension comes in for a follow-up accompanied by his daughter, who says he has "not been himself" lately. He has withdrawn from the family, has gotten very "grumpy," and has lost weight. On further questioning, the patient admits that he has had some headaches but "doesn't know what all the fuss is about."

137.   All of the following pieces of historical information are important EXCEPT

(A)   visual changes.

(B)   muscle pain.

(C)   joint pain.

(D)   family history.

(E)   fevers and chills.

138.   You test the patient's muscle strength and find that it is normal throughout, although he does have tenderness in his proximal musculature. This finding makes which of the following conditions least likely?

(A)   Polymyositis

(B)   Polymyalgia rheumatica

(C)   Rheumatoid arthritis

(D)   Depression

(E)   Occult malignancy

139.   Which one of the following tests is likely to be the most useful diagnostically?

(A)   CPK

(B)   Aldolase

(C)   Westergren sedimentation rate

(D)   Urinalysis

(E)   Electromyogram

140.   The patient's sedimentation rate is very high at 92. Your working diagnosis is now

(A)   dermatomyositis.

(B)   radiculopathy.

(C)   myasthenia gravis.

(D)   polymyalgia rheumatica.

(E)   amyotrophic lateral sclerosis.

Questions 141-144 refer to the following:

A 44-year-old female presents to the emergency room with tachycardia, a widened pulse pressure, a fine tremor, and moist skin.

141.   Your differential diagnosis includes all of the following EXCEPT

(A)   septic shock.

(B)   hyperthyroidism.

(C)   hypothyroidism.

(D)   malignant hyperthermia.

(E)   insulin shock.

142.   All of the following symptoms would go along with your differential diagnosis EXCEPT

(A)   increased sweating.

(B)   decreased sweating.

(C)   increased appetite.

(D)   weight loss.

(E)   frequent bowel movements.

143.   All of the following would be appropriate tests to order EXCEPT

(A)   SMA-7.

(B)   CBC with differential.

(C)   liver-function tests.

(D)   thyroid-function tests.

(E)   EKG.

144.   The thyroid tests come back abnormal. Examination of this patient's eyes would reveal

(A)   nothing abnormal.

(B)   wide angle glaucoma.

(C)   narrow angle glaucoma.

(D)   conjunctival injection.

(E)   blindness.

145. At her annual well-care examination, a 70-year-old female patient has no complaints. Physical examination and routine laboratory test results are normal. As part of your counseling about her risks for cardiovascular diseases, you tell her that

(A)   death rates attributable to heart disease continued to increase over the past three decades.

(B)   heart disease is no longer the most common cause of death.

(C)   health education has been the major contributing factor for the recent decline in the death rate of heart disease.

(D)   increased numbers of deaths from coronary artery disease have resulted in a decreased proportion of the elderly in the United States.

(E)   lifestyle modification is the major cause of the recent decline of death rates from cardiovascular diseases.

For Questions 146-149, match the high-risk groups with the screening tests for the conditions listed below.

(A)   Syphilis and gonorrhea

(B)   Gonorrhea

(C)   Chlamydial infection and gonorrhea

(D)   Hepatitis B

(E)   HSV-2 infection

146. Individuals who regularly attend clinics to be checked on sexually transmitted diseases (STD)

147. Individuals with multiple sexual partners

148. Prostitutes

149. Homosexual men

Questions 150 and 151 refer to the following:

A 62-year-old noninsulin-dependent diabetic returns for his yearly examination to your office and reports that he is doing well and nothing is bothering him.

150. Questions that should be asked include all of the following EXCEPT

(A)   "How is your vision?"

(B)   "How is your appetite?"

(C)   "Are you more thirsty?"

(D)   "Are you going to the bathroom to void more often?"

(E)   "Are you having breathing problems?"

151. Screening laboratory tests would include

(A)   a CBC.

(B)   pulmonary function tests.

(C)   liver function tests.

(D)   an EKG.

(E)   a chest X-ray.

Questions 152 and 153 refer to the following:

Your 66-year-old patient develops a pleural effusion. You perform a diagnostic tap and you determine that the fluid is a transudate.

152. A transudate will have a protein level of

(A)   1.0 g/dL or less.

(B)   1.5 g/dL or less.

(C)   2.0 g/dL or less.

(D)   2.5 g/dL or less.

(E)   3.0 g/dL or less.

153. All of the following represent a transudate EXCEPT

(A) CHF.

(B) nephrotic syndrome.

(C) cirrhosis.

(D) infection.

(E) advanced liver disease.

154. A 50-year-old obese black female presents with new onset polyuria, polydipsia, weakness, and fatigue. Her fasting glucose level is 301 mg/dl. She has a family history of diabetes mellitus. All of the following statements are true EXCEPT

(A) type II diabetes is strongly inherited and complications are usually present at diagnosis.

(B) the results of the diabetes control and complications trial show that a decrease in HbA1c by 2% will result in 60% less retinopathy.

(C) diabetes is a cardiovascular risk factor.

(D) the goal should be to control glucose, lower cholesterol (LDL) below 130 mg/dl, and keep the HbA1c below 10%.

(E) 60-70% of all diabetics in the United States have non-insulin-dependent diabetes mellitus.

For Questions 155-159, you are covering the coronary intensive care unit and need to interpret EKG rhythms. Match the disease with the following rhythms.

(A) Atrial flutter

(B) Sinus bradycardia

(C) Premature ventricular contraction

(D) Ventricular tachycardia

(E) First-degree block

155. An early beat arising in the ventricle; P-wave may be present but unrelated to the QRS of the early beat.

156. A regular rhythm with a ventricular rate of 52 beats per minute

157. Three or more premature ventricular contractions in a row

158. PR interval greater than 0.2 seconds

159. Sawtooth waves with an atrial rate around 300 beats per minute and a variable ventricular rate

160. Angular kyphosis resulting from collapse of one or more vertebral bodies forms a protruding angle known as a

(A) singultus.

(B) torus.

(C) gibbus.

(D) tragus.

(E) conus.

161. Angular kyphosis may be secondary to all of the following EXCEPT

(A) Pott's disease.

(B) compression fracture.

(C) syphilis.

(D) AIDS.

(E) neoplasm of the bodies.

162. An 18-year-old man presents to your office with shortness of breath. He complains of shortness of breath and wheezing in the spring and in the autumn. He has been previously diagnosed with asthma and is taking Albuterol inhalers as needed. Currently, he says that he is needing them more often than usual and occasionally waking up at night with some shortness of breath. He denies fevers, chills, sputum production, or chest pain. Physical examination reveals that he is afebrile and his respiratory rate is 14, and he is not in any acute distress. His lungs have mild expiratory wheezes diffusely. The most appropriate intervention would be to

(A) begin oral corticosteroids immediately.

(B) begin a course of antibiotics.

(C) begin inhaled corticosteroids immediately.

(D) begin theophylline.

(E) order a chest radiograph.

163. A 73-year-old male was admitted with the acute onset of epigastric pain and abdominal distention. A computed tomographic scan, done as part of his diagnostic evaluation, is shown in the figure. You diagnose

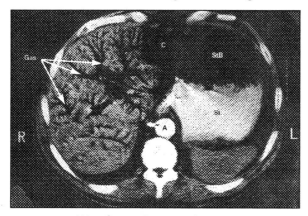

(A) fungating gastric mass.

(B) gas in the portal venous system.

(C) asplenia.

(D) colon carcinoma.

(E) aortic aneurysm.

164. An intravenous pyelogram, shown in the figure, was performed to evaluate left flank pain and hematuria in a 37-year-old female with long-standing regional enteritis. The most likely predisposing factor for this lesion in this patient is

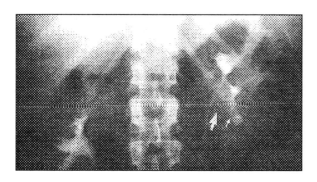

(A) dehydration secondary to diarrhea.

(B) steatorrhea.

(C) inflammatory reaction due to ileal disease.

(D) fistula secondary to ileal disease.

(E) amyloid deposition due to chronic inflammation.

165. Endocarditis infected with *Streptococcus bovis* is pathognomonic for

(A) intravenous drug use.

(B) colon cancer.

(C) idiopathic hypertrophic subaorticstenosis.

(D) diabetes mellitus.

(E) peptic ulcer disease.

166. Which one of the following operations is associated with the highest incidence of postoperative nausea?

(A) Laparoscopic cholecystectomy

(B) Partial small bowel resection

(C) Coronary artery bypass grafting

(D) Carotid endarterectomy

(E) Transurethral prostate resection

167. The bulk of health care expenditures in the U.S. is attributed to

(A) HMOs.

(B) health insurance.

(C) on-site payments.

(D) Medicare and Medicaid.

(E) None of the above.

168. The prevalence rate of a certain disease is defined as

(A) the number of new cases divided by the mean of population during a given time period.

(B) the number of all existing cases of a disease diagnosed during a certain time period, divided by the mid-interval population.

(C) the number of all new cases of a disease during a given period of time, divided by the mid-interval population.

(D) the number of existing cases, divided by the mean of population.

(E) the number of all existing cases of a disease at a single moment in time, divided by the population at the same time.

169. Upon examining a 65-year-old male, you notice a nodular umbilicus. You are suspicious of

(A) umbilical hernia.

(B) aortic aneurysm.

(C) metastatic gastric carcinoma.

(D) fecal impaction.

(E) an ileus.

170. You find a breast mass during the course of a routine physical exam of one of your patients. You tell her she needs a biopsy because of the risk of cancer. She refuses any further workup. You must

(A) call her husband.

(B) try to change her mind but respect her decision if you cannot dissuade her.

(C) commit her.

(D) refuse to see her again.

(E) tell her she is stupid.

171. A 40-year-old man presents to his primary care physician for a routine check-up. He was found to have a subperiosteal xanthoma over the upper tibia, orange-yellow tuberous xanthomas on the lower third of the forearm, elbows and knees, and bilateral arcus senilis. He has a strong family history of premature coronary artery disease. His serum cholesterol level was 304 mg/dl. This patient was otherwise asymptomatic and with no other

physical findings. What would be the initial management plan for this patient?

(A) Step I diet therapy

(B) Biopsy of the xanthomas

(C) Allopurinol

(D) HMG-CoA reductase inhibitor

(E) Gemfibrozil and niacin combination

Questions 172-175 refer to the following:

A mother brings her 17-year-old son to your office because of concern over the son's hand, which has fingers that are long and slender as well as having hyperextendable joints.

172. This is classically known as

(A) normal variant.

(B) arachnodactyly.

(C) Mongoloid hand.

(D) trident hand.

(E) claw hand.

173. The hand described above may be associated with which one of the following diseases?

(A) Down's syndrome

(B) Cerebral palsy

(C) Marfan's syndrome

(D) Hypothyroidism

(E) Carpel tunnel syndrome

174. Marfan's syndrome is passed on as

(A) sporadic.

(B) autosomal dominant.

(C) autosomal recessive.

(D) X-linked.

(E) Y-linked.

175. All of the following are seen with the above-described disease EXCEPT

(A) fused vertebrae.

(B) short and wide skull.

(C) high arched palate.

(D) elongation of the globe.

(E) deformities of the cardiac valve cusps.

176. Tenderness of the walls of the vagina and a discharge from the introitus is characteristic of

(A) vaginitis.

(B) bartholinitis.

(C) colpocele.

(D) cystocele.

(E) rectocele.

For Questions 177-180, match the serologic test associated with each disease with each numbered case question.

(A) Anti-smooth muscle antibody

(B) Anti-nuclear cytoplasmic antibody

(C) Anti-histone antibody

(D) Anti-mitochondrial antibody

(E) Anti-parietal cell antibody

177. A 35-year-old male presents to the Veterans Administration Hospital with severe anemia. His hematocrit was 20% and his MCV was 106.

178. A 56-year-old male, with a long-standing arrhythmia and on procainamide, presents with arthralgias and a left-sided pleural effusion.

179. A 46-year-old obese female nurse comes to the medical clinic complaining of nighttime pruritus, fatigue, and malaise. On exam, she has mild jaundice. Lab data reveals an elevated alkaline phosphatase level and a very high cholesterol level.

180. A 30-year-old male, with a history of chronic sinusitis, presents to the emergency room with severe shortness of breath and oliguria. His chest X-ray revealed nodular densities, and a kidney biopsy revealed rapidly progressive glomerulonephritis.

USMLE STEP 3
PRACTICE TEST 3

Day One – Afternoon Session

(Answer sheets appear in the back of this book.)

TIME: 3 Hours
180 Questions

> **DIRECTIONS:** Each of the following numbered items or incomplete sentences is followed by an answer or a completion of the statement. Choose the **ONE** choice that **BEST** answers the question or completes the sentence.

1. A 22-year-old white female with no past medical history presents with several years of crampy abdominal pain associated with diarrhea, a feeling of incomplete evacuation, and a bloated feeling. She sometimes has alternating constipation with diarrhea and achieves relief of the abdominal cramps subsequent to evacuation. She has no other systemic symptoms and there is no blood or mucous in the stool. The barium enema and sigmoidoscopy tests are normal. All of the following would be steps in managing this patient EXCEPT

    (A) ask the patient to keep a diary of foods that consistently bother her.

    (B) treatment with an antispasmodic agent.

    (C) behavioral modification.

    (D) ampicillin.

    (E) fiber supplementation when constipation occurs.

2. A 34-year-old black male presents to the emergency room with complaints of shortness of breath, fever, weight loss, and pleuritic chest pain. The CD4 count was 50 cells. Chest X-ray reveals bilateral interstitial infiltrates, and the LDH was elevated to 450 mg/dL. What would be the next step in treating this patient?

    (A) IV penicillin

    (B) IV trimethoprim-sulfamethoxazole

    (C) Transbronchial biopsy

    (D) IV Ganciclovir

    (E) Corticosteroids only

3. A 25-year-old infertile female presents to the gynecology clinic with complaints of dyspareunia, pelvic pain, dysmenorrhea, and rectal pain, which is cyclical in nature and associated with her menses. On exam, she has a tender, nodular cul-de-sac, a fixed, tender retroverted uterus, and a mass palpated in the rectovaginal septum. Which one of the following tests confirms the diagnosis?

    (A) Ultrasound of the pelvis

    (B) CT of the pelvis

    (C) Laparoscopy

    (D) Serum CA-125

    (E) Endometrial secretory protein-PP14

4. A middle-aged homeless man is brought into the emergency room after being found unresponsive on a heating grate in the snow. He's hypotensive with a blood pressure of 60/palpable, and has a respiratory rate of 2, a temperature of 83.5°F, and a heart rate of 50. Of the following statements, the true one regarding the patient's prognosis is

   (A) the patient has expired and is only exhibiting brainstem function.

   (B) the patient's prognosis for any meaningful recovery is nil and should be treated as such.

   (C) the patient should be resuscitated only for a few minutes, after which resuscitation efforts should be stopped.

   (D) the patient should be treated aggressively until the temperature returns to body temperature.

   (E) None of the above.

5. A 36-year-old Chinese female presents to the clinic without an appointment. She states she feels very weak with a poor appetite over the last week. She also has dark, amber urine and grayish color stools. On examination, she has mild hepatomegaly, right upper quadrant tenderness, scleral icterus, and jaundice. Lab data reveals elevated aminotransaminase levels and bilirubin in the urine. Hepatitis profile shows hepatitis B surface antibody positive, hepatitis A IgM positive, and negative hepatitis C antibody. What would be the next step in the initial management of this patient?

   (A) Interferon alpha

   (B) Steroids

   (C) Bed rest and encourage oral hydration

   (D) Hepatitis B vaccine

   (E) Liver biopsy

6. A 30-year-old male with known HIV disease presents to the infectious disease clinic complaining of symptoms of diarrhea, weakness, fatigue, weight loss, loss of appetite, and high fevers. He was found on examination to have diffuse lymphadenopathy and a hematocrit of 17%. His T-cell count was 20. Chest X-ray showed bilateral hilar adenopathy. Blood cultures grew *Mycobacterium avium intracellulare*. What would be the treatment?

   (A) Sulfadiazine and pyrimethamine

   (B) Clarithromycin, rifampin, and clofazimine

   (C) Azithromycin alone

   (D) Clarithromycin alone

   (E) Isoniazid, pyrazinamide, ethambutol, and rifampin

7. A 31-year-old woman is brought to the ER by her husband. The patient is unconscious and does not respond to external stimuli. You suspect drug overdose and immediately start resuscitation procedures. Your action

   (A) may result in a lawsuit since you do not have the husband's informed consent.

   (B) is appropriate under these circumstances.

   (C) may result in suspension of your license since you do not have the court's decision.

   (D) is appropriate only if you save the patient's life.

   (E) is an example of professional malpractice.

8. The authors of a highly reputable research study have found that autopsies reveal that 70% of all people over 65 years of age who die from nonmalignancy-associated conditions have evidence of an occult, newly-starting malignancy or a premalignant condition. Subsequently, they concluded that cancer is the leading cause of death for people over 70 years of age. This conclusion

   (A) is valid because selection bias has been eliminated.

   (B) could be valid if the level of results of the t-test would have been included in the study.

(C) is invalid because of lead-time bias.

(D) is invalid because of possibility of random error.

(E) is invalid because of ecologic fallacy.

9. Your postoperative cholecystectomy patient has a temperature on the first postoperative day. The most likely reason is

(A) wound infection.

(B) atelectasis.

(C) urinary tract infection.

(D) phlebitis.

(E) pharyngitis.

10. An intubated 75-year-old black female in the intensive care unit has a new fever of 103°F, an increase in her white blood cell count from 10,000 to 15,000, as well as a new radiographic infiltrate in the right middle lobe on the chest X-ray. Gram stain of an endotracheal aspirate demonstrates many WBCs. Which one of the following statements regarding treatment of this patient is FALSE?

(A) Empiric antibiotic coverage with a beta-lactam antibiotic and an aminoglycoside will be inappropriate in at least 25% of cases of ventilator-associated pneumonia.

(B) Combination therapy is required for *Pseudomonas* ventilator-associated pneumonia.

(C) Most of the excess mortality of ventilator-associated pneumonia is due to *Pseudomonas*.

(D) Clindamycin monotherapy should be initiated.

(E) Sending tracheal aspirate cultures and sensitivities to the microbiology lab is important in management of this patient.

11. You are asked to evaluate a patient in the emergency room with a blunt injury to his upper extremity and you diagnose a Madelung's deformity, which is

(A) dorsal angulation of the wrist.

(B) volar angulation of the wrist.

(C) dorsal angulation of the elbow.

(D) radial deviation of the elbow.

(E) ulnar deviation of the elbow.

12. A 47-year-old white male is seen in the ER for recurrent palpitations and pounding chest pain. He does not smoke or use alcohol. Family history is remarkable for coronary artery disease. Auscultation reveals a harsh systolic murmur in the left sternal border, which increases when the patient assumes a standing position. The long-term management of this patient's condition should include

(A) diuretics.

(B) digitalis.

(C) beta-blockers.

(D) nitrates.

(E) procainamide.

13. All of the following may be seen with myasthenia gravis EXCEPT

(A) increased fatigue.

(B) weakness.

(C) weakness worsened by neostigmine injection.

(D) abnormal speech.

(E) ptosis.

14. A 25-year-old gravida 2, para 1 female presents with vaginal bleeding at 27 weeks gestation. What would be the LEAST likely cause of bleeding?

(A) Placenta previa

(B) Abruptio placenta

(C) Active labor

(D) Placenta accreta

15. Acute left lower quadrant pain may be indicative of

    (A) acute appendicitis.

    (B) Meckel's diverticulitis.

    (C) regional ileitis.

    (D) colonic diverticulitis.

    (E) perforated duodenal ulcer.

16. A 67-year-old man with a history of sustained ventricular tachycardia has been placed on amiodarone. Appropriate follow-up should include all of the following EXCEPT

    (A) routine pulmonary function tests.

    (B) routine chest radiograph.

    (C) routine thyroid function tests.

    (D) routine complete blood counts.

    (E) routine hepatic transaminase levels.

17. A 15-year-old black teenager presents to the emergency room complaining of severe joint pain and shortness of breath. She has had sickle cell anemia all of her life with three "sickling crises" in the past year. On exam, she has a low-grade fever and lab data reveals a hematocrit of 18%. All of the following should be included in the management of this patient EXCEPT

    (A) oxygen.

    (B) blood transfusions.

    (C) intravenous hydration.

    (D) pain medication.

    (E) hydroxyurea.

18. A 54-year-old man with acute myelogenous leukemia was admitted to the hospital and given a course of chemotherapy. Neutropenia and fever developed after treatment was completed. Soon tense, grouped hemorrhagic pustules appeared on the patient's buttocks. The pustules ruptured and evolved into round ulcers with necrotic black eschars. On exam, there were several gangre-

nous ulcers with gray-black eschars surrounded by an erythematous halo. Blood cultures revealed *Pseudomonas aeruginosa*. What is the most likely diagnosis of the skin lesions?

    (A) *Pyoderma gangrenosum*

    (B) *Ecthyma gangrenosum*

    (C) Necrotizing vasculitis

    (D) Cryoglobulinemia

    (E) Erythema multiforme

19. A 68-year-old cowboy presents to the emergency room with severe shortness of breath. He has been a chronic smoker for 50 years. He was found to have chronic obstructive pulmonary disease with a bronchospastic component. The chest X-ray was negative. His forced expiratory volume in one second was less than one liter. All of the following can be used to manage this patient's case EXCEPT

    (A) steroids.

    (B) bronchodilators.

    (C) inhaled ipratropium bromide.

    (D) antibiotics.

    (E) theophylline.

20. A 72-year-old female patient presents with a two-hour history of cyanosis, shortness of breath, and substernal chest pain. She has a history of severe, deforming osteoarthritis and had been discharged from a local hospital a week ago after having a total hip replacement. Your examination shows a patient in acute respiratory distress. Her blood pressure is 100/65 and respiratory rate is 45/min. Auscultation reveals decreased breath sounds in the left lower lobe. What is your choice of diagnostic procedure for this patient's condition in the outpatient setting?

    (A) Ventilation/perfusion scan

    (B) Pulmonary angiography

    (C) Radionuclide scanning

    (D) Impedance plethysmography

    (E) Pelvic vein ultrasound

21. A 60-year-old male with a known cardiomyopathy was admitted last evening with congestive heart failure. His ejection fraction one month ago was 12%. The electrocardiogram, phonocardiogram, and carotid-pulse tracing, shown in the figure, confirm your findings on physical examination. Your diagnosis is

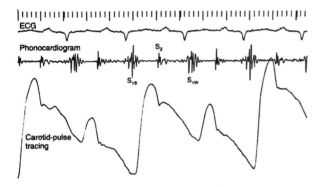

   (A) bigeminy.

   (B) Mobitz type I second-degree AV block.

   (C) pulsus alternans.

   (D) first-degree AV block.

   (E) pulsus paradoxus.

22. A previously healthy 70-year-old female was admitted last evening with complaints of nocturnal fever, weight loss, malaise, and diarrhea. She had been doing missionary work in East India, returning to the United States four months ago. Physical examination reveals a temperature of 104°F, pulse of 120, blood pressure of 110/70, respiration of 18, nontoxic appearance hepatomegaly, and marked splenomegaly. The bone marrow aspirate, performed to evaluate pancytopenia, is shown in the figure at the top of the next column. You diagnose

   (A) aplastic anemia.

   (B) acute myelogenous leukemia.

   (C) malaria.

   (D) visceral leishmaniasis.

   (E) plasma cell leukemia.

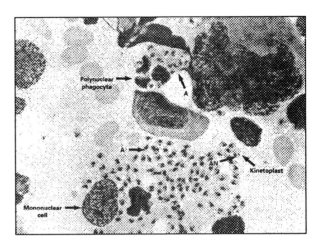

23. You are called to see a 54-year-old male patient in the emergency room for a complaint of stomach pain. The patient describes the pain as a stabbing epigastric pain, associated with nausea and vomiting, which has been occurring intermittently over the past several years. On further history, he drinks 10-15 beers a day and has been drinking for 30 years. The pain generally improves when he stops eating and drinking for a few days. Physical examination reveals marked epigastric tenderness. Which one of the following tests would NOT be useful in making a diagnosis in this patient?

   (A) Abdominal ultrasound

   (B) Serum amylase/lipase

   (C) Abdominal CT scan

   (D) Mesenteric angiogram

   (E) Abdominal X-ray

24. A 75-year-old man presents to your office with one day of fevers to 102.5°F associated with nasal stuffiness and clear rhinorrhea and with myalgias and arthralgias. He denies any cough. He has a past medical history of congestive heart failure, chronic obstructive pulmonary disease, and diabetes mellitus. His vital signs show that he has a temperature of 101.9°F, blood pressure of 130/70, heart rate of 90, and a respiratory rate of 14. His lungs are clear and his cardiac exam reveals no gallops or murmurs. There is no edema on physical examination. The most appropriate medication for his symptoms is

(A) azithromycin.

(B) amoxicillin.

(C) furosemide.

(D) amantadine.

(E) None of the above.

25. A 35-year-old white female with breast cancer presents to her oncologist's office for a routine follow-up appointment. She had received chemotherapy ten days ago, and her total white blood cell count is 214. On examination she has a temperature of 100.5°F. All of the following should be performed in this neutropenic cancer patient EXCEPT

(A) full set of blood cultures.

(B) granulocyte colony stimulating factor injections.

(C) respiratory isolation.

(D) intravenous antibiotics.

(E) reverse isolation precautions.

26. A 69-year-old Hispanic male who has been hospitalized with a gastric ulcer presents suddenly with severe, right-sided thoracic pain radiating across the back and associated with fever. On examination, the T12 dermatomal skin lesion shows vesicular lesions, which are tender and pruritic in nature. The nurse calls the medical resident to evaluate this patient's complaints. What would be the next step in making the diagnosis?

(A) Biopsy of the skin lesion

(B) Topical corticosteroids

(C) Empiric treatment with acyclovir

(D) Tzanck prep

(E) Electrocardiogram

27. While making hospital rounds on his patients, the attending physician was told by one of his patients that she had severe, watery diarrhea associated with abdominal cramps that has been occurring over the course of three days. This patient is on intravenous antibiotics for ten days for treatment of a community-acquired pneumonia. What is the next step in managing this patient?

(A) Flexible sigmoidoscopy

(B) Check stool for ova and parasites

(C) Treat empirically with oral metronidazole

(D) Treat empirically with trimethoprim-sulfamethoxazole

(E) Discontinue the antibiotics and check stool for culture and sensitivities

28. A 23-year-old gravida 1 para 0 at 36 weeks gestation, to whom you have been providing prenatal care, comes to your office for a scheduled appointment. You notice that her face and hands are moderately edematous. She has also gained five pounds over the last week. You suspect that she might have

(A) gestational diabetes.

(B) changes normally observed toward the end of pregnancy.

(C) preeclampsia.

(D) eclampsia.

(E) a complete placenta previa.

29. A 26-year-old female comes to your office with dysuria, frequency, and a mild temperature. Physical examination reveals CVA tenderness and suprapubic tenderness. The most likely diagnosis is

(A) intrauterine pregnancy.

(B) urinary tract infection.

(C) kidney stones.

(D) bladder tumor.

(E) ovarian cyst.

30. A 65-year-old navy captain is referred to your office for progressive memory impairment, personality alterations, and an increasing inability to orient himself to his surroundings. A presumptive diagnosis of Alzheimer's disease was made after an evaluation for other causes of dementia was negative. After ten years, the patient progressed to a near-vegetative state and died of pneumonia. A postmortem examination of the brain was done.

What pathology of the brain is NOT usually found in a patient with Alzheimer's disease?

(A)   Neurofibrillary tangles derived in part of bundles of microtubules and neurofilaments occurring within neurons.

(B)   Amyloid plaques occurring within the cerebral cortex, hippocampus, and amygdala.

(C)   Depigmentation of cells in the substantia nigra and locus ceruleus.

(D)   Intracytoplasmic proximal dendritic eosinophilic inclusions consisting of actin.

31.   A 64-year-old male was seen in your clinic because of palpitations. The most appropriate admission for this patient is to admit him to

(A)   the operating room for an emergent pacemaker.

(B)   the intensive care unit.

(C)   telemetry.

(D)   the ward.

(E)   home with instructions to come back to the clinic in the morning.

32.   A 51-year-old female with chronic hepatitis C complains of fatigue, ankle pain, and recurrent skin lesions on both lower extremities. Physical examination reveals hepatomegaly and superficial vasculitic lesions of both lower extremities with palpable purpura. An uncentrifuged serum specimen, obtained as part of the initial evaluation and stored at 4°C for 48 hours, is shown in the figure in the next column. All of the following are true of the illustrated precipitate EXCEPT

(A)   it dissolves when heated.

(B)   if monoclonal, it is most commonly of the IgG or IgM class.

(C)   if polyclonal (type III), it is of no clinical significance in the presence of an underlying infectious process.

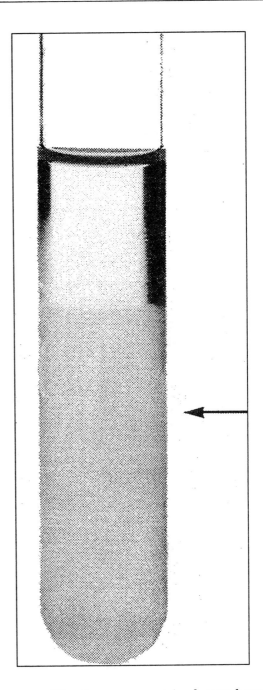

(D)   the serum protein electrophoresis may be normal in the mixed, type II variety.

(E)   when associated with hepatitis C, it usually exceeds 20 g/dL.

33.   A 30-year-old woman without significant past medical history presents with symptoms of palpitations, tremors, and anxiety. She denies any chest pain, shortness of breath, nausea, or vomiting. She denies any

previous medical illnesses and is not taking any medications. On physical examination, her blood pressure is 150/70, heart rate is 140, respiratory rate is 24, and temperature is 99°F. Her lungs are clear and her cardiac exam is regular with a normal S1 and S2 without murmurs and S3. Her abdominal exam is benign and she has no peripheral edema. Chest radiograph reveals a normal cardiac silhouette and no infiltrates or effusions. Electrocardiogram reveals sinus tachycardia without evidence of ischemia or infarction. Her laboratory results are all within normal limits except it is noted that she is severely hyperthyroid. Of the following, what is an appropriate immediate medication to treat her symptoms?

(A)   Radioactive iodine

(B)   Propylthiouracil

(C)   Propranolol

(D)   Methimazole

(E)   Iodide

Questions 34-37 refer to the following:

You are called to the emergency room to see a 34-year-old gentleman with a fusiform swelling of his right long finger.

34.   All of the following should be obtained EXCEPT

(A)   complete blood count.

(B)   finger X-ray.

(C)   culture and sensitivity of the drainage.

(D)   arterial blood gas.

(E)   detailed history and physical.

35.   Admission orders for this patient should include all of the following EXCEPT

(A)   warm soaks.

(B)   antibiotics.

(C)   elevation of hand.

(D)   nothing by mouth status.

(E)   serial examinations.

36.   The best route of antibiotic administration for this patient is

(A)   IV.

(B)   IM.

(C)   PO.

(D)   topical.

(E)   through irrigation catheters.

37.   The most important discharge criteria for this patient is

(A)   one week of antibiotics.

(B)   absence of pain.

(C)   clinical resolution of the infection.

(D)   improvement on X-ray.

(E)   sterile wound.

Questions 38-40 refer to the following:

A 17-year-old teenager is hospitalized by her primary care physician. The doctor admitted her electively to the hospital to evaluate her extensive weight loss, which was below 85% of her ideal body weight. This patient has been reported by family and friends to have not been eating for the last three to four months, and the patient's mother found laxatives in her daughter's bedroom.

38.   All of the following signs and symptoms are found in patients with anorexia nervosa EXCEPT

(A)   amenorrhea.

(B)   high T3 concentrations.

(C)   binge eating.

(D)   osteoporosis.

(E)   hypokalemia.

39.   Several weeks later, this young female is still hospitalized because she refuses to eat and is continuing to lose weight. Her blood pressure is low and she has an elevation of her creatinine phosphokinase level consistent with myopathy. She is talking about suicide. All of the following management items need

to be considered at this point in time EXCEPT

    (A)   intravenous fluids.

    (B)   estrogen replacement.

    (C)   psychiatric counseling.

    (D)   nasogastric tube feedings.

    (E)   cardiac monitoring for arrhythmias.

40.   Three months later, this patient is discharged home and she resumes her normal daily activities at school. Her weight has been stabilized, and she has been eating her meals with her friends and family. What is the most important treatment recommended at this point in time?

    (A)   Psychiatric outpatient follow-up

    (B)   Estrogen replacement

    (C)   Antidepressants

    (D)   Nutritional counseling

    (E)   High-protein diet

41.   You are walking in the grocery store and see an elderly gentleman clutch his chest and pass out. Upon arrival, he has no pulse and has no spontaneous respirations. The most appropriate initial intervention is

    (A)   a precordial thump.

    (B)   chest compressions.

    (C)   mouth-to-mouth resuscitation.

    (D)   asking nearby family members about his medical history.

    (E)   brief absence from the scene to telephone the paramedics for help.

42.   All of the following should be performed during a breast examination EXCEPT

    (A)   compression of the breast to show dimpling.

    (B)   palpation of supraclavicular nodes.

    (C)   palpation of axillary nodes.

    (D)   transillumination of any masses.

    (E)   percussion of palpated masses.

Questions 43-50 refer to the following:

The supervisor of the hospital laboratory refers his technician to the clinic for evaluation of persistent anorexia, nausea, malaise, arthralgias, myalgias, and cough. He consumes alcohol socially and does not smoke. He denies illicit or prescription drug use. There is no family history of liver disease, and he denies fever. Physical examination is significant for hepatomegaly and right upper quadrant tenderness.

43.   You consider the possibility of acute viral hepatitis and discuss all of the following EXCEPT

    (A)   in acute hepatitis B, elevation of serum transaminases precedes the rise in serum bilirubin.

    (B)   in acute hepatitis A, elevation of serum transaminases follows the rise in serum bilirubin.

    (C)   jaundice is usually visible in the sclera or skin when the serum bilirubin exceeds 2.5 mg/dL.

    (D)   acute viral hepatitis may be mimicked by other acute infectious and noninfectious disease processes.

    (E)   all five types of hepatitis (A-E) produce clinically similar illnesses in the acute phase.

44.   In acute hepatitis B infection, all of the following are true EXCEPT

    (A)   HBsAg is the first virologic marker detectable in the serum.

    (B)   circulating HBsAg precedes elevations of serum aminotransferase activity.

    (C)   antibody to HBsAg (anti-HBs) becomes detectable in the serum following the disappearance of HBsAg.

(D) HBcAg is routinely detectable in the serum two to four weeks following the onset of jaundice.

(E) IgM anti-HBc predominates during the first six months following acute infection.

45. Which one of the following is true regarding the clinical usefulness of the "e" antigen in hepatitis?

(A) It is a serologic marker of hepatitis A infection.

(B) It is a serologic marker of hepatitis B infection.

(C) It is a serologic marker of hepatitis C infection.

(D) It is a serologic marker of hepatitis E infection.

(E) Its appearance heralds the termination of viral replication.

46. Which one of the following is NOT true of the delta agent in hepatitis?

(A) IgM anti-HDV predominates in acute HDV infection.

(B) The titer of anti-HDV is low in self-limited infections.

(C) In self-limited infections, anti-HDV is usually not detectable after HBsAg is cleared from the serum.

(D) Anti-HDV is usually undetectable in the serum in chronic HDV infections.

(E) IgG anti-HDV is present in the serum in chronic HDV infection

47. Which one of the following is true of serologic tests for acute hepatitis C infection?

(A) First-generation enzyme-linked immunoassays become positive two to three weeks following infection.

(B) Second-generation enzyme-linked immunoassays do not become positive until the clinical incubation period has passed.

(C) Second-generation enzyme-linked immunoassays may become positive as early as two to three weeks following infection.

(D) The first-generation enzyme-linked immunoassay (EIA-1) is more sensitive than the second-generation RIBA assay.

(E) Second-generation RIBA assays correlate poorly with the presence of HCV-RNA

48. The patient is lost to follow-up, but returns two years later with complaints of easy bruisability, difficulty concentrating, anxiety, restlessness, and increasing abdominal girth. Physical examination is significant for spider angioma, palmer erythema, hepatomegaly, splenomegaly, ascites, and asterixis. A paracentesis is performed. All of the following are consistent with a transudate EXCEPT

(A) protein less than 25 g/dL.

(B) specific gravity less than 1.016.

(C) plasma ascites albumin gradient (PAAG) greater than 1.1 g/dL.

(D) 100 polymorphonuclear cells (PMN) /mm^3.

(E) triglyceride greater than 200 mg/dL.

49. Although compliant with your medical regimen, his ascites remain refractory to treatment. A transjugular intrahepatic portosystemic shunt was placed following an episode of minor variceal bleeding. The Doppler sonogram of the liver, shown in the figure on the following page, demonstrates all of the following EXCEPT

(A) characteristic echogenicity of the shunt.

(B) intense blue signal from shunted blood.

(C) intense blue signal from shunt throsis.

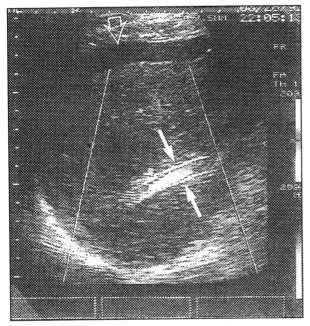

(D) hypointense signal due to ascites.

(E) successful placement of the shunt.

50. One year later he was admitted following a variceal hemorrhage. Azotemia, hyponatremia, and oliguria developed during his hospital stay. There is no evidence of intravascular volume depletion. To exclude hepatorenal syndrome, which one of the following tests is most helpful?

(A) Analysis of the urine sediment

(B) Urine specific gravity

(C) Urinary sodium

(D) Urine creatinine

(E) Urine potassium

Questions 51-54 refer to the following:

A 60-year-old recently widowed farmer, who was working on his fall harvest in October, presents to the emergency room with severe shortness of breath, chest tightness, and burning of his eyes after filling his silo with freshly cropped corn. He subsequently noticed a "chlorine-like odor." The chest X-ray revealed bilateral diffuse alveolar infiltrates. The patient was afebrile with a blood pressure of 90/70 mm/HG and a respiratory rate

of 36/min. He had bilateral conjunctivitis on examination.

51. Which one of the following diagnostic tests is inappropriate?

(A) Bronchoalveolar lavage for cultures and acid-fast bacilli

(B) Serologic tests for identification of possible exposure to *Aspergillus, Candida, Histoplasma,* and *Blastomyces*

(C) Serologic tests for identification of possible exposures to micropolyspora and thermoactinomyces

(D) Pulmonary function tests

(E) Alcohol and drug toxicology screening

52. Which one of the following is most likely to have caused this patient's pulmonary disease?

(A) Pulmonary embolism

(B) Dermal absorption of chemicals from the silage

(C) Infection with thermophilic fungal spores

(D) Chemical injury from inhalation of oxides of nitrogen (silo filler's disease)

(E) *Legionella* pneumonia

53. In light of the clinical diagnosis, which one of the following measures is most likely to help prevent similar episodes?

(A) Education of agricultural workers at risk

(B) Wearing of a face mask and gloves at the workplace

(C) Inspection of the ventilation systems in silos

(D) Use of oxygen-monitoring devices in silos

(E) Screening of workers by routine chest X-rays and pulmonary function tests

54. On the basis of the clinical diagnosis, which one of the following complications is more likely than the others to occur in this patient?

    (A) Lymphocytic interstitial pneumonitis

    (B) Pulmonary fibrosis

    (C) A chronic systemic autoimmune disease

    (D) Recurrence of symptoms without further exposure to the offending agent

    (E) Bronchiolitis obliterans

Questions 55-58 refer to the following:

A 43-year-old man comes to the walk-in clinic complaining of substernal discomfort, especially after eating. He has noticed a sour, burning sensation in his throat in association with this. He has been taking a nonsteroidal anti-inflammatory agent for three months because of low back pain.

55. All of the following questions would be important in your evaluation at this point EXCEPT

    (A) "Do you taste or feel sour material in your mouth when you bend over to tie your shoes?"

    (B) "What relieves the discomfort?"

    (C) "Have you ever vomited blood?"

    (D) "Does anyone in your family have similar problems?"

    (E) "Does the pain radiate anywhere?"

56. All of the following should be obtained at this point EXCEPT

    (A) stool hemoccult.

    (B) abdominal palpation.

    (C) electrocardiogram.

    (D) chest radiograph.

    (E) upper GI series.

57. The patient has noticed sour material in his mouth when he bends over. He has never had hematemesis. The hemoccult is negative and the electrocardiogram is normal. Your leading diagnosis now is

    (A) angina pectoris.

    (B) peptic ulcer disease.

    (C) gastroesophageal reflux disease.

    (D) gastric cancer.

    (E) pancreatitis.

58. Which one of the following conditions should also be suspected in this patient?

    (A) Esophageal stricture

    (B) Mallory-Weiss tear

    (C) Hirshsprung's disease

    (D) Diverticulitis

    (E) Pancreatitis

For Questions 59-62, select the most appropriate intervention.

    (A) Immediate transvenous pacing

    (B) Immediate transcutaneous pacing

    (C) Immediate permanent pacing

    (D) Immediate cardioversion

    (E) Immediate adenosine administration

59. A 48-year-old man without known past medical history is noted to be without a pulse or respirations. Chest compressions are begun and his airway is secured. Monitor reveals asystole.

60. An 82-year-old woman with hypertension and congestive heart failure presents with a congestive heart failure exacerbation. She denies any chest pain, but has noted shortness of breath upon lying down and with exertion. Physical examination reveals a temperature of 98°F, a blood pressure of 170/80, a heart rate of 40, and a respiratory rate of 20. Her lungs reveal bilateral inspiratory rales and her cardiac exam reveals a normal S1

and S2 and a notable S3. On electrocardiogram, she is noted to be in third-degree atrioventricular block.

61. A 27-year-old woman without significant past medical history presents with feelings of palpitations. She denies any shortness of breath or chest pain. She is taking no medications and denies any past medical illnesses. Physical examination reveals a temperature of 98°F, a blood pressure of 130/70, a heart rate of 180, and a respiratory rate of 20. The remainder of her examination is without abnormalities. Electrocardiogram reveals a narrow complex tachycardia.

62. A 50-year-old man with a history of atrial fibrillation is noted to be tachycardiac to 150. He complains of chest pain, shortness of breath, and nausea. His past medical history is significant for paroxysmal atrial fibrillation and coronary artery disease. His temperature is 98°F, blood pressure is 90/60, heart rate is 150, and respiratory rate is 30. His lungs are clear, his heart exam reveals an irregular rate and rhythm, and his abdominal exam is benign. Electrocardiogram reveals atrial fibrillation with a rapid ventricular response.

63. When counseling your patients about smoking cessation, all of the following are true EXCEPT

    (A) smoking is associated with a higher incidence of coronary atherosclerotic disease.

    (B) smoking interacts with oral contraceptives in significantly increasing the incidence of myocardial infarction.

    (C) even if one discontinues smoking, the damage to the upper respiratory tract has already been done and one will always be at significantly increased risk of upper respiratory tract infections.

    (D) smoking by pregnant women is associated with an increased incidence of fetal death.

    (E) smoking is associated with an increased incidence of several cancers including lung, cervical, and gastric.

For Questions 64-67, select the most likely diagnosis.

    (A) Gout

    (B) Osteoarthritis

    (C) Rheumatoid arthritis

    (D) Pseudogout

    (E) Infective arthritis

64. A 47-year-old woman comes to the clinic complaining of low-grade fevers and joint pains involving both knees. Physical examination reveals bilateral synovitis of the metacarpophalangeal and proximal interphalangeal joints, in addition to bilateral ballottable patellae.

65. A 56-year-old female comes to the emergency room complaining of severe pain in the left wrist. White blood cell count is 16.4. Joint aspiration reveals needle-shaped crystals which appear negatively birefringent under a polarized light microscope.

66. A 50-year-old female complains of bilateral pain in the fingers. Physical examination reveals nodes in the proximal and distal interphalangeal joints. X-ray of the hands show a loss of joint space narrowing.

67. A 55-year-old alcoholic man complains of severe pain in the right big toe. Joint aspiration reveals rhomboid crystals which are positively birefringent.

68. A middle-aged man is brought to the ER in full cardiac arrest. He collapsed while at work. His wife says he had been having chest pain. You try to resuscitate him. He does not respond to electric shock, chest compression, or intubation and ventilation. His EKG is flat-line despite all your efforts. After 20 minutes of a full code and continued flat-line EKG, you

    (A) call the cardiac surgeons.

    (B) call the transplant team.

(C)   admit him to the CCU.

(D)   declare him dead.

(E)   ask a colleague to continue trying to resuscitate him.

Questions 69-72 refer to the following:

A 54-year-old white male with a long history of alcoholism presents with severe abdominal pain associated with nausea and vomiting. There was no history of trauma. On examination, he has abdominal distension with fever and mild ascites. Lab data reveals a serum amylase level of 400 U/L and lipase level of 250 U/L. His glucose level was 100 mg/dL, hematocrit was 43%, and he showed no evidence of jaundice.

69.   The most likely diagnosis is

(A)   pancreatic carcinoma.

(B)   chronic pancreatitis.

(C)   cholecystitis.

(D)   acute pancreatitis.

(E)   bowel perforation.

70.   The most useful test to make the correct diagnosis would be

(A)   laparoscopy.

(B)   CT scan of the abdomen.

(C)   ultrasound of the abdomen.

(D)   X-rays of the abdomen.

(E)   clinical examination.

71.   What could be the most likely cause for this disorder?

(A)   Biliary sludge

(B)   Medications

(C)   Alcoholism

(D)   Gallstones

(E)   Infection

72.   How would the physician manage this patient?

(A)   Intravenous antibiotics

(B)   Oxygenation

(C)   Morphine for pain

(D)   Peritoneal lavage

(E)   Nasogastric tube placement and hydration

73.   Your patient is a 30-year-old woman. Her pulse is 120 beats/min and her blood pressure is 180/100 mm Hg. Her temperature measures 39.2°C. The medical records received from her family physician show that she has been on methimazole for hyperthyroidism. To prevent this patient from possible development of intraoperative thyrotoxic crisis, you should decide on a right dose of the antithyroid drug. To do so, which of the following laboratory tests should you order to evaluate this patient's thyroid problem?

(A)   Total plasma T4 and T3 levels

(B)   Thyroid resin uptake

(C)   Radioactive iodine uptake

(D)   Serum TSH

(E)   All of the above.

74.   A 21-year-old schoolteacher presents to the physician's office with complaints of a rash on her thigh after having been bitten by a tick. She also has symptoms of lethargy, malaise, and a headache. On examination, the rash is typical of erythema migrans. All of the following should be carried out by the physician EXCEPT

(A)   lumbar puncture.

(B)   start doxycycline.

(C)   culture for *Borrelia burgdorferi*.

(D)   ELISA serologic test for *Borrelia burgdorferi*.

(E)   careful search on the patient's body for the tick.

75. A 74-year-old obese white female with NIDDM during the last eight years, treated with sulfonylureas, is admitted for an elective cholecystectomy. Her blood pressure immediately before surgery is 190/120 mm Hg, pulse is 100 bm regular, and temperature is 98.9°F. Physical examination is not clinically remarkable. ECG is unrevealing. Blood pressure measured after surgery reads 170/100 mm Hg.

Post-Surgery Laboratory Data

Blood		Urine	
Sodium	149 mEq/L	Proteins	+++
Potassium	3.6 mEq/L	Ketones	-
Chloride	94 mEq/L		
Glucose	300 mg/dL		
Creatinine	1.0 mg/dL		
BUN	9.0 mg/dL		
LDL	200 mg/dL		
HDL	30 mg/dL		
Hemoglobin	16 g/dL		
Hematocrit	44%		

Which one of the following risk factors should you address first in the primary treatment and prevention of this patient's diabetes?

(A) High HDL/LDL ratio

(B) Obesity

(C) Hypertension

(D) Sedentary lifestyle

(E) Smoking

76. During a routine visit to the geriatric clinic, an 87-year-old white female presents with symptoms of right temporal headache associated with a low-grade fever and malaise. Her ESR is 100 mm/hr. What would be the immediate management in this case?

(A) Temporal artery biopsy

(B) Nonsteroidal anti-inflammatory drugs

(C) Antibiotics

(D) Steroids

(E) CT of the brain

77. Causes of prerenal oliguria include all of the following EXCEPT

(A) glomerular disease.

(B) volume depletion.

(C) renal artery compromise.

(D) shock.

(E) heart failure.

78. A 54-year-old man who gets an occasional transient backache when he lifts too many boxes has a negative radiograph of his lumbosacral spine. His physical examination is completely normal. He demands a magnetic resonance imaging scan of his back "because my brother-in-law had one." You do not think this is medically indicated. You

(A) order the MRI.

(B) explain your reasoning to the patient.

(C) call the insurance company so they can refuse coverage and you can blame them.

(D) tell the patient he has no right to tell you what to do.

(E) tell the patient to find another doctor.

79. A 70-year-old white male with stage C prostate cancer recently returned from a Brazilian vacation. His wife found him unconscious in the bathroom this morning, with blood in his mouth. She also brought the specimen shown in the figure on the following page. She inquires whether or not it is related to her husband's illness. You inform her of all of the following EXCEPT

(A) immunosuppressed states predispose to hyperinfection by this organism.

(B) the condition may be fatal.

(C) there is no association between the organism and her husband's illness.

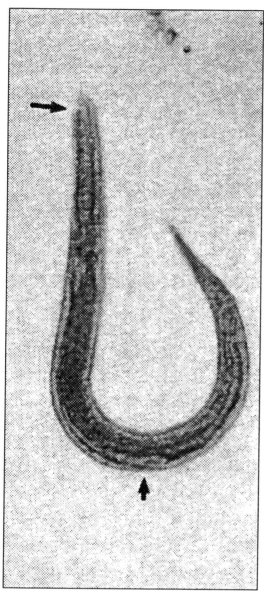

(D)   the organism may invade the central nervous system.

(E)   Gram-negative sepsis is common in this setting.

80.   Of the five patients below, the one who should be seen first is

(A)   a 17-year-old male with an upper respiratory tract infection.

(B)   a 35-year-old woman with a urinary tract infection.

(C)   a 22-year-old female with an acute asthma attack.

(D)   a 44-year-old male with a broken thumb.

(E)   a six-month-old child with otitis media.

81.   A 31-year-old male is brought by his girlfriend to the ER unconscious, hypoventilating, and tachycardiac. Appropriate resuscitation maneuvers are begun and his initial room air ABG is as follows

$$pH = 7.14 \qquad pCO_2 = 80 \qquad pO_2 = 40$$

$$HCO_3- = 26 \qquad O_2 \text{ Sat.} = 58\%$$

Which one of the following clinical situations best fits this ABG?

(A)   Acute anxiety reaction

(B)   Prolonged vomiting

(C)   ARDS

(D)   Heroin overdose

Questions 82-88 refer to the following:

A 31-year-old male presents with sharp abdominal pain in the right upper quadrant. There is some associated vomiting. There is tenderness under the liver. You call for a general surgeon and he diagnoses acute cholecystitis. After much discussion, the surgeon opts for surgery and the gall bladder is removed uneventfully.

82.   You take care of the patient postoperatively. Your pain medicine postoperatively should avoid the use of

(A)   Demerol.

(B)   morphine.

(C)   aspirin.

(D)   Tylenol.

(E)   ibuprofen.

83. Preoperatively, concerning the patient's diet, it is best to

    (A) keep the patient NPO with a nasogastric tube.

    (B) just keep the patient NPO.

    (C) allow the patient clear liquids only.

    (D) allow the patient to have full liquids.

    (E) allow the patient to have a regular diet.

84. On post-op day 2, the patient develops abdominal distention. The most likely cause is

    (A) abdominal perforation.

    (B) ileus.

    (C) infection.

    (D) dead bowel.

    (E) bleeding.

85. The patient's distention resolves, but two days later he develops sharp abdominal pain with peritoneal signs. A flat plate of the abdomen suggests free air under the diaphragm. The patient most likely is suffering from a(n)

    (A) bleeding ulcer.

    (B) perforated viscous.

    (C) abdominal infection.

    (D) recurrent cholecystitis.

    (E) jaundice.

86. The most appropriate management for this patient is

    (A) close observation.

    (B) placement of a nasogastric tube.

    (C) an enema.

    (D) an exploratory laparotomy in the operating room.

    (E) a CAT scan to determine the location of the problem.

87. Three days later, the patient is feeling much better and is enjoying a regular diet. He is ready for discharge and asks what he can and can't do. You inform him

    (A) he is free to do anything he wants.

    (B) he should lie in bed for three weeks.

    (C) he should lift nothing greater than ten pounds for three weeks.

    (D) he should lift nothing greater than ten pounds for six weeks.

    (E) he can lift as much as he wants as soon as he wants.

88. Two months later, the patient returns to your clinic because of some separation of the wound edges. Your next step is to

    (A) take the patient back to the operating room for exploration.

    (B) prescribe hyperbaric oxygen.

    (C) apply topical antibiotics.

    (D) debride the wound and allow it to heal by secondary intention.

    (E) close the wound primarily.

89. A male physician who performs gynecologic exams should

    (A) do the procedures by himself.

    (B) stop doing these exams and send patients to female colleagues.

    (C) have a female assistant in the room with him when he examines patients.

    (D) tell his patients a nurse is watching through a one-way mirror.

    (E) date attractive patients.

90. A sexually active 20-year-old female was admitted last evening with acute swelling of the right knee. She denies pharyngeal or anogenital symptoms. Physical examination reveals: Temperature of 101°F, pulse of 98, blood pressure of 120/80, and respiration of 16. There are no cutaneous lesions; the

pharynx is benign; there is a painful, swollen, hot, red right knee. Other joints are unremarkable; the patient refuses a pelvic exam due to menses. Arthrocentesis is cloudy, with 80,000 neutrophils/cc. The Gram-stain is most likely to show

(A) Gram-positive cocci in chains.

(B) Gram-negative intracellular diplococci.

(C) Gram-negative cocci in clusters.

(D) Gram-positive cocci in clusters.

(E) Gram-negative rods.

91. A paraplegic patient develops a pressure sore. The most likely location for this sore is

(A) sacral.

(B) trochanteric.

(C) occipital.

(D) ischial

(E) heel.

92. You are seeing one of your patients in the emergency department because his family has brought him in since he has been threatening to commit suicide. His wife recently left him and he has been very depressed. He refuses hospitalization, but his family says he has a plan to kill himself and has a gun. You

(A) call a psychiatrist to arrange an involuntary 72-hour psychiatric admission.

(B) call the police to get him arrested.

(C) refer him to a psychiatrist for outpatient follow-up.

(D) tell the family they are overreacting.

(E) admit the patient to the ICU.

93. A 29-year-old Asian male presents to the clinic with symptoms of severe pain on the tips of his fingers and along the veins of both his lower and upper extremities. On examination, he has erythema, edema, and ten-

derness along the superficial veins of both his forearms and lower calves. He is a heavy smoker. There is no associated fever and the ESR is 30 mm/hr. What would be the initial management in this patient?

(A) Venography

(B) Steroids

(C) Antibiotics

(D) Discontinuing smoking

(E) Local heat and aspirin

Questions 94-101 refer to the following:

A 56-year-old man who has been your patient for over ten years presents for his yearly physical. You notice a 6-by-6 millimeter black lesion on his ankle. The patient states that it has slowly enlarged, and when you examine your notes, you read that last year it was tan-brown and only 3-by-3 millimeters, and that was unchanged over the years.

94. Further examination should include all of the following EXCEPT

(A) the skin for other lesions.

(B) palpation of inguinal lymph nodes.

(C) abdomen.

(D) rectosigmoid.

(E) eyes.

95. You suspect malignant melanoma. All of the following characteristics of the lesion are important EXCEPT

(A) the size of the lesion.

(B) the border of the lesion.

(C) the color of the lesion.

(D) the depth of the lesion.

(E) the vascularity of the lesion.

96. The melanoma that appears on the face of elderly patients is

(A) superficial spreading melanoma.

(B) nodular melanoma.

(C) acral lentiginous melanoma.

(D) lentigo maligna melanoma.

(E) mucocutaneous melanoma

97. The presence of inguinal lymphadenopathy is worrisome because it may signal

(A) lymphoma.

(B) Hodgkin's disease.

(C) regional spread.

(D) venereal disease.

(E) regional infection and lymphad-enitis.

98. Appropriate management of this patient would be

(A) close observation.

(B) biopsy.

(C) surgery

(D) radiation therapy.

(E) chemotherapy.

99. The patient sees an oncologist, is treated and cured, and presents back to your office six months later. You now are performing your physical examination and note no abnormalities and feel comfortable that your patient is free of disease. You schedule your next history and physical in

(A) three months.

(B) one year.

(C) two years.

(D) five years.

(E) No more follow-up since he is now free of disease.

100. The patient asks you what he could have done to avoid this and what to do in the future. You advise him to

(A) do nothing.

(B) stop smoking.

(C) stop drinking.

(D) lower cholesterol and eat more healthily.

(E) avoid sunlight.

101. Five years after his treatment, the patient comes to you with a swollen leg on the side of his ankle melanoma. You attribute this to

(A) congestive heart failure.

(B) varicose veins.

(C) lymphedema.

(D) recurrent tumor.

(E) weight gain.

102. A 45-year-old man comes in for acute bronchitis. While you are examining him, he suddenly admits to you that he is bisexual. He has only two partners: his wife and his male lover of seven years, neither of whom has other partners. He has recently been found to be HIV-negative. You should

(A) tell him if he does not practice safe sex with his wife and lover you will tell his wife about his lover.

(B) promise him not to tell his wife if he gives you money.

(C) call the Board of Health.

(D) advise him to use a condom with both partners.

(E) refuse to see him again because you do not approve of bisexuality.

103. A 47-year-old man with a history of alcohol abuse came to the emergency room complaining of severe pain and swelling of the first left toe. These symptoms started the day before and became worse at night. On exam, the patient's first metatarsophalangeal joint was deeply erythematous and exquisitely tender, particularly the medial portion. Extensive soft-tissue edema on the dorsum of the foot and his ankle was warm to touch. His temperature was 100°F and the WBC was 10,000 cells/UL. The uric acid level was normal. The X-ray of the joint was negative. This

patient has had no significant past medical history. All of the following are acute management options for this patient EXCEPT

    (A)   colchicine.

    (B)   prednisone.

    (C)   allopurinol.

    (D)   corticotropin.

    (E)   indomethacin.

Questions 104-111 refer to the following:

A 42-year-old man with a history of hypertension presents to the emergency room with severe crushing substernal chest pain. He says that he awoke this morning with that pain and that it hasn't changed since then. He notes no associated radiation of the pain, diaphoresis, shortness of breath, or vomiting, but does feel nauseated. He denies any recent fevers, chills, cough, shortness of breath, sick contacts, nausea, vomiting, or abdominal pain. His past medical history is significant for hypertension, for which he used to take blood pressure medications, but has stopped taking them on his own. He has had no surgeries and is taking no medications. He denies alcohol or smoking or illicit drug use.

104. Of the following, all need to be considered in the initial differential diagnosis EXCEPT

    (A)   acute myocardial infarction.

    (B)   aortic dissection.

    (C)   pulmonary embolism.

    (D)   acute gastritis.

    (E)   gastric ulcer perforation.

105. Of the following, all need to be immediate interventions EXCEPT

    (A)   nasogastric tube lavage.

    (B)   12-lead electrocardiogram.

    (C)   chest radiograph.

    (D)   monitor.

    (E)   physical examination.

106. All of the above interventions are done and the physical exam reveals vital signs with a temperature of 99°F, a heart rate of 70, a blood pressure of 100/60, and a respiratory rate of 30. The patient appears in severe distress with his pain. Lungs are clear, and cardiovascular exam reveals a regular rate and rhythm with a normal S1 and S2 and without S3 or murmurs. Abdominal examination reveals normoactive bowel sounds and no pain to palpation nor any rebound tenderness. Rectal examination reveals guaiac-negative brown stool, and extremities reveal no edema. Based on physical examination alone, the diagnosis that can safely be excluded would be

    (A)   acute myocardial infarction.

    (B)   aortic dissection.

    (C)   pulmonary embolism.

    (D)   acute gastritis.

    (E)   gastric ulcer perforation.

107. A nasogastric tube lavage reveals minimal bilious fluid. A 12-lead electrocardiogram reveals sinus rhythm at 70 and 3 millimeter ST elevations in leads II, III, avF and 2 mm ST depression in V2 and V3. Chest radiograph reveals a normal cardiac silhouette, no infiltrates or effusions, and a widened mediastinum. Monitor reveals sinus rhythm at 70, and pulse-oximetry reveals a room air saturation of 98%. The next most appropriate intervention is

    (A)   transesophageal echocardiogram.

    (B)   initiation of thrombolytics.

    (C)   immediate call to the cardiac catheterization lab.

    (D)   computed tomography scan of the abdomen.

    (E)   esophagogastroduodenoscopy.

108. All of the following are absolute contraindications to the use of thrombolytics EXCEPT

    (A)   known intracranial tumor.

    (B)   recent surgery, within ten days.

(C) history of intracranial hemorrhage within the previous year.

(D) hypotension.

(E) prolonged cardiopulmonary
resuscitation.

109. Of the following medical interventions, with
the information above, all of the following
are appropriate EXCEPT

(A) aspirin.

(B) intravenous heparin.

(C) streptokinase.

(D) oxygen.

(E) nitroglycerin.

110. Based on the appropriate tests, the diagnosis of an ascending dissecting aortic aneurysm is made. Of the following, which is NOT
an appropriate diagnostic test for an aortic
aneurysm?

(A) Magnetic resonance imaging of
the chest

(B) Computed tomography scan of
the chest

(C) Aortogram

(D) Transesophageal echocardiogram

(E) All of the above are appropriate
tests.

111. The most appropriate treatment for the
above situation is

(A) immediate cardiac catheterization and percutaneous transluminal angioplasty.

(B) immediate cardiac catheterization to assess the need for
coronary artery bypass surgery.

(C) immediate treatment with tissue
plasminogen activator.

(D) immediate surgery.

(E) None of the above.

112. A 22-year-old woman presents to your office
with a complaint of vaginal discharge. You

make the diagnosis of bacterial vaginosis
and prescribe metronidazole. Appropriate
precautions regarding the administration of
this drug would be

(A) that it can cause urine to turn
orange.

(B) that it can cause a disulfiram-
type reaction.

(C) that it can cause *Clostridium
difficile* colitis.

(D) that it can cause a dry taste in
one's mouth.

(E) that it can cause a rash in some
patients.

113. A nine-year-old boy states he was playing
and "may" have stepped on a rusty nail.
There is a puncture wound on the foot. All
of the following need to be done EXCEPT

(A) closure of the wound.

(B) irrigation of the wound.

(C) X-ray of the foot.

(D) antibiotic administration.

(E) tetanus administration.

Questions 114-116 refer to the following:

A 79-year-old farmer visits his physician for
a routine annual physical examination. He
has no complaints and no past medical history. The physical examination was within
physical normal limits and all lab data were
normal except for an elevated alkaline phosphatase level of 249 mg/dL. The aminotransferase levels were normal, as well as the bilirubin level.

114. What would be the appropriate management at this point?

(A) Liver biopsy

(B) Hepatitis profile

(C) Follow-up alkaline phosphatase
level in six months

(D) Bone biopsy

(E) CT scan of the spine

115. Six months later, this patient comes into the office with an elevated alkaline phosphatase of 2,908 mg/dL and symptoms of severe low back pain and shortness of breath. His physician notices an elevation of jugular veins, tinnitus, and vertigo. All of the following tests can be used to make the diagnosis of this disorder EXCEPT

    (A) bone scan.

    (B) skull X-ray.

    (C) calcitonin level.

    (D) urinary hydroxyproline excretion.

    (E) CT scan of the spine.

116. All of the following are treatment options for this disease EXCEPT

    (A) biphosphonates.

    (B) surgery.

    (C) calcitonin.

    (D) mithramycin.

    (E) radiation therapy.

Questions 117–119 refer to the following:

A 67-year-old nursing home resident is brought in for evaluation because of severe weight loss, depression, jaundice, and weakness. These symptoms have been going on for approximately three to six months, according to the nursing staff. His appetite has also decreased. On examination by the nursing home physician, this patient is severely jaundiced with cachexia and ascites.

117. All of the following tests can be used to detect pancreatic carcinoma EXCEPT

    (A) CT of the abdomen.

    (B) gallium scan.

    (C) ultrasound of the pancreas.

    (D) endoscopic retrograde cholangiopancreatography (ERCP).

    (E) serum CA19-9.

118. Which one of the following is associated with adenocarcinoma of the pancreas?

    (A) The most common site of cancer is the body and tail of the pancreas.

    (B) Migratory venous thrombophlebitis is associated with pancreatic cancer.

    (C) The Philadelphia chromosome (chromosome 9, 22) is associated with the pathogenesis of pancreatic carcinoma.

    (D) The amylase level is the most frequent enzyme elevated in pancreatic carcinoma.

    (E) Serologic markers for pancreatic cancer, such as the CEA level and the CA19-9 level, are highly sensitive and highly specific for the tumor.

119. This patient has an imaging test and was found to have Stage II disease of pancreatic cancer. Which one of the following treatment options would be best suited for him?

    (A) Surgical resection of the tumor

    (B) Radiation therapy

    (C) Chemotherapy

    (D) Biliary stent placement

    (E) Hormone therapy

120. You would expect to see some or all of the following in your elderly diabetic patients EXCEPT

    (A) hypertension.

    (B) coronary artery disease.

    (C) renal disease.

    (D) visual changes.

    (E) osteosarcoma.

121. Acute idiopathic immune thrombocytopenia

    (A) is the most common cause of thrombocytopenia in children.

    (B) occurs most often in adults after a viral infection.

    (C) is commonly associated with a life-threatening hemorrhage.

    (D) usually lasts for years.

    (E) is treated by bone-marrow transplantation.

For Questions 122-125 choose one lettered answer for each numbered question. Each letter may be used once, more than once, or not at all.

    (A) Honor patient's requests

    (B) Brain death

    (C) Mentally impaired

    (D) Parental permission not needed prior to medical intervention

122. An unresponsive patient with flat-line EEG for 72 hours

123. A 35-year-old patient with an IQ of 50 and a non-life-threatening condition

124. A minor with a life-threatening condition

125. A 72-year-old woman with metastatic cancer and a living will and advanced directives for no heroic measures

For Questions 126-129, match the volumes with the lines from the tracings shown below.

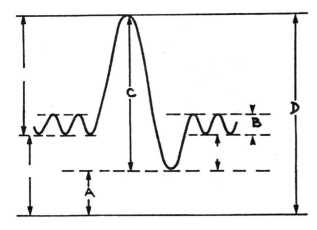

A third-year medical student is doing a clerkship in your office. In preparation for scheduled patients today, all of whom have pulmonary disease, you request that he discuss pulmonary function tests with you. The ventilatory tracing, shown in the figure, displays normal resting ventilation, followed by a typical forced inhalation/exhalation. You ask him to match the volumes, as indicated by the lines, from the tracing.

    (A) Line A

    (B) Line B

    (C) Line C

    (D) Line D

126. Vital capacity

127. Total lung capacity

128. Residual volume

129. Tidal volume

130. A patient is brought to the hospital by the police because he is found in a confused state. He cannot give his name or address and does not know what happened to him. Which one of the following statements is true?

    (A) You must obtain consent from the patient's family before you can do anything.

    (B) You must identify the patient first.

    (C) You must send the police out to find his next-of-kin.

    (D) You can perform any procedure that is medically necessary for the patient's well-being.

    (E) You must wait until the patient can give his consent.

Questions 131-136 refer to the following:

You are consulted to evaluate a patient with a possible deep vein thrombosis.

131. Some of the risk factors for the development of a deep vein thrombosis include all of the following EXCEPT

    (A)   length of surgery.

    (B)   type of surgery.

    (C)   emergent versus elective surgery.

    (D)   type of anesthesia.

    (E)   history of a previous deep vein thrombosis.

132. The most serious problem with a deep vein thrombosis is the development of

    (A)   a pulmonary embolus.

    (B)   a myocardial infarction.

    (C)   an ischemic lower extremity.

    (D)   malignant hyperthermia.

    (E)   a deep artery thrombosis.

133. Ways to prevent a primary deep vein thrombosis (DVT) include all of the following EXCEPT

    (A)   sequential compression devices.

    (B)   compression stockings on the legs and thighs.

    (C)   heparin.

    (D)   low molecular weight heparin.

    (E)   Coumadin.

134. Ways to diagnose a deep vein thrombosis include all off the following EXCEPT

    (A)   clinical examination.

    (B)   ultrasound.

    (C)   venogram.

    (D)   plethysmography.

    (E)   radiograph.

135. You are also asked to treat the thrombosis. All of the following are acceptable means to do so EXCEPT

    (A)   heparin.

    (B)   antithrombotic therapy.

    (C)   surgical interruption of the vena cava.

    (D)   leg physical therapy.

    (E)   Coumadin.

136. Medical treatment for the deep vein thrombosis should last for

    (A)   one month.

    (B)   two months.

    (C)   six months.

    (D)   one year.

    (E)   the rest of the patient's life.

137. A 58-year-old woman has had an uneventful hospital course after an acute myocardial infarction treated successfully with thrombolytic therapy. She asks what her long-term prognosis is. You tell her that

    (A)   long-term mortality is closely associated with ejection fraction.

    (B)   long-term mortality is closely associated with incidence of arrhythmias during the first 48 hours after the myocardial infarction.

    (C)   long-term mortality is closely associated with control of hypertension.

    (D)   long-term mortality is closely associated with her adherence to a low cholesterol diet.

    (E)   there is no information that we have regarding how to predict long-term mortality.

Questions 138 and 139 refer to the following:

You are on call when a 65-year-old woman is brought to the ER by her husband. The patient has a temperature of 103.9°F, sore throat, rhinorrhea, cough, headache, myalgia, and malaise. Physical examination reveals pharyngeal erythema and bilateral rales.

138. What is a usual mode of transmission of this patient's condition?

    (A) Sexual intercourse

    (B) Blood transfusions

    (C) Contaminated food

    (D) Sneezing and coughing

    (E) Oral-fecal route

139. Concerning influenza prophylaxis, which one of the following statements is INCORRECT?

    (A) Influenza vaccine should be administered to all patients in chronic care facilities.

    (B) Amantadine is equally effective in preventing both influenza A and influenza B.

    (C) Influenza vaccine is equally effective in revealing both influenza A and influenza B.

    (D) Vaccinated persons experience less severe symptoms.

    (E) Vaccination produces the best results if administered in early to mid-Fall.

140. You are reviewing the barium enema performed on a 70-year-old male, who was admitted with complaints of left lower abdominal colicky pain. Based on the CT scan of the pelvis and the spot films of the barium enema, both done on the same day and shown below, you

    (A) request an oncology consult.

    (B) discharge the patient.

    (C) request radiotherapy consultation.

    (D) initiate treatment with a cephalosporin and metronidazole.

    (E) initiate treatment with ketoconazole.

Panel A

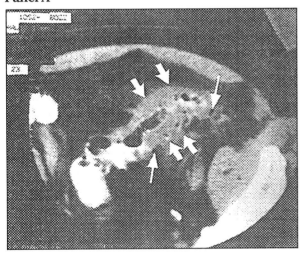

Panel B

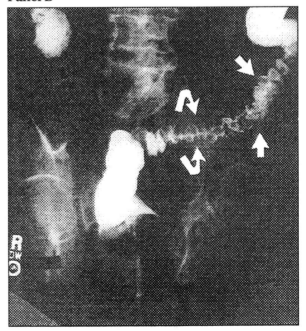

Questions 141-144 refer to the following:

As an expert witness, you are reviewing the clinical record in a malpractice case. The deceased is a 47-year-old male intravenous drug user with AIDS, who presented with complaints of fever, weakness, fatigue, anorexia, nausea, vomiting, weight loss, and abdominal pain. Admission physical examination revealed a temperature of 104°F, pulse of 100, respiration of 20, blood pressure of 80/50. The patient was an ill-appearing male, mildly icteric, with rales in the lung apices, a Gr II/VI systolic ejection murmur at the left sternal border, diffuse abdominal tenderness to palpation, with decreased bowel sounds, guarding, and no rebound. Stool guaiac was negative; there was skin pigmentation but no recent "tracks." One section of a computed tomographic scan of the abdomen is shown in the figure below.

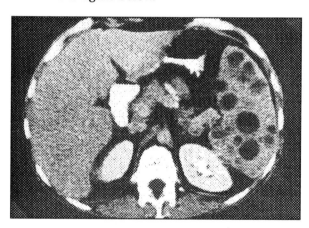

141. You agree with the clinical diagnosis of

    (A) polycystic renal disease.

    (B) perforated peptic ulcer.

    (C) multicentric hepatocellular carcinoma.

    (D) multiple splenic abscesses.

    (E) vertebral osteomyelitis.

142. You review the Ziehl-Neelsen-stained bone marrow biopsy specimen, shown in the figure below. In order to confirm your clinical impression, you search the laboratory results section of the clinical record for a positive culture result of which one of the following organisms?

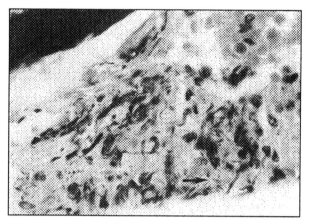

    (A) *Mycobacterium*

    (B) *Staphylococcus*

    (C) *Cryptosporidium*

    (D) *Pneumocystis*

    (E) *Entamoeba*

143. Admission laboratory tests include all of the following results

    Na: 120 mEq/L

    K: 5.9 mEq/dL

    Cl: 87 mEq/dL

    BUN: 30 mg/dL

    Gluc: 60 mg/dL

In an attempt to most parsimoniously explain these results, you search the clinical record for which test result?

    (A) Urinary renin

    (B) Thyroid-stimulating hormone

    (C) Plasma cortisol

    (D) Serum insulin

    (E) Serum vasopressin

144. In reviewing the urine toxicology report, you take all of the following into consideration EXCEPT

   (A) traces of morphine may be present in the urine up to 48 hours following an intravenous injection of heroin.

   (B) traces of heroin may be present in the urine up to 48 hours following an intravenous injection of heroin.

   (C) quinine in the urine may suggest recent opiate abuse, even in the absence of illicit drugs.

   (D) quinine in the urine may result from ingestion of legal substances, such as tonic water.

   (E) cannabis may be detected in the urine for up to one week following smoking.

145. A 23-year-old athlete comes to the emergency room after twisting his ankle. Films are negative and the ankle is swollen yet stable by exam. Appropriate treatment is to

   (A) take to surgery.

   (B) treat conservatively.

   (C) do nothing.

   (D) repeat the X-ray, as it is unlikely there is no fracture.

   (E) allow the patient to "walk it off."

For Questions 146-149, match the following terms with their appropriate scenarios.

   (A) Vicarious liability

   (B) Professional malpractice

   (C) Professional liability

   (D) Intentional tort

   (E) None of the above.

146. A physician omits to obtain consent for an invasive diagnostic procedure.

147. A baby damaged negligently during delivery sues the obstetrician 18 years later.

148. The hospital is held liable if an employee physician commits a negligent act leading to damages.

149. A physician does not accept a patient.

Questions 150-153 refer to the following:

A 60-year-old woman with a history of hypertension presents to your office with an episode of right facial numbness and weakness. This started the night previously and has resolved by the time she comes into your office. She notes no other symptoms. This happened once previously about two months ago. Besides her hypertension, she has no other medical illnesses. She is taking enalapril for her hypertension, but has been non-compliant. She also smokes one pack of cigarettes each day. She denies alcohol or illicit drug use.

150. The most likely diagnosis is

   (A) acute stroke.

   (B) transient ischemic attack.

   (C) panic episode.

   (D) Bell's palsy.

   (E) migraine headache.

151. Pertinent findings on physical examination consistent with the diagnosis would be all EXCEPT

   (A) cholesterol plaques in the fundus.

   (B) carotid bruits.

   (C) diminished carotid upstrokes.

   (D) palmar erythema.

   (E) xanthomas.

152. Appropriate initial treatment includes

   (A) aspirin.

   (B) warfarin.

   (C) lorazepam.

   (D) acetaminophen.

   (E) imitrex.

153. Of the following statements regarding possible surgical treatments for carotid stenosis, which one is correct?

    (A) Asymptomatic patients with a carotid stenosis greater than 70% should be treated with surgery.

    (B) Asymptomatic patients with a carotid stenosis greater than 90% should be treated with surgery.

    (C) Symptomatic patients with a carotid stenosis greater than 70% should be treated with surgery.

    (D) Symptomatic patients with a carotid stenosis greater than 90% should be treated with surgery.

    (E) None of the above are true.

Questions 154 and 155 refer to the following:

A forty-year-old woman whom you have treated for over 20 years comes to your office with complaints of dysuria. A urinalysis is obtained with the presence of RBCs and WBCs.

154. You diagnose

    (A) a vaginal yeast infection.

    (B) a urinary tract infection.

    (C) kidney stones.

    (D) a bladder tumor.

    (E) a coagulopathy.

155. After your diagnosis, you prescribe

    (A) an antifungal medication.

    (B) an antibiotic.

    (C) an intravenous pyelogram.

    (D) a CAT scan.

    (E) bleeding studies.

156. After reviewing the temporal artery biopsy (shown in the figures below) of a 77-year-old female who was admitted for headaches, scalp tenderness, amaurosis fugax, and jaw fatigue after chewing, you begin treatment with

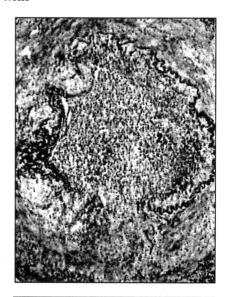

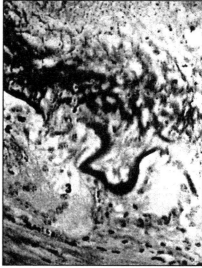

    (A) cyclophosphamide, 2 mg/kg/day.

    (B) cyclophosphamide, 10 mg/kg/day.

    (C) prednisone, 10 mg/day.

    (D) prednisone, 60 mg/day.

    (E) interferon alpha-2b, 3 million units.

157. The Perthes' test is examining for

    (A) competence of the sapheno-femoral complex.

    (B) obstruction of the deep veins.

    (C) deep vein thrombophlebitis.

    (D) A-V fistulas.

    (E) muscle atrophy.

158. Which one of the following statements is in accord with the United States Preventive Services Task Force?

    (A) There is ample evidence to assess the effectiveness of various preventive services.

    (B) Interventions that address lifestyle choices tend to decrease in importance.

    (C) Preventive services should only be rendered during scheduled visits.

    (D) All of the above.

    (E) None of the above.

Questions 159-161 refer to the following:

A 76-year-old English professor presents to the clinic with an unscheduled appointment. He complains of symptoms of urinary frequency, hesitancy, terminal dribbling, and nocturia. These symptoms have been going on for several months, and he is now unable to prepare his lectures for the students at college. He denies any significant past medical history, and his physical exam is normal except for an enlarged prostate gland.

159. A urologic consultation is obtained. All of the following management strategies should be suggested by the consultation service at this point in time EXCEPT

    (A) measurement of voiding pressure and urine flow.

    (B) transrectal biopsy.

    (C) transrectal sonogram.

    (D) prostatic specific antigen.

    (E) digital rectal examination.

160. Two months later, this patient presents to the urologist with complete inability to void and bladder fullness. A Foley catheter is inserted and 2 liters of urine are drained. He is subsequently hospitalized. What would now be the recommended treatment of choice?

    (A) Initiation of alpha-antagonist drugs

    (B) Insertion of a suprapubic catheter

    (C) Placement of nephrostomy tubes bilaterally

    (D) Transurethral resection of the prostate

    (E) Initiation of the drug finasteride

161. The prostatic specific antigen level comes back as 6.0 mg/ml. The transrectal biopsy specimen shows carcinoma in-situ. The alkaline phosphatase level is normal and there is no bone pain. What would be the appropriate management at this time?

    (A) Orchiectomy

    (B) Radiation therapy

    (C) Follow-up prostatic specific antigen level in six months

    (D) Radical prostatectomy

    (E) Luteinizing hormone-releasing hormone agonists

For Questions 162-165, match the condition with the appropriate patient.

    (A) Gonococcal infection

    (B) Herpes simplex

    (C) Papillomavirus

    (D) Syphilis

    (E) Chlamydial infection

162. A 74-year-old male with ataxia and forgetfulness.

163. A sexually active 20-year-old male with acute arthritis of the knee and erythematous papules.

164. A 34-year-old woman with infertility.

165. A 40-year-old woman with cervical cancer.

166. A three-year-old child is brought to the emergency department by his aunt because he has had a high fever for over a week, has had a few seizures in the last day, and the parents have refused to seek medical attention because of their religious preferences. You should

   (A) do nothing without their permission.

   (B) call the police.

   (C) treat the patient without their permission.

   (D) tell the aunt to convince the parents to change their minds

   (E) call the family's minister.

167. Tic douloureux can be diagnosed by the testing of which cranial nerve?

   (A) III

   (B) V

   (C) VII

   (D) IX

   (E) X

168. You suspect acute pancreatitis in a 55-year-old male patient that you have treated on and off for the past 15 years. You would do all of the following EXCEPT

   (A) admit to a hospital.

   (B) send home and schedule a follow-up appointment in one week.

   (C) keep NPO.

   (D) place a nasogastric tube.

   (E) watch amylase levels.

Questions 169-172 refer to the following:

A two-year-old male whom you saw once in the well-baby clinic is brought to the emergency department by his mother at 2 a.m. She states that he has been cranky and fussy all day and that she "finally couldn't take it any more." Your examination of the child reveals a thin, whimpering boy who seems younger than his age and who has several large bruises on his arms and legs. His right ulna has a protrusion that you can palpate on the dorsal surface but is not painful. The mother says he was "born with it."

169. Your working diagnosis is

   (A) child abuse.

   (B) hemophilia.

   (C) hemoglobinopathy.

   (D) malabsorption.

   (E) idiopathic thrombocytopenic purpura.

170. In addition to routine blood tests, you order

   (A) a toxicology screen.

   (B) a bleeding time.

   (C) an abdominal CT.

   (D) radiographs of the right forearm.

   (E) MRI of the brain.

171. The patient's chart has arrived from medical records and shows all of the following EXCEPT

   (A) multiple emergency room visits for episodes similar to this.

   (B) a normal uncomplicated delivery.

   (C) regular pediatric visits for shots, etc.

   (D) radiographs showing fractures in several different bones.

   (E) normal hemoglobin profile.

172. You now decide to

    (A) confront the mother and accuse her of abuse.

    (B) admit the patient for observation.

    (C) obtain a brain MRI.

    (D) make an appointment for a social worker to visit the home.

    (E) call an orthopedist to set the patient's fracture so he can go home.

173. A 47-year-old male presents to your office complaining of severe pounding headaches and occasional palpitations. His main concern, however, is the shortness of breath that he had three hours ago in his workplace where he works as CEO. Physical examination is normal. Blood pressure measures 125/85 mm Hg, and pulse is 72/min. Given the history and risk factors for this patient, you decide to start low-dose aspirin prophylaxis. Your decision is justified because the patient has which one of the following risk factors?

    (A) Age over 40

    (B) Male sex

    (C) Employment in a high-pressure environment

    (D) All of the above.

    (E) Your decision would result in malpractice; the patient's PE is normal and all he needs is reassurance.

Questions 174-180 refer to the following:

You examine a nine-month-old infant. She developed an upper respiratory tract infection three days ago and had a temperature of 37.9°C. Suddenly, this evening, she developed a barky cough and difficulty breathing. PE reveals a child in respiratory distress. You record nasal flaring and intercostal retractions. While she is coughing, you manage to hear breath sounds transmitted from the upper airway. Respiratory rate is 42/min and temperature is 38.6°C.

174. This child is most likely experiencing

    (A) bronchial asthma.

    (B) bacterial pneumonia.

    (C) reinfection of her present condition.

    (D) acute epiglottitis.

    (E) acute laryngotracheobronchitis.

175. The most likely etiology of this child's condition is

    (A) H. influenzae.

    (B) RSV.

    (C) parainfluenza virus.

    (D) adenovirus.

    (E) mixed viral and bacterial flora.

176. Two days later you see this child's five-year-old brother who is brought to the ER in acute respiratory distress. His respiratory rate is 50/min and temperature is 37.7°C. On auscultation the child has bilateral wheezes. He is using the accessory muscles to breathe. The most likely etiologic agent of the child's present condition is

    (A) H. influenzae.

    (B) RSV.

    (C) parainfluenza virus.

    (D) Any two of the above.

    (E) None of the above.

177. Which of the following pulmonary function parameters is going to remain unchanged after bronchodilator administration?

    (A) Total lung capacity

    (B) Maximum expiratory flow

    (C) FEV1/FVC

    (D) Both (B) and (C).

    (E) All of the above.

178. The child is stabilized with IV corticosteroids, a nebulized beta-agonist, and ipratropium bromide. Now you have to choose

a prophylactic agent to prevent further attacks. The prophylactic agent of your choice is

- (A) corticosteroid PO.
- (B) inhaled corticosteroid.
- (C) theophylline PO.
- (D) a nebulized beta-agonist.
- (E) cromolyn.

179. The prophylactic agent of choice in Question 178 has replaced which one of the following medications, used previously?

- (A) Corticosteroid PO
- (B) An inhaled corticosteroid
- (C) Theophylline PO
- (D) A nebulized beta-agonist
- (E) Cromolyn

180. Regarding wheezing in infants and children, which one of the following statements is FALSE?

- (A) Wheezing in infancy and childhood can be caused by conditions other than asthma.
- (B) Asthma and bronchitis are the most common causes of diffuse wheezing.
- (C) Airway obstruction may result in localized wheezing.
- (D) Wheezing may be absent in children with asthma.
- (E) All of the above.

USMLE STEP 3
PRACTICE TEST 3

Day Two – Morning Session

(Answer sheets appear in the back of this book.)

TIME: 3 Hours
180 Questions

DIRECTIONS: Each of the following numbered items or incomplete sentences is followed by an answer or a completion of the statement. Choose the **ONE** choice that **BEST** answers the question or completes the sentence.

For Questions 1-4, match the patient with the most likely diagnosis.

- (A) Pyelonephritis
- (B) Ankylosing spondylitis
- (C) Mechanical back syndrome
- (D) Dissecting aortic aneurysm
- (E) Pancreatitis

1. A 42-year-old male alcoholic with abdominal pain

2. A 33-year-old woman with fever, chills, low-back pain, and vaginal burning

3. A 35-year-old male with low-back pain that hurts most in the morning

4. A 35-year-old male with low-back pain that is worse after being active all day

5. A 30-year-old white woman presents to your office with symptoms of generalized weakness and "not having enough energy" to do the things she could previously do. She is currently taking no medications. She denies any fevers, chills, or easy bruising. On physical examination, she is slightly tachycardiac at 108, and her blood pressure is 130/70. She is afebrile. Her lungs are clear. Her cardiac exam reveals a slightly hyperdynamic precordium with a III/VI systolic ejection murmur. Her abdominal exam reveals no hepatosplenomegaly and is otherwise normal. Her stool exam is hemoccult-negative for blood. Labs reveal a normal white count and a normal platelet count. Her blood chemistries are within normal limits and her ferritin, folate, and B12 levels are pending. Her hematocrit is 25% with an MCV of 68fL. The most likely etiology for this patient's symptoms is

- (A) iron deficiency anemia from menses and poor dietary supplements.
- (B) vitamin B12 deficiency secondary to pernicious anemia.
- (C) acute leukemia.
- (D) sickle cell anemia.
- (E) None of the above.

Questions 6-8 refer to the following:

A 32-year-old male was in a house fire and sustained third-degree burns over 20% of his body, as well as inhalation injury.

6. The most appropriate step to do first is

    (A)   start intravenous antibiotics.

    (B)   intravenous fluid administration.

    (C)   chill the patient's body temperature.

    (D)   administer tetanus prophylaxis.

    (E)   start massive steroids.

7. This patient will most likely have

    (A)   a normal carboxyhemoglobin level.

    (B)   a depressed carboxyhemoglobin level.

    (C)   an elevated carboxyhemoglobin level.

    (D)   an increased urine output.

    (E)   an increased O_2 level.

8. The fastest way to treat the above abnormality is

    (A)   hypobaric oxygen.

    (B)   hyperbaric oxygen.

    (C)   intubation.

    (D)   chest tube.

    (E)   Foley catheterization.

9. All of the following groups of people can participate in clinical trials with appropriate consent EXCEPT

    (A)   men.

    (B)   women.

    (C)   adults.

    (D)   prisoners.

    (E)   the elderly.

10. Regarding epidemiology of cardiovascular diseases, which one of the following statements is true?

    (A)   For each one percent reduction in serum cholesterol, there is an eight percent reduction in the risk of heart disease death.

    (B)   Cigarette smoking accounts for approximately 20% of deaths from cardiovascular diseases.

    (C)   Mean serum cholesterol levels of the population are increasing in the United States.

    (D)   The percentage of hypertensive patients whose blood pressure is under control is approximately 10%.

    (E)   Physical inactivity may be as strong a risk factor for cardiovascular disease as several other risk factors taken together.

For Questions 11-14, match a lettered answer with each numbered question.

    (A)   Honor patient's requests

    (B)   Do necessary procedure

    (C)   Get spouse's approval

    (D)   Get guardian's permission

11. A 10-year-old boy with a severe asthma attack while in the hospital

12. A 14-year-old girl who needs a non-emergent ophthalmologic examination during hospitalization

13. An 82-year-old man with end-stage renal failure and advanced directives stating he does not want to be resuscitated if he arrests

14. A 52-year-old female Jehovah's Witness who is mentally alert and has diverticulosis with bleeding

15. A 35-year-old Indian male comes to the emergency department complaining of left facial weakness and bilateral parotid swelling for the past two days. He also has a

low-grade fever, excessive lacrimation, and inability to swallow. His tuberculin skin test was non-reactive, and he was anergic to mumps skin testing. His chest X-ray shows bilateral hilar adenopathy. How does one determine the definitive diagnosis in this case?

    (A)   CT of the chest

    (B)   Angiotensin-converting enzyme levels

    (C)   Kveim test

    (D)   Gallium scan

    (E)   Mediastinal biopsy

16.   A 26-year-old man comes to the office complaining of swelling under his armpits. On physical examination you note that there are swollen lymph nodes in several locations including the groin, axilla, and the subclavicular area. All of the following conditions may result in these signs and symptoms EXCEPT

    (A)   HIV disease.

    (B)   syphilis.

    (C)   lymphoma.

    (D)   infectious mononucleosis.

    (E)   polycythemia vera.

17.   A 78-year-old white male nursing home resident is visited by his geriatrician. The patient is found to be mildly demented with a masked facial expression, seen with "pill-rolling" tremors, and a shuffling, slow gait. This patient denies any symptoms and is not incontinent. What would be the next best intervention?

    (A)   Brain biopsy

    (B)   Lumbar puncture

    (C)   Thyroid function tests

    (D)   Spinal-cord MRI scan

    (E)   Watchful waiting

18.   A 19-year-old college basketball player was brought in to see the cardiologist after feeling light-headed during basketball try-outs. His pulse was bounding and irregular at that time. An echocardiogram showed asymmetric septal hypertrophy and marked anterior systolic motion of the mitral valve. Physical findings included an increased left ventricular impulse, a bifid carotid pulse, a fourth heart sound, and a systolic murmur which increases in intensity when the patient stands. All of the following should be suggested by the cardiologist EXCEPT

    (A)   the patient's first-degree relatives should undergo a cardiovascular workup.

    (B)   advise the patient not to participate in strenuous sports.

    (C)   calcium-channel blockers such as diltiazem or verapamil.

    (D)   myectomy.

    (E)   diuretics.

19. An unusual case caused by *Ascaris lumbricoides* is presented. Shown below, the worm was evident at upper endoscopy. Case discussion includes all of the following EXCEPT

Panel A

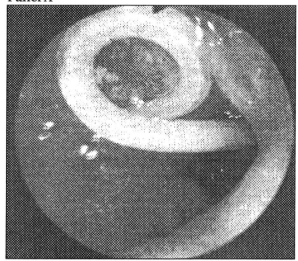

Panel B

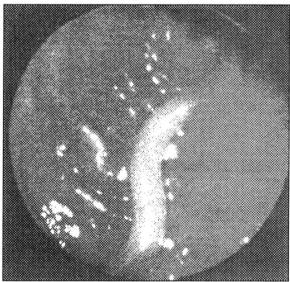

Panel C

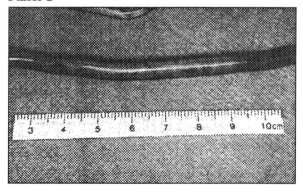

(A) it is unusual to find the worm on upper endoscopy because the worms normally reside in the lower intestine.

(B) intestinal infection is diagnosed by finding oval, thick-shelled ascaris eggs in thick fecal smears.

(C) eosinophilia occurs during the lung phase of larval migration.

(D) chest X-rays may reveal evidence of eosinophilic pneumonitis.

(E) pulmonary ascariasis can be diagnosed by identifying ova in the feces.

20. A 60-year-old female with temporal arteritis returns for follow-up evaluation, complaining of pain in both knees. X-rays of the knees are shown in the figures below and on the following page. You diagnose

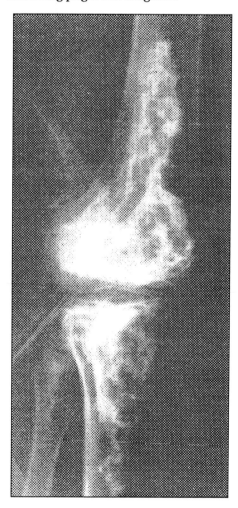

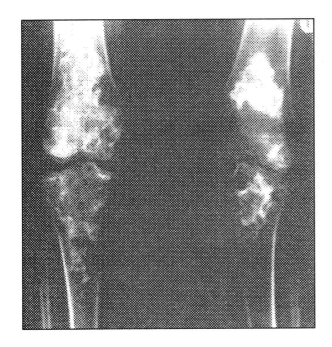

(A) scleroderma.

(B) osteopetrosis.

(C) osteonecrosis.

(D) osteomyelitis.

(E) hyperparathyroidism.

21. Upon examining the joints of an 18-year-old athlete, a grating sound is auscultated whose vibrations may also be palpated. This physical finding is known as

(A) cracking.

(B) emphysema.

(C) articular crepitus.

(D) popping.

(E) creaking.

22. You see your 50-year-old male patient in clinic for follow-up of gout. He had a recent episode of gouty arthritis, which has resolved with colchicine and is currently asymptomatic. His uric acid is 12.5 mg/dL. Which one of the following agents will NOT reduce this patient's uric acid level?

(A) Allopurinol

(B) Probenecid

(C) Thiazide diuretics

(D) Large doses of salicylate

(E) Sulfinpyrazone

23. A 12-year-old boy is bitten by a dog with unknown rabies status. In addition to possible rabies toxoid, appropriate management includes

(A) watertight skin closure of the wound.

(B) thorough irrigation and debridement.

(C) amputation of the involved body part.

(D) treatment of all family members.

(E) observation of the child for two weeks in the intensive care unit.

Questions 24 and 25 refer to the following:

A 41-year-old primigravida pregnant pianist presents to her obstetrician for a routine prenatal visit in her 29th week of gestation. She complains of increased swelling of her feet bilaterally. On examination, her blood pressure is 160/105 mm/Hg. She also has signs of edema, proteinuria, and excessive weight gain.

24. All of the following are appropriate measures that should be undertaken by the obstetrician EXCEPT

(A) start aspirin.

(B) bed rest.

(C) start methyldopa.

(D) start ACE inhibitors.

(E) electively delivering the baby.

25. This patient is hospitalized and kept on strict bed rest. Her urine output is closely monitored as well as her blood pressure and weight. Twelve hours later, the nurse finds the patient in a convulsive seizure and rushes to call the obstetrician. The blood pressure is now 180/115 mm/Hg. What would be the immediate management of choice?

(A) Deliver the baby

(B) Intravenous phenytoin

(C) Intravenous magnesium sulfate

(D) Calcium gluconate

(E) Sodium nitroprusside

Questions 26-29 refer to the following:

An elderly man is brought to the ER by his family. He is comatose and the family does not want anything done. There is no living will and there are no advanced directives. The patient has no known medical illnesses.

26. You listen to the family, examine the patient, review the chart, and

    (A) agree to do nothing.

    (B) send him to a hospice.

    (C) admit him to the ICU.

    (D) tell the family you must try to find the cause of his coma since it may well be reversible.

    (E) treat him empirically with antibiotics.

27. The family argues against doing anything, but you prevail. No one has guardianship of him since he has been perfectly competent until two days ago. Your workup reveals that he is dehydrated and hyperglycemic. He also is acidotic. The family denies any history of diabetes mellitus. You

    (A) do nothing.

    (B) treat him for hyperglycemic coma.

    (C) call a surgeon.

    (D) send him to a hospice.

    (E) accuse the family of neglect.

28. The patient wakes up after appropriate treatment. He recalls being very thirsty, going to the bathroom a lot, and vomiting a few days ago, but does not remember anything since then. He does think he had a flu like illness before these symptoms began. You

    (A) send him home without further treatment.

    (B) tell him his family does not care about him.

    (C) send him to a nursing home.

    (D) further evaluate the etiology of his illness.

    (E) give him an antiemetic to use as needed.

29. Your evaluation reveals that he has diabetes mellitus. He responds well to a relatively low dose of insulin. You

    (A) teach him how to administer insulin and send him home with office follow-ups in a week or two.

    (B) tell the family they have to take care of him.

    (C) send him to a nursing home.

    (D) send him home without treatment.

    (E) send him to a hospice.

30. With respect to cancer epidemiology in the United States, which one of the following statements is FALSE?

    (A) During the last two decades, the overall death rate from all cancers has increased.

    (B) Mass screening for many cancers is promising to dramatically decrease cancer mortality in the near future.

    (C) Lung cancer has become the number one cause of cancer mortality among both men and women.

    (D) At this time, science does not have a clear answer as to the cause of the increase in cancer mortality.

    (E) Certain lifestyle choices have been implicated in the etiology and pathogenesis of some malignancies.

31. A 19-year-old white female presents to the physician's office with complaints of arthralgias, malaise, headaches, pleuritis, and a malar rash on the face. Her urine analysis showed red blood casts. Her lab tests revealed leukopenia. All of the following serologic tests are useful to determine systemic lupus erythematosus as the diagnosis EXCEPT

    (A) antinuclear antibody.

    (B) anti-double stranded DNA antibody.

    (C) false-positive VDRL titer.

    (D) anti-sm antibody.

    (E) antinuclear ribonucleoprotein antibody.

32. Your 76-year-old hypertensive patient returns to the office for her regular physical and the blood pressure is elevated. Your next step is to

    (A) repeat it again.

    (B) increase her medication.

    (C) admit her to the hospital for a 24-hour urine.

    (D) admit her to the telemetry ward.

    (E) admit her to the ICU for IV hypertension control.

Questions 33-36 refer to the following:

You have a 75-year-old female patient that lives on a diet of tea and toast. She comes to your office with pallor and maceration of the mucosa of the mouth.

33. This is known as

    (A) angular stomatitis.

    (B) macrocheilia.

    (C) xerostomia.

    (D) gingivitis.

    (E) periodontitis.

34. This disease will result from a deficiency of which one of the following vitamins?

    (A) Riboflavin

    (B) Niacin

    (C) Pyridoxine

    (D) Cobalamin

    (E) Folic acid

35. All of the following may cause this condition EXCEPT

    (A) liver disease.

    (B) chronic alcoholism.

    (C) chronic diarrhea.

    (D) poor diet.

    (E) lack of vitamin C.

36. Treatment for this consists of

    (A) surgery.

    (B) PO and IM vitamin supplementation.

    (C) total parenteral nutrition.

    (D) nasogastric tube feeding.

    (E) intestinal bypassing.

37. You follow a 30-year-old man with an IQ of 60 who meets the medical criteria for a clinical trial that you are conducting. You explain the study to him and he seems to understand. You

    (A) can enroll him in the study if he agrees.

    (B) can enroll him if his guardian agrees.

    (C) can enroll him only if the IRB has approved the enrollment of mentally impaired individuals with appropriate consent.

    (D) cannot enroll him under any circumstances.

    (E) can use him as a historical control.

Questions 38-41 refer to the following:

A 52-year-old woman is referred to your endocrinology clinic with a suprasternal mass. Match the characteristics of the mass with the disease entity.

 (A) Pulsatile mass

 (B) Non-pulsatile, fluctuant mass

 (C) Non-pulsatile, non-fluctuant mass

 (D) Fatty mass

 (E) Draining mass

38. Innominate artery

39. Dewlap tumor

40. Tuberculous abscess

41. Dermoid cyst

For Questions 42-45, select the tumor marker associated with the disease for each numbered case question.

 (A) Carcinoembryonic antigen

 (B) Prostatic specific antigen

 (C) Alpha-fetoprotein

 (D) Beta2-microglobulin

 (E) Lactic dehydrogenase

42. A 42-year-old male has been followed up in the oncology clinic for several years to monitor the status of his tumor. His serum calcium level is 14 mEq/L, and his rib films reveal lytic lesions. Bone marrow shows plasma cells.

43. A 57-year-old resident of the Veterans Administration Hospital, who has chronic active hepatitis B and cirrhosis, presents with symptoms of weight loss, increasing ascites, and jaundice. A liver sonogram reveals an echogenic mass.

44. A 34-year-old teacher presents with fevers, weight loss, malaise, anorexia, and a non-mobile, non-tender lymph node detected in her axilla and groin.

45. A 78-year-old nursing home resident presents to the clinic with symptoms of urinary tract obstruction, microscopic hematuria, and symptoms of hesitancy voiding.

Questions 46-49 refer to the following:

A 44-year-old woman is referred to you for evaluation of possible hyperthyroidism.

46. You expect to find all of the following signs EXCEPT

 (A) tachycardia.

 (B) goiter.

 (C) moist skin.

 (D) dry skin.

 (E) widened pulse pressure.

47. The eye signs associated with hyperthyroidism include

 (A) lid retraction.

 (B) entropion.

 (C) ectropion.

 (D) blepharitis.

 (E) conjunctivitis.

48. You order laboratory tests including T3 and T4. Which one of the following is true?

 (A) T3 and T4 are normal.

 (B) T3 and T4 are decreased.

 (C) T3 and T4 are increased.

 (D) T3 is increased and T4 is decreased.

 (E) T3 is decreased and T4 is increased.

49. Treatment for this woman includes all of the following EXCEPT

 (A) surgery.

 (B) iodine.

 (C) propylthiouracil.

 (D) methimazole.

 (E) L-thyroxine.

50. Which one of the following conditions has an increased incidence rate with the use of estrogen-containing oral contraceptives?

    (A) Cirrhosis

    (B) Thromboembolism

    (C) Breast cancer

    (D) Cancer of the cervix

    (E) All of the above.

Questions 51 and 52 refer to the following:

A 44-year-old laborer comes to your minor medical clinic with an abscess of his right index finger. The abscess is drained and sent for culture and sensitivity.

51. The most likely organism is

    (A) *Bacteroides.*

    (B) *Streptococcus.*

    (C) *Staphylococcus.*

    (D) *Clostridium.*

    (E) *Herpes.*

52. The most appropriate antibiotic is

    (A) penicillin.

    (B) first-generation cephalosporin.

    (C) second-generation cephalosporin.

    (D) third-generation cephalosporin.

    (E) erythromycin.

53. A 43-year-old male comes to the clinic without an appointment complaining of a whitish penile discharge occurring over the course of seven days after unprotected sexual intercourse. He denies any previous medical history, and he does not complain of any pain. On exam, he is afebrile and there is no evidence of penile warts, vesicles, or rash. What is the next step in making the diagnosis?

    (A) CT scan of the pelvis

    (B) Culture of the penile discharge

    (C) Urine culture

    (D) Prostate exam

    (E) Checking the serum VDRL

54. A patient of yours who just arrived home from a cross-country airline trip complains of a spontaneous, sharp pain radiating to the cervical area with severe dyspnea and cyanosis. You suspect

    (A) angina.

    (B) myocardial infarction.

    (C) pneumothorax.

    (D) fractured rib.

    (E) bronchitis.

For Questions 55-58, match the appropriate type of lung cancer with the appropriate patient presentation.

    (A) Small-cell carcinoma

    (B) Adenocarcinoma

    (C) Squamous cell carcinoma

    (D) Large-cell carcinoma

    (E) Carcinoid tumor

55. A 65-year-old male with a history of tobacco abuse presents with complaints of cough and fatigue. His wife notes that he appears to be more confused as of late. Blood tests reveal a serum Ca of 13.5 and albumin of 2.0.

56. A 70-year-old female with a history of tobacco abuse presents with complaints of weakness in the distal extremities. Physical examination reveals muscle weakness that is maximal with first effort, but improves with repeated tries.

57. A 65-year-old male presents with symptoms of cough and diarrhea. He has no history of tobacco use.

58. A 71-year-old female with a history of 100 pack years of tobacco use is found to have a peripheral lesion on chest X-ray. Biopsy is performed and histopathologic studies reveal gland formation and mucin production.

Questions 59-66 refer to the following:

A 37-year-old woman is scheduled for an outpatient diagnostic pelvic laparoscopy for suspected endometriosis. She has arrived one hour before the scheduled surgery with her 14-year-old daughter and appears to be extremely apprehensive. Her past medical history is significant for long-standing stable asthma that has been successfully controlled with inhaled sympathomimetics and steroids, and also juvenile-onset diabetes mellitus, presently controlled with regular insulin injections.

59. All of the following are advantages of outpatient surgical procedures EXCEPT

  (A) it is cost-effective due in part to a decrease in the number of laboratory tests requested and medical consultations obtained.

  (B) it is cost-effective due in part to a decrease in the number of post-intervention complications.

  (C) the patient returns much more quickly to the familiar home environment.

  (D) the chance of acquiring nosocomial infections is significantly reduced.

  (E) the incidence of medication errors related to either faulty prescribing or dispensing of drugs has decreased.

60. With respect to the candidacy of this patient for outpatient surgical intervention, which one of the following statements is NOT true?

  (A) She is at high risk for developing perioperative complications in contrast to patients with adult-onset diabetes.

  (B) Because of the critical nature of glucose homeostasis, it may be advisable to hospitalize the patient.

  (C) Preoperative assessment for end-organ damage should be an integral part of her surgical treatment.

  (D) It is recommended that she receive insulin along with a continuous infusion of dextrose upon arrival.

  (E) Early-morning scheduling of the surgery is preferable.

61. Patients that can be considered as acceptable candidates for outpatient surgery include all of the following categories EXCEPT

  (A) preterm infants.

  (B) pediatric patients.

  (C) geriatric patients.

  (D) organ transplant recipients.

  (E) cancer patients who receive chemotherapy.

62. Which one of the following is NOT a guideline for safe discharge after same-day surgery?

  (A) Stabilized vital signs

  (B) Orientation to time, place, and person

  (C) Ability to void independently

  (D) Capability of walking independently

  (E) Tolerable nausea

63. Functions of the escort in ambulatory surgery include

  (A) accompanying the patient during transport home.

  (B) being available to summon medical assistance in the event of a medical, surgical, or anesthetic complication.

  (C) receiving and comprehending postoperative instructions.

  (D) Both (A) and (C).

  (E) All of the above.

64. Although the patient had been scheduled to return home after laparoscopy, she is hospitalized. What could be the reason(s) for this sudden change of plans?

    (A) Patient refuses to leave for home.

    (B) Unrelenting nausea or vomiting

    (C) Uncontrollable pain

    (D) Both (B) and (C).

    (E) All of the above.

65. Concerning the role of and indications for aftercare centers for same-day surgery patients, which one of the following is NOT a true statement?

    (A) Aftercare center may be needed for significant postoperative pain that cannot be readily controlled with PO narcotics.

    (B) Some skilled nursing observation or specialized care may be accomplished outside the setting of an acute care hospital at lower cost and with greater comfort for the patient and her family.

    (C) This health-care model is a relatively new category of inpatient postsurgical care.

    (D) It integrates ambulatory surgery with overnight or extended care outside of a hospital.

    (E) If this type of facility is unavailable, arrangements should be made to hospitalize a patient with significant postsurgical complications.

66. Quality assurance and continuous quality improvement for ambulatory surgery can be accomplished by which one of the following means of communication with the discharged patient?

    (A) Follow-up telephone calls

    (B) Sending postage-paid postcards requesting information

    (C) Visiting patient's home

    (D) Both (A) and (B).

    (E) All of the above.

67. A 20-year-old male college student presents to the student health center with complaints of severe, generalized headache, high fever, joint and muscle pain, and excessive diaphoresis. He recently underwent a splenectomy secondary to a motor vehicle accident three weeks ago. This patient took a trip to India one year ago. Lab data reveals a white blood cell count of 14,500 cells/uL with 10% bands and HCT of 43%. Blood cultures were negative, and there were no toxic granulations seen on the peripheral smear. The LDH was normal. The ESR was 70 mm/hr. The blood smear with Giemsa stain showed diffuse red dots in the erythrocytes. What is the most likely diagnosis and management?

    (A) *Streptococcus pneumoniae* abscess in the splenic bed treated with penicillin

    (B) Splenic hematoma diagnosed by CT of the abdomen

    (C) *Plasmodium vivax* infection treated with chloroquine

    (D) Hemolytic anemia treated with blood transfusions

    (E) Lymphoma treated with chemotherapy

68. A 53-year-old asymptomatic female presents for a routine physical check-up. She has a history of two packs of cigarettes a day for 15 years. You should tell her that she is at increased risk of all of the following malignancies EXCEPT

    (A) carcinoma of the breast.

    (B) carcinoma of the liver.

    (C) carcinoma of the pharynx.

    (D) carcinoma of the brain.

    (E) carcinoma of the colon.

69. Cardiac output is dependent on all of the following variables EXCEPT

    (A) vagal stimulation to the heart.

    (B) beta-adrenergic input to the heart.

    (C) systemic vascular resistance.

(D) myocardial-contractility.

(E) ventricular end-diastolic volume.

Questions 70-77 refer to the following:

A 41-year-old man is brought to the emergency department with a fractured femur after falling down the stairs in his backyard. While you are evaluating him, he tells you how angry he is at his wife because she was not at home at the time of his injury. He says that she is having an affair and that he plans to kill her and her boyfriend. You try to calm him down and send off his blood for labs before he goes to surgery to have his fracture set by open reduction and internal fixation. You visit him on the ward to see how he is feeling. He reiterates his intention to kill his wife and her boyfriend and shows you a hunting knife that he has secreted in his boot. He also tells you he has a gun at home.

70. This interaction troubles you. The patient is not expected to be discharged for another two days. You

   (A) call the hospital chaplain to talk to the patient.

   (B) discuss the case with your chief of medicine.

   (C) call a lawyer.

   (D) call a psychiatric consult.

   (E) do nothing.

71. You decide to talk to the patient again because you think he may change his mind with the passage of time. He has not. You

   (A) tell the patient he cannot kill people.

   (B) tell him you will call the police.

   (C) tell him you will get him committed to the psychiatric ward.

   (D) try to suggest alternative solutions.

   (E) do nothing.

72. As the patient's discharge approaches, you feel that you must do something definitive. You do all of the following EXCEPT

   (A) call the patient's wife to warn her.

   (B) call the police.

   (C) notify hospital security.

   (D) nothing.

   (E) urge the patient not to harm anyone.

73. Your obligation in this situation is called

   (A) duty to prevent.

   (B) duty to stop.

   (C) duty to warn.

   (D) abrogation of privacy.

   (E) loss of privacy.

74. This is not considered a breach of doctor-patient confidentiality because

   (A) a person's life is at stake.

   (B) doctor-patient confidentiality is not a physician's obligation.

   (C) a physician has no duty to his patient.

   (D) privacy is not important.

   (E) medical records should be public knowledge.

75. You cannot get this patient committed to a psychiatric ward because

   (A) you would need to convince three psychiatrists to agree to this.

   (B) threats to do harm do not constitute a committable state.

   (C) no one else agrees that he is a threat.

   (D) psychiatrists do not take care of potentially violent people.

   (E) the patient probably won't hurt anyone.

76. Because of your warning, the patient's wife and her friend leave town safely. The police

    (A) arrest the patient.

    (B) observe him for a while.

    (C) warn him not to leave town.

    (D) put him on probation.

    (E) confiscate his gun.

77. The wife could

    (A) have a restraining order placed on the patient.

    (B) get 24-hour police protection indefinitely.

    (C) shoot the man in self-defense even if he does not try to harm her.

    (D) call the police and have him arrested if he does not do anything.

    (E) go into the federal witness protection program.

78. Which one of the following signs is NOT characteristic of cretinism?

    (A) Tall stature

    (B) Thick lips

    (C) Obesity

    (D) Short hands

    (E) Thick fingers

79. With respect to the ethical and legal considerations of discontinuing life support, which one of the following statements is INCORRECT?

    (A) If the patient is conscious, competent, and totally dependent on a mechanical ventilator for survival, the patient can request that the ventilator be discontinued.

    (B) Discontinuing life support in an unconscious, but not brain-dead, patient may be unethical but is medically and legally justified.

    (C) If the patient is going to be served as a donor for heart, lung, or kidney, and the Harvard criteria of brain death are established, the organ(s) may be removed prior to discontinuing the ventilator.

    (D) Before making decisions on discontinuing life support in a terminally ill patient, the court takes into consideration medical testimony, which should indicate that there is no reasonable chance of the patient recovering consciousness.

    (E) When making decisions on discontinuing life support, the family's consent is not required.

80. A 33-year-old male complains of dysuria for the last three days. He has no frequency and no suprapubic pain. He is sexually active. You obtain cultures and treat him presumptively for

    (A) pyelonephritis.

    (B) bladder infection.

    (C) syphilis.

    (D) chlamydia.

    (E) chancroid.

81. A 52-year-old man who has recently moved here from Sweden has an acutely swollen right ankle. He has had painful episodes of diarrhea for several months. He has had some visual pain and blurring recently, too. You consider all of the following to be likely diagnoses EXCEPT

    (A) *Yersinia* enterocolitis.

    (B) Reiter's syndrome.

    (C) chlamydial infection.

    (D) inflammatory bowel disease.

    (E) Behçet's syndrome.

82. A 54-year-old obese diabetic woman comes in because her family has noticed that her right leg is red and swollen. On examination, you find a puncture wound in the sole of the right foot that is draining purulent material. The patient does not know how this occurred. You conclude that

    (A) the patient is not mentally competent.

    (B) she has diabetic peripheral neuropathy.

    (C) she has thrush.

    (D) she is demented.

    (E) someone has been abusing her.

83. A 50-year-old woman comes in with heavy vaginal bleeding associated with some cramping. She says she thought she went through menopause last year. You are most likely to find

    (A) she is pregnant.

    (B) she has uterine cancer.

    (C) she has endometriosis.

    (D) she has fibroids.

    (E) she has a hydatiform mole.

84. A 60-year-old man with diabetes mellitus, hypercholesterolemia, and hypertension presents to your office with three weeks of substernal chest discomfort, especially noted with exertion. He has had a previous stress test that is consistent with ischemia. On physical examination, his blood pressure is 130/70, his heart rate is 90, his respiratory rate is 16, and his temperature is 98.7°F. His lungs are clear and his cardiac examination reveals normal S1 and S2 without murmurs or gallops. He has no peripheral edema. You tell him that all of the following medications have been noted to decrease mortality in patients similar to him EXCEPT

    (A) aspirin.

    (B) metoprolol.

    (C) nitroglycerin.

    (D) nifedipine.

    (E) simvastatin.

For Questions 85-88, match the most INAPPRO-PRIATE choice for a first-line medication for mild hypertension with the symptoms presented.

    (A) ACE inhibitor

    (B) Clonidine

    (C) Beta-blocker

    (D) Calcium-channel blocker

    (E) All of the above would be appropriate.

85. A 38-year-old woman with a history of non-compliance with office visits and diet is noted to have mild hypertension on physical examination. She has no other medical problems.

86. A 30-year-old woman with a history of type I diabetes mellitus that has been very difficult to control is noted to have mild hypertension on physical examination. Her only medical problem is type I diabetes mellitus, for which she takes 70/30 insulin, 48 units in the a.m. and 24 units in the p.m.

87. A 60-year-old man with a history of renal artery stenosis is noted to have mild hypertension on physical examination. He otherwise doesn't have any medical problems.

88. A 48-year-old woman with severe rheumatoid arthritis is noted to have mild hypertension on physical examination. She has no other medical problems other than her rheumatoid arthritis, for which she is taking high doses of NSAIDs.

For Questions 89-92, match the vasculitic syndrome with each numbered case question.

(A) Temporal arteritis

(B) Behçet's disease

(C) Takayasu's disease

(D) Classic polyarteritis nodosa

(E) Churg-Strauss disease

89. A 79-year-old female on the geriatric ward at the University Hospital suddenly complains of right-sided headache associated with weakness, malaise, and weight loss. At times, she has intermittent right-sided visual loss. On exam, she has right scalp tenderness with jaw claudication. The ESR is 100 mm hr.

90. A 21-year-old marathon runner presents to the emergency room because of numbness, tingling, and loss of sensation of the left upper extremity. There was no history of trauma. After being hospitalized for a workup, she suddenly developed a transient ischemic attack. On examination, she had diminished pulses in the right brachial and radial arteries.

91. An 18-year-old male Turkish foreign exchange student is hospitalized for evaluation of fever and weight loss of unknown etiology. He was found to have phlebitis of the lower extremities. Upon further examination, he is found to have painful oral ulcers, uveitis, and genital ulcers.

92. A 42-year-old man is walking his dog outside in the snow and suddenly becomes short of breath. The emergency medical technicians come to the scene and examine him. He is found to have diffuse wheezing on lung exam. He is hospitalized on the rheumatology service in the hospital. On further history, he is allergic to pollen. Lab data reveals an elevated ESR and eosinophilia.

93. Routine urine testing is NOT recommended for

(A) asymptomatic persons with DM.

(B) pregnant women with DM.

(C) asymptomatic adults with childhood history of bacteriuria, hematuria, and proteinuria in the absence of DM.

(D) pregnant women without DM.

(E) a family history of lupus nephritis.

94. A 24-year-old woman presents to your clinic with spotting and cramping pain occurring after her first missed period. You later discovered that the pregnancy occurred outside the endometrium. This is known as a(n)

(A) spontaneous abortion.

(B) threatened abortion.

(C) hyperemesis gravidarum.

(D) preeclampsia.

(E) ectopic pregnancy.

95. A 43-year-old woman with a history of mild osteoarthritis presents to your office with severe right knee pain. She also notes fevers to 103°F, but denies chills or other constitutional symptoms. Her past medical history is significant only for osteoarthritis, for which she occasionally takes acetaminophen. On physical examination, you note that her right knee is swollen compared to the left side and is erythematous and warm. Joint aspiration reveals 90,000 cells, 45,000 of them being nucleated and 90% of them neutrophils. Negatively birefringent crystals are noted. The most likely diagnosis is

(A) gonococcal septic joint.

(B) nongonococcal septic joint.

(C) rheumatoid arthritis.

(D) gout.

(E) pseudogout.

For Questions 96-99, match the most likely diagnosis with each numbered question.

    (A)   Acute myeloid leukemia (AML)

    (B)   Acute lymphocytic leukemia (ALL)

    (C)   Chronic myeloid leukemia (CML)

    (D)   Chronic lymphocytic leukemia (CLL)

    (E)   Hairy cell leukemia

96. A 50-year-old male with fatigue. Physical examination reveals splenomegaly. Blood count reveals WBC of 100,000, HCT of 8.8, and PLT of 900,000. Cytogenetic evaluation reveals a reciprocal translocation of part of the long arm of chromosome 22 to chromosome 9.

97. An 80-year-old male with recurrent infections. Physical exam reveals hepatosplenomegaly and generalized lymphadenopathy. Peripheral and bone marrow smears reveal small, well-differentiated lymphocytes. Type and screen of blood reveals a Coombs-positive hemolytic anemia.

98. A 10-year-old female with symptoms of fever and bruising. Physical examination reveals lymphadenopathy and splenomegaly. Blood count reveals WBC of 88,000, HCT of 9.0, and PLT of 30. Blood smear reveals large primitive cells with prominent nucleoli. Histochemical staining reveals myeloperoxidase negativity, and Auer rods are not present.

99. A 52-year-old female with symptoms of gum bleeding. Physical exam reveals purpuric skin lesions and gingival hemorrhage. Blood smear reveals Auer rods in numerous blast cells.

100. You are a passenger on a transcontinental flight. The crew calls for a physician over the intercom because a passenger is ill. You

    (A)   identify yourself and do whatever is necessary for the patient.

    (B)   do not identify yourself.

    (C)   see the patient but refuse to do anything except tell the pilot to land.

    (D)   hide in the lavatory.

    (E)   should be willing to perform any procedure the patient needs even if you are not comfortable with it.

Questions 101-104 refer to the following:

A 74-year-old male patient with a history of chronic stable angina comes to the clinic complaining of shortness of breath and diaphoresis for the past day. On physical exam, his BP is 90/58, pulse is 140, and respirations are 25. There is no fever. Cardiac exam reveals an irregular rhythm. Pulmonary exam is normal.

101. Which of the following factors is LEAST likely to predispose to the development of atrial fibrillation?

    (A)   Hypothyroidism

    (B)   Pulmonary embolism

    (C)   Pericarditis

    (D)   Ethanol ingestion

    (E)   Hypertension

102. All of the following are medications which have a role in the treatment of atrial fibrillation EXCEPT

    (A)   amiodarone.

    (B)   digitalis.

    (C)   propranolol.

    (D)   quinidine.

    (E)   Bretylium.

103. Which one of the following is an EKG characteristic of multifocal atrial tachycardia?

    (A)   Variable P-P interval

    (B)   Variation in QRS wave morphology

    (C)   Atrial rates of 200

    (D)   Retrograde P-wave

    (E)   Shortened P-R interval

104. Multifocal atrial tachycardia is associated with which one of the following conditions?

    (A)   Pulmonary disease

    (B)   Zollinger-Ellison syndrome

    (C)   Pericarditis

    (D)   Atrial myxoma

    (E)   None of the above.

105. A 50-year-old Japanese man presents with a chief complaint of easy fatiguability for several weeks. He denies any medical illnesses and is not taking any medications. His physical examination is only remarkable for guaiac-positive stool. Esophagogastroduodenoscopy reveals a gastric ulcer, which by biopsy reveals gastric adenocarcinoma. Of the following possible findings on physical examination, which one would give you a clue to the diagnosis?

    (A)   Unilateral testicular enlargement

    (B)   Bilateral inguinal adenopathy

    (C)   Left supraclavicular adenopathy

    (D)   Spider angiomatas

    (E)   Pitting of the nails

106. A 42-year-old executive comes to your office complaining of a "constant stomach pain." All of the following are consistent with a diagnosis of a peptic ulcer EXCEPT

    (A)   epigastric pain.

    (B)   one to four hours postprandial.

    (C)   increasing pain with food.

    (D)   relief with H2 blockers.

    (E)   rhythmic and periodic pain.

107. A 61-year-old woman is admitted for shortness of breath. She has a history of chronic obstructive pulmonary disease, for which she is on corticosteroids and inhaled bronchodilators. She is placed on corticosteroids, inhaled bronchodilators, antibiotics, and supplemental oxygen upon admission. Shortly after she is admitted, she is noted to be somnolent and difficult to arouse. Her arterial blood gas shows a pH of 7.15, a pO_2 of 190, a pCO_2 of 102, and a calculated HCO_3 of 43. The most likely etiology of the patient's decompensation is

    (A)   lactic acidosis.

    (B)   carbon dioxide narcosis.

    (C)   bacterial meningitis.

    (D)   acute stroke.

    (E)   anaphylaxis to the antibiotic.

108. A wife and her husband are in your office and have questions about breast disease. You tell them that the median age for fibrocystic breast disease is

    (A)   13.

    (B)   20.

    (C)   30.

    (D)   40.

    (E)   54.

Questions 109-112 refer to the following:

A 65-year-old man is brought to the emergency room by a family member with complaints of cough and fever. Sputum appears rust-colored. Vital signs are

Temperature: 102°F
Pulse: 110
Blood Pressure: 90/60
Respirations: 30

109. Physical examination is most likely to reveal

    (A)   rales in the right base.

    (B)   bilateral wheezing.

    (C)   crepitus over the anterior clavicle.

    (D)   absent breath sounds and hyperresonance in the left upper lung.

    (E)   normal breath sounds.

110. Sputum Gram stain is most likely to reveal

    (A) Gram-positive cocci in pairs and chains.

    (B) Gram-positive cocci in clusters.

    (C) intracellular Gram-positive bacilli.

    (D) Gram-negative bacilli and cocci.

    (E) acid-fast bacilli.

111. If the pathologic organism was found to be *S. aureus*, this patient should be treated with

    (A) intravenous oxacillin.

    (B) intravenous penicillin.

    (C) intravenous vancomycin.

    (D) oral vancomycin.

    (E) oral first-generation cephalosporin.

112. After three days of therapy, the X-ray is unchanged from admission.

    (A) Sputum should be obtained for cytology.

    (B) The spectrum of antibiotic coverage should be broadened.

    (C) Chest X-ray should be followed on a daily basis for the next three days.

    (D) Consultation should be obtained for open lung biopsy.

    (E) Current management should be continued.

Questions 113-116 refer to the following:

A 28-year-old woman presents to your office with symptoms of fevers, chills, and cough productive of purulent sputum for three days. She has no other medical problems and denies taking any medications. Her physical examination reveals a temperature of 103°F and a respiratory rate of 18. She is tachycardiac at 114 and is normotensive. Her lungs reveal decreased breath sounds at the left base.

113. All of the following are likely organisms causing community-acquired pneumonia in this patient EXCEPT

    (A) *Streptococcus pneumoniae.*

    (B) *Mycoplasma pneumoniae.*

    (C) *Legionella spp.*

    (D) *Haemophilus influenzae.*

    (E) *Chlamydia pneumoniae.*

114. Of the following factors, the one that would most increase the chance of *Haemophilus influenzae* as the etiology would be

    (A) history of smoking.

    (B) history of ethanol intake.

    (C) history of cystic fibrosis.

    (D) history of night sweats.

    (E) history of diabetes mellitus.

115. Appropriate initial antibiotics for outpatient treatment of this patient would be

    (A) cipronoxacin.

    (B) penicillin.

    (C) clarithromycin.

    (D) one dose of intramuscular third-generation cephalosporin.

    (E) vancomycin.

116. Of the following, the true statement regarding chest radiograph findings is

    (A) abnormalities on chest radiograph resolve as clinical symptoms do.

    (B) abnormalities on chest radiograph resolve within a week of initiating antibiotics.

    (C) abnormalities on chest radiograph can resolve up to six weeks after the treatment of pneumonia.

    (D) abnormalities on chest radiograph ten weeks after treatment are likely due to scar of pneumonia.

    (E) None of the above.

Questions 117 and 118 refer to the following:

A three-year-old boy is brought to your office by his mother because of a gradually worsening barking cough over the past three days. On physical exam you note he is sitting up and is tachypneic with significant inspiratory stridor. He also has a low-grade temperature to 100.4°F.

117. All of the following are causes of stridor in a child EXCEPT

   (A)   foreign body aspiration.

   (B)   croup.

   (C)   epiglottis.

   (D)   laryngomalacia.

   (E)   asthma.

118. All of the following are true about croup EXCEPT

   (A)   viral croup is most often caused by infection with parainfluenza or RSV.

   (B)   spasmodic croup may resolve with exposure to humidified air.

   (C)   radiographs of the frontal neck show the classic steeple sign.

   (D)   viral croup is an emergency. No blood work should be drawn until the airway has been visualized and secured.

   (E)   racemic epinephrine is often used in the management of croup.

119. The death rate from which of the following malignancies has increased to the greatest extent over the last 30 years?

   (A)   Colon cancer

   (B)   Kaposi's sarcoma

   (C)   Breast cancer

   (D)   Lung cancer

   (E)   Prostate cancer

120. Diastolic hypertension may be observed with all of the following EXCEPT

   (A)   pheochromocytoma.

   (B)   acromegaly.

   (C)   adrenalcortical hyperfunction.

   (D)   adrenalcortical hypofunction.

   (E)   carcinoid.

121. A complete history and physical examination done yesterday on a previously healthy 20-year-old female was unremarkable. Laboratory results are within normal limits, except the platelet count, which is reported as 44,000/mm^3. After an examination of the patient's peripheral smear, shown here, you discuss all of the following with the patient EXCEPT

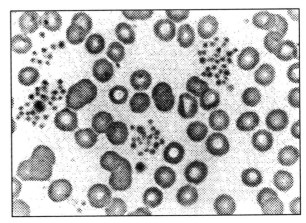

   (A)   the condition is benign.

   (B)   this may occur if the blood is collected in a heparinized tube.

   (C)   the actual in vivo platelet count is normal.

   (D)   in this condition, platelets agglutinate or adhere to leukocytes.

   (E)   the condition is a laboratory artifact.

Questions 122-129 refer to the following:

A 53-year-old woman who comes in once a year for a check-up has missed the last two years but presents now for her examination. She has noticed some weight loss but has attributed it to a diet she has tried. She has some fatigue but thinks she is working harder. On examination she is very thin and has a slightly protuberant abdomen. She weighs 30 pounds less than she did the last time you saw her. Your examination reveals that she has some ascites. She is afebrile. She does not drink alcohol.

122. You decide to

(A) perform a paracentesis.

(B) get an abdominal ultrasound.

(C) order colposcopy.

(D) get a chest radiograph.

(E) give her a diuretic.

123. The patient has not had a menstrual cycle for three years. As a result, you

(A) do a pelvic exam.

(B) do not do a pelvic exam.

(C) order assays of vaginal estrogen.

(D) prescribe a douche.

(E) order a serum HCG.

124. Your testing confirms that the patient has a significant amount of ascites. You perform a paracentesis. It is critical to send some of the fluid for

(A) lactose levels.

(B) LDH.

(C) glucose.

(D) fungal cultures.

(E) cytology.

125. Your pelvic examination is unremarkable. All of the following tests would be useful in this patient EXCEPT

(A) abdominal CT.

(B) chest radiograph.

(C) CBC.

(D) EEG.

(E) electrolytes.

126. The abdominal CT reveals multiple small masses as well as a large mass in the right adnexa. The chest radiograph shows a few small nodules in the lower lung fields. Your working diagnosis is

(A) pancreatic cancer.

(B) miliary tuberculosis.

(C) Meigs' syndrome.

(D) Stein-Leventhal syndrome.

(E) histoplasmosis.

127. This patient should

(A) have immediate emergency surgery.

(B) be referred to a gynecologic oncologist.

(C) be started on high-dose chemotherapy.

(D) be seen by a priest.

(E) be sent to a hospice.

128. The patient asks you about the risk of the same disease developing in her daughters. You tell her

(A) they are at risk but there is nothing to do.

(B) they are at risk and you will have a genetic counselor talk to the family.

(C) they are at no risk.

(D) they probably already have ovarian cancer.

(E) the daughters will be at greater risk than she.

129. Before the patient leaves your office, you

    (A) say good-bye and wish her luck.

    (B) tell her she only needs to see the oncologist.

    (C) give her a follow-up appointment with you.

    (D) tell her to call the gynecologist if she has any questions.

    (E) tell her how long you think she will live.

130. One of your patients is applying for a job with the FBI that requires a security clearance. You receive a telephone call from someone identifying himself as a member of the FBI who asks you for medical information regarding the patient. You

    (A) ask him to send you his credentials.

    (B) tell him you will have to see him in person.

    (C) tell him you cannot discuss the patient with him without the patient's written permission.

    (D) tell him you do not talk to the authorities about patients.

    (E) ask him to submit written questions.

131. A 28-year-old woman presents to the emergency room with feelings of palpitations. She says that she has had four similar episodes to this during the last two years. Her vital signs show that she is tachycardiac to 180 and has a blood pressure of 120/80. Electrocardiogram reveals a regular narrow-complex tachycardia. The most appropriate initial therapy would be

    (A) intravenous adenosine.

    (B) electrical cardioversion.

    (C) intravenous lidocaine.

    (D) intravenous procainamide.

    (E) intravenous amiodarone.

132. Which one of the following vaccines contain live viruses?

    (A) MMR—measles/mumps/rubella

    (B) IPV—inactivated polio vaccine

    (C) Hepatitis B vaccine

    (D) DTP—diptheria/tetanus/ pertussis vaccine

    (E) Hib—hemophilus influenzae type B

133. A pneumoperitoneum presents with

    (A) dull abdomen with absent bowel sounds.

    (B) dull abdomen with hyperactive bowel sounds.

    (C) tympanitic abdomen with absent bowel sounds.

    (D) tympanitic abdomen with hypoactive bowel sounds.

    (E) tympanitic abdomen with hyperactive bowel sounds.

134. A 55-year-old female reports to you that her bowels have recently become tarry. In your workup, you should perform all of the following EXCEPT

    (A) stool hemoccult.

    (B) rectal exam.

    (C) sigmoidoscopy.

    (D) barium enema.

    (E) CAT scan of the abdomen.

135. You are to perform a spinal tap on a 34-year-old male with confusion. You are informing his wife of the possible complications, which include all of the following EXCEPT

    (A) infection.

    (B) headache.

    (C) nerve injury.

    (D) herniation.

    (E) aortic rupture.

136. A 58-year-old man comes in for his annual physical examination. You find that his stool tests positive for blood. He has had no symptoms. You order

    (A) serum iron.

    (B) serum ferritin.

    (C) upper endoscopy.

    (D) sigmoidoscopy.

    (E) colonoscopy.

137. A 33-year-old female with rheumatoid arthritis has been receiving a nonsteroidal anti-inflammatory agent. She comes in for a routine follow-up visit and complains of dyspepsia. Her HGB has dropped from 14 to 12 since her last visit two months earlier. The likeliest cause of these symptoms and findings is

    (A) peptic ulcer disease.

    (B) Barrett's esophagus.

    (C) gastric cancer.

    (D) Crohn's disease.

    (E) Mallory-Weiss tear.

138. A 15-year-old boy was brought into the pediatrician's office because of pain in his left finger. His brother had similar complaints. On examination, there were vesicles and vesiculopustules on an erythematous base present on the third digit. There were no associated fever, chills, headache, or diarrhea. What would be the treatment?

    (A) Steroids

    (B) Antibiotics

    (C) Antifungal cream

    (D) Acyclovir

    (E) Irrigate with saline

Questions 139-146 refer to the following:

A 58-year-old man presents to your office with increasing shortness of breath for three weeks. He denies any fevers, chills, chest pain, or cough. His past medical history includes a recent myocardial infarction three months previously, diabetes mellitus previously treated with oral hypoglycemics, and hypertension. His medications are aspirin, an oral hypoglycemic, and a calcium channel blocker. He denies any alcohol use or smoking.

139. Of the following symptoms by history, which one would be LEAST likely to be consistent with congestive heart failure?

    (A) Lower extremity edema

    (B) Cough productive of yellow sputum

    (C) Dyspnea on ambulation of two blocks

    (D) Orthopnea requiring him to sleep on three pillows

    (E) Complaint of waking up several times a night with shortness of breath

140. Of the patient's medical history and medications, which one is most likely to be causing his symptoms?

    (A) Recent myocardial infarction

    (B) Diabetes mellitus

    (C) Hypertension

    (D) Aspirin

    (E) Calcium channel blocker

141. Of the following physical findings, which one would be LEAST likely to be suggestive of congestive heart failure?

    (A) A third heart sound

    (B) A systolic flow murmur

    (C) Inspiratory rales on ausculation of the lungs

(D) Elevated jugular venous distension

(E) Hepato-jugular reflex

142. The patient's history and physical findings support the diagnosis of congestive heart failure. His vital signs reveal a blood pressure of 160/95, heart rate of 95, respiratory rate of 16, and a temperature of 98.6°F. Appropriate initial testing to confirm your diagnosis and to assist in management include all of the following EXCEPT

(A) two-dimensional echocardiogram.

(B) serum electrolytes and creatinine.

(C) cardiac catheterization.

(D) stress test.

(E) resting electrocardiogram.

143. The studies you order confirm the diagnosis of congestive heart failure, likely secondary to his recent myocardial infarction. The studies reveal an ejection fraction of 25% with segmental wall motion abnormalities. Blood tests reveal a sodium of 131, potassium of 4.4, bicarbonate of 22, and creatinine of 3.8. Urinalysis reveals 1+ albumin and is otherwise normal. All of the following antihypertensive medications have been shown to have additional benefits for a patient like ours EXCEPT

(A) beta-blocker.

(B) ACE inhibitor.

(C) calcium channel blocker.

(D) nitrates.

(E) hydralazine.

144. In this patient, all of the following are benefits of beginning the use of an ACE inhibitor EXCEPT

(A) it slows down the progression of renal disease in diabetics with proteinuria.

(B) it slows down the progression of renal disease secondary to all causes.

(C) it decreases mortality in patients with congestive heart failure.

(D) it decreases mortality in patients after a myocardial infarction.

(E) it has the fewest side effects.

145. You begin an ACE inhibitor for hypertensive control in place of his calcium channel blocker. All of the following are possible side effects of ACE inhibitors EXCEPT

(A) renal failure.

(B) hyperkalemia.

(C) cough.

(D) pruritus.

(E) cholestatic jaundice.

146. In two weeks, your patient comes back for follow-up. His symptoms are markedly improved, and he is able to sleep flat and walk several blocks without getting short of breath. He continues to deny any shortness of breath. His physical examination reveals a blood pressure of 160/95, heart rate of 100, and no signs of congestive heart failure. His serum creatinine is 2.0. Of the following, which one would be most appropriate to begin, in addition to his ACE inhibitor, for further blood pressure control?

(A) Beta-blocker

(B) Calcium channel blocker

(C) Diuretic

(D) Nitrates

(E) Clonidine

147. Histopathologic studies from a periorbital lesion are shown in the figures below. In addition to obtaining an immediate surgical consultation, you

Panel A

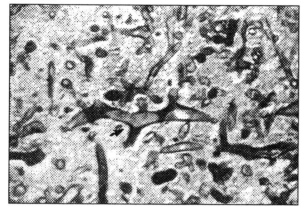

Panel B

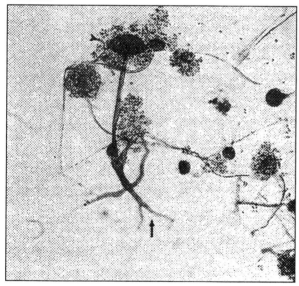

(A)   begin amphotericin.

(B)   begin penicillin and gentamicin.

(C)   begin cephalosporin, metronidazole, and gentamicin.

(D)   begin acyclovir.

(E)   begin cyclophosphamide.

Questions 148-151 refer to the following:

A 72-year-old female presents to your office with a persistent, throbbing headache with tenderness of the arteries of her head. She also has some visual disturbance. You suspect temporal arteritis.

148. Which one of the following is characteristic of temporal arteritis?

(A)   Strictly unilateral

(B)   Lasts only one to three days

(C)   Often associated with polymyalgia rheumatica

(D)   Jaw claudication is infrequent.

(E)   Never lasts more than two years

149. All of the following are physical signs EXCEPT

(A)   the artery involved feels hard and nodular.

(B)   the artery is tender.

(C)   the artery is pulsatile.

(D)   overlying skin is normal.

(E)   there is associated weakness, malaise, and prostration.

150. Which is (are) associated eye findings?

(A)   Impaired vision

(B)   Ophthalmoplegia

(C)   Retinal changes

(D)   Unilateral or bilateral eye involvement

(E)   All of the above.

151. Temporal arteritis is known as a vascular headache. Which one of the following is not in that category?

(A)   Fever headache

(B)   Hypertensive headache

(C)   Cluster headache

(D)   Atypical migraine

(E)   Brain tumor

For Questions 152-155, choose a lettered answer for each numbered question.

    (A)   Competent patient

    (B)   Spouse

    (C)   Legal guardian

    (D)   Physician

152. Able to decide course of medical action in an emergency situation in a minor when no appropriate adults available

153. Able to give permission for nonemergency procedure in a minor

154. Able to give permission for postmortem organ donation in a patient

155. Able to refuse treatment

156. A 35-year-old East Indian male presents to the emergency room with symptoms of high fevers, diarrhea, and anorexia. On exam, he has blanching, macular erythematous spots on the thorax, and a temperature of 104°F. He also has a pulse of 64. His white blood cell count is 5.0. He has just returned from a trip to India. What would be the initial step in management of this patient?

    (A)   Stool cultures for ova and parasites

    (B)   Blood cultures

    (C)   Bone marrow aspirate

    (D)   Look at the peripheral smear

    (E)   Chest X-ray

157. Postexposure prophylaxis should be considered for selected individuals who have a history of exposure to all of the following EXCEPT

    (A)   TB.

    (B)   hepatitis B.

    (C)   meningococcal infection.

    (D)   salmonellosis.

    (E)   Hib.

For Questions 158-161, match the hematologic disorder with each numbered case question.

    (A)   Chronic myelogenous leukemia

    (B)   Essential thrombocythemia

    (C)   Hairy cell leukemia

    (D)   Agnogenic myeloid metaplasia

    (E)   Polycythemia vera

158. A 50-year-old male is playing with his grandchild and suddenly feels left upper quadrant abdominal pain. He visits his primary care physician who discovers an enlarged spleen, severe anemia, monocytopenia, and a positive tartaric acid level. There is no palpable lymphadenopathy.

159. A 58-year-old female feels increasing fatigue over the course of several months and decides to visit her primary care physician for a routine check-up. On examination, she has splenomegaly and weight loss. Her white blood cell count is 100,000 per microliter.

160. A 70-year-old male is found unconscious during a baseball game. He is brought by ambulance to the emergency room and is found to have right-sided hemiplegia. His physical examination reveals right-sided hemiparesis, splenomegaly, and skin plethora. Lab data reveals a hematocrit of 57%, platelet count of 110,000/uL, and an elevated leukocyte alkaline phosphatase.

161. A 48-year-old mechanic is brought into the emergency room by his collagues because he felt a sudden onset of numbness and loss of sensation in his left upper extremity. These symptoms resolved over the course of three hours. He has no other significant past medical history, and he has never been seen by a physician before. His physical examination was normal. Lab results revealed a platelet count of 700,000/uL. Bone marrow biopsy showed normal iron stores and absence of collagen fibrosis.

162. Macroglossia, hypertension, hepatosplenomegaly, edema, and muscle and joint pain may be seen with

    (A) angioneurotic edema.

    (B) hyperthyroidism.

    (C) hypothyroidism.

    (D) amyloidosis.

    (E) Down's syndrome.

163. Screening for diminished visual acuity is recommended for all of the following EXCEPT

    (A) children at age three.

    (B) children before entering school.

    (C) adolescents with IDDM.

    (D) the elderly as a component of their routine physical examination.

    (E) all adults with advancing NIDDM.

164. The presence of rales and hyperresonant percussion is most consistent with a diagnosis of

    (A) closed pneumothorax.

    (B) open pneumothorax.

    (C) emphysema.

    (D) hydropneumothorax.

165. Current indications for tetanus toxoid comprise all of the following EXCEPT

    (A) as a component of DTP in pediatric patients.

    (B) booster injections with ten-year intervals.

    (C) a clean wound in a person who has received his last shot less than ten years ago.

    (D) a dirty wound in a person regardless of his or her immune status and unconfirmed date of last booster.

    (E) a wound in a person with no records of immunization history.

166. A 30-year-old woman is admitted for ethylene glycol ingestion. She is normotensive and afebrile, although she is somewhat somnolent. Appropriate treatments include all of the following EXCEPT

    (A) gastric lavage.

    (B) intravenous ethanol.

    (C) treatment with flumazenil.

    (D) thiamine.

    (E) hemodialysis.

Question 167 refers to the following:

A 50-year-old man presents to the emergency room with days of nausea, vomiting, and abdominal pain. He has not been able to keep anything down and has had emesis of undigested food and bile without blood. He describes the pain as intermittent and crampy. His past medical history is significant for a partial colectomy for diverticulosis. He is not taking any medications. His vital signs reveal a temperature of 101°F, a blood pressure of 130/80, a heart rate of 100, and a respiratory rate of 14. His lungs are clear and his heart exam is without murmurs or gallops. Abdominal exam reveals decreased bowel sounds throughout and significant distension that is tympanitic. Obstructive series reveals multiple dilated loops of small bowel.

167. The most likely etiology for this patient's obstruction is

    (A) hernia.

    (B) cancer.

    (C) adhesions.

    (D) volvulus.

    (E) intussusception.

168. The chest X-ray, shown in the figure below, was obtained to further evaluate the patient. You diagnose

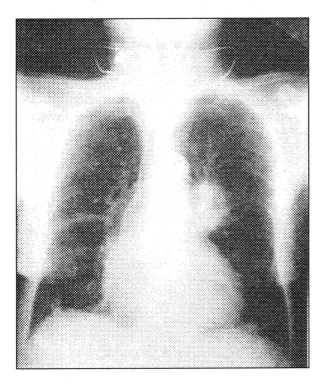

    (A)   primary pulmonary hypertension.

    (B)   sarcoidosis.

    (C)   lung carcinoma.

    (D)   lung abscess.

    (E)   metastatic breast cancer.

Questions 169 and 170 refer to the following:

A 38-year-old female with rheumatoid arthritis comes to the office complaining of cough and shortness of breath.

169. All of the following are pulmonary complications of rheumatoid arthritis EXCEPT

    (A)   small-cell carcinoma.

    (B)   pulmonary nodules.

    (C)   obliterative bronchiolitis.

    (D)   pleural effusion.

    (E)   fibrosing alveolitis.

170. In addition to pulmonary disease, other extra-articular features of rheumatoid arthritis include all of the following EXCEPT

    (A)   vasculitis.

    (B)   episcleritis.

    (C)   splenomegaly.

    (D)   pericarditis.

    (E)   urethral discharge.

171. A 32-year-old female smoker presents to the clinic complaining of moderate pain on the tips of her fingers after exposure to cold weather. On exam, there is blanching of the fingers, followed by cyanosis and then redness: a triphasic color response. This occurred in an air-conditioned office. Which one of the following should be the initial management?

    (A)   Discontinue cigarette smoking

    (B)   Calcium-channel blockers

    (C)   Steroids

    (D)   No treatment available

    (E)   Sympathectomy

172. A complete physical examination in a 28-year-old female patient is normal. However, laboratory evaluation shows IgM against HAV. Which one of the following statements is true regarding your intervention at this time?

    (A)   Refer the patient to an infectionist.

    (B)   Advise her to request a sick leave from her employer and have bed rest.

    (C)   Do nothing at this time, but urge her to call you later for an appointment when she is symptomatic.

    (D)   Consider immunization against HAV.

    (E)   Administer additional tests to exclude other causes of this patient's present condition.

173. A 63-year-old white female presents with a 30-lb. weight loss, bright red blood per rectum, decreased appetite, and weakness. A double contrast lower GI series revealed an "apple-core" lesion in the transverse colon. A CT scan of the abdomen showed metastatic lesions to the liver. Colonoscopy with biopsy showed adenocarcinoma of the colon. This patient was diagnosed with Dukes stage D metastatic colon carcinoma. All of the following are treatments used for metastatic colon cancer EXCEPT

    (A) 5-fluorouracil.

    (B) surgery.

    (C) 5-fluorouricil and levamisole hydrochloride.

    (D) 5-fluorouricil and leucovorin calcium.

    (E) hepatic artery infusion of floxuridine and dexamethasone.

174. A 30-year-old woman presents to your office with symptoms of urinary frequency and dysuria for two days. She denies any fevers, chills, or flank tenderness. On urinalysis, of the following, which is LEAST commonly associated with acute cystitis?

    (A) Leukocyte esterase

    (B) Nitrites

    (C) White blood cells

    (D) Red blood cell casts

    (E) Bacteria

175. A 29-year-old man presents to your office with concerns of esophageal cancer. He tells you that his father and two of his uncles had it, and he will do anything to avoid it. You tell him that he should appropriately avoid all of the following EXCEPT

    (A) alcohol usage.

    (B) smoking.

    (C) gastroesophageal reflux.

    (D) low-fiber diet.

    (E) ingestion of lye.

176. The incidence of male breast carcinoma is closest to

    (A) 1% of that in women.

    (B) 5% of that in women.

    (C) 10% of that in women.

    (D) 25% of that in women.

    (E) 98% of that in women.

177. A 32-year-old female has missed her menstrual period for three consecutive cycles. Her serum pregnancy test was negative. She is otherwise in good health and has no other complaints. What would be the next step in managing this patient?

    (A) Endometrial biopsy

    (B) Colposcopy

    (C) Oral medroxyprogesterone

    (D) Oral estrogen

    (E) Obtaining serum prolactin

178. A 27-year-old female presents with acute chest pain and shortness of breath. She has livedo reticularis on her trunk and lower extremities. She is diagnosed as having a pulmonary embolus and is appropriately treated. Which of the following tests would be most likely to diagnose her underlying disease process?

    (A) Rh typing

    (B) Anti-smooth muscle antibodies

    (C) Anti-phospholipid antibodies

    (D) Anti-mitochondrial antibodies

    (E) Rheumatoid factor

179. Cor pulmonale is associated with

    (A) pulmonary hypertension.

    (B) mitral regurgitation.

    (C) pulmonary hypotension.

    (D) cardiac hypotension.

    (E) None of the above.

180. A 58-year-old woman who is on several medications is noted to have decreasing platelet levels over several days. Of the following medications, all are well known to potentially cause thrombocytopenia EXCEPT

    (A) heparin.

    (B) famotidine.

    (C) gold salts.

    (D) aspirin.

    (E) quinidine.

USMLE STEP 3
PRACTICE TEST 3

Day Two – Afternoon Session

(Answer sheets appear in the back of this book.)

TIME: 3 Hours
180 Questions

DIRECTIONS: Each of the following numbered items or incomplete sentences is followed by an answer or a completion of the statement. Choose the **ONE** choice that **BEST** answers the question or completes the sentence.

---

1. A 30-year-old woman presents to the emergency room in severe distress. She notes intermittent severe right flank pain for the last six hours. She also feels nauseous, although she has not vomited. She describes this pain as the worst pain in her life and colicky in nature. She has no past medical problems. Her vital signs show a temperature of 100°F, a heart rate of 110, a blood pressure of 150/70, and a respiratory rate of 20. Her lungs are clear, and her cardiac exam is without murmurs or gallops. Her abdominal exam reveals normoactive bowel sounds and no tenderness or distension. She localizes the pain to the right costovertebral area, but when you palpate, she doesn't note any exacerbation of the pain. She feels that she just can't get comfortable. Urinalysis reveals >50 RBCs per high-power field. The test of choice to confirm the likely diagnosis is

    (A) CT scan of the abdomen and pelvis.

    (B) urine culture and sensitivity.

    (C) renal artery angiogram.

    (D) lumbar spine films.

    (E) intravenous pyelogram.

Questions 2-7 refer to the following:

A 67-year-old woman comes to your office with a chief complaint of chest pain at rest that resolves quickly.

2. This is known as

    (A) stable angina.

    (B) unstable angina.

    (C) myocardial infarction.

    (D) heart attack.

    (E) None of the above.

3. You work the patient up and the EKG is abnormal and cardiac enzymes are elevated. Your next step is

    (A) discharge to home.

    (B) admit to floor.

    (C) admit to coronary ICU.

    (D) schedule an appointment with a cardiologist.

    (E) start the patient on aspirin and nitroglycerin.

4. The patient gets a further work-up and an echocardiogram is ordered. You expect to see

   (A) a normal echo.

   (B) decreased wall motion.

   (C) increased wall motion.

   (D) no wall motion at all.

   (E) None of the above will be seen.

5. The patient is scheduled for surgery. Before surgery, which one of the following must be obtained?

   (A) CT of the chest

   (B) MRI of the chest

   (C) Cardiac catheterization

   (D) Chest X-ray

   (E) Left ventricular end diastolic pressure readings

6. A successful three-vessel bypass is performed. You inform the patient that the results of surgery should be expected to last for

   (A) one to two years

   (B) three to five years

   (C) five to ten years

   (D) 15-20 years

   (E) life.

7. Prior to discharge from the hospital, it is important to teach the patient all of the following EXCEPT

   (A) exercise.

   (B) diet.

   (C) smoking cessation.

   (D) stress and lifestyle modification.

   (E) avoiding pressure sores.

8. A three-month-old child presents with a temperature of 103.5°F and is tugging at his ears. The most likely diagnosis is

   (A) otitis externa.

   (B) otitis media.

   (C) otitis interna.

   (D) sinusitis.

   (E) meningitis.

9. The return of the bulbocavernosus reflex following spinal cord injury indicates

   (A) the patient should reach a full recovery.

   (B) the patient will not recover.

   (C) the patient is in spinal shock.

   (D) the patient is no longer in spinal shock.

   (E) lower extremity reflexes should return to normal.

For Questions 10-13, select the most likely diagnosis.

   (A) Alcoholic liver disease

   (B) Viral hepatitis

   (C) Cholangiocarcinoma

   (D) Acute cholangitis

   (E) Acute cholecystitis

10. A 60-year-old male presents with right upper quadrant pain for 15 hours. Physical examination reveals scleral icterus and a temperature of 102°F. Liver function tests show SGOT of 147, SGPT of 150, total bilirubin of 4.5, and alkaline phosphatase of 350.

11. A 27-year-old female presents with right upper quadrant discomfort, nausea, fatigue, and muscle ache. Liver function tests show SGOT of 188, SGPT of 277, total bilirubin of 1.0, and alkaline phosphatase of 66.

12. A 68-year-old female presents with weight loss, anorexia, and fatigue. Physical examination reveals jaundice and muscle wasting and spider angiomata. Liver function tests show SGOT of 150, SGPT of 62, total bilirubin of 5.2, and alkaline phosphatase of 88.

13. A 50-year-old male presents with severe epigastric and right upper abdominal pain. On physical examination, temperature is 102°F. Liver function tests show SGOT of 41, SGPT of 36, total bilirubin of 1.0, and alkaline phosphatase of 61.

14. A previously healthy, athletic male was brought in by ambulance because of fever, pain, and erythema in the left forearm, decreased strength in the left forearm, and diminished pulses in that extremity. He also had a decreased sensation and swelling in that arm. Blood cultures grew *Strep. pyogenes*. What would be the immediate intervention needed in this case?

    (A) Surgical fasciotomy

    (B) Clindamycin

    (C) Hyperbaric oxygen chamber

    (D) CT of the head

    (E) Thrombolytic agents

15. A 50-year-old man presents to the emergency room with three episodes of bright red blood per rectum. His past medical history is significant for hypertension, diabetes mellitus, and an abdominal aortic aneurysm repair four years previously. His vital signs reveal that he is tachycardiac to 120, and his blood pressure is 140/80, but he is orthostatic. His abdominal exam reveals decreased bowel sounds throughout and diffuse mild abdominal tenderness. His rectal examination reveals bright red blood. The most appropriate initial intervention is

    (A) abdominal CT to rule out diverticulosis.

    (B) tagged red cell scan to assess the site of bleeding.

    (C) colonoscopy to visualize the source of bleeding.

    (D) immediate laparotomy to rule out aorto-enteric fistula.

    (E) admission and observation for 24 hours.

16. A 42-year-old homeless, demented male is brought into the emergency room by ambulance after he was found lying down in the street. The patient stated he drank a quart of antifreeze and he felt light-headed. Lab data revealed a BUN of 110 mg/dL and a creatinine level of 9.0 mg/dL. There were oxalate crystals found in his urine. What would be the next step in management of this patient?

    (A) Hemoperfusion

    (B) Dialysis

    (C) Activated charcoal

    (D) Gastric lavage

    (E) Forced alkaline diuresis

Questions 17-24 refer to the following:

A 57-year-old obese man comes to your office with a complaint of excessive daytime sleepiness. You suspect a diagnosis of obstructive sleep apnea (OSA).

17. Which one of the following is NOT a symptom commonly associated with OSA?

    (A) Snoring

    (B) Cataplexy

    (C) Poor sleep quality

    (D) Intellectual deterioration

    (E) Personality changes

18. Which one of the following is another condition associated with excessive daytime sleepiness?

    (A) Nocturnal myoclonus

    (B) Schizophrenia

    (C) Somnambulism

    (D) Sleep terrors

    (E) None of the above.

19. Further history from the patient and his wife supports your diagnosis of OSA. Which one of the following is NOT a pathophysiological surgical mechanism related to the development of OSA?

    (A) Increased upper airway muscle activity

    (B) Structural compromise of airway patency

    (C) High airway compliance

    (D) High nasal resistance

    (E) Increased subatmospheric pressure generated in the pharynx during inspiration

20. You decide to further investigate this patient's symptoms with the definitive diagnostic test for OSA. Which one of the following is the definitive test for the diagnosis of OSA?

    (A) Holter monitoring

    (B) Electroencephalography

    (C) Polysomnography

    (D) Pharyngeal nerve conduction studies

    (E) None of the above.

21. Which one the following is a diagnostic finding in the evaluation of OSA?

    (A) Episodes of airflow cessation that are not accompanied by respiratory effort

    (B) Falls in oxygen saturation during apneic episodes

    (C) Direct wake-to-REM sleep transitions

    (D) Seizure activity during non-REM sleep

    (E) None of the above.

22. Which one of the following is NOT indicated as a first-line therapy in patients with OSA?

    (A) Weight reduction

    (B) Avoidance of alcohol

    (C) Nasal CPAP

    (D) Tracheostomy

    (E) Uvulopalatopharyngoplasty

23. The patient is lost to your follow-up. However, he returns several years later with several new medical problems, including systemic hypertension, right-sided heart failure, dysrhythmias, chronic hypoxemia, and anemia. Which one of the patient's medical problems is LEAST likely to be related to his untreated OSA?

    (A) Systemic hypertension

    (B) Right-sided heart failure

    (C) Dysrhythmias

    (D) Chronic hypoxemia

    (E) Anemia

24. You discuss with the patient his increased risk of sudden death during sleep if he continues to avoid treatment for his OSA. Which one of the following is thought to be the most likely mechanism of nocturnal sudden death in patients with OSA?

    (A) Myocardial infarction

    (B) Pulmonary embolus

    (C) Stroke

    (D) Pneumothorax

    (E) None of the above.

25. The bleeding of dysentery is due to

    (A) ulcerative erosions into arterial feed vessels.

    (B) colonic mucosal invasion of the pathogen.

    (C) a systemic coagulopathy.

    (D) thrombosis of submucosal capillaries.

    (E) bowel necrosis.

26. A 65-year-old postmenopausal white female presents to the emergency room after having fallen in her apartment and injuring her right hip. X-rays revealed a right trochanter

fracture, and the orthopedic surgeons performed an open reduction and internal fixation of the hip. Dual-photon imaging studies revealed that the patient had a very low bone-mineral density suggestive of osteoporosis. To prevent future fractures, her primary physician can suggest all of the following EXCEPT

- (A) alendronate.
- (B) adequate lighting at home.
- (C) plain sodium fluoride.
- (D) transdermal estrogen patch.
- (E) salmon calcitonin nasal spray.

27. Which one of the following is a feature of Plummer-Vinson syndrome?

- (A) Moist oral membranes
- (B) Dysphagia
- (C) Hypertension
- (D) Osteoporosis
- (E) Hypercholesteremia

28. A 49-year-old female comes to the emergency room complaining of severe pain in the left knee. Physical exam reveals reduced range of motion and a large effusion. Synovial fluid analysis is as follows: yellow fluid, 120,000 WBC with 80% polymorphonuclear cells; glucose: 50 (blood glucose of 130). Which one of the following diagnoses is most consistent with this synovial fluid analysis?

- (A) *S. aureus* infection in the knee
- (B) Rheumatoid arthritis
- (C) Factor negative spondylo-arthropathy
- (D) Traumatic injury to the knee
- (E) None of the above.

29. A 45-year-old archeologist visits his primary care physician for advice. He is traveling to several remote areas in the world such as India, Panama, and Africa and he wants to know what health precautions to take when such travel is undertaken. All of the follow-

ing should be the advice given by the physician EXCEPT

- (A) three days of cipronoxacin and loperamide for traveler's diarrhea.
- (B) avoid unboiled water, raw vegetables, and seafood.
- (C) cover exposed skin with a long-sleeved shirt and long pants.
- (D) travelers should take blood with them in case of an overseas emergency.
- (E) use bottled carbonated beverages whenever possible.

30. A 16-year-old woman comes to the ER complaining of vaginal discharge. You obtain culture proof of gonorrhea. You must

- (A) tell her parents.
- (B) report the case to the Board of Health.
- (C) tell her boyfriend.
- (D) identify and trace all her contacts.
- (E) not tell anyone.

Questions 31-34 refer to the following:

A 58-year-old male comes to your office with a 15-pound weight loss and complains of having difficulty swallowing.

31. Questions you should ask during your history include all of the following EXCEPT

- (A) "Is swallowing painful or painless?"
- (B) "Has the weight loss been intentional?"
- (C) "Do you smoke or drink?"
- (D) "Does the difficulty occur with solids or liquids?"
- (E) "Do you have any difficulty tasting foods?"

32. Difficulty in swallowing is known as

    (A) odynophagia.

    (B) dysphagia.

    (C) regurgitation.

    (D) obstruction.

    (E) emesis.

33. The patient states that swallowing is painful and points to the neck where the pain localizes. The pain, therefore, originates from the

    (A) nasopharynx.

    (B) oropharynx.

    (C) esophagus.

    (D) stomach.

    (E) duodenum.

34. Possible diagnoses for the above include all of the following EXCEPT

    (A) tonsillitis.

    (B) angioneurotic edema.

    (C) carcinoma.

    (D) esophagitis.

    (E) pharyngitis.

35. A 25-year-old male whom you have seen once a year for eczema walks into your clinic with a hacking cough and weight loss. All of the following are pertinent to your history at this point EXCEPT

    (A) questions regarding sexual preferences.

    (B) questions regarding sexual activities.

    (C) questions regarding intravenous drug use.

    (D) family history.

    (E) questions regarding bleeding disorders.

36. A 32-year-old male presents to the doctor's office with complaints of persistent low back pain for the last six months, which is worse in the morning and gradually improves after

activity. The physical examination is normal except for decreased flexion of the lumbar spine. The HLA-B27 test is positive. Which one of the following tests will also assist us in arriving at the correct diagnosis and subsequent management?

    (A) Plain X-rays of the sacroiliac joint

    (B) Serum rheumatoid

    (C) Arthrocentesis of the first metatarsophalangeal joint

    (D) Spinal films

    (E) Straight-leg testing

37. A 33-year-old male presents for a periodic health examination. He is planning on traveling to Mexico. Physical examination is unremarkable. He requests prophylaxis against diarrhea, which his friend had had two years ago after returning from Mexico. What is your proper mode of action?

    (A) Given the obvious risk of developing traveler's diarrhea, you should immediately administer Ciprofloxin.

    (B) Given the obvious risk of developing traveler's diarrhea, you should try to have the patient change his mind.

    (C) Explain to the patient the importance of personal hygiene and recommend that he eat only properly cooked food.

    (D) Prescribe one of the quinoline derivatives and recommend that the patient use it as symptoms begin to develop.

    (E) Do nothing at this time; wait for your patient's next visit after he returns from his trip to Mexico.

For Questions 38-41, match each of the following numbered conditions with the correct answer.

    (A) Sepsis

    (B) Somogyi

(C) Lupus flare

(D) Drug reaction

38. A 47-year-old man hospitalized for hyperglycemia who has now developed morning hypoglycemia on inpatient insulin regimen

39. A 25-year-old primigravida who has phenomenon polyarthralgias, pleurisy, rising creatinine, and has just delivered a baby

40. A 63-year-old woman receiving antibiotics for pneumonia who develops truncal rash

41. A 73-year-old man with pneumonia who develops spiking fever and confusion

Questions 42-45 refer to the following:

An 18-year-old male with known sickle cell anemia comes to the emergency room with acute abdominal pain. He was last seen in the ER a month earlier with severe left humerus pain.

42. All of the following should be initiated immediately EXCEPT

(A) intravenous hydration.

(B) abdominal radiograph.

(C) IVP.

(D) oxygen.

(E) surgical consult.

43. The KUB shows some distended loops of bowel, but no air-fluid levels. The surgical resident does not think this patient has a surgical abdomen. The patient is feeling a little better. The likeliest diagnosis is

(A) acute appendicitis.

(B) diverticulitis.

(C) ruptured viscus.

(D) malingering.

(E) sickle crisis.

44. All of the following laboratory abnormalities would be expected in this patient EXCEPT

(A) hypomagnesemia.

(B) sickled cells on peripheral smear.

(C) elevated amylase.

(D) leukocytosis.

(E) elevated BUN.

45. Which one of the following statements is true?

(A) This patient's next crisis will probably be abdominal.

(B) This patient's next crisis cannot be predicted.

(C) The next crisis will occur in another month.

(D) All of the patient's siblings probably have sickle cell anemia.

(E) The patient's next crisis will be aplastic.

46. Which one of the following is associated with increased lead absorption from the gastrointestinal tract?

(A) Anorexia nervosa

(B) Iron deficiency

(C) Hypercalcemia

(D) Measles

(E) Ulcerative colitis

47. A 44-year-old man is on your service after a mitral valve replacement for rheumatic heart disease. He has been receiving heparin postoperatively, but is now being switched to Coumadin prior to discharge. Which is the best test to use to monitor his Coumadinization?

(A) Bleeding time

(B) Activated partial thromboplastin time

(C) Partial thromboplastin time

(D) Prothrombin time

(E) Platelet count

For Questions 48-51, match each of the numbered conditions with one of the following answers.

    (A)   Pregnancy

    (B)   Pulmonary embolus

    (C)   Cellulitis

    (D)   Acute bronchitis

48.   A 33-year-old woman taking birth control pills who develops acute shortness of breath and pleuritic chest pain

49.   A 45-year-old man with diabetes and large area of erythema and warmth on his right leg

50.   A 52-year-old male with COPD who smokes cigarettes and develops acute productive cough

51.   A 27-year-old woman with well controlled lupus who has not had a menstrual period for eight weeks

Questions 52-55 refer to the following:

A 44-year-old male is brought to the ER because of severe agitation, confusion, and tremulousness. He is disheveled and has a faint odor of alcohol about him. He has a low-grade fever, tachycardia, mild tachypnea, and mild leukocytosis.

52.   All of the following must be included in the differential diagnosis at this point EXCEPT

    (A)   alcohol withdrawal.

    (B)   pneumonia.

    (C)   sepsis.

    (D)   Wernicke-Korsakoff syndrome.

    (E)   meningitis.

53.   The patient's radiograph is normal. Blood cultures are obtained and an LP is attempted, but cannot be successfully completed because of the patient's increasing combativeness. You decide to

    (A)   send him home because of lack of cooperation.

    (B)   sedate him with ativan.

    (C)   give him morphine.

    (D)   give him general anesthesia.

    (E)   put him in restraints and wait for him to calm down.

54.   Once the patient is calmed down, you perform an LP and send the fluid for culture. The patient's family arrives and tells you he has a long history of binge consumption of alcohol and has been drinking vodka and beer for the last week. You decide to

    (A)   admit him to the hospital.

    (B)   send him home with his family.

    (C)   send him to a detoxification unit.

    (D)   talk to him about joining Alcoholics Anonymous.

    (E)   call a priest.

55.   The patient subsequently develops hallucinations and seizures. This patient's condition is

    (A)   benign.

    (B)   self-limited even without treatment.

    (C)   potentially life-threatening.

    (D)   always fatal.

    (E)   usually hereditary.

56.   A 66-year-old man with steroid-dependent asthma comes in with blurred vision. He has had no headaches or neurological complaints. His general physical exam is normal except that you cannot visualize his fundi. The likeliest cause of his visual complaints is

    (A)   chlamydial infection.

    (B)   iritis.

    (C)   conjunctivitis.

    (D)   presbyopia.

    (E)   cataracts.

57. A 55-year-old woman with a history of asthma had a cholecystectomy yesterday. Today she has fever, chills, a productive cough, and a right upper lobe infiltrate on chest radiograph. Your assessment and plans are

    (A) she is having an asthma attack and needs theophylline.

    (B) she has pneumonia and needs antibiotics.

    (C) she has a pulmonary neoplasm.

    (D) she has tuberculosis and needs treatment.

    (E) she has a viral infection that can be treated symptomatically.

Questions 58-60 refer to the following:

A 72-year-old woman is going to be transferred to a nursing home for rehabilitation after a stroke. Her routine pre-transfer PPD is positive. No one knows if she has ever had a PPD before.

58. The first thing you do is

    (A) begin isoniazid.

    (B) call for an infectious disease consult.

    (C) call the health department.

    (D) get a sputum for culture.

    (E) get a chest radiograph.

59. A chest radiograph is obtained and is unremarkable except for a small calcification in the left upper lobe. You

    (A) give the patient isoniazid.

    (B) obtain sputum samples for culture.

    (C) order a chest CT.

    (D) write transfer orders.

    (E) discharge the patient to home.

60. While waiting for the results of sputum cultures, you

    (A) begin the patient on isoniazid.

    (B) put the patient in isolation.

    (C) send the patient home.

    (D) explain the situation to the family.

    (E) call the health department.

Questions 61-64 refer to the following:

A 50-year-old woman comes to the clinic because of recent onset of headaches, joint and muscle pain, and an episodic rash. She and her family went camping in Minnesota a few months ago and she has been feeling tired ever since. The rest of her family is healthy. She has had no other medical problems.

61. On physical exam you see no rash, but you do find a small raised reddish lesion on the patient's right thigh. You suspect

    (A) drug abuse.

    (B) Munchausen syndrome with self-injection.

    (C) allergic reaction.

    (D) insect bite of some sort.

    (E) a splinter.

62. You should ask the patient and her family all of the following questions EXCEPT

    (A) Was she bitten by a tick?

    (B) What does the rash look like?

    (C) Has she ever had anything like this before?

    (D) When was her last PPD?

    (E) Has she had any swollen joints?

63. The patient remembers pulling a tick from her thigh. Her husband says the rash comes and goes and is reddish. Your working diagnosis now is

    (A) rheumatoid arthritis.

    (B) sporotrichosis.

(C) trichinosis.

(D) histoplasmosis.

(E) Lyme disease.

64. The treatment of choice is

(A) tetracycline.

(B) amphotericin.

(C) fluconazole.

(D) Flagyl.

(E) trimethoprim-sulfa.

Questions 65-71 refer to the following:

A 55-year-old woman comes to see you because of a cough productive of yellow sputum for about two weeks. She has a 90-pack-year history of cigarette smoking. She has had similar episodes in the past, which have been successfully treated with antibiotics. However, her family physician gave her a prescription for trimethoprim-sulfa about ten days ago and she is no better. On physical exam, she has diffuse rhonchi and some rales over her right posterior thorax. She has a low-grade fever and looks very tired. The patient would like you to give her a different antibiotic and let her go home.

65. A chest radiograph is obtained. It shows a 10-cm perihilar mass extending into the right upper lobe. You

(A) send the patient to a surgeon.

(B) admit her for antibiotic therapy.

(C) tell her the radiograph is not normal and needs to be evaluated further.

(D) give her oral antibiotics and send her home without saying anything about the radiograph.

(E) call her family physician and tell him to tell her about the radiograph.

66. You now do all of the following EXCEPT

(A) schedule a CT scan of the chest.

(B) call to arrange for a biopsy.

(C) give the patient a prescription for a different antibiotic.

(D) admit the patient to the ICU.

(E) explain to the patient and her husband what you are arranging.

67. A CT scan is done three days later and not only confirms the radiographic findings but also shows enlargement of regional lymph nodes and some pleural thickening. The patient is feeling somewhat better on the antibiotic and is afebrile. The most important thing to do now is

(A) obtain tissue for histology.

(B) remove the mass.

(C) prepare the patient for her likely death.

(D) admit her to a hospice.

(E) get her home oxygen.

68. The cytopathologist is able to perform a needle biopsy with CT guidance. Which one of the following is most likely to be related to the tissue diagnosis?

(A) The patient's family history

(B) The fact that the patient's husband worked in a coal mine years ago

(C) The patient's cigarette consumption

(D) The patient's menopausal status

(E) The patient's weight

69. The histology reveals a non-small-cell cancer that appears to be primary to the lung. You discuss the patient with the oncologists and find that the best you can offer her is

(A) high-dose chemotherapy.

(B) a bone marrow transplant.

(C) oxygen.

(D) morphine.

(E) palliative radiotherapy.

70. You feel that you must discuss the prognosis with the patient and her family. You tell them

    (A) she will probably die in six weeks.

    (B) a new therapeutic regimen could be "around the corner."

    (C) she could live for as much as a year or two.

    (D) no one can tell how long she will live but you will do everything to keep her comfortable.

    (E) she should try a course of high-dose vitamin therapy.

71. All of the following are appropriate EXCEPT

    (A) you give the patient a prescription for a strong pain medicine.

    (B) you give her a prescription for antibiotics to take if the cough recurs.

    (C) you tell her to go back to her family physician and not come to see you again since you can offer her nothing.

    (D) you make her an appointment to see the radiation oncologist.

    (E) you answer her questions about "alternate" therapies to the best of your ability.

72. A nine-year-old boy is brought to your office because of severe headaches and vomiting. He has had these symptoms for a week or two. He is afebrile. His mother volunteers that he has been more irritable and argumentative than usual in the last few months. She had attributed it to a "growth spurt." You tell her that

    (A) there is nothing to worry about; this is a phase that will pass.

    (B) it is necessary to obtain a CT scan of the head.

    (C) you have to do a lumbar puncture right away.

    (D) you will refer the child to a psychiatrist.

    (E) you will call in a surgeon to evaluate his stomach.

Questions 73-76 refer to the following:

A three-year-old girl has been admitted because of wheezing and cough. She apparently had several similar episodes in the past, all managed in the emergency department. This episode has been associated with mild hypoxia and lack of response to nebulizers and, thus, resulted in admission.

73. The likeliest diagnosis is

    (A) pneumonia.

    (B) asthma.

    (C) bronchitis.

    (D) obliterative alveolitis.

    (E) tuberculosis.

74. Appropriate management of this condition may include all of the following EXCEPT

    (A) aminophylline.

    (B) oxygen.

    (C) epinephrine.

    (D) beta-blockers.

    (E) steroids.

75. Appropriate evaluation of a child with asthma may include all of the following EXCEPT

    (A) allergy tests.

    (B) pulmonary function tests.

    (C) lung scan.

    (D) chest radiograph.

    (E) arterial blood gases.

76. The long-term prognosis for young children with asthma is

    (A) development of early COPD.

    (B) good.

    (C) Goodpasture's syndrome.

(D) transfusion dependence.

(E) necrotizing bronchiolitis.

77. A 45-year-old woman with steroid-dependent asthma comes to see you because she had a PPD during her job physical and it was negative. The plant nurse assured her not to worry and told her she did not need a chest radiograph. She is concerned because she has known people who had tuberculosis. You

(A) reassure her.

(B) place another PPD.

(C) obtain a chest radiograph.

(D) treat her with INH empirically.

(E) tell her to get plenty of rest.

78. A 14-year-old boy slipped this morning at home as he was getting ready to go to school. He braced his fall with his hands. His mother brings him to your clinic because his right forearm is painful and slightly swollen. After examining the patient, the first thing you do is

(A) call an ambulance.

(B) send the patient for a radiograph of his arm.

(C) prescribe a splint for his arm.

(D) give him an analgesic and send him home.

(E) tell him not to worry and send him home.

For Questions 79-82, match the numbered condition with the best answer.

(A) Hemorrhoids

(B) Peptic ulcer

(C) Varices

(D) Mallory-Weiss tear

79. Acute hematemesis

80. Hematemesis after prolonged retching

81. Blood streaking on toilet paper

82. Melena

83. A 36-year-old woman who is in her 14th week of pregnancy comes in with severe abdominal cramps and some bloody discharge. The likeliest diagnosis is

(A) renal colic.

(B) miscarriage.

(C) ulcerative colitis.

(D) pyelonephritis.

(E) irritable colon.

84. A 50-year-old man is brought in by the paramedics because of chest discomfort and a rapid pulse. He is conscious, although uncomfortable, and has a normal blood pressure. His ECG shows ventricular tachycardia with a rate of 140. You should

(A) electrically cardiovert him.

(B) call Anesthesia to intubate him.

(C) begin digoxin.

(D) start an antiarrhythmic.

(E) order an angiogram.

Questions 85-88 refer to the following:

A 33-year-old man was admitted to your service the previous evening for severe abdominal pain and mild hematemesis. He was described as alert and oriented and cooperative. On morning rounds today he is clearly confused and combative. The nurses on duty during the night have restrained him because he pulled out two intravenous lines.

85. You ask for the results of several tests that you had ordered. Which one of the following tests do you expect will be abnormal?

(A) Serum alcohol level

(B) Serum lead level

(C) Urinalysis

(D) ECG

(E) Serum ferritin

86. All of the following tests come back abnormal EXCEPT

(A) serum amylase.

(B)   stool hemoccult.

(C)   serum lipase.

(D)   fibrin split products.

(E)   albumin.

87.   You decide to

(A)   send the patient home so he can resume drinking and get over his withdrawal symptoms.

(B)   send him to surgery for pancreatic resection.

(C)   treat him with ativan and hydration.

(D)   send him home with a daily visit from home health care.

(E)   transfer him to the ICU.

88.   All of the following statements regarding this patient's condition are true EXCEPT

(A)   it can cause death.

(B)   it can result in pneumonia.

(C)   it can be associated with seizures.

(D)   it is benign.

(E)   it is treatable.

89.   All of the following can be complications of otitis media EXCEPT

(A)   mastoiditis.

(B)   meningitis.

(C)   cavernous sinus thrombosis.

(D)   sepsis.

(E)   erythema nodosum.

90.   A patient with lupus erythematous develops severe hemolytic anemia. Recommended treatment may include all of the following EXCEPT

(A)   corticosteroids.

(B)   gammaglobulin.

(C)   immunosuppressive drugs.

(D)   splenectomy.

(E)   blood transfusion.

91.   Treatment of acute pancreatitis in a patient that is euglycemic and hypocalcemic may include all of the following EXCEPT

(A)   volume replacement.

(B)   narcotics.

(C)   nasogastric suction.

(D)   insulin.

(E)   calcium.

92.   A 26-year-old female presents with a copious, yellow-green vaginal discharge and dysuria. Wet mount shows a large amount of WBCs and whiff test is positive. Treatment consists of

(A)   tetracycline for patient only.

(B)   tetracycline for patient and sexual contacts.

(C)   metronidazole for patient only.

(D)   metronidazole for patient and sexual contacts.

(E)   miconazole.

93.   In most cases of recurrent dislocation of the shoulder, the dislocation is

(A)   posterior.

(B)   anterior.

(C)   asymptomatic.

(D)   lateral.

(E)   medial.

94.   Neonatal mortality most correlates with

(A)   birth weight.

(B)   maternal age.

(C)   sex.

(D)   maternal diabetes.

(E)   maternal cigarette smoking.

95.   A 50-year-old male complains of bone pain with increasing deafness. Serum laboratory

analyses demonstrate a normal calcium and phosphate level, yet alkaline phosphatase levels are elevated. Urinalysis reveals an elevated level of hydroxyproline and roentengram studies demonstrate dense, enlarged bones. Finally, an osteocalcin study is performed, indicating an increase. Which one of the following represents the most likely diagnosis?

(A) Pott's disease

(B) Osteogenic sarcoma

(C) Fibrogenesis imperfect ossium

(D) Hyperparathyroidism

(E) Paget's disease

96. A patient's profile seven shows a Na+ = 135 mEq/L, HCO3- = 15.0 mEq/L, and Cl- = 100 mEq/L. What is the anion gap?

(A) 0 mEq/L

(B) 10 mEq/L

(C) 20 mEq/L

(D) 30 mEq/L

(E) 40 mEq/L

97. All of the following are associated with hyperthyroidism EXCEPT

(A) exogenous thyroid hormone.

(B) TSH excess.

(C) iodine deficiency.

(D) toxic struma ovarii.

(E) toxic thyroid carcinoma.

98. Which one of the following is NOT important in the transmission of *Corynebacterium diphtheriae*?

(A) Humans are the only natural reservoir.

(B) Spread occurs in close-contact settings via respiratory droplets.

(C) The organism survives for several weeks on environmental surfaces and in dust.

(D) Asymptomatic carriers are important.

(E) Diphtheria immunization prevents carriage.

99. Which one of the following is NOT true of malignant hyperthermia?

(A) Sudden massive muscle contractions lead to a rapid rise in body temperature.

(B) A linkage to mutations of the skeletal muscle ryanodine receptor has been observed in some cases.

(C) Muscle biopsies from susceptible individuals may contract when exposed to caffeine.

(D) Screening with CPK is the best way to identify susceptible individuals.

(E) Triggering anesthetics release calcium from the membrane of the muscle cell's sarcoplasmic reticulum.

100. A 57-year-old woman comes to the emergency department with diarrhea. Her history is significant for a recent urinary tract infection, which was treated with antibiotics. No one else in her environment has a diarrheal illness, and she has not eaten anything unusual recently. You suspect

(A) ulcerative colitis.

(B) *C. difficile.*

(C) hepatitis A.

(D) appendicitis.

(E) shigellosis.

101. A six-year-old girl had a sore throat, which you treated with an antibiotic about seven days earlier just before Thanksgiving. Her mother now brings her in because, while her throat is fine, she has now developed an urticarial eruption. You tell the mother that this is most likely due to

(A)   drug reaction.

(B)   poison ivy.

(C)   rubella.

(D)   chicken pox.

(E)   pyoderma.

Questions 102-105 refer to the following:

A 45-year-old woman comes to your office with a six-year history of episodic flank pain, abdominal cramping, and associated fevers. She has never been evaluated for this because she did not have any insurance. She now has insurance and wants to find out what is wrong with her. Her last bout of this condition was about four months ago.

102.   She is likely to have a history of

    (A)   peptic ulcer disease.

    (B)   recurrent urinary tract infections.

    (C)   migraines.

    (D)   premenstrual syndrome.

    (E)   diabetes.

103.   Other members of her family are likely to have

    (A)   diverticulosis.

    (B)   diabetes.

    (C)   intermittent claudication.

    (D)   diarrhea.

    (E)   renal calculi.

104.   You obtain all of the following tests EXCEPT

    (A)   complete blood count.

    (B)   creatinine.

    (C)   blood urea nitrogen.

    (D)   24-hour urine for protein.

    (E)   urinalysis.

105.   You tell the patient that if she develops a recurrence she should

    (A)   try to wait it out.

(B)   come to see you in the daytime or go to the emergency department if the attack occurs at night or when you are not in the office.

(C)   go to a walk-in clinic.

(D)   ignore it.

(E)   take acetaminophen.

Questions 106-113 refer to the following:

A 53-year-old woman is admitted to the hospital during the night because of dyspnea, tachycardia, and chest pain. She has been monitored by telemetry all night and has had tachycardia on the monitor. Serial CPKs have been normal. Serial ECGs have been obtained and demonstrate atrial fibrillation.

106.   The ECG

    (A)   shows RSR' complexes.

    (B)   lacks P waves.

    (C)   has poor R-wave progression.

    (D)   has Q waves in the inferior leads.

    (E)   shows first-degree AV block.

107.   On questioning the patient, she tells you that she has been nervous lately and has also felt quite warm. You order

    (A)   a PPD.

    (B)   an EEG.

    (C)   thyroid function tests.

    (D)   serum prolactin.

    (E)   sputum cultures.

108.   Other tests that should be ordered at this point include

    (A)   a bone scan.

    (B)   a streptococcal throat culture.

    (C)   a head CT.

    (D)   arterial blood gases.

    (E)   antiphospholipid antibodies.

109. Common causes of atrial fibrillation include all of the following EXCEPT

    (A) mitral valve disease.

    (B) hypothyroidism.

    (C) hyperthyroidism.

    (D) pulmonary embolus.

    (E) rheumatic heart disease.

110. The patient's blood gases show a pO$_2$ of 65 on 2L of oxygen. She has a 60-pack-year history of cigarette smoking. You decide

    (A) the relatively low pO$_2$ is due to her cigarette ingestion and does not need to be further evaluated.

    (B) to increase her oxygen flow.

    (C) to order a ventilation-perfusion scan of the lungs.

    (D) to order a chest CT.

    (E) to give her CPAP.

111. The patient's labs return and you find that her T4 level is high and her TSH is low. Your working diagnosis is

    (A) primary hyperthyroidism.

    (B) pituitary adenoma.

    (C) adrenal adenoma.

    (D) pheochromocytoma.

    (E) medullary thyroid cancer.

112. The long-term treatment of choice for this patient is

    (A) implants of radioiodine.

    (B) a beta-blocker.

    (C) theophylline.

    (D) thyroidectomy.

    (E) hydrochlorothiazide.

113. Short-term treatment for this patient's condition may require

    (A) cardioversion.

    (B) cardiac catheterization.

    (C) lidocaine.

    (D) furosemide.

    (E) hydralazine.

114. A four-year-old child is brought into the emergency room by his mother. He has an obvious fracture of his ulna. The child is not willing to talk to you, but the mother says he fell down some stairs while playing. You obtain a radiograph of the arm and discover, in addition to the acute fracture, evidence of old, healed, but maligned, fractures. Your assessment of this case is

    (A) this may be a case of child abuse.

    (B) the child is clumsy.

    (C) the child probably has osteogenesis imperfecta.

    (D) the child has rickets.

    (E) the child is malnourished.

115. A 78-year-old woman whom you admitted for severe dysphagia fell on her way to the bathroom the night before rounds. You insist that she have

    (A) appropriate radiographs.

    (B) bone densitometry.

    (C) colonoscopy.

    (D) EEG.

    (E) ECG.

116. A 33-year-old man admitted for pneumonia develops confusion, shakiness, and tachycardia. You inquire about

    (A) his family history.

    (B) his alcohol consumption.

    (C) his drug allergies.

    (D) history of migraines.

    (E) his antinuclear antibody titer.

117. A woman who is in her 32nd week of pregnancy comes in because of vaginal bleeding. The bleeding has been increasing for an hour or so. The first thing you do is

(A) draw a CBC.

(B) call her husband.

(C) arrange for an outpatient transfusion if necessary.

(D) send the patient to the emergency department via ambulance.

(E) tell her to go home and lie down.

Questions 118-121 refer to the following:

A diabetic 28-year-old woman gives birth after 30 weeks of gestation to a two-pound baby who has severe respiratory distress requiring resuscitation immediately after delivery. The mother has had minimal prenatal care.

118. The likeliest diagnosis in this newborn is

(A) streptococcal pneumonia.

(B) hyaline membrane disease.

(C) empyema.

(D) congenital histoplasmosis.

(E) congenital syphilis.

119. This condition results from

(A) a deficiency of pulmonary surfactant.

(B) a viral infection.

(C) cardiomyopathy.

(D) rubella.

(E) phenylketonuria.

120. All of the following are predisposing factors for this condition EXCEPT

(A) prematurity.

(B) maleness.

(C) maternal diabetes.

(D) maternal asthma.

(E) maternal history of similarly affected babies.

121. All of the following are helpful in the management of this condition EXCEPT

(A) oxygen.

(B) CPAP.

(C) assisted mechanical ventilation.

(D) penicillin.

(E) administration of surfactant.

122. A 36-year-old woman comes to your office because of recent onset of seizures. She had been in excellent health until she was in a motor vehicle accident about two months ago. She was the restrained driver of a car that was sideswiped. Her head bumped the windshield, but X-rays were negative for fractures. She had her first seizure about a week ago and has since had two more. They have been tonic-clonic in nature. You explain to her that you think her seizures are due to

(A) meningitis.

(B) a congenital malformation.

·(C) a brain tumor.

(D) head trauma from the accident.

(E) anxiety.

123. A 35-year-old woman comes to the walk-in clinic because of hematuria. She has had a sense of pressure over her bladder but has no other symptoms. The likeliest diagnosis is

(A) urinary tract infection.

(B) pyelonephritis.

(C) renal stone.

(D) ovarian cyst.

(E) ectopic pregnancy.

124. A 63-year-old patient calls you because she has had five episodes of chest pain, some of which have been associated with shortness of breath, in the last 48 hours. You tell her to

(A) take more nitroglycerine.

(B) call an ambulance.

(C) ignore it.

(D) take acetaminophen with codeine.

(E) do more exercise.

125. A 26-year-old male with classical hemophilia comes to the emergency department with a swollen knee. He noticed this after walking downstairs at home. It is not painful but "stiff," and it is neither warm nor red. An arthrocentesis is necessary for the diagnosis, but you suspect you will find

(A) septic arthritis.

(B) monosodium urate crystals.

(C) hemarthrosis.

(D) chylous fluid.

(E) hydroxyapatite crystals.

126. A 51-year-old woman complains of drenching nightsweats. Her appetite is good and her weight has been stable. You tell her

(A) she needs a PPD and chest radiograph to rule out tuberculosis.

(B) she needs blood cultures.

(C) she is probably perimenopausal.

(D) she probably has influenza.

(E) she needs more rest.

127. A tall 16-year-old male is seen because of blurred vision. Your ophthalmologic colleague diagnoses ectopia lentis. You hear a heart murmur when you examine him. You ask the patient and his family about a family history of

(A) polyarthritis.

(B) back pain.

(C) blindness.

(D) Marfan's syndrome.

(E) chondroepiphyseal dysplasia.

128. A 62-year-old man with chronic hypertension comes in for a routine follow-up appointment. He has no complaints, but you find that his blood pressure is elevated on the same medications he has been taking for a long time, which have previously controlled his pressure. The first thing you should do is

(A) get an IVP.

(B) change his medications.

(C) give him IM clonidine to lower his blood pressure acutely.

(D) give him a new diet.

(E) ask him if he has taken his morning doses of medicine.

129. A 47-year-old man admitted for a severe urinary tract infection develops hematuria and colicky lower abdominal pain while receiving appropriate antibiotic therapy. Your working diagnosis is

(A) diverticulitis.

(B) sepsis.

(C) renal adenocarcinoma.

(D) renal calculi.

(E) malingering.

130. A 53-year-old man comes in because of episodic headaches. He is having a particularly bad one today. These have been occurring for several years but have been getting progressively more severe. He describes a "pounding" sensation over his left parietal region with occasional radiation elsewhere. He has no neurological findings, is afebrile, and has no papilledema. You should

(A) give him an analgesic and tell him to come back in one month with a diary of episodes of headache.

(B) schedule a brain MRI as soon as possible.

(C) order an EEG.

(D) order skull films.

(E) perform a lumbar puncture.

131. A seven-year-old boy is brought to the walk-in clinic because of a several-month history of complaints of pain and swelling in his knees and wrists. He has been seen in the past and cultures of his synovial fluid have been negative, as has his rheumatoid factor. You perform an arthrocentesis and tell the patient's mother that you think he has

    (A) septic arthritis.

    (B) juvenile rheumatoid arthritis.

    (C) pseudogout.

    (D) repetitive trauma.

    (E) osteogenesis imperfecta.

132. A 33-year-old man with AIDS comes in because of recent onset of a pruritic rash on his trunk and extremities. He takes a number of medicines, the names of which he cannot remember, but he knows one is "for pneumonia." You suspect that the rash represents

    (A) erysipelas.

    (B) poison ivy.

    (C) psoriasis.

    (D) allergic reaction to sulfa.

    (E) a reaction to HIV.

133. A 56-year-old woman who has not seen you or any other physician for about three years comes in because she has noticed a change in the skin of one of her breasts. On exam she has thickened skin overlying a 3-cm mass on the right breast. Your assessment is

    (A) fibrocystic breast disease.

    (B) moderately advanced breast cancer.

    (C) early breast cancer.

    (D) lipoma.

    (E) scleroderma.

For Questions 134-137, match the numbered condition with the best answer.

    (A) Pleurisy

    (B) Unstable angina

    (C) Acute myocardial infarction

    (D) Cervical disk disease

134. Chest pain at rest

135. Sharp chest pain with breathing

136. Neck pain radiating to left arm

137. Acute severe substernal chest pain

138. A 23-year-old man comes in because of a severe headache for the last day or two, associated with photophobia and neck pain. His temperature is 38°C. His eye-rounds reveal no evidence of papilledema. The next thing you should do is

    (A) schedule an angiogram.

    (B) begin intravenous antibiotics in your office.

    (C) perform a lumbar puncture.

    (D) give him acetaminophen and tell him he will feel better soon.

    (E) obtain blood cultures.

139. A 26-year-old woman who had camped in the Wisconsin woods a few months ago comes in because of severe headache, joint pain, and fever. She has no joint effusions or rash. Her neurologic exam is nonfocal. You should ask her about

    (A) a family history of rheumatoid arthritis.

    (B) recent colic.

    (C) history of tick bites.

    (D) exposure to a rabid dog.

    (E) recent ingestion of uncooked pork.

140. A 53-year-old woman is brought to the walk-in clinic by her family because she has not been eating, has been awakening early, and has not shown any interest in her usual activities. Her CBC and chemistries are all within normal limits. Your leading diagnosis is

(A) pancreatitis.

(B) colon cancer.

(C) depression.

(D) peptic ulcer disease.

(E) obsessive-compulsive disorder.

141. A 64-year-old man has been hospitalized for repair of a femoral shaft fracture sustained after he fell from a ladder. Three days after surgery he develops acute tachypnea, tachycardia, and chest pain. The likeliest diagnosis is

(A) pneumonia.

(B) lung cancer.

(C) acute bronchitis.

(D) pulmonary embolus.

(E) arrhythmia.

142. A 15-year-old boy comes to your office with a warm, swollen, and tender ankle. It began when he was tackled during a school football game this afternoon. The first test you should order is

(A) a radiograph of the affected site.

(B) a bone scan.

(C) a blood culture.

(D) serum uric acid level.

(E) a toxicology screen.

For Questions 143-146, match each numbered condition with the best answer.

(A) Diabetes mellitus

(B) Diuretic ingestion

(C) Acute renal failure

(D) Aminophylline ingestion

143. Hyperosmolarity

144. Hypermagnesemia

145. Hypokalemia

146. Hypoglycemia

147. A 35-year-old woman with chronic rheumatoid arthritis is found to have a hemoglobin of 10. You decide to

(A) give her a transfusion.

(B) give her iron therapy.

(C) give her vitamin B12 injections.

(D) evaluate her blood smear.

(E) order a bone marrow biopsy.

Questions 148-155 refer to the following:

A 50-year-old woman is brought to the emergency room by her husband because of chest pain. The pain has been occurring on and off for several days but has gotten much worse in the last six hours. The patient is clearly uncomfortable and is sitting up in the gurney, breathing shallowly. She has never smoked, has no family history of heart disease, and takes Premarin for her postmenopausal symptoms.

148. Your initial decision is to

(A) admit the patient to the CCU.

(B) evaluate her carefully in the emergency department.

(C) give her IV morphine.

(D) give her a nonsteroidal and send her home.

(E) get a pulmonary angiogram.

149. The patient describes her pain as a "sharp pressure." It is less painful when she sits up and more painful when she lies down or moves or takes a deep breath. You anticipate that the ECG will show

(A) T-wave inversion.

(B) ST segment elevation.

(C) bundle branch block.

(D) left axis deviation.

(E) inverted P waves.

150. Your expectation of the ECG is correct. Meanwhile, the initial CPK returns and is

    (A) elevated.

    (B) normal.

    (C) all MB.

    (D) all BB.

    (E) zero.

151. A more careful review of the patient's medical history is likely to reveal

    (A) a history of asthma.

    (B) a history of idiopathic pneumothoraces.

    (C) a recent flu-like illness.

    (D) a history of lupus.

    (E) cyanotic congenital heart disease.

152. This condition is most likely to respond to

    (A) ibuprofen.

    (B) fluconazole.

    (C) nitroglycerine.

    (D) lidocaine.

    (E) fibrinolytics.

153. You admit the patient for short-term observation. In the morning, her physical examination has changed, and you now hear

    (A) a heart murmur.

    (B) an aortic bruit.

    (C) a water hammer pulse.

    (D) mitral valve prolapse.

    (E) a rub.

154. You order a chest radiograph, which is most likely to show

    (A) a large heart.

    (B) a solitary lung nodule.

    (C) bilateral infiltrates.

    (D) a completely normal chest.

    (E) a hiatal hernia.

155. The prognosis of this condition is

    (A) poor.

    (B) certain death.

    (C) benign.

    (D) transformation to another condition.

    (E) guarded due to bleeding.

156. A 53-year-old man with hypertension is sitting in the waiting room to see you because of a cough when he develops acute severe substernal chest pain and diaphoresis. The nurse comes running into your examining room. You

    (A) scold her for interrupting you.

    (B) tell her to call an ambulance and go out to the waiting room.

    (C) tell her to call an ambulance and continue examining the patient you are with.

    (D) tell her to begin resuscitation.

    (E) tell her to reassure the patient that he will be seen shortly.

157. Which one of the following is NOT true of systemic lupus erythematosus?

    (A) It is increased in monozygotic as compared to dizygotic twins.

    (B) It is increased in women during childbearing years.

    (C) The relative risk of developing it increases as the number of susceptibility genes increases.

    (D) Ultraviolet light produces disease flares.

    (E) Drug-induced and spontaneous disease have the same clinical and autoantibody picture.

For Questions 158-161, match the numbered condition with the best answer.

    (A) Wernicke-Korsakoff psychosis

    (B) Manic-depressive

(C)　Paranoid schizophrenia

(D)　Situational depression

158.　A 22-year-old woman who works as a janitor and has just spent $5,000 on clothes

159.　A 37-year-old woman who is contemplating suicide because her husband has just left her

160.　A 55-year-old man with a long history of alcohol consumption who is sure he saw you in the local bar a few hours ago

161.　A 40-year-old man who says that the FBI is following him

Questions 162-169 refer to the following:

A 16-year-old girl comes in with a two-month history of diarrhea associated with cramping abdominal pain, occasional bleeding, and low-grade fever. She has lost some weight and feels tired. She has done no recent traveling, eaten nothing unusual, and no one else in her family or among her friends is sick.

162.　All of the following tests should be ordered EXCEPT

(A)　CBC.

(B)　stool culture.

(C)　barium enema.

(D)　chest radiograph.

(E)　stool hemoccult.

163.　The stool culture comes back negative. The barium enema shows a thickened bowel wall with a suggestion of ulcerations. A more definitive test at this point would be

(A)　upper GI endoscopy.

(B)　colonoscopy with biopsy.

(C)　proctoscopy.

(D)　a KUB.

(E)　a paracentesis.

164.　A biopsy of the descending colon is performed and shows acute and chronic inflam-mation and cryptitis. You suspect that the correct diagnosis is

(A)　ulcerative colitis.

(B)　diverticulitis.

(C)　peptic ulcer disease.

(D)　Hirschsprung's disease.

(E)　Meckel's diverticulum.

165.　In this setting, another condition must be ruled out. The best way to determine the presence of that condition is

(A)　CT scan of the abdomen.

(B)　pelvic ultrasound.

(C)　arteriography.

(D)　upper GI endoscopy.

(E)　barium swallow.

166.　The upper GI endoscopy is negative. The treatment of choice at this point is

(A)　steroids.

(B)　cyclophosphamide.

(C)　colectomy.

(D)　plasmapheresis.

(E)　chelating agents.

167.　To evaluate her disease, this patient should have annual

(A)　mammography.

(B)　Pap smear.

(C)　gastric brushing.

(D)　colonoscopy.

(E)　barium enema.

168.　This patient is at higher risk than the general population for the development of

(A)　myocardial infarction.

(B)　morbid obesity.

(C)　colon cancer.

(D)　esophageal cancer.

(E)　COPD.

169. Ultimately, the curative treatment for this disease is

    (A) steroid therapy.

    (B) colectomy.

    (C) a cytotoxic agent.

    (D) biofeedback.

    (E) chronic antidiarrheal agents.

Questions 170 and 171 refer to the following:

A 52-year-old woman comes to your office because of irregular menses. She is otherwise in good health. She has no constitutional symptoms. Blood tests are unremarkable except for a hemoglobin of 10.5.

170. All of the following should be done or arranged based on this information EXCEPT

    (A) a pelvic exam.

    (B) oral iron therapy.

    (C) dilatation and curettage.

    (D) history of bleeding from any site.

    (E) review of past blood tests.

171. The likeliest diagnosis for this patient is

    (A) uterine fibroids.

    (B) perimenopause.

    (C) uterine cancer.

    (D) cervicitis.

    (E) cervical cancer.

172. A 48-year-old man presents with severe hypertension. He has a long history of hypertension with many fluctuations up and down. He has been given medicine for his blood pressure on many occasions. He is an occasional drinker. The most likely cause of his hypertension in this setting is

    (A) a pheochromocytoma.

    (B) anxiety.

    (C) abdominal pain.

    (D) noncompliance with his medicine.

    (E) the drugs are incorrect.

173. A 35-year-old woman with a history of psychiatric hospitalizations comes in because of amenorrhea for four months. She is convinced she has felt "the baby kicking." Your examination reveals a slightly distended abdomen and no fetal sounds. An HCG drawn a few months earlier had been negative. Your leading diagnosis is

    (A) intrauterine fetal death.

    (B) teratoma.

    (C) hydatidiform mole.

    (D) pseudocyesis.

    (E) ectopic pregnancy.

174. A 45-year-old woman with a history of chronic depression is brought in because of presumptive ingestion of cleaning solvent in a suicide attempt. You should do all of the following EXCEPT

    (A) hydrate the patient.

    (B) try to obtain the bottle of cleaning solvent.

    (C) administer charcoal.

    (D) administer ipecac.

    (E) administer a cathartic.

Questions 175-178 refer to the following:

A 35-year-old man who indulges in binge consumption of alcohol comes to see you because of nausea, vomiting, and abdominal pain. On abdominal exam, he is tender and has decreased bowel sounds.

175. You order all of the following tests EXCEPT

    (A) amylase.

    (B) barium swallow.

    (C) lipase.

    (D) KUB.

    (E) CBC.

176. The amylase is significantly elevated. The KUB shows an air-filled loop of bowel. The

peripheral white count is elevated. Your working diagnosis is

   (A) peptic ulcer disease.

   (B) irritable colon.

   (C) ulcerative colitis.

   (D) perforated viscus.

   (E) acute pancreatitis.

177. You admit the patient to a hospital and order all of the following EXCEPT

   (A) NPO status.

   (B) liquid diet.

   (C) intravenous hydration.

   (D) analgesia.

   (E) nasogastric tube drainage.

178. Despite treatment, the patient's pain continues. You order an ultrasound to evaluate the possibility of

   (A) ileus.

   (B) retroperitoneal lymphoma.

   (C) intussusception.

   (D) pseudocyst.

   (E) colon polyps.

179. A 25-year-old woman with a history of multiple sexual contacts has been admitted because of a pulmonary infiltrate. She has a cough and low-grade fever. She denies other medical history. On rounds you notice that she has a white coating on her tongue, and upon questioning she admits to a sore throat. You ask her if you can order

   (A) a chest CT.

   (B) histoplasma titers.

   (C) an HIV test.

   (D) an STS.

   (E) a psychiatric consult.

180. A 64-year-old man has been transferred to your service after undergoing a colectomy for colon cancer. Three days after surgery he develops a swollen painful great toe. While examining him, he tells you that all of his usual medicines were discontinued prior to surgery. You ask him if one of the medications was

   (A) penicillin.

   (B) allopurinol.

   (C) acetaminophen.

   (D) theophylline.

   (E) propoxyphene.

USMLE STEP 3 – PRACTICE TEST 3

Day One – Morning Session

ANSWER KEY

1. (E)	31. (C)	61. (B)	91. (A)
2. (E)	32. (A)	62. (B)	92. (B)
3. (D)	33. (E)	63. (B)	93. (D)
4. (D)	34. (D)	64. (B)	94. (E)
5. (E)	35. (B)	65. (D)	95. (B)
6. (A)	36. (B)	66. (D)	96. (B)
7. (B)	37. (B)	67. (B)	97. (B)
8. (D)	38. (D)	68. (B)	98. (B)
9. (A)	39. (B)	69. (B)	99. (A)
10. (E)	40. (B)	70. (D)	100. (A)
11. (E)	41. (E)	71. (A)	101. (A)
12. (B)	42. (C)	72. (D)	102. (E)
13. (B)	43. (B)	73. (B)	103. (E)
14. (C)	44. (C)	74. (C)	104. (D)
15. (D)	45. (D)	75. (A)	105. (C)
16. (C)	46. (D)	76. (D)	106. (A)
17. (B)	47. (B)	77. (E)	107. (D)
18. (C)	48. (B)	78. (C)	108. (C)
19. (B)	49. (C)	79. (C)	109. (B)
20. (A)	50. (C)	80. (A)	110. (C)
21. (B)	51. (E)	81. (E)	111. (C)
22. (D)	52. (E)	82. (C)	112. (D)
23. (B)	53. (A)	83. (D)	113. (C)
24. (B)	54. (D)	84. (B)	114. (C)
25. (C)	55. (D)	85. (C)	115. (B)
26. (D)	56. (C)	86. (A)	116. (C)
27. (A)	57. (D)	87. (C)	117. (D)
28. (A)	58. (B)	88. (B)	118. (C)
29. (B)	59. (A)	89. (C)	119. (A)
30. (B)	60. (B)	90. (C)	120. (D)

121.	(C)	136.	(D)	151.	(D)	166.	(A)
122.	(C)	137.	(D)	152.	(D)	167.	(D)
123.	(D)	138.	(A)	153.	(D)	168.	(E)
124.	(E)	139.	(C)	154.	(D)	169.	(C)
125.	(D)	140.	(D)	155.	(C)	170.	(B)
126.	(C)	141.	(C)	156.	(B)	171.	(D)
127.	(B)	142.	(B)	157.	(D)	172.	(B)
128.	(C)	143.	(C)	158.	(E)	173.	(C)
129.	(D)	144.	(D)	159.	(A)	174.	(B)
130.	(D)	145.	(E)	160.	(C)	175.	(B)
131.	(E)	146.	(C)	161.	(D)	176.	(A)
132.	(C)	147.	(C)	162.	(C)	177.	(E)
133.	(D)	148.	(A)	163.	(B)	178.	(C)
134.	(D)	149.	(E)	164.	(A)	179.	(D)
135.	(E)	150.	(E)	165.	(B)	180.	(B)

USMLE STEP 3 – PRACTICE TEST 3

Day One – Afternoon Session

ANSWER KEY

1.	(D)	31.	(C)	61.	(E)	91.	(D)
2.	(B)	32.	(E)	62.	(D)	92.	(A)
3.	(C)	33.	(C)	63.	(C)	93.	(D)
4.	(D)	34.	(D)	64.	(C)	94.	(D)
5.	(C)	35.	(D)	65.	(A)	95.	(E)
6.	(B)	36.	(A)	66.	(B)	96.	(D)
7.	(B)	37.	(C)	67.	(D)	97.	(C)
8.	(D)	38.	(B)	68.	(D)	98.	(B)
9.	(B)	39.	(B)	69.	(D)	99.	(A)
10.	(D)	40.	(A)	70.	(B)	100.	(E)
11.	(A)	41.	(A)	71.	(C)	101.	(C)
12.	(C)	42.	(E)	72.	(E)	102.	(D)
13.	(C)	43.	(B)	73.	(E)	103.	(C)
14.	(D)	44.	(D)	74.	(C)	104.	(D)
15.	(D)	45.	(B)	75.	(B)	105.	(A)
16.	(D)	46.	(D)	76.	(D)	106.	(E)
17.	(E)	47.	(C)	77.	(A)	107.	(A)
18.	(B)	48.	(E)	78.	(B)	108.	(D)
19.	(D)	49.	(C)	79.	(C)	109.	(C)
20.	(D)	50.	(C)	80.	(C)	110.	(C)
21.	(C)	51.	(D)	81.	(D)	111.	(D)
22.	(D)	52.	(D)	82.	(B)	112.	(B)
23.	(D)	53.	(A)	83.	(A)	113.	(A)
24.	(D)	54.	(E)	84.	(B)	114.	(C)
25.	(C)	55.	(D)	85.	(B)	115.	(C)
26.	(D)	56.	(E)	86.	(D)	116.	(E)
27.	(C)	57.	(C)	87.	(D)	117.	(B)
28.	(C)	58.	(A)	88.	(D)	118.	(B)
29.	(B)	59.	(B)	89.	(C)	119.	(A)
30.	(C)	60.	(C)	90.	(B)	120.	(E)

121.	(A)	136.	(C)	151.	(D)	166.	(C)
122.	(B)	137.	(A)	152.	(A)	167.	(B)
123.	(C)	138.	(D)	153.	(C)	168.	(B)
124.	(D)	139.	(B)	154.	(B)	169.	(A)
125.	(A)	140.	(D)	155.	(B)	170.	(D)
126.	(C)	141.	(D)	156.	(D)	171.	(C)
127.	(D)	142.	(A)	157.	(B)	172.	(B)
128.	(A)	143.	(C)	158.	(E)	173.	(D)
129.	(B)	144.	(B)	159.	(B)	174.	(E)
130.	(D)	145.	(B)	160.	(D)	175.	(B)
131.	(C)	146.	(D)	161.	(C)	176.	(A)
132.	(A)	147.	(E)	162.	(D)	177.	(A)
133.	(E)	148.	(A)	163.	(A)	178.	(D)
134.	(E)	149.	(E)	164.	(E)	179.	(D)
135.	(D)	150.	(B)	165.	(C)	180.	(B)

USMLE STEP 3 – PRACTICE TEST 3

Day Two – Morning Session

ANSWER KEY

1. (E)	31. (E)	61. (A)	91. (B)
2. (A)	32. (A)	62. (D)	92. (E)
3. (B)	33. (A)	63. (E)	93. (C)
4. (C)	34. (A)	64. (E)	94. (E)
5. (A)	35. (E)	65. (E)	95. (D)
6. (B)	36. (B)	66. (D)	96. (C)
7. (C)	37. (C)	67. (C)	97. (D)
8. (B)	38. (A)	68. (E)	98. (B)
9. (D)	39. (D)	69. (C)	99. (A)
10. (E)	40. (C)	70. (B)	100. (A)
11. (B)	41. (B)	71. (D)	101. (A)
12. (D)	42. (D)	72. (D)	102. (E)
13. (A)	43. (C)	73. (C)	103. (A)
14. (A)	44. (E)	74. (A)	104. (A)
15. (E)	45. (B)	75. (B)	105. (C)
16. (E)	46. (D)	76. (B)	106. (C)
17. (E)	47. (A)	77. (A)	107. (B)
18. (E)	48. (C)	78. (A)	108. (C)
19. (E)	49. (E)	79. (B)	109. (A)
20. (C)	50. (B)	80. (D)	110. (A)
21. (C)	51. (C)	81. (E)	111. (A)
22. (C)	52. (B)	82. (B)	112. (E)
23. (B)	53. (B)	83. (D)	113. (C)
24. (D)	54. (C)	84. (D)	114. (A)
25. (C)	55. (C)	85. (B)	115. (C)
26. (D)	56. (A)	86. (C)	116. (C)
27. (B)	57. (E)	87. (A)	117. (E)
28. (D)	58. (B)	88. (A)	118. (D)
29. (A)	59. (B)	89. (A)	119. (D)
30. (B)	60. (A)	90. (C)	120. (D)

121.	(B)	136.	(D)	151.	(E)	166.	(C)
122.	(B)	137.	(A)	152.	(D)	167.	(C)
123.	(A)	138.	(D)	153.	(C)	168.	(C)
124.	(E)	139.	(B)	154.	(A)	169.	(A)
125.	(D)	140.	(A)	155.	(A)	170.	(E)
126.	(C)	141.	(B)	156.	(B)	171.	(A)
127.	(B)	142.	(C)	157.	(D)	172.	(E)
128.	(B)	143.	(C)	158.	(C)	173.	(B)
129.	(C)	144.	(E)	159.	(A)	174.	(D)
130.	(C)	145.	(D)	160.	(E)	175.	(D)
131.	(A)	146.	(A)	161.	(B)	176.	(A)
132.	(A)	147.	(A)	162.	(D)	177.	(C)
133.	(C)	148.	(C)	163.	(D)	178.	(C)
134.	(E)	149.	(D)	164.	(C)	179.	(A)
135.	(E)	150.	(E)	165.	(C)	180.	(D)

USMLE STEP 3 – PRACTICE TEST 3

Day Two – Afternoon Session

ANSWER KEY

1. (E)	31. (E)	61. (D)	91. (D)
2. (B)	32. (B)	62. (D)	92. (D)
3. (C)	33. (B)	63. (E)	93. (B)
4. (B)	34. (D)	64. (A)	94. (A)
5. (C)	35. (D)	65. (C)	95. (E)
6. (C)	36. (A)	66. (D)	96. (C)
7. (E)	37. (C)	67. (A)	97. (C)
8. (B)	38. (B)	68. (C)	98. (E)
9. (D)	39. (C)	69. (E)	99. (D)
10. (D)	40. (D)	70. (D)	100. (B)
11. (B)	41. (A)	71. (C)	101. (A)
12. (A)	42. (C)	72. (B)	102. (B)
13. (E)	43. (E)	73. (B)	103. (E)
14. (A)	44. (A)	74. (D)	104. (D)
15. (D)	45. (B)	75. (C)	105. (B)
16. (B)	46. (B)	76. (B)	106. (B)
17. (B)	47. (D)	77. (C)	107. (C)
18. (A)	48. (B)	78. (B)	108. (D)
19. (A)	49. (C)	79. (C)	109. (B)
20. (C)	50. (D)	80. (D)	110. (C)
21. (B)	51. (A)	81. (A)	111. (A)
22. (D)	52. (D)	82. (B)	112. (D)
23. (E)	53. (B)	83. (B)	113. (A)
24. (E)	54. (A)	84. (D)	114. (A)
25. (B)	55. (C)	85. (A)	115. (A)
26. (C)	56. (E)	86. (D)	116. (B)
27. (B)	57. (B)	87. (C)	117. (D)
28. (A)	58. (E)	88. (D)	118. (B)
29. (D)	59. (B)	89. (E)	119. (A)
30. (B)	60. (D)	90. (E)	120. (D)

121. (D)	136. (D)	151. (C)	166. (A)
122. (D)	137. (C)	152. (A)	167. (D)
123. (A)	138. (C)	153. (E)	168. (C)
124. (B)	139. (C)	154. (D)	169. (B)
125. (C)	140. (C)	155. (C)	170. (C)
126. (C)	141. (D)	156. (B)	171. (B)
127. (D)	142. (A)	157. (E)	172. (D)
128. (E)	143. (A)	158. (B)	173. (D)
129. (D)	144. (C)	159. (D)	174. (D)
130. (B)	145. (B)	160. (A)	175. (B)
131. (B)	146. (A)	161. (C)	176. (E)
132. (D)	147. (D)	162. (D)	177. (B)
133. (B)	148. (B)	163. (B)	178. (D)
134. (B)	149. (B)	164. (A)	179. (C)
135. (A)	150. (B)	165. (D)	180. (B)

DETAILED EXPLANATIONS
OF ANSWERS

USMLE Step 3 – Practice Test 3
Day One – Morning Session

1.   **(E)**   Multidrug resistance (MDR) has been well characterized in vitro. The clinical role still remains to be defined. MDR denotes the ability of malignancies to withstand exposure to lethal doses of several structurally and functionally un-related antineoplastics (A). Several mechanisms of MDR have been identified. The "classic" MDR in-volves overexpression of P-glycoprotein. Many normal tissues express P-glycoprotein. This pro-tein functions as an energy-dependent pump, which decreases the intracellular concentrations of some antineoplastics by actively extruding them across the cell membrane (B). Another mechanism of MDR is through overexpression or mutation of genes than control-cell cycle kinetics. Inherent multidrug resistance occurs in those tu-mors which arise from tissues that normally ex-press the MDR1 gene (C). Another mechanism of MDR is programmed cell death, also known as "apoptosis" (D). Still another means of MDR is through alterations of topoisomerase II. These nuclear enzymes modulate topologic structure of DNA. Only certain classes of antineoplastics are affected by topoisomerase alterations (E).

2.   **(E)**   Surface components and extracellular products produced by Group A streptococci are important in the development of infection. The M protein (A) is the major surface protein of Group A streptococci. This protein acts as a membrane anchor and correlates with the capacity of a strain to resist phagocytic killing. The extracellular en-zyme, hyaluronidase (B), facilitates the spread of infection along fascial planes by hydrolyzing hy-aluronic acid in deeper tissues. Pyrogenic exotox-ins (C) types A, B, and C induce lymphocyte blas-togenesis, potentiate endotoxin-induced shock, induce fever, and suppress antibody synthesis.

Streptolysins (D) O and S damage cell membranes and account for the hemolysis produced by the bacterium. CAMP factor (E) is a phospholipase produced by Group B streptococci, which causes hemolysis synergistically with beta-lysins.

3.   **(D)**   Alcoholic liver disease and hepatitis C are two of the most common indications for liver transplantation. The one-year survival rate has risen from around 50% to greater than 80%. The development of prognostic criteria for various pa-tients such as age, prothrombin time, and jaun-dice can predict the success of the transplanta-tion. Being HIV-positive (A) is a contraindication for liver transplantation because of the relatively shortened life span. Life span would be shortened dramatically as a result of the immunosuppress-ing drugs required to prevent host rejection of the liver transplant, as it would exacerbate the immu-nosuppression induced by HIV. Extrahepatic ma-lignancies (B), such as breast and lung cancer, are absolute contraindications for transplantation because of the shortened life span and the lack of available donors for liver transplantation. Ad-vanced cardiac disease (C) such as triple-vessel coronary artery disease and end-stage congestive heart failure are contraindications for transplan-tation because of the very high risk of mortality during the surgery. Emphysema (E) and pulmo-nary fibrosis are also diseases associated with a poor prognosis during liver transplantation sur-gery and thus are absolute contraindications.

4.   **(D)**   A likely explanation for this patient's symptoms is apathetic hyperthyroidism, which tends to occur in older individuals and which of-ten lacks some of the classical attributes of hyper-thyroidism in younger people. These individuals tend to present more with a picture consistent

with depression than with the seeming hyperactivity of a younger patient with hyperthyroidism. Antinuclear antibodies (A) would not be helpful in the initial evaluation of this patient, nor would a urinalysis (B), CT scan (C), or antimitochondrial antibodies (E), which are associated with primary biliary cirrhosis. Some of these tests, especially a urinalysis and CT scan, might ultimately be needed if thyroid disorders are ruled out. Similarly, if the patient does have thyroid dysfunction, antinuclear antibodies might be appropriate in the evaluation of a possible autoimmune basis for this condition.

5.   **(E)**   A six-week-old with projectile vomiting will usually have pyloric stenosis. It is common in this age range.

6.   **(A)**   A urinary tract infection will present with pain over the bladder or anywhere along the genitourinary tract. The pain from the kidneys will be present by the costovertebral angles (CVA).

7.   **(B)**   A patient with a deep-vein thrombosis will usually have calf tenderness, as the deep veins of the lower extremity are usually involved. The calf may be swollen, as well.

8.   **(D)**   A patient with a basilar skull fracture may leak cerebrospinal fluid through his nose (rhinorrhea) or his ear (otorrhea). He may also have severe neurologic signs with a decreased Glasgow coma scale score.

9.   **(A)**   This patient has benign prostatic hypertrophy (BPH) with mild symptoms of urinary frequency and hesitancy. A prostatic biopsy is not indicated at this time because a "blind" biopsy of the prostate gland is useless and would not reveal any relevant information. Invasive tests are not indicated at this point in the workup. A serum PSA or prostate-specific antigen test (B) is a screening test to determine if prostate cancer is present. If the PSA test is moderately elevated, then a biopsy is indicated along with a sonogram. Terazosin (C) is an alpha-adrenergic antagonist, which alleviates the symptoms of BPH by relaxing the smooth muscle around the prostate gland. It has been proven effective and safe in the study from the Veterans Affairs Cooperative Studies Benign Prostatic Hyperplasia Trial. Finasteride (D) is a 5-alpha-reductase inhibitor, which has been shown in clinical trials to decrease the progression of prostatic hyperplasia and, thus, prevent early transure-

thral resection of the prostate. An ultrasound of the prostate gland (E) is a non-invasive test, which helps identify the nodules and their location in the prostate gland. It can guide us when performing a biopsy.

10.   **(E)**   None of the statements are correct. Exercise alone (A) rarely results in significant weight loss without dietary modification. A proper weight reduction regimen should result in a reduction of one to two lbs per week (B). Five to ten lbs per week is excessive. Diuretics, thyroid hormone, and digitalis use are inappropriate methods of supplementing weight loss (C). Gastric stapling procedures (D) should be considered only in patients with marked obesity who are 200% or more of their ideal body weight.

11.   **(E)**   An HIV test is not a routine preoperative test and also cannot be obtained without a patient's permission.

12.   **(B)**   The association of occult chlamydia infection with gonococcal infection is about 40% in females and 25% in males. Patients who are treated for a known gonococcal infection should be treated for chlamydia empirically. Considerations should be made for testing for syphilis and HIV, but treatment doesn't need to be started empirically.

13.   **(B)**   Interleukin-1 is also known as the "endogenous pyrogen" due to its role of acting upon the hypothalamus to raise the temperature set point. Nitric oxide (A) is a molecule that plays a role in numerous physiologic and cellular processes, such as blood flow regulation and angiogenesis. Fibroblast growth factor (C) plays a role in cellular proliferation and cellular responses. Vascular endothelial growth factor (D) stimulates endothelial cells to proliferate. Atrial natriuretic peptide (E) plays a role in intravascular volume regulation.

14.   **(C)**   Cryptosporidiosis is more likely to occur in an immunocompromised host, but is also seen in previously healthy individuals exposed to the organism via fecal contamination by means of animal-human or person-to-person contact in closed environments, especially day care centers, and among household members and health care providers. Contaminated water (A) appears to be responsible for infection in travelers and swim-

mers, and in sewage tanks. Several outbreaks in the United States have been reported. Cryptosporidium has been found in the pharynx, esophagus, stomach, duodenum, and gallbladder (B). Microscopic studies reveal the organism adherent to the enterocyte surface and enveloped by a membrane. Studies have shown that the antibiotic paramomycin (D) ameliorates infection with cryptosporidium and reduces the symptoms of diarrhea and abdominal pain. Cryptosporidium belongs to the class *Sporozoa* (E). It is a parasite that has the ability to develop completely within one host. This factor may contribute to the refractory nature of the illness and the tremendous potential for reinfection.

15. **(D)** Chronic hepatitis B infection is not associated with eosinophilia, but rather a lymphocytosis and neutrophilia. Allergic reactions to any medications, including sulfa compounds (A), can cause eosinophilia. Loffler's syndrome (B) is a condition associated with peripheral eosinophilia and pulmonary infiltrates. Hodgkin's disease (C) and other hematological malignancies can be associated with eosinophilia. *Strongyloides* (E) and other parasitic infections can be a cause of eosinophilia.

16. **(C)** Biopsy of the lesion is the only accurate way to get a tissue diagnosis. A CT scan (A) may show enlarged nodes without the etiology. Similarly, a panendoscopy (B), which examines the nasopharynx, the oropharynx, the esophagus and larynx, and a barium swallow (D), may show abnormalities, but will not accurately diagnose a cancer. Liver-function tests (E) may show metastatic spread to the liver, but they may be elevated for other reasons.

17. **(B)** The social history, which includes a smoking and drinking history, is the most important risk factor for head and neck cancer, which attacks the aerodigestive system. The other components of the history are important, but not as essential.

18. **(C)** BUN and creatinine may not rise with metastasis from head and neck cancer. A chest X-ray (A) will detect a metastasis to the lungs, and a bone scan (D) and brain scan (E) will detect spread to the bones and brain, respectively. Liver-function tests (B) will rise with metastasis to the liver, which is not uncommon with head and neck cancer.

19. **(B)** This patient should be admitted and have further tests. Immediate surgery (A) may not be indicated. Smoking and drinking cessation should be encouraged, but the patient should not be sent away for one month (C); he should certainly not be asked to return in three months (D) or six months (E), especially when cancer is a possibility.

20. **(A)** Although the lateral decubitus position for subarachnoid block is used most commonly, the sitting position is more appropriate for this obese patient with a flattened lumbar spine (E). Sitting also prevents rotation or distortion of the vertebral bodies [(C) and (D)]. Also, fat is a problem in obese patients and may obscure landmarks used for injection. The disadvantage of the sitting position is possible aggravation of the pain that is associated with this procedure (A).

21. **(B)** In a patient with an acutely swollen, painful joint, fluid aspiration is the most important first step in the evaluation. Fluid should be sent for white count and differential, Gram stain and culture, microscopic examination for crystals, and glucose. A sedimentation rate (A) would probably confirm the inflammatory nature of the joint process but would not be specific. Electrolytes (C) would not be helpful in the acute evaluation of the knee fluid. Blood cultures (D) and urinalysis (E) will probably be necessary in the workup of this febrile patient, but do not take precedence over the evaluation of the synovial fluid. A septic joint is a medical emergency and should be identified as soon as possible.

22. **(D)** While it would be useful to know if the patient's father or any other relatives has had a similar type of problem (E), it is immaterial to the patient's immediate condition whether his father is alive or not. A history of a similar episode (A) could be helpful in suggesting certain kinds of conditions, especially crystal-induced arthritides. Recent surgeries, dental extractions, or trauma (B) might suggest a portal of entry for an infectious agent. Certain medications (C), such as diuretics, which the patient may be taking for his hypertension, might precipitate certain kinds of arthritis.

23. **(B)** Similar attacks in the past and diuretic use, especially with a recent increase in dose, indicate the possibility that this patient might have gout. Previous episodes can be consistent with

pseudogout (A), but diuretic usage would not induce an attack. The symptoms and history are not consistent with osteoarthritis (C), rheumatoid arthritis (D), or Reiter's syndrome (E).

24. **(B)** A serum uric acid would be indicated in a patient presenting in this fashion. A spot uric acid (A) would not be helpful. This setting is not consistent with diseases associated with positive rheumatoid factors (C) or antinuclear antibodies (D), which would not be available on an emergency basis anyway. The patient's condition does not suggest Lyme disease (E).

25. **(C)** Occasionally, a tibial or femoral plateau fracture might present in this fashion. You would not expect to see osteomyelitis (A) after such a brief illness. Loose bodies (B) would not usually cause a febrile illness such as this.

26. **(D)** Despite the negative Gram stain, a joint infection is still possible and is the single potentially life-threatening condition likely to cause this scenario. A septic joint is considered a medical emergency. It is not wise to assume that the lab has made a mistake (A). The setting is not consistent with rheumatoid arthritis (B). Pseudogout is a remote possibility, but does not usually produce such high white counts and fever (C). Monosodium urate crystals are found in fewer than 50% of joint fluids from patients with gout, so a negative fluid analysis does not eliminate the diagnosis of gout (E).

27. **(A)** It is appropriate to treat this patient empirically with antibiotics until the culture results definitively prove or disprove an infection. Steroids are contraindicated because of the possibility of worsening an infection [(B) and (C)]. Indomethacin (D) would not be used until the diagnosis is clear because it can mask the febrile manifestations of an infection. Allopurinol (E) is not indicated in an acute episode such as this.

28. **(A)** It is quite likely that this patient has gout. Intravenous colchicine is both a diagnostic and therapeutic intervention. Few diseases other than gout (e.g., Familial Mediterranean Fever, which is unlikely in this setting) respond to intravenous colchicine. Pseudogout rarely improves with this treatment. If the patient has gout, colchicine should alleviate his symptoms. Changing antibiotics (B) is not indicated in the setting of a

negative Gram stain and negative cultures. Intravenous prednisone (C) is still contraindicated. Agents which can alter the uric acid equilibrium, such as allopurinol (D) or probenecid (E), are contraindicated in the setting of acute gout.

29. **(B)** The buffy coat preparation of the blood shows a typical, large, polyhedral Gaucher cell, with cytoplasm resembling crinkled tissue paper, indicating Gaucher's disease. Clinical studies indicate that most extraskeletal symptoms respond to debulking doses of alglucerase, 30-60 IV/kq intravenously every other week. Alglucerase is a modified form of beta-glucosidase and is prepared from human placenta (B). Hexosaminidase A is the enzyme deficiency found in Tay-Sachs disease (A). Persons with Fabry's disease, another of the lipid-storage diseases, may develop renal failure. These persons are acceptable candidates for renal transplantation because the donor kidney is not affected by the disease process (C). Niemann-Pick disease is characterized by accumulation of sphingomyelin and cholesterol in lysosomes of macrophage monocytic cells. Both orthotopic liver and bone marrow transplantation have been unsuccessfully attempted in the treatment of the disease [(D) and (E)].

30. **(B)** This patient has symptoms of benign prostatic hypertrophy and he is also hypertensive. The best medication for this patient is an alpha 1 adrenergic blocker such as terazosin. This drug will relax the smooth muscle wall lining the blood vessels as well as relax the smooth muscles lining the prostate gland, resulting in fewer symptoms of urgency and frequent micturition. Verapamil (A) is a calcium-channel blocker which is used in hypertension. It also causes constipation. This drug should not be used in patients with systolic dysfunction of the heart because it has a negative inotropic effect. Clonidine (C) is a centrally acting alpha 2 blocker which is used in hypertension. It can cause dry mouth and dizziness. It should be avoided in stroke patients because its effects occur centrally. Nifedipine (D) is also a calcium channel blocker, which acts through vasodilation of the blood vessels by relaxing the smooth muscle of the vasculature. It does not alleviate symptoms of benign prostatic hypertrophy. Hydrochlorothiazide (E) is a diuretic, which acts by increasing salt-loss and, thus, plasma volume. This, in turn, decreases blood pressure in certain patients with high plasma volume hypertension and

salt-retainers. This drug would make the symptoms of increased urinary frequency worse in this patient.

31. **(C)** Hypertension is usually not a reaction to a blood transfusion. The other notable reactions are fever (A), hypotension (B), tachycardia (D), and diaphoresis (E). Patients receiving transfusions are often prophylaxed to minimize these complications.

32. **(A)** Barrett's esophagus is a complication of gastroesophageal reflux disease, in which squamous epithelium is replaced by intestinal metaplasia. Barrett's esophagus is a premalignant lesion for both adenocarcinoma of the esophagus and adenocarcinoma of the gastric cardia. Endoscopic ablation by argon or YAG laser of the metaplastic epithelium, along with addition of a proton-pump inhibitor, has been shown to regenerate the squamous epithelium and reverse the Barrett's esophagus. H2 blockers (B) can alleviate the symptoms of acid reflux disease, but it cannot change the histology of the Barrett's esophagus. Proton-pump inhibition alone (C) cannot reverse the metaplastic lesion of Barrett's esophagus. It can only alleviate the symptoms of reflux disease by decreasing the acid load. Repeating the upper endoscopy (D) is an excellent way to see the progression of the metaplasia and to take a biopsy to determine if adenocarcinoma has developed. The upper endoscopy should be performed yearly, not every three years. ERCP (E) is an invasive procedure to visualize the biliary tree and pancreatic ducts. This procedure is not useful for Barrett's esophagus.

33. **(E)** This patient has classic Parkinson's disease, which is diagnosed by history and physical exam. Eventually, sinemet, amantadine, and bromocriptine can be added to the drug regimen to alleviate some of the symptoms of tremors and bradykinesia. A CT of the head, EEG, and MRI of the brain are usually normal. This disease process is severely debilitating and can eventually result in bed sores, incontinence, and wasting. A brain biopsy (A) would be too invasive and not diagnostic for this disease. A lumbar puncture (B) would be normal in Parkinson's disease patients. A lumbar puncture would yield diagnostic results in multiple sclerosis, meningitis, and pseudotumor cerebri. This patient does not have hypothyroidism, and thyroid function tests (C) would not give

us the diagnosis of Parkinson's disease. A spinal cord imaging study such as MRI or CT scan (D) would be normal in a Parkinson's disease patient. It would not be a good test to perform unless one suspects a spinal cord lesion. This patient does not exhibit any specific signs of spinal cord damage.

34. **(D)** Third-degree burns are full thickness, including the nerve endings, and are, therefore, insensate. First- (A) and second-degree burns are partial thickness, and they are painful because the nerve endings are intact. Superficial burns (A), if partial thickness in the epidermis, are usually similar to first-degree burns and are, therefore, sensate. Fourth-degree burns (E) are deep into the muscle or bone and are also insensate.

35. **(B)** Normal urine output for an adult is $1/2$ to 1 cc of urine per kg body weight per hour. Therefore, one-half to one times 80 equals anywhere between 40 to 80 cc an hour, and 60 cc is the closest.

36. **(B)** This patient has disseminated MAC infection, which is associated with a T-cell count below 50 in HIV individuals. The treatment of choice is any number of combinations of drugs such as cipronoxacin, ethambutol, rifampin, and clarithromycin. Any drug given alone will lead to resistance. Sulfadiazine and pyrimethamine in combination (A) are useful for life-long treatment of CNS toxoplasmosis encephalitis. Another new macrolide, azithromycin (C), given alone, has been shown in one study to be used for prophylaxis, and not treatment, of MAI infection. Clarithromycin (D) alone has been shown to rapidly induce resistance in the prophylaxis for MAI infection. Thus, this macrolide should be used in combination with rifabutin or other medications. Isoniazid, pyrazidamide, ethambutol, and rifampin (E) have been used for the treatment of mycoplasma tuberculosis and not *Mycobacterium avium* infection.

37. **(B)** Hyperventilating the patient (A) to lower the pCO_2 to 25-30 mm Hg causes vasoconstriction, reduced cerebral blood flow, and immediate reduction in intracerebral blood volume resulting in a decrease of intracranial pressure. Mannitol (D) is an osmotic dehydrating agent useful in decreasing intracranial pressure by drawing intracerebral water into the intravascular space

because of its hypertonicity. Lasix is usually given in conjunction with mannitol. Steroids are used to treat the vasogenic edema associated with brain tumors (C). The mechanism of this action is poorly understood. Benzodiazepines (B) do not decrease intracranial pressure.

38. **(D)** The patient needs to be anticoagulated for his heart valve, but also needs to have clotting ability to extract a tooth. This is best accomplished by changing the patient over to heparin and stopping his Coumadin. You can more finely titrate the anticoagulation with a patient on heparin because of its quicker onset and termination of action. You need to stop Coumadin for about two days to have its effect wear off. Switching the patient to aspirin is insufficient (E).

39. **(B)** Heparin should be stopped four hours before surgery. The PTT should normalize by then, and the dentist should be able to safely extract the tooth. Don't forget that this patient will need SBE prophylaxis because of the mechanical heart valve.

40. **(B)** Coumadin should be started the day of surgery. It takes about two days to reach therapeutic levels, and, as such, it could be started the day of surgery without affecting bleeding times during surgery.

41. **(E)** Heparin is used here as a substitute when Coumadin is not being used. When the PT level returns to the patient's adequate level, then the heparin may be safely discontinued.

42. **(C)** Primary infection with rubella induces lifelong immunity after an initial infection (A). Active immunization with live, attenuated rubella vaccines induces antibodies that persist for at least 16 years in more than 95% of immunocompetent recipients (B). Postpartum immunization of persons found to be seronegative during pregnancy is recommended (C). Congenital transplacental rubella infection usually results from maternal infection during the first trimester (D). The initial IgG antibody response changes during the first several months to an IgM antibody response (E).

43. **(B)** Redundant walls of the vagina protruding through the vaginal orifice is a colpocele. A cystocele (A) is bladder prolapse. A rectocele (C)

is rectal prolapse. A uterine prolapse (D) is prolapse of the uterus where it is lower than normal. An enlarged introitus (E) is usually the result of pelvic relaxation secondary to childbirth.

44. **(C)** This does not prevent you from admitting a patient under emergency conditions, but does require you to inform the company within 24 hours.

45. **(D)** Hydroxyurea (A) has been shown to decrease the frequency of sickle cell crisis attacks. Folic acid (B) should be taken for baseline mild anemia. Patients should be immunized (C) when young against encapsulated organisms because they often autoinfarct their spleens and are left functionally asplenic. Intense exercise (E) can sometimes cause sudden death in patients with sickle cell disease and should be avoided. There is no evidence that suppression antibiotics (D) have any benefit in patients with sickle cell disease.

46. **(D)** When someone presents with an upper gastrointestinal bleed, plans for transfusion and treatment with acid suppression medications should be the initial treatment. Also, an NG tube should be inserted to ensure that the bleeding has stopped and a consult should be called immediately for an upper endoscopy that evening.

47. **(B)** When a patient loses up to about 15% of his blood volume, he usually is not symptomatic from it, but may sometimes be orthostatic. When he loses 15 to 25% of his blood volume, he is usually baseline tachycardiac and usually is orthostatic. A loss of 25 to 35% of his blood volume usually results in supine hypotension and tachycardia. Finally, a loss of greater than 35% of his blood volume usually results in decreased mental status.

48. **(B)** When a gastric ulcer is found on EGD, it always needs to be biopsied to rule out gastric carcinoma. However, in an actively bleeding ulcer, biopsies can be confusing. The patient should be stabilized and treated for his ulcer and return for a repeat EGD in a few weeks for a biopsy to rule out gastric carcinoma.

49. **(C)** Although pickled foods have been associated with a higher incidence of gastric carcinoma, there has not been an association shown between pickled foods and peptic ulcer disease.

However, all of the other things, including alcohol, smoking, *Helicobacter pylori* infection, and chronic NSAID use, can be associated with peptic ulcer disease and may exacerbate symptoms.

50. **(C)**   This patient meets the definition of no higher cortical function.

51. **(E)**   Systolic hypertension in any age group, including the elderly, is as important as diastolic hypertension (A). Recent data obtained from the Systolic Hypertension in the Elderly Program showed a significant reduction in morbidity and mortality rates of myocardial infarction in elderly patients. Diagnosis of essential hypertension requires at least two more readings two weeks apart. Therefore, at this time, you should not consider any type of antihypertensives either alone or in combination [(C) and (D)]. After counseling about diet and exercise, the patient should be scheduled for the next visit.

52. **(E)**   While awaiting the results of diagnostic testing, it is essential to begin treatment of conditions that are potentially reversible. Diphenylhydantoin is not indicated either to treat or prevent seizures secondary to alcohol withdrawal. If seizures are documented, underlying medical causes must be excluded (E). Thiamin is administered to prevent either the precipitation or exacerbation of Wernicke's encephalopathy (A). Dextrose is administered to treat an underlying hypoglycemia. This dose will not significantly affect hyperglycemia, if it is subsequently found to be present. It should not be administered until after thiamin has been given, since glucose may precipitate a Wernicke's syndrome if thiamin stores are borderline (B). Naloxone is administered whenever narcotic overdose is a remote possibility (C). Flumazenil is administered to reverse sedative overdose. Although it may precipitate seizures, this occurs primarily in persons with seizures secondary to chronic treatment with benzodiazepines or sedatives (D).

53. **(A)**   Although a laboratory error is a possibility in this emergent clinical situation, it is important to attempt to better define the etiology of the hyponatremia [(A) and (D)]. Hyponatremia secondary to myxedema is typically associated with characteristic clinical findings (C). Addison's disease may also cause hyponatremia. However, one would expect an associated hyperkalemia (B).

Severe hyperlipidemia, in which the plasma is grossly milky, may produce a pseudohyponatremia. In such cases, part of any unit volume of plasma used for analysis will be lipid, which is free of sodium. Consequently, a low sodium concentration is reported by the laboratory (E).

54. **(D)**   On average, a typical 70-kg adult male is able to eliminate approximately one ounce of 85-proof alcohol, or its equivalent, per hour. Once the blood alcohol has attained its peak value, it can be expected to decrease approximately 10-25 mg% each hour, with a mean drop of 18 mg% each hour (D). The blood alcohol level will continue to decrease over the next several hours only if absorption is complete (A). In nonalcoholics, an alcohol level between 200-300 mg% is associated with lethargy and stupor. Coma typically does not occur until levels of 300 mg% (C). In alcoholics, due to tolerance to the effects of alcohol, only drowsiness occurs at alcohol levels of 300 mg% (B). When a small, nonsodium solute is distributed in total body water, such as occurs in ethanol intoxication, the serum sodium concentration remains normal (E).

55. **(D)**   The reduced serum osmolality, in the presence of an increased urine sodium, decreased serum uric acid, and less than maximally dilute urine, suggest that the hyponatremia is caused by the syndrome of inappropriate ADH secretion. Treatment in the acute setting is controversial. In the presence of seizures or other evidence of increased intracranial pressure, hypertonic saline is indicated to raise the serum sodium by 4-5 mM/L per hour (D). In the asymptomatic patient, hypertonic saline is not indicated. Treatment with isotonic saline, which is 154 mM/L, is indicated to raise the serum sodium. Several formulas are available to calculate the free water excess (C). If the condition is chronic, and the patient is asymptomatic, water restriction may be adequate (A). Demeclocycline, which antagonizes the effects of ADH, is also used in chronic conditions (B). Thiazide diuretics frequently produce hyponatremia, particularly in older females. These drugs must be discontinued in the presence of hyponatremia (E).

56. **(C)**   Alcohol withdrawal seizures may occur at this blood level, particularly if the alcoholic maintains consistently higher blood alcohol levels. In such situations, an alcohol level of 100-200 mg% may be a significant reduction from

"normal" levels. When acute medical problems arise, alcohol consumption ceases abruptly, setting the stage for a withdrawal syndrome to develop [(C) and (A)]. Alcohol withdrawal seizures typically occur early in the withdrawal syndrome, as early as 7-24 hours after abrupt cessation of alcohol (B). Seizures typically occur as an isolated phenomenon, although multiple seizures may occur. It is extremely rare for more than six seizures to occur solely due to alcohol withdrawal (D). Focal seizures are rare and should suggest a focal lesion, as should focal neurologic findings (E).

57. **(D)** Increased plasma MB-CK activity reaches a peak in 12-20 hours following the onset of chest pain in persons with a myocardial infarction. Depending on the extent of myocardial damage, the CK returns to normal within 36-48 hours (A). Sometimes, an increased MB-CK occurs in noncardiac conditions. Such causes should be considered when elevations of MB-CK persist without change over serial samples. Noncardiac muscle injury may produce elevations in MB-CK activity. With both extensive muscle trauma and rhabdomyolysis, the percentage of MB-CK relative to total CK activity is low (D). However, with muscular dystrophy, myopathies, polymyositis, and vigorous exercise in trained athletes, the percentage of MB-CK to total CK is high (E). Intracerebral hemorrhage, extensive intracerebral infarction, prostatic carcinoma, and bowel infarction all produce elevations of the BB-CK fraction (B).

58. **(B)** The magnetic resonance imaging study shows central pontine myelinolysis, with a region of prominent low signal intensity. Vigorous and rapid correction of severe hyponatremia has been incriminated in the pathogenesis of this lesion (B). The MRI picture of hemorrhage depends on the age of the hemorrhage. T1-weighted images done within 24 hours typically display more marked hyperintensity when compared to studies done at 72 hours (A). Consciousness is typically initially preserved in cerebellar hemorrhage because the brainstem is spared. The location of the lesion on this scan also excludes a cerebellar hemorrhage (D). Likewise, the location of the lesion excludes a putaminal hemorrhage (C). Marchiafava-Bignami disease, a rare disorder, is characterized by demyelination of the corpus callosum and adjacent white matter (E).

59. **(A)** Central pontine myelinolysis is an osmotic demyelination syndrome, which results from the selective loss of myelin and sparing of the neurons and axial cylinders [(D) and (E)]. It is thought to result from too rapid correction of hyponatremia (B). It occurs more frequently in someone who develops hyponatremia slowly (C). In nonfatal cases, recovery is slow. Even after many weeks, there may be residual sequelae (A).

60. **(B)** Cluster headaches are common in young males and occur episodically. They are characterized by periorbital and, sometimes, temporal pain that is accompanied by reddening of the eye, excessive lacrimation, and facial flushing on the affected side. Most patients are awakened about two hours after sleep onset. These patients are in so much pain that they cannot lie still and the pains are described as "boring" in nature. These headaches last from 15 minutes to three hours each day. Migraine headaches (A) are more common in females. They are associated with throbbing pain which can be bilateral or unilateral. Migraines are associated with nausea, vomiting, and photophobia. Cerebral emboli (C) would present initially with neurologic deficits, not headache. Temporal arteritis (D) is a giant cell vasculitis that is more common in the elderly population. It is associated with jaw claudication, malaise, and an elevated ESR. The pain is described as burning in nature. (E) Trigeminal neuralgia pain is usually unilateral and in the fifth nerve distribution. There is usually a trigger zone located cutaneously or inside the mouth. The pain lasts from seconds to minutes.

61. **(B)** Since his wife is readily available, it is appropriate to discuss the situation with her and determine her current wishes.

62. **(B)** A child this age cannot complain of an earache, but the clinical symptoms and the observation that she has some discomfort on the right side of her head should suggest the ear as a source of infection.

63. **(B)** This is a typical history for an individual with sickle cell anemia.

64. **(B)** A cardiac thrill, or vibrations over the precordium, may be detected with mitral

stenosis during diastole and presystole. In mitral regurgitation (A), myocardial infarct (C), and pulmonary hypertension (D), there is no cardiac thrill palpated.

65. **(D)** The treatment for diabetic ketoacidosis includes intravenous insulin and hydration. Also, replacement of electrolytes, particularly potassium and phosphate, is important. The precipitation factors for DKA include any infection, but antibiotics don't need to be started unless a source of infection is found.

66. **(D)** Severe illnesses, such as myocardial infarction and sepsis, can cause DKA, as can dehydration. Also, patients with insulin-dependent diabetes mellitus should take insulin every day, even if oral intake of foods decreases.

67. **(B)** Patients usually are total body potassium-deficient and with correction of the acidosis can become very hypokalemic. If patients are kept on intravenous insulin and hydration without close monitoring, hypoglycemia and fluid overload can occur. Once patients are treated for DKA, they should be monitored closely to ensure that DKA does not recur. The treatment of DKA with insulin usually causes a hypophosphatemia, not hyperphosphatemia.

68. **(B)** Patients can continue to have some ketones in their serum and urine after DKA is corrected. Fluid status does not always correlate to correction of DKA. Accuchecks within normal limits can occur while the patient is still in DKA after treatment with hydration, so this should not be a measurement of when to stop intravenous insulin.

69. **(B)** The single most important factor for patients with chronic renal insufficiency is to slow down the progression of the disease by controlling the hypertension. ACE inhibitors (D) should be considered as a cause of acute renal failure, but did not cause renal failure in the patient in this question.

70. **(D)** It is best for you to talk to each individual separately, trying to maintain an open mind until you learn the truth. After all, it is possible the intern copied the write-up from the student. Whoever copied the document is at fault.

71. **(A)** This patient consumes large amounts of vegetables containing vitamin K. Vitamin K can negate the action of warfarin. The large dose of 12.5 mg of warfarin a day was adequate enough, but the effect of vitamin K on anticoagulation was detrimental. Thus, this patient was advised by a dietician to limit the amount of broccoli, brussels sprouts, and spinach he consumed. Cardioversion (B) is not effective in chronic atrial fibrillation. Cardioversion would be more useful if used in acute atrial fibrillation to convert to normal sinus rhythm. The risk of bleeding would be high with continued increases at the dose of warfarin (C) without counteracting the effect of vitamin K. The reason for the TIAs is embolism from atrial fibrillation and not from carotid artery thrombosis. Thus, performing a carotid endarterectomy (D) would be futile. Aspirin (E) is not as effective an anticoagulant as warfarin.

72. **(D)** In surveillance studies, 5-40% of women are rectal or vaginal carriers of group B streptococci. Almost half of the infants delivered vaginally from carrier mothers become colonized. One to two percent of these colonized infants develop clinically evident infection. Early onset infection, occurring within the first week of life, is characterized by respiratory distress, lethargy, and hypotension. Virtually 100% of infants with early onset infection are bacteremic (D). *Corynebacterium diptheriae* in an infant is unlikely, due to transplacental transfer of maternal IgC antitoxin (E). Group A streptococci were commonly implicated in puerperal sepsis in the preantibiotic era (A). *Candida albicans* is most likely to be isolated from an immunocompromised host (B). Predisposing factors for the development of *Mycobacterium avium intracellulare* include advanced age, collagen vascular disease, immunocompromised status, and underlying pulmonary disease. Pulmonary infection typically follows an indolent or slowly progressive course (C).

73. **(B)** Thirty to forty percent of infants with early onset group B streptococcal infection have meningitis. By contrast, meningitis occurring in 80-90% of infants presenting with late onset infection occurring from one week to three months of age.

74. **(C)** The incidence of group B streptococcal infection is increased in premature infants (A).

Prolonged labor, maternal fever, and chorio-amnionitis all increase the risk of infection [(B), (D), and (E)]. Prolonged rupture of the membranes for more than 18 hours also increases the risk of infection (C).

75. **(A)** Prophylactic administration of ampicillin (A) to high-risk women during delivery has been shown to prevent infection in the newborn [(A), (E), and (B)]. Indiscriminate use of antibiotics is not to be condoned, however, since the risk of adverse reactions to antibiotics outweighs the benefit to the infant (C). Vancomycin is used to treat infections in penicillin-allergic patients (D).

76. **(D)** This patient most likely has an elevation of his liver enzymes secondary to chronic alcohol use. His cirrhosis is also most likely secondary to alcohol use. A liver biopsy would not be the initial procedure in this case. It is an invasive procedure that is not needed at this time. This patient should be advised to stop drinking alcohol and subsequently come in for follow-up serum liver tests after discontinuation of alcohol. Any immunocompromised patient, such as alcoholics, diabetics, and dialysis patients, should have a baseline PPD and anergy panel skin test (A). If the test is positive (greater than 10 mm), than prophylactic isoniazid should be started to prevent active tuberculosis. This patient has elevation of liver function tests; therefore, isoniazid should be started cautiously if the PPD is positive. A baseline hepatitis B and C antigen and antibody test should be taken in any patient with elevation of liver transaminase (B). If the patient has a negative hepatitis B antibody status, then he should be given the hepatitis B vaccine. This patient should avoid Nyquil, Tylenol, and other over-the-counter medications that affect the liver (C). This patient should be encouraged to join an Alcoholics Anonymous self-help counseling group that would assist him in giving up alcoholic beverages (E).

77. **(E)** Only a small proportion of CMV-infected newborns will go on to develop the classic signs of CMV infection, which are microcephaly, chorioretinitis, deafness, hepatosplenomegaly (D), thrombocytopenia (B), and jaundice.

78. **(C)** The computed axial tomographic study of the abdomen demonstrates air in the biliary tree. In the absence of prior biliary tract surgery, this uncommon finding suggests a choledocho-duodenal fistula (C). There is no evidence of granulomatous disease in the liver (A). Metastatic lesions appear as one or more discreet lesions within the hepatic parenchyma, not within the biliary tract (B). Varices due to liver disease are typically esophageal or gastric (D). In polycystic liver disease, numerous cysts are apparent within the hepatic parenchyma (E).

79. **(C)** Panel A of the upper gastrointestinal series demonstrates a cholecystoduodenal fistula between the duodenal bulb and the gallbladder. In panel B, the biliary tree, the corkscrew-shaped cystic duct, and the common bile duct are also visualized (C). Gastric ulcers appear as craters on upper gastrointestinal X-rays. If the ulcer is present within a mass, it suggests a malignancy [(A) and (E)]. On upper gastrointestinal X-rays, typical duodenal ulcers appear as discrete craters in the proximal portion of the duodenal bulb. Chronic, recurrent ulcers may cause marked deformity of the bulb (B). There is no evidence of diverticular outpouchings of the duodenum (D). Incidentally, multiple radiolucent gallstones are also evident in the gallbladder.

80. **(A)** The most significant lesion demonstrated on these diagnostic studies is the cholecystoduodenal fistula, which requires surgical correction. Simultaneously, cholecystectomy should be performed to remove the remaining gallstones (A). Treatment of gallstones with ursodeoxycholic acid requires several years to completely dissolve all the stones. Patients must be selected carefully for this treatment (B). Extracorporeal shock wave lithotripsy is considered an experimental therapy for gallstones (C). There is no evidence of peptic ulcer disease on these studies [(D) and (E)].

81. **(E)** Uncomplicated acute cholecystitis is a clinical diagnosis, which has no specific plain abdominal radiographic findings. Ultrasound studies of the abdomen demonstrate gallstones in more than 90% of patients (E). Porcelain gallbladder refers to the eggshell appearance on X-rays, which result from the deposition of calcium in the fibrotic gallbladder wall (A). Air in the biliary tree, in the absence of prior biliary surgery or gas-producing organisms, suggests choledochoduodenal fistula (B). Limey bile, also known as milk of calcium bile, occurs when calcium precipitates, producing a diffuse, hazy opacification of bile or a layering effect on plain abdominal radiographs.

Although innocuous in itself, it commonly occurs in the setting of a hydropic gallbladder (C). Gallstone ileus commonly results when a large gallstone becomes impacted in the ileum, producing a mechanical obstruction (D).

82. **(C)** Nonketotic hyperosmolar coma is characterized by hyperosmolarity (>320 mOsmol/L), hyperglycemia (>600 mg/dL), and dehydration (C). Note that the glucose value in this case is presented in mmol/L, rather than mg/dL. Most often a complication of non-insulin-dependent diabetes, it represents a state of profound dehydration caused by hyperglycemic diuresis in situations where the affected person is unable to consume sufficient water (D). The lack of accompanying acidosis remains an enigma [(A) and (B)]. Drug overdose is unlikely to present with this degree of hyperosmolality and hyperglycemia (E).

83. **(D)** This patient's symptoms are classic for gastroesophageal reflux disease. Suggestions to decrease symptoms include decreasing alcohol usage, smaller meals, avoidance of foods before bedtime, antacids, elevation of the head when sleeping, and acid suppression medications.

84. **(B)** Any patient with an unknown neck injury should have the neck immobilized until the diagnosis is known. The patient should not be allowed to move the neck (A). He does not need immediate fusion (C) nor the placement of tongs (D). A cervical block to decrease pain should not be performed (E).

85. **(C)** A complete C-spine series should always be obtained prior to removal of a collar. There should also be absence of clinical symptoms. The cervical collar should not be removed any sooner (A), and the neck should not move (B). The patient should not go home with a soft collar (D) until the diagnosis is known. A steroid dose pack may not be necessary (E).

86. **(A)** There should always be lack of clinical findings prior to the removal. Remember, you are treating the patient, not the X-ray. Movement of extremities is only part of the criteria (D). Although we like to listen to our patients' wishes, we can't let them guide us to do something that may harm them (E).

87. **(C)** Embolization of cholesterol crystals occurs most often in elderly persons with widespread atherosclerosis. Renal insufficiency, hypertension, visual impairment, and gangrene of the extremities are common manifestations of cholesterol embolization. The histopathologic section of the amputated digit demonstrates an arteriole with characteristic needle-shaped clefts resulting from atheroemboli (C). There is no evidence of a vasculitis or inflammation on this slide (A). There is no evidence of infectious emboli (D). Although Gram-negative sepsis may produce multiorgan failure, this histologic picture is not compatible with that diagnosis (B).

88. **(B)** You should not order a test that you do not consider medically necessary just because a patient wants it done.

89. **(C)** Sodium fluoride improves bone-mineral density by stimulating osteoblasts. High doses of plain sodium fluoride have been shown to decrease spine fractures, but increase the incidence of new hip fractures by increasing bone fragility. Recently, slow-release sodium fluoride has been associated with an increased formation of normal bone. Alendronate (A) is a biphosphonate, which has been shown to decrease bone turnover and inhibit osteoclast activity. This drug is now available and approved by the FDA for treatment of postmenopausal osteoporosis. It is extremely important that there is adequate lighting (B) and fall-proof carpets and furniture along with adequate bathroom fixtures that can prevent future falls and fractures in this elderly female. Estrogen replacement (D) can protect postmenopausal women against osteoporosis and decrease the incidence of hip and spine fractures by 50% in some studies. Adding progesterone to estrogen decreases the incidence of endometrial carcinoma. Nasal salmon calcitonin (E) in a dose of 200 IU per day has been shown to increase bone-mineral density and reduce the rate of new fractures. Nausea and nasal dryness are some of the side effects of this new drug.

90. **(C)** Before you do anything further, you should ascertain if he intends to operate on patients that day.

91. **(A)** You should try to reason with him about his condition.

92. **(B)** Since he is not amenable to reason at this point, you need to notify others to keep him from operating on anyone.

93. **(D)** A physician who abuses any substance, including alcohol, is considered impaired.

94. **(E)** This patient has nephrolithiasis, or kidney stones, and he is in severe pain. Antibiotics are not necessary unless the stone causes obstruction of the ureters and subsequent kidney infection. There is no sign of infection because no white blood cells or leukocyte esterase are found in the urine sample. It is unusual for a male to obtain a urinary tract infection unless there is a structural abnormality involved. Intravenous hydration (A), along with pain medications such as Demerol, are the treatment of choice for acute nephrolithiasis. An IVP (B) would demonstrate if hydronephrosis is present and where the location of the stone is. Sometimes the stone would pass when the dye is introduced with the intravenous pyelogram. Renal sonogram (C) is a very useful noninvasive test to demonstrate the location of the stone and if obstruction is present. An elevation of the BUN and creatinine (D) would tell us if the kidney stone has done intrinsic damage to the kidneys. This is important in the prognosis of this disorder and to determine if surgical intervention is needed.

95. **(B)** Epidemiologic investigations show that epidemics of meningococcal disease directly correlate with low socioeconomic conditions. Thus, improvement of life standards leads to the reduced number of outbreaks. Vaccines (A), increased patient compliance (C), a lower patient/physician ratio (D), and lower cost of vaccinations (E) may prevent sporadic occurrences of the disease, but are less contributory to reducing the overall occurrence of epidemics from all pathogens combined.

96. **(B)** Among other medications, sulfa drugs can cause hemolytic anemia in patients with G6PD deficiency. The other mentioned medications haven't been shown to have the same problems.

97. **(B)** Retained CO_2 will lead to elevated levels and this, as well as decreased CO_2, are problems of ventilation (B). Oxygenation problems will lead to changes in O_2 (A).

98. **(B)** Mechanical ventilation on a ventilator would correct this woman's problem. The ventilator will take over the work of breathing. Sedation (A) will lead to an increased CO_2. Increasing (C) or decreasing (D) the inspired O_2 will change the oxygenation, not the ventilation. Incentive spirometry (E) is used to prevent atelectases by preventing alveolar collapse.

99. **(A)** The patient described appears to have pneumonia. Auscultation often reveals rales in the affected lung field. Bilateral wheezing is a more common finding in patients with asthma or congestive heart failure ("cardiac asthma") (B). Subcutaneous emphysema may present with crepitus over the anterior clavicle and is not a common finding in pneumonia (C). The ausculatory findings of pneumothorax include absent breath sounds and hyperresonance in the area of the collapsed lung (D). Although there may be normal breath sounds in patients with pneumonia, rales in the affected area are more common (E).

100. **(A)** The most common organism causing community-acquired pneumonia is the *Pneumococcus*. Gram stain reveals Gram-positive diplococci and chains. *S. aureus* is commonly seen as Gram-positive cocci in clusters. This organism is not as common a cause of community-acquired pneumonia as the *Pneumococcus* (B). Diptheroids are not common causes of pneumonia (C). Gram-negative organisms are more common in nosocomial pneumonia rather than community-acquired pneumonia (D). Acid-fast bacilli suggest tuberculous infection, a less common cause of community-acquired pneumonia (E).

101. **(A)** The patient should be treated with in-hospital intravenous antibiotics due to his age, fever, and tachypnea. Oxacillin is an active agent against most *S. aureus* organisms and should be used in this situation. There is a significant resistance of *S. aureus* to penicillin due to the ability of this organism to produce beta-lactamase (B). Intravenous vancomycin should be limited to cases of oxacillin-resistant *S. aureus* due to the increasing development of vancomycin-resistant organisms with injudicious use of this agent (C). Oral vancomycin is not well absorbed and is not effective for pneumonia (D). First-generation cephalosporins are active against *S. aureus;* however, intravenous antibiotics are indicated in the patient described (E).

102. **(E)** Pulmonary examination and X-ray findings lag behind clinical improvement and may take weeks to months before resolving. Therefore, management should be based on clinical improvement rather than improvement on X-ray. Malignancy is not yet a consideration based on a five-day interval chest X-ray (A). If there is clinical improvement, broadening of antibiotic coverage is not indicated (B). Daily chest X-rays are not indicated for management of community-acquired pneumonia (C). Open lung biopsy is not indicated based on these X-ray findings (D).

103. **(E)** Pleurodynia caused by coxsackievirus is often preceded by a nonspecific upper respiratory syndrome and presents as severe pleurisy.

104. **(D)** Testicular cancer reaches its peak in males in the third decade. Early diagnosis, as with other cancers, is vital in improved survival rates.

105. **(C)** This patient may be sufficiently depressed as to be unable to make sound judgments about her condition. Consulting with a psychiatrist is the proper thing to do.

106. **(A)** The patient is being properly treated. Her family needs to be informed of her condition.

107. **(D)** The patient's psychiatric condition appears to have changed. The psychiatrist needs to re-evaluate her.

108. **(C)** It is appropriate and mandatory in this case to call in another psychiatrist.

109. **(B)** Mild to moderate metastatic bone pain is manageable with first-line agents such as NSAIDs. Fentanyl (A), levorphanol (C), and leritine (D) are third-line agents, and hydrocodone (E) is a second-line agent on the World Health Organization's analgesic ladder.

110. **(C)** Patients with lupus who are subjected to excessive sun exposure can develop visceral flares, such as pancytopenia or even renal disease, due to the ultraviolet rays.

111. **(C)** Ingestion of excessive quantities of antacids and milk can cause hypercalcemia, especially in older people.

112. **(D)** In hemolysis, from any etiology, the bone marrow would try to compensate for the anemia and produce excess red blood cells, and thus reticulocytosis. This patient has antibody-induced Coomb's positive hemolysis, secondary to mycoplasma pneumonia infection. A low haptoglobin level (A) indicates active hemolysis by high protein binding to the red blood cells. Lactate dehydrogenase levels (B) would be elevated in hemolysis from cell lysis. Elevated potassium levels (C) would occur from cell lysis. The urate level (E) would be elevated from increased cell turnover.

113. **(C)** His weight loss is ominous because it has signified advanced disease affecting other organ systems. His voice (A) is a result of the local tumor, and hoarseness may result from a very early treatable disease. His age (B) is not a prognostic factor. The smoking and drinking (D) are risk factors and are not as important prognostically. Unless it was a rare environmental oral cancer that both husband and wife were exposed to, the wife's death (E) is noncontributory.

114. **(C)** A systolic ejection murmur is not associated with any local, regional, or metastatic spread of oral cancer. A soft palate lesion (A) can arise as a synchronous lesion. One must always inspect the local areas for other primary cancers. Cervical lymphadenopathy (B) signifies regional disease. Decreased breath sound (D) and hepatomegaly (E) can herald metastatic disease to the lungs and liver, respectively.

115. **(B)** Lingual thyroid is a round, smooth, red mass at the base of the tongue which arises from the remnants of the thyroglossal duct. Trauma (A) leads to a hyperkeratosis (E) of the mucosa, which appears leukoplakic. An aphthous ulcer (C), as well as lichen planus (D), are benign oral conditions that also appear as white or leukoplakic lesions.

116. **(C)** Stable, asymptomatic, calcified cysts do not require intervention, but should be monitored periodically (A). When technically feasible, expanding, infected, or symptomatic cysts are best treated by *in toto* excision. Isolation and killing of the cysts with hypertonic saline or scolicidal agents, such as iodophor or ethanol, is necessary

prior to excision in order to prevent secondary spread of cysts (B). Hypernitremia or ethanol intoxication may result from this therapy [(C) and (D)]. Leakage of fluid at the time of surgery may result in anaphylaxis (E).

117. **(D)** Tracheoesophageal fistulas are a potential complication of lung cancer and esophageal cancer. They should be suspected when a patient with known lung or esophageal cancer presents with recurrent pneumonia or bronchitis, respiratory failure, or symptoms of reflux with aspiration. Reflux disease (A) may cause symptoms of cough, asthma, and, therefore, shortness of breath. However, they are not typically associated with meals; they may occur after a meal while in a recumbent position. A patient with CHF (B) may present with this, however, not typically solely with eating. Pneumocystis pneumonia (C) is an HIV-associated illness.

118. **(C)** Although bronchoscopy (A) and esophagoscopy (B) may contribute to the diagnosis, tracheoesophageal fistula is most easily confirmed by an esophagram. Bronchoscopy has limitations in visualizing fistulas and may miss some. However, it can often detect airway invasion by tumor and extrinsic compression of the lumen; both can suggest fistulization. Endoscopy has similar limitations as bronchoscopy.

119. **(A)** Prolonged intubation can lead to abnormalities of the posterior wall of the trachea, thus eroding into the esophagus and leading to tracheoesophageal fistulization (TEF). Other risk factors include trauma, Wegener's granulomatosis, infections in immunocompromised hosts, mycobacterial (fungal and viral), and esophageal carcinoma, particularly after radiotherapy. Stenting of the esophagus for luminal obstruction has also been known to be complicated by TEF. (B), (C), and (D) are not known to be associated with TEF.

120. **(D)** Esophagectomy alone is risky and is associated with an unreasonably high mortality and morbidity. Esophageal stenting (A) appears to be the safest, most effective, and best-tolerated procedure. The expandable coated metal stents are the least technically challenging of all stents. However, they are associated with a reasonably high morbidity. (B) would allow for reasonable

palliation; however, the patient's saliva may produce respiratory problems and would be less satisfactory to the patient. (C) has been done and is technically difficult. There is no advantage over esophageal stenting. (E) will provide palliation, but the least patient satisfaction.

121. **(C)** N-acetylcysteine is a specific antidote for acetaminophen hepatotoxicity by serving as a glutathione substitute in detoxifying hepatotoxic metabolites. It should be used for any acetaminophen overdose with a toxic serum acetaminophen level within the first 24 hours after ingestion. It is especially effective if used within the first eight hours after ingestion.

122. **(C)** The treatment for trichomoniasis is oral metronidazole (B). The presence of trichomonads shows that the patient has been having unprotected sexual intercourse (A), and that testing and counseling about sexually transmitted diseases is necessary [(D) and (E)].

123. **(D)** Less than 5% of falls result in hip fractures. A low body mass index, thin body habitus, and low bone mineral density at the femoral neck can all predispose to a hip fracture after a fall. Osteoporosis is a major public health concern; it affects more than 25 million American men and women (A). The aim of primary prevention is to achieve optimal bone mass at maturity and maintain bone mass in adulthood so that fractures can be prevented after a fall. Prevention of falls (B) can occur through exercise and rehabilitation programs. Exercise fitness programs and musculoskeletal rehabilitation programs can improve skeletal strength and decrease the risk of falling. Lack of estrogen in postmenopausal women (C), low body mass index, low bone mineral density and thinness can all contribute to an increased incidence of hip fractures after a fall. About 50% of fall injuries occur in and around the house. Biphosphonates, such as etidronate and alendronate, can decrease osteoclastic activity and, thus, decrease bone resorption. They have been shown to slow down the progression of osteoporosis along with estrogen, calcium, sodium fluoride, and nasal calcitonin (E). Optimal vitamin D intake maximizes the absorption of calcium from the gastrointestinal tract and, thus, appears effective in limiting bone loss.

124. **(E)** The infant has fever without a focus. It usually has an acute onset and should persist for no more than one week. It is a pediatric disease and occurs in infants who are under two years of age. Typically, history and physical examination are unrevealing.

125. **(D)** The cause of the disease is a microbial agent, which is identifiable in most cases and is responsible for an occult bacteremia.

126. **(C)** The most likely microorganism that causes the occult bacteremia is *Streptococcus pneumoniae*. It is identifiable in about 65% of cases. In the remaining cases, the occult bacteremia is associated with *Haemophilus influenzae* type b and *Neisseria meningitidis*.

127. **(B)** An infant under two years of age with a temperature > 40°C, severe leukopenia (i.e., WBCs < 5,000/mm^3) or severe leukocytosis (i.e., WBCs > 15,000/mm^3), and positive exposure history without lateralizing signs and symptoms is most likely experiencing fever with no focus.

128. **(C)** Management of fever with no focus includes keeping in touch with the infant's parents, repeating examinations, using antibiotics cautiously, and using acetaminophen if antipyretic therapy is considered. Blood cultures should be obtained prior to the rise in temperature.

129. **(D)** Febrile seizures may last as long as 15 minutes. They are tonic-clonic in character, with no focal signs. Only a small proportion of infants with febrile convulsions develop epilepsy in later life. It is common between the ages of six months and five years.

130. **(D)** Fever of unknown origin is a diagnostic entity that must be distinguished from the fever with no focus. By definition, fever must persist for at least one week and must be documented in a hospital setting. Regardless of all possible investigations, no origin is identified.

131. **(E)** Prophylactic antibiotic treatment in presumptive bacteremia is controversial. It is often up to a treating physician to include or exclude antibiotics from the treatment plan of fever in a child who is experiencing occult bacteremia.

132. **(C)** Rheumatoid arthritis has multisystem organ involvement, but the pancreas is not usually affected. Hoarseness, pain radiating to the ears, speech discomfort, and a sensation of illness in the throat are all manifestations of laryngeal involvement in rheumatoid arthritis. Arthritis of the cricoarytenoid joints (A) leading to narrowing of the glottis and fixed adduction of the vocal cords can occur and lead to problems during endotracheal intubation during anesthesia. Felty's syndrome is a form of rheumatoid arthritis associated with both splenomegaly and leukopenia (B). The upper cervical spine (D) may be affected by rheumatoid arthritis. Cardiovascular disease (E) is in the form of pericarditis or coronary arteritis, is seen in some patients with rheumatoid arthritis, but rarely results in serious conditions such as cardiac tamponade, angina pectoris, or myocardial infarction.

133. **(D)** Severe salicylate intoxication unresponsive to other treatment in children is an indication for hemodialysis. Overdoses of tricyclic antidepressants (A), digitalis (B), and opiates (C) are not treated by dialysis. Methemoglobinemia (E) also is not an indication for hemodialysis.

134. **(D)** Malaria prevention is possibly the most important consideration for travelers, because malaria is common throughout the tropical and subtropical regions of the world and because infections with *Plasmodium falciparum* are frequently fatal in nonimmune persons. Chloroquine-resistant *P. falciparum* is now found in all malarious areas around the world. Therefore, mefloquine (C), and not chloroquine (D), is now recommended as prophylaxis for malaria prevention in travelers. Use of mosquito repellent (B), mosquito netting (A), and wearing long-sleeve shirts and pants (E) are also recommended to prevent mosquito bites.

135. **(E)** This patient has just returned from an endemic area where malaria and typhoid fever are common infections. Blood (A) and stool (B) cultures should be taken immediately to verify salmonella typhi sepsis, and intravenous hydration (D) should be instituted because this patient could be volume-depleted from poor appetite and high fevers. The thick and thin blood film after staining with Giemsa stains should be reviewed

under the microscope to look for red blood cells infested with parasites if malaria is suspected (C). A chest X-ray is not needed at this point in time, because this patient has no respiratory symptoms, such as cough and pleuritic chest pain.

136. **(D)** Human diploid (killed virus) vaccine is infrequently recommended to travelers unless the risk of pre-exposure is very high. This patient is going to be stationed in an agricultural environment, and thus the pre-exposure risk of being bitten by a rabid animal is small. Thus, it would not be prudent at this time to recommend a rabies vaccine. Water and food are common vehicles for many of the pathogens acquired by travelers to developing nations, and all the necessary precautions should be taken (E). Hepatitis A vaccine is now available and should be given to travelers going to endemic areas (C). Chronic hepatitis B is potentially fatal, and this vaccine should be given in scheduled three doses prior to travelling (A). Typhoid fever (B) is common in India, and it is acquired by ingestion of dairy products, cold food, and eggs. An oral typhoid vaccine is available (attenuated bacteria), and it is good for up to five years.

137. **(D)** A family history is not likely to help explain the patient's recent deterioration, although it should be obtained as part of a complete history.

138. **(A)** Polymyositis is characterized by proximal muscle weakness. The other conditions can occur in the presence of normal muscle strength.

139. **(C)** Though nonspecific, the sedimentation rate is nearly always elevated in the disease that this patient has. The absence of an elevation essentially rules out this condition.

140. **(D)** This patient's disease is most consistent with polymyalgia rheumatica, with an elevated sedimentation rate, constitutional symptoms, proximal muscle tenderness without weakness, and weight loss.

141. **(C)** Septic shock (A), hyperthyroidism (B), malignant hyperthermia (D), and insulin shock (E) will all present with tachycardia, widened pulse pressure, and moist skin. The opposite is seen with hypothyroidism (C) where the body is acting "slowed down" rather than "speeded up."

142. **(B)** Decreased sweating will not be seen here. Rather, signs of increased metabolism will be seen, such as increased sweating (A), increased appetite (C), weight loss (D), and frequent bowel movements (E).

143. **(C)** Liver-function tests would not give you as much useful information as the others. An SMA-7 (A) will tell you about electrolytes, BUN, creatinine, and glucose, and it may give you information about insulin shock. The CBC with differential (B) may give you information regarding sepsis or anemia. Thyroid-function tests (D) will tell you about the thyroid and the possibility of hyperthyroidism or hypothyroidism. The EKG (E) will tell you about the heart and any sympathetic effects on it.

144. **(D)** You suspect hyperthyroidism because of the abnormal test results and presenting symptoms. With hyperthyroidism, there is conjunctival injection due to excessive adrenergic stimulation.

145. **(E)** Exercising and modifying certain risk factors, such as smoking and a high-cholesterol diet, are considered to be the major contributions to declining mortality rates among high-risk groups. Death rates from heart disease continued to decrease over the past 30 years (A). Health education (C) is certainly very important, but it is not the best choice for this problem. The proportion of the chronically ill elderly (D) has been increased and continues to increase due to improved life conditions, improved pharmacology, and high technology.

146. **(C)** Testing for concomitant chlamydial infection and gonorrhea is indicated in persons who regularly attend clinics for the treatment of sexually transmitted diseases. Chlamydial infection is more common in women, whereas men are more frequently asymptomatic carriers.

147. **(C)** Persons with multiple sexual partners are always at higher risk for developing both gonococcal and chlamydial infections. As a general rule, when screening for gonorrhea, it is advisable to screen for the presence of chlamydial infection, as well.

148. **(A)** Syphilis has a long latent period and, therefore, it is prevalent in prostitutes who are

likely to continue their life-style for many years. Their choice for multiple sexual partners places them at a higher than normal risk for developing gonococcal infection.

149. **(E)** Although HIV infection is still a major risk in homosexual men, it is not listed as one of the choices. Given the serious nature of the disease and associated life-threatening complications, screening for HSV is indicated in all homosexual and bisexual men.

150. **(E)** Breathing problems will not affect a noninsulin-dependent diabetic. However, ocular problems and retinopathy will occur and, therefore, vision (A) must be assessed. Common problems with the three "polys" occur with diabetics; specifically—polyphagia, polydipsia, and polyuria. Therefore, changes in appetite (B), thirst (C), and voiding (D) are important.

151. **(D)** An EKG would be a good screen because diabetics often have coronary artery disease and silent myocardial infarctions. A CBC (A), pulmonary function tests (B), liver function tests (C), and a chest X-ray (E) may be ordered as the exam dictates, but for a screening test they are not initially appropriate.

152. **(D)** A transudate of pleural effusion by definition has a protein <2.5 g/dL. An exudate represents a protein content >3.0 g/dL.

153. **(D)** A transudate may result from CHF (A), nephrotic syndrome (B), cirrhosis (C), and advanced liver disease (E). It does not arise from infection. An infection results in an exudate, as does a malignant state, pneumothorax, chest trauma, or pneumonia.

154. **(D)** The goal in diabetes control should be to keep the hemoglobin A1c level below 8%. By the time one presents with symptoms of type II diabetes (A), some end-organ damage has been done. The diabetes control and complications trail (B) has been one of the largest diabetes trails in the nation. It showed that tight control of glucose will result in slow progression of retinopathy and nephropathy. Diabetes is a strong risk factor for myocardial infarction (C), stroke, peripheral vascular disease, and generalized atherosclerosis. Three to five percent of the United States population have diabetes. Sixteen million people (diag-

nosed and undiagnosed) have diabetes. Diabetes is two to five times more common in minorities. Sixty to seventy percent of all diabetics are non-insulin-dependent (E) and 10% are juvenile onset diabetics.

155. **(C)** A premature ventricular contraction occurs with an early beat arising within the ventricle. P-waves may be present, but are unrelated to the QRS complex of the early beat.

156. **(B)** Sinus bradycardia is a sinus rhythm with a ventricular rate of less than 60 beats per minute.

157. **(D)** Ventricular tachycardia, or V Tach, is the presence of three or more PVCs (premature ventricular contractions) in a row.

158. **(E)** First-degree block occurs when the PR interval of the beat is greater than 0.2 seconds.

159. **(A)** Atrial flutter appears as sawtooth waves with an atrial rate of between 250 and 350 beats per minute and a variable ventricular rate.

160. **(C)** A gibbus is the protruding angle seen from collapse of one or more vertebral bodies. A singultus (A) is a hiccup. A torus (B) is an exostosis of the maxilla or mandible. A tragus (D) is a cartilaginous projection in front of the ear. A conus (E) is an anatomic term for a cone, such as the conus orbitalis.

161. **(D)** AIDS does not lead to kyphosis. Pott's disease (A) or TB of the bodies may, as it leads to weakening and compression. Compression fracture (B) obviously will lead to a kyphosis. Syphilis (C) and neoplasm (E) will lead to compression, as there is invasion in both, leading to a weakening and collapse of the bodies.

162. **(C)** First-line therapy for asthma is inhaled corticosteroids. If someone is very ill, systemic steroids may be needed; however, in this patient, the mild symptoms warrant inhaled corticosteroids.

163. **(B)** The computed tomographic scan of the abdomen demonstrates gas in the portal venous system (B). The stomach is partially filled with contrast and partially filled with gas (A). The spleen is present (C). There is no evidence of a

carcinoma of the colon or an aortic aneurysm on this section [(D and (E)].

164. **(A)** The intravenous pyelogram illustrates radiolucent filling defects in the renal pelvis. In inflammatory bowel disease, radiolucent uric acid stones are associated with dehydration in persons with diarrhea or ileostomies (A). Calcium oxalate stones are associated with steatorrhea (B). Obstructive uropathies may result from inflammatory masses compressing the ureter (C). Ileal-sigmoid bladder fistulas may produce sterile pyuria (D). Rarely, amyloidosis may complicate long-standing chronic inflammation (E).

165. **(B)** When a patient presents with *Streptococcus bovis* endocarditis, he/she needs to undergo colonoscopy to screen for colon cancer.

166. **(A)** Laproscopic procedures are notorious for having a high incidence of postoperative nausea. Although the exact etiology is uncertain, it is thought to be caused by intra-abdominal organ distention and peritoneal stretching produced by the carbon dioxide used to inflate the peritoneal cavity.

167. **(D)** According to the Department of Health and Human Services, in 1987, the estimated share of government expenditures on health care constituted 41%. HMOs and other forms of health insurance paid for 31%, while on-site payments or self-pay was 26%.

168. **(E)** The prevalence rate is equal to the number of existing cases at a single moment of time, divided by the population at the same moment. It is not to be confused with incidence rate (C) or period prevalent rate (B). Answer choices (A) and (D) do not represent an epidemiological value.

169. **(C)** A nodular umbilicus is known as Sister Mary Joseph's nodule and is significant for abdominal carcinoma, especially gastric carcinoma, which may metastasize to the navel. An umbilical hernia (A) may present with a reducible or non-reducible mass around the umbilicus. An aortic aneurysm (B) may present as a pulsatile abdominal mass. Fecal impaction (D) may present as a tender, solid abdomen. An ileus (E) may present with tympany and absent or decreased bowel sounds.

170. **(B)** If the patient is mentally competent and understands what you are telling her, all you can ethically do is try to convince her to change her mind. Since her refusal to obtain treatment does not allow a contagious disease to spread in this case, you cannot tell anyone else in her environment about her condition without her permission (A). You could, however, ask one of your colleagues to give her his/her opinion.

171. **(D)** This patient has hypercholesterolemia and a strong family history of coronary artery disease. He also manifests signs of hypercholesterolemia such as tuberous xanthomas and arcus senilis. This patient should immediately be started on a lipid-lowering regimen, which includes the statin drugs such as pravastatin and lovastatin (HMG-CoA reductase inhibitors). These drugs work by inhibiting the rate-limiting step in the production of cholesterol in the liver. Pravastatin sodium has been shown to reduce the risk of a first myocardial infarction by 31%. Keeping the patient on a low cholesterol diet (A) is helpful also, but it cannot be the only choice of treatment in the initial management of this patient because of his high risk profile of coronary disease. Biopsy (B) of the xanthoma would only reveal cholesterol plaques, and this would not give us any other information that can aid in the management of this patient. Allopurinol (C) is the treatment of choice for hyperuricemia and tophaceous gout, which can mimic xanthomas. Gemfibrozil and niacin (E) can both lower the serum triglyceride levels, but they are not ideal to lower the serum LDL and serum cholesterol levels. These two drugs combined can, in rare instances, cause myopathy.

172. **(B)** Arachnodactyly is characterized by long, slender fingers and hyperextendable joints. It is seen in Marfan's syndrome. Mongoloid hand (C) is characterized by short digits and is seen in trisomy 21 or Down's syndrome. Trident hand (D) occurs in achrondroplasia, and the fingers are short and almost equal in length. The index and middle fingers are widely separated. Claw hand (E) is a configuration of the hand seen with types of paralysis.

173. **(C)** Arachnodactyly may be seen in Marfan's syndrome. Down's syndrome (A) may have an associated Mongoloid hand. Cerebral palsy (B) may have an associated claw hand. Carpel tunnel

syndrome (E) may show signs of median nerve compression such as thenar wasting and a positive Tinel's sign or Phalen's sign.

174. **(B)** Marfan's syndrome is passed on as an autosomal dominant trait.

175. **(B)** The skull in Marfan's syndrome is long and narrow, not short and wide. Other characteristics include the fused vertebrae (A), a high arched palate (C), elongation of the globe (D), and deformities of the cardiac valve cusps (E).

176. **(A)** Vaginitis is characteristic of tenderness of the walls of the vagina and a discharge. Bartholinitis (B) is inflammation of the Bartholin's glands. A colpocele (C) is vaginal prolapse. Cystocele (D) is bladder prolapse. Rectocele (E) is rectal prolapse.

177. **(E)** This patient has pernicious anemia secondary to vitamin B12 deficiency and, thus, he has anemia and an elevated mean corpuscular volume. An antibody binds to the parietal cell in the stomach, which prevents vitamin B12 from being absorbed in the small intestine. This is an autoimmune process.

178. **(C)** This patient has been on procainamide for an extended period of time. This drug has been known to cause drug-induced lupus. Drug-induced lupus causes arthralgias and pleural effusions. Hydralazine can also cause drug-induced lupus-like syndrome. Usually, drug-induced lupus is not associated with renal disease, and it is associated with the anti-histone antibody.

179. **(D)** This patient has classic symptoms of primary biliary cirrhosis, which is associated with inflammation of the small intrahepatic bile ducts and is an autoimmune process. It occurs mainly in middle-aged women and is associated with an elevated cholesterol level, elevated bilirubin level, and nighttime pruritus. Xanthomas are also present. Therapy includes rifampin, cholestyramine, or ursodeoxycholic acid. The definitive cure is a liver transplant. The antimitochondrial antibody titer is elevated in primary biliary cirrhosis.

180. **(B)** This patient has Wegener's granulomatoses, which is a necrotizing vasculitis. This disorder is more common in men. It is usually preceded by an upper respiratory tract infection in 90% of cases. Wegener's granulomatoses is associated with both pulmonary and renal disease and the treatment of choice is cyclophosphamide. The antinuclear cytoplasmic antibody titer would be elevated in patients with this disorder, and the titers would fall when the disease abates.

USMLE Step 3 – Practice Test 3
Day One – Afternoon Session

1. **(D)** This patient has irritable bowel syndrome, which is a functional disorder rather than an infectious or structural cause for diarrhea. Ampicillin should not be used because no documented infection has been the etiology for this disorder. Ampicillin impairs colonic fermentation of carbohydrates, resulting in higher stool weight and greater stool frequency and a greater percentage of unformed stool. Dietary intervention (A) can be helpful in irritable bowel syndrome patients in one-third of the cases. Restricting intake of sugars and gasogenic foods can alleviate symptoms, and generally rice, chicken, and lamb are well tolerated in these patients. Antispasmodic agents (B) such as dicyclomine hydrochloride and hyoscyamine sulfate may help the symptoms of cramping. Patients who are anxious and depressed have a high prevalence of this disorder. Thus, studies have shown that psychologic therapy, behavioral modification, and even antidepressants are useful for this disorder (C). The patient should be reassured that the disorder is benign. Fiber supplementation (E) is useful if the clinical spectrum of the disorder is constipation and not diarrhea.

2. **(B)** This patient most likely has pneumocystis pneumoniae carinii infection because he is immunocompromised, and the treatment of choice would be intravenous trimethoprim-sulfamethoxazole and oxygen. An elevation of the A-a gradient, an elevation of the LDH, and bilateral interstitial infiltrates on an X-ray suggest PCP. Intravenous penicillin (A) is used to treat penicillin-sensitive Strep, pneumoniae, or severe Strep throat infection. Penicillin is not a good antibiotic of choice because of the emergence of penicillin-resistant organisms. A bronchial lavage and transbronchial biopsy (C) would be a diagnostic tool to identify the organism responsible for the pneumonia, but it is not useful for treatment. Intravenous Ganciclovir (D) would be useful to treat cytomegalovirus pneumonia, but the initial presumptive diagnosis in an immunocompromised individual should be PCP first. CMV pneumonia should first be diagnosed by a transbronchial biopsy before treatment is initiated. Steroids (E) are given in conjunction with intravenous trimethoprim-sulfamethoxazole if the patient is severely hypoxic with PCP.

3. **(C)** This patient has endometriosis, which is associated with implantation of the endometrial tissue on the pelvic viscera and other remote sites such as the GI tract, pulmonary system, and even the urinary tract system. Usually the patients are premenopausal and have cyclic, recurrent symptoms. Endometrial implants can migrate by direct extension, hematogenous routes, or by lymphatic channels. It tends to be a highly familial disease. After an initial pelvic examination is performed, a definitive diagnosis of endometriosis is made in 90% of cases by laparoscopy. This will give a tissue biopsy of the lesion and confirm the diagnosis. Endometriosis is a common cause of infertility in young women. An ultrasound of the pelvis (A) can identify solid or cystic lesions in the pelvis, but it offers no etiology of the masses, which can be neoplasms, fibromas, or benign lesions. A CT scan (B) or MRI is useful to evaluate adenomyosis, but neither imaging studies offer significant information in women who have endometriosis. Serum CA-125 is useful to screen women for ovarian carcinoma, and it is under investigation as a test to monitor therapy in patients with endometriosis. It has a very low sensitivity and specificity for diagnosis of this disorder. Serum markers, such as antiendometrial antibody test (PP14) (E), are currently being investigated as a potential tool to screen for endometriosis.

4. **(D)** It's impossible to make any assessment of a patient's status until the temperature is brought back to body temperature.

5. **(C)** This patient has acute hepatitis A infection, which is self limiting and associated with malaise and anorexia. This infection is acquired by the fecal-oral route, such as contaminated shellfish. This viral infection has no chronicity and thus

the only treatment is rest, hydration, and vitamins until the symptoms resolve. Interferon alpha (A) is the treatment of choice for chronic hepatitis B infection. This drug is given subcutaneously and has been shown to decrease the viral load and prevent relapse. Once interferon therapy is discontinued, the alanine transaminase levels start to increase again. This patient does not have hepatitis B because she is protected by the hepatitis B antibody. Steroids (B) will exacerbate this infection and prevent recovery. Steroids are only indicated in lupoid autoimmune hepatitis, which is common in lupus patients. The hepatitis B vaccine (D) is given in three doses at zero, two, and six months. It is a preventive step given to patients who are hepatitis B surface-antibody negative and who are at risk for developing hepatitis B infection—such as health care workers. This patient has already had the hepatitis B surface-antibody protection and therefore does not need the vaccine. Liver biopsy (E) is only indicated in chronic hepatitis B or chronic hepatitis C infection to see how much damage has been done.

6. **(B)** This patient has disseminated MAC infection, which is associated with a T-cell count below 50 in HIV individuals. The treatment of choice is any number of combinations of drugs such as cipronoxacin, ethambutol, rifampin, and clarithromycin. Any drug given alone will lead to resistance. Sulfadiazine and pyrimethamine in combination (A) are useful for life-long treatment of CNS toxoplasmosis encephalitis. Another new macrolide, azithromycin (C), given alone, has been shown in one study to be used for prophylaxis, and not treatment, of MAI infection. Clarithromycin (D) alone has been shown to rapidly induce resistance in the prophylaxis for MAI infection. Thus, this macrolide should be used in combination with rifabutin or other medications. Isoniazid, pyrazidamide, ethambutol, and rifampin (E) have been used for the treatment of mycoplasma tuberculosis and not *Mycobacterium avium* infection.

7. **(B)** Patients of legal age may give consent for themselves. In general, no person may consent on behalf of another person unless the patient is a nonemancipated minor or a legally incompetent person. Consent given by a relative has no legal validity. If the competent patient of legal age is unconscious and his or her condition is life-threatening, medical care should be given assuming that the patient would have consented had he or she been able to do so.

8. **(D)** The study should be large enough to avoid random error, while only relatively few people undergo autopsy. Therefore, a possibility of random error is obvious. Selection bias (A) would have made this conclusion invalid if only selected people were investigated. The t-test (B) is used to compare the means of two small ($n<30$) samples or groups. Lead-time bias (C) refers to an increase in survival rates of people who are diagnosed by screening procedures. The ecologic fallacy (E) occurs when associations among groups of subjects are mistakenly assumed to hold for individuals. Conversely, random error is made when findings in a small sample are assumed to hold true for the whole population.

9. **(B)** Atelectasis, collapse of the alveoli, occurs with postoperative patients undergoing anesthesia. It can be prevented by incentive spirometry. It will usually cause a fever in the early post-op course. Wound infection (A), unless streptococcus, usually occurs two to three days post-op. A urinary tract infection (C) occurs several days post-op and usually only with retention or with prolonged catheterization. Phlebitis (D) also occurs several days post-op and usually in patients that have not been ambulating. Pharyngitis (E) is unlikely to occur in a post-op patient as a result of either the surgery or the anesthesia.

10. **(D)** This patient has a nosocomial, iatrogenic pneumonia acquired in the intensive care unit and it is probably secondary to a Gram-negative organism. Clindamycin is an antibiotic that covers Gram-positive organisms and anaerobes. Less than five percent of pneumonias in a mechanically ventilated patient are due to anaerobes. Thus, clindamycin would be an inappropriate treatment. The other 25% of organisms can be from anaerobes secondary to aspiration or polymicrobial organisms, which are resistant to beta-lactams (A). *Pseudomonas* is the most virulent Gram-negative organism and requires combination therapy. Even the best single agents alone (cipro) have an unacceptable rate of failure and, thus, dual therapy is best (B). *Pseudomonas* is a highly lethal organism and the mortality rate of ventilator-associated pneumonias with pseudomonas is high. Sinusitis and catheter-related infections should also not be overlooked in the

intensive care unit. Tracheal colonization with pathogenic bacteria occurs in 75% of cases, and tracheal aspiration with cultures (E) has a good diagnostic yield.

11. **(A)** Madelung's deformity is a dorsal angulation of the wrist caused by a dorsal subluxation of the distal end of the ulna. It is usually seen in adolescent girls. It is not caused by a volar angulation of the wrist (B), nor is it caused by any dorsal (C), radial (D), or ulnar (E) deviation of the elbow.

12. **(C)** Hypertrophic obstructive cardiomyopathy is characterized by left ventricular hypertrophy with the asymmetrically hypertrophied interventricular septum. The latter is responsible for obstructive signs and elevated diastolic filling pressure. Additional signs and symptoms include dyspnea on exertion, angina, a brisk carotid upstroke with pulsus bisferans, S4, and a blowing murmur of mitral regurgitation. Murmurs change with changing positions and Valsalva maneuver. ECG shows left ventricular hypertrophy with prominent Q-waves in leads I, aVL, and V5-6. In addition to beta-adrenergic blockers, the treatment plan should include verapamil and disopyramide. Positive inotropic agents (e.g., digoxin), diuretics (A), and vasodilators (e.g., nitrates) (D) would aggravate the pathophysiology of this condition and, therefore, are contraindicated.

13. **(C)** With myasthenia gravis, there is an autoantibody binding of acetylcholine receptors at the neuromuscular junction. There is increased fatigue (A), weakness (B), abnormal speech (D), and ptosis (E). The weakness is relieved, not worsened, by neostigmine injections.

14. **(D)** Twenty-five percent of patients with mid-trimester bleeding will have placenta previa (A) or abruptio placenta (B). Placenta previa is an attachment of the placenta to the lower uterine segment. Abruptio placenta is the premature separation of the placenta. Also, slight bleeding through the vagina is common during active labor (C) and may indicate premature labor in this patient. Placenta accreta (D) is attachment of the placenta directly to the myometrium. The decidual layer is defective. It is manifested clinically by impaired placental separation, sometimes with massive hemorrhage after delivery, not before delivery as in this patient.

15. **(D)** Colonic diverticulitis presents with left lower quadrant pain. Acute appendicitis (A), Meckel's diverticulitis (B), regional ileitis (C), and a perforated duodenal ulcer (E) all present with acute right lower quadrant pain.

16. **(D)** Although the possible side effects of amiodarone include hepatic and pulmonary toxicity and thyroid dysfunction, it usually does not involve the bone marrow.

17. **(E)** This patient has an acute sickle cell crisis, probably secondary to a viral infection. The latest data reveals that hydroxyurea, which is a chemotherapeutic drug, can prevent crises from recurring because this drug increases the fetal hemoglobin in the blood. This drug is used for chronic, long-term use and not in an acute crisis situation. Oxygen (A) is supplemented to increase the oxygen content and the oxygen saturation. This will alleviate tissue ischemia and decrease the symptom of dyspnea. Whole blood transfusions (B) will increase the hematocrit and decrease the severity of the anemia. This anemia is from hemolysis from sickling of the red blood cells. Transfusions will alleviate the shortness of breath also. The mainstay of treatment is to start intravenous hydration (C) as soon as possible to decrease the stasis of the sickling red blood cells in the joint spaces and increase circulation. These patients are usually in severe pain and, thus, they need subcutaneous or intramuscular Demerol or morphine (D) to relieve the painful crisis.

18. **(B)** *Ecthyma gangrenosum* is considered to be pathognomonic of pseudomonas septicemia. These purple-black lesions begin as bullae or hemorrhagic pustules and evolve into necrotic ulcers. It is associated with a poor prognosis and usually occurs in immunocompromised individuals. Tissue culture after skin biopsy can make the diagnosis. *Pyoderma gangrenosum* (A) is associated with ulcerative colitis and presents as weeping, purulent lesions, usually on the lower extremities. Necrotizing vasculitis lesions (C) also present as cutaneous ulcers. They can be secondary to Wegener's granulomatosus or polyalteritis nodosa. These patients are usually not neutropenic or have pseudomonas bacteremia. Cryoglobinemia (D) usually presents as palpable purpura and is secondary to a vasculitis reaction. Eschars and bullous lesions are not usually present. Erythema multiforme (E) usually pre-

sents as target lesions of the skin. It is secondary to a drug reaction or infection with *Mycoplasma pneumoniae*. Skin biopsy would reveal heavy infiltration with neutrophil and eosinophil leucocytes. The small blood vessels are dilated and surrounded by lymphocytes.

19. **(D)** This patient has an exacerbation of COPD, and his chest X-ray reveals no evidence of an underlying pneumonia. Thus, antibiotics are not necessary and would not alleviate the patient's immediate symptoms. Steroids (A) are very effective and have been shown to decrease the inflammatory component of asthma and COPD and, thus, decrease the smooth muscle edema in the bronchioles. Bronchodilators (B) via nebulizers or metered-dose inhalers are the main treatment in COPD to dilate the airways in bronchospasm. This alleviates the immediate symptoms of wheezing and shortness of breath. Ipratropium bromide (C) is an anticholinergic drug which is especially useful in COPD patients. This drug also relieves the airway edema and decreases the inflammatory component to a certain extent. Theophylline (E) is not used often anymore, but some physicians still keep the patient on this medication. It is said that theophylline can help the diaphragm contract better and more efficiently. Theophylline or aminophylline levels need to be checked routinely to prevent toxic levels from accumulating.

20. **(D)** Impedance plethysmography is readily available in most outpatient settings and is revealing in most cases with deep venous thrombosis. It can be used either to establish the diagnosis or increase the index of suspicion regarding the diagnosis of deep venous thrombosis. Plethysmography is a very sensitive test and is used to detect proximal deep vein thrombi. Pulmonary angiography (B) is the gold standard procedure in the presence of strong clinical suspicion for pulmonary embolism and in the absence of contributory results on V/Q scan. Radionuclide scanning (C) is very sensitive and is performed for detecting thromboemboli in the calves. Pelvic vein ultrasound (E) is not currently very common in the diagnostic evaluation of deep venous thrombosis. Instead, ascending venography is regarded as the gold standard for the diagnosis of deep venous thrombosis and is performed in a hospital setting.

21. **(C)** Shown here in pulsus alternans, pulse waves alternate between those of greater and lesser volume, occurring in conditions of a weakened myocardium, such as cardiomyopathy. Although pulsus alternans often follows an atrial or ventricular premature beat, the cardiac rhythm, as well as the interval between beats, is normal (C). This must be distinguished from pulsus bigeminus, in which the intervals between beats of the couplet are shorter than the time between pairs (A). At rest, there is normally an inspiratory fall of less than 10 mm Hg in the arterial systolic pressure and an accompanying inspiratory fall in venous pressure, usually not detectable on physical examination. In pulsus paradoxus, the inspiratory decrease in arterial pressure exceeds 10 mm Hg, and the inspiratory venous pressure remains steady or increases. These exaggerated changes are usually detectable by palpation. Such changes are significant only if they occur during normal cardiac rhythm (E). First-degree AV block prolongs the PR interval, but does not affect the intensity of the cardiac sounds nor the intensity of the pulse (D). In Mobitz type I second-degree AV block, there is a progressive prolongation of the PR interval on the electrocardiogram, eventually resulting in the failure to conduct an atrial beat. At slow cardiac rates, each beat has the same intensity (B).

22. **(D)** The bone marrow aspirate, which is positive in more than 50% of cases, demonstrates both intracellular and extracellular amastigotes, the form of the *Leishmania* organism that lacks an exteriorized flagellum. The kinetoplast, also shown, is an independently replicating organelle in the mitochondrion of the organism (D). Malaria is a consideration in this clinical situation. Diagnosis requires the demonstration of asexual forms of the parasite in thick or thin smears of peripheral blood, stained with Giemsa (C). Plasma cell leukemia, a variant of multiple myeloma, is a consideration if the peripheral blood smear contains more than 20% plasma cells (E). Although persons with acute myelogenous leukemia may present with pancytopenia without circulating blasts, the bone marrow aspirate in this case is not suggestive of an acute leukemic process, in which the marrow is typically hypercellular. The Auer rod, which is a slender, fusiform cytoplasmic inclusion that stains red with Wright-Giemsa stain, is a distinguishing feature of acute myelogenous leukemia (B). In aplastic anemia, the bone marrow

aspirate may yield either a "watery" marrow or a "dry tap." A bone marrow biopsy often reveals severely hypocellular or aplastic marrow, replaced by fat. Reduction of myeloid precursors is common (A).

23. **(D)** The patient described has a history suggestive of acute pancreatitis or an exacerbation of chronic pancreatitis. Mesenteric angiography is not useful in making this diagnosis, though it would be useful in making the diagnosis of mesenteric ischemia. The history in this case is not suggestive of this diagnosis. Abdominal ultrasound (A) and CT scan (C) often reveal parenchymal changes in the pancreas seen in pancreatitis. Serum amylase/lipase (B) are usually elevated in acute pancreatitis and sometimes in chronic pancreatitis. Abdominal X-ray (E) reveals calcification in the pancreas in chronic pancreatitis.

24. **(D)** This patient's symptoms are most consistent with influenza. Viral illnesses cannot be treated with antibiotics such as amoxicillin (B) or azithromycin (A). Furosemide (C) doesn't change viral illness, either. In patients with numerous comorbidities, treatment with amantadine (D) is reasonable. In younger, healthy patients, anti-viral treatment is probably not necessary, and treatment consists of supportive measures.

25. **(C)** This patient has absolute neutropenia secondary to reaching a nadir from chemotherapy for her breast cancer. She is extremely immunosuppressed and has a very low white blood cell count to fight off infection. She is at risk of acquiring infection from others and not transmitting infection. Thus, respiratory isolation is not needed for this patient. On the contrary, a mask and gloves would be prudent for visitors who come near her in order to prevent transmission of any viral or bacterial infection from the visitor to the patient. A full set of blood, urine, and sputum culture (A) is necessary in order to rule out sepsis. Granulocyte colony stimulating factor (Neupogen) (B) is an immunomodulating agent, which stimulates the bone marrow to produce granulocytes and, thus, increase the white blood cell count in this patient. Empiric treatment with anti-pseudomonal and anti-staphylococcus antibiotics (D) is a medical emergency whenever a neutropenic patient spikes a temperature. This rapid institution of antibiotics can prevent disseminated sepsis. Reverse isolation precautions (E) include

strict hand-washing, no fresh fruits and vegetables, no fresh flowers, no rectal temperatures, and even gloves and masks for visitors. These reverse isolation precautions would prevent the patient from being exposed to a possible infectious source. These precautions should be maintained until the white blood cell count is over 500 cells.

26. **(D)** This patient has shingles or herpes zoster. The lesions are self-limiting over time but very painful. A Tzanck prep is obtained by taking a swab from the vesicular fluid off the lesion and looking under the microscope. In herpes zoster, multinucleated giant cells and ballooning of the epidermal cells are seen under the Tzanck prep slide. Biopsy of the skin vesicles (A) would not give us a very quick diagnosis. The procedure would also be invasive and painful to the patient. Topical steroids (B) applied to the dermatomal lesions would exacerbate the shingles and cause replication of the virus. Acyclovir (C) is the treatment of choice in immunocompromised individuals to prevent dissemination. It has also been shown to prevent post-herpetic neuralgia pain in zoster patients. An electrocardiogram (E) is not necessary because the cause of the thoracic pain is not related to the cardiovascular system, but to nerve root involvement by the herpes virus.

27. **(C)** This patient most probably has *C. difficile*-associated diarrhea, which would be detected by a positive *C. difficile* toxin in the stool. This infectious diarrhea is associated with intravenous antibiotics secondary to a change in the intestinal bacterial milieu. Treatment is discontinuation of antibiotics and oral vancomycin or metronidazole. An invasive procedure (A) is not necessary at this point. It is very unlikely that this patient has rectosigmoid cancer or needs a biopsy. If her symptoms are still persistent after empiric treatment, then a flexible sigmoidoscopy can be done. If *C. difficile* colitis is present, then pseudomembranous plaques would be visible on colonoscopy. It is very unlikely that this patient has diarrhea secondary to a parasitic infection (B). Eosinophilia would occur as well as fever and chronicity of the diarrhea. Empiric treatment with trimethoprim-sulfamethoxazole (D) is given only if the diarrhea is secondary to a bacterial infection such as isospora belli, salmonella, and shigella. Discontinuation of the intravenous antibiotics is an appropriate choice, especially after a full ten days of treatment for pneumonia; but checking

the stool for cultures and sensitivities is not appropriate (E). It would be better to check the stool for C. *difficile* toxin since this is the most likely cause of the diarrhea.

28. **(C)** Nondependent edema of the hands and face and excessive weight gain over a short period time in a pregnant woman should lead one to suspect preeclampsia. Other criteria for the diagnosis of preeclampsia include the development of significant hypertension or a significant rise in either diastolic or systolic blood pressure over baseline. Significant proteinuria and oliguria is also noted. Gestational diabetes (A) is not associated with nondependent edema or significant weight gain over a short period of time. While pregnant women can also experience nondependent edema, the edema and weight gain need to be investigated and preeclampsia either ruled in or out (B). Eclampsia (D) is the occurrence of seizures in a patient with preeclampsia. A complete placenta previa (E) is diagnosed when the placenta overlies the cervical os.

29. **(B)** A urinary tract infection will occur anywhere along the GU tract and classically presents with dysuria, frequency, and CVA tenderness. A fever may or may not be present. Pregnancy (A) may be associated with frequency. Kidney stones (C) are usually painful and they may be associated with hematuria. Bladder tumors (D) may present with nothing or may have hematuria or pain. An ovarian cyst (E) may also present in many ways, but usually not in the way a urinary tract infection may present.

30. **(C)** All of the pathologies stated in the answer are found in Alzheimer's patients except the depigmentation of cells in the substantia nigra and locus ceruleus, which occurs in patients with Parkinson's disease.

31. **(C)** Any patient with palpitations who is stable should be monitored in a telemetry bed. If the patient is unstable, then the intensive care unit (B) is more appropriate. There is no emergent need for the operating room for a pacemaker (A) at this moment. The ward (D) does not suitably monitor the patient, and by no means should this patient be sent home (E) until he is adequately worked up.

32. **(E)** Cryoglobulins, illustrated here, are proteins that precipitate when cooled and dissolve when warm (A). Three types occur. Monoclonal (type I) cryoglobulins are usually of the IgG or IgM class. They are associated with multiple myeloma and macroglobulinemia (B). Type II cryoglobulinemia (mixed) usually consists of a monoclonal IgM protein and a polyclonal IgG. The serum protein electrophoresis usually shows either a normal pattern or a diffuse, polyclonal hypergammaglobulinemic pattern (D). The quantity of mixed cryoglobulin is usually less than 0.2 g/dL. This pattern is associated with vasculitis, glomerulonephritis, lymphoproliferative disease, chronic infections, and hepatitis C infection (E). Type III (polyclonal) cryoglobulinemia is associated with infections and inflammatory diseases, but has no clinical significance (C).

33. **(C)** Beta-blockers such as propranolol can be used immediately to decrease the symptoms of hyperthyroidism. The other treatments of radioactive iodine (A), propylthiouracil (B), and methimazole (D) are all longer term possibilities to decrease the chance that this will happen again.

34. **(D)** This man appears to have a bad infection of his finger. There is no need to obtain an arterial blood gas unless he is in severe respiratory distress, which is unlikely. By obtaining a CBC (A), you can look for an elevated white blood count. A finger X-ray (B) will tell you if there is any bone involvement or the presence of a foreign body. Culturing the drainage (C) will guide your antibiotic coverage. As with any patient, a detailed history and physical (E) is paramount.

35. **(D)** Unless this patient is being taken emergently to the operating room, he may eat and, therefore, does not have to have nothing by mouth (NPO) status. Warm soaks (A), antibiotics (B), and elevation of the hand (C) all are indicated for an infected extremity. By performing serial examinations of the hand (E), you can monitor your treatment and make sure it is working.

36. **(A)** With an infection of this type and the fact that the patient is hospitalized, the best route of antibiotic administration is IV. IM (B) and PO (C) are not as effective. Topical (D) antibiotics would not work well to get to the infection in an

acutely infected hand. Irrigation catheters (E) may act as an adjunct to IV antibiotics, but are not as effective as the primary treatment modality.

37.   **(C)**   Before this patient can leave the hospital, there must be clinical resolve of the infection. One week of antibiotics (A) may or may not be enough, and you must make a clinical decision as to the discontinuance of the antibiotic. Pain (B) may be absent either before or after the resolution and should not be the sole decisionmaker. X-ray changes (D) may lag behind the clinical picture, and a sterile wound (E) may take weeks to achieve even after there is significant clinical resolve.

38.   **(B)**   The lifetime prevalence of anorexia nervosa is 0.5%. Most surveys show greater preponderance among upper socioeconomic classes. Women are more prone to this disorder than men. One-half of those with anorexia nervosa develop bulimic behavior with binge eating (C) and purging during the course of the disease. Women with anorexia nervosa usually have amenorrhea (A) for at least three months, failure to maintain ideal body weight, and osteoporosis if the starvation goes on for a long period of time (D). Hypokalemia (E) can occur if diuretics and laxatives are abused in order to lose weight. Thyroid function in anorexia nervosa resembles that of the euthyroid sick syndrome with a low T3 concentration in the blood.

39.   **(B)**   At this point of hospitalization, this patient is in critical condition with hypotension and myopathy. She does not need estrogen replacement to prevent osteoporosis at this point in time because osteoporosis is not life-threatening, and neither is resuming her menses. Intravenous fluids (A) are needed to maintain her blood pressure and replace electrolytes. Psychiatric counseling (C) is needed immediately because this patient is contemplating suicide. A cardiac monitor (E) should be placed on this patient to prevent fatal arrhythmias. Tube feedings (D) or parenteral nutrition should be considered to maintain nutrition and weight.

40.   **(A)**   Although it seems that this patient has recovered fully from her disorder, anorexia nervosa has a high prevalence of recurrence and, thus, mandatory psychiatric follow-up is necessary to prevent a relapse. Estrogen replacement (B) is not needed if she is menstruating normally and there

is no evidence of osteoporosis. Antidepressants (C) have side effects and are not needed if this patient shows no present signs and symptoms of depression. Nutritional counseling (D) should have been done while the patient was an inpatient in the hospital. A high-protein diet (E) or any other type of special diet has not been shown to prevent a relapse of anorexia nervosa. Some studies show that 30% of patients with anorexia nervosa remain chronically ill with the disorder.

41.   **(A)**   In a witnessed cardiac arrest, the most appropriate initial intervention is a precordial thump. If that doesn't work, activate EMS and start basic life support with cardiopulmonary resuscitation.

42.   **(E)**   A thorough breast examination should be performed on all women in a variety of sitting and lying positions so as to adequately examine the breast. During this examination, it is important to compress the breast to show dimpling (A), palpate both the supraclavicular (B) and axillary (C) nodes, and transilluminate any masses (D) that may be cysts. There is no role for percussion of breast masses (E). Breast masses are important and should be noted and worked up separately.

43.   **(B)**   In acute hepatitis A and B, elevation of serum transaminases precedes the rise in bilirubin. Jaundice normally is visible in the sclera or skin when the serum bilirubin exceeds 2.5 mg/dL (C). All five types of viral hepatitis produce clinically similar illnesses, which range from an asymptomatic carrier state to fulminant and fatal acute infections (E). Other acute infectious and noninfectious disease processes may mimic acute viral hepatitis (D).

44.   **(D)**   Following infection with hepatitis B, the first virologic marker detectable in the serum is HBsAg (A). Serum HBsAg precedes both the elevation of serum aminotransferase levels and the onset of clinical symptoms (B). Following the disappearance of HBsAg from the serum, antibody to HBsAg (anti-HBs) becomes detectable in the serum and remains present indefinitely (C). Because HBcAg is sequestered within an HBsAg coat, it is not routinely detectable in the serum of infected persons (D). By contrast, antibody to HBcAg (anti-HBc) appears in the serum within one to two weeks after the appearance of HBsAg. IgM anti-HBc predominates during the first six months

following acute hepatitis B infection. IgG anti-HBc predominates beyond six months (E).

45. **(B)** Hepatitis B antigen is a readily detectable serologic marker of hepatitis B infection. HBeAg is detectable in the serum concurrently or shortly after the appearance of HBsAg. Its appearance occurs simultaneously with high levels of virus replication, reflecting the presence of circulating intact virions (E). Serologic testing for hepatitis E is still in the investigational stages. Following an acute infection, both IgM and IgG anti-HEV can be detected (D).

46. **(D)** Infection with hepatitis D (HDV, delta agent) requires antecedent or concomitant infection with hepatitis B. The HDV antigen is expressed predominantly in the hepatocyte nuclei. During acute hepatitis D infection, IgM anti-HDV predominates in the serum (A). In self-limited infections, the titer of anti-HDV is low and rarely present after HBsAg has been cleared from the serum (B). In chronic infections, anti-HDV is present in the serum in high titers (D). IgG anti-HDV can be detected in the serum in chronic infections (E).

47. **(C)** First-generation enzyme-linked immunoassays (EIA-1) for hepatitis C usually do not become positive until 12 or more weeks following infection (A). By contrast, second-generation enzyme-linked immunoassays (EIA-2) usually becomes positive five to six weeks following infection, but may be positive as early as two weeks following infection. Thus, these tests become positive before the end of the clinical incubation period [(B) and (C)]. Second-generation assays (EIA-2, RIBA) are both more sensitive and more specific than first-generation enzyme-linked immunoassays (D). In most cases, second-generation RIBA assays correlate well with the presence of HCV-RNA (E).

48. **(E)** Diagnostic paracentesis is recommended for all persons with new onset ascites. Transudative ascites are characterized by a protein concentration of less than 25 g/dL (2.5 g/dL) and a specific gravity of less than 1.016 [(A) and (B)]. Instead of using the total protein count, the ratio of protein in plasma to ascites is sometimes used. This PAAG is greater than 1.1 in transudates (C). A white blood cell count of less than 250 polymorphonuclear cells is consistent with a transudate (D). New onset chylous ascites, due to leakage of lymph into the peritoneal cavity, is most often caused by an underlying malignancy, especially a lymphoma. The triglyceride concentration is greater than 200 mg/dL and often greater than 1,000 mg/dL (E).

49. **(C)** The hepatic Doppler sonogram shows successful placement of a transjugular intrahepatic portosystemic shunt (E). The characteristic echogenicity of the shunt, indicated by the solid white lines, is evident (A). Ascites is demonstrated by the hypointense signal (D). The intense blue signal represents shunted blood [(B) and (C)].

50. **(C)** Hepatorenal syndrome (functional renal failure) is renal failure occurring in the presence of severe liver disease, without evidence of an intrinsic abnormality of the kidney. Hallmarks of the syndrome include hyponatremia, progressive azotemia, and worsening oliguria. Hypotension is common. The syndrome may be precipitated by gastrointestinal bleeding, overly aggressive diuresis, or sepsis. The diagnosis is supported by the demonstration of avid sodium retention, with urinary sodium concentrations less than 10 mEq/L (C). The urine sediment is unremarkable. However, other causes of prerenal azotemia must be excluded [(A), (B), and (D)]. Urine potassium concentrations are usually of limited value due to the wide range of values, which are affected by diet (E).

51. **(D)** This patient is too unstable with abnormal vital signs to cooperate for a pulmonary function test. He needs to be stabilized. This patient has silo filler's disease, which is a hypersensitivity pneumonitis of the lungs caused by inhalation of organic proteins that were produced by the bacteria in the silo fermenting the corn. A bronchoscopy (A) would give a definitive answer to see if the pulmonary process is of an infectious nature or an immune-mediated process. Serologic blood tests (B) for various fungi would reveal if exposure to a fungal organism was responsible for this acute process. Inhalation of spores (C) from certain bacteria can also produce similar symptoms, and this needs to be ruled out by serologic testing and a rise in titers. These spores can also be inhaled on farms. This patient was a recent widower and thus he could have been depressed and ingested a toxic substance or alcohol. Thus, toxicology screening (E) is prudent in the emergency room.

52. **(D)** This patient has acute hypersensitivity pneumonitis secondary to inhalation of gaseous oxides of nitrogen produced by bacteria in freshly cut silage. Hypersensitivity pneumonitis is an agricultural lung disease mediated by a cellular process. The smell of a "chlorine-like" odor is typical in silo filler's disease. This patient has atypical features of pulmonary embolism (A), and it is unlikely because this patient was active and did not have risk factors for hypercoagulation. Dermal absorption (B) of chemicals is unlikely, especially since this patient inhaled the toxic gas and presented with pulmonary symptoms—not a rash. This patient did not recall exposure to any dusts or molds while working in the silo. Thermophilic fungal spore lung injury (C) is an immune-mediated rather than an infectious process. *Legionella* pneumonia (E) would present with cough, fever, and an insidious onset. This patient was afebrile. He did not have *Legionella* pneumonia.

53. **(A)** Farmers should be aware of the locations where oxides are likely to accumulate, and they should be alert for the early symptoms of exposure. Thus, the key element in the prevention of silo filler's disease is the education of farmers and other agricultural workers at risk to avoid exposure and to recognize the signs of silo gas. Face masks and gloves (B) would not provide adequate protection against a toxin with a small molecular structure, such as oxides of nitrogen. Even with an adequate ventilation system in the silo and a working blower in place, this would only provide secondary protection (C). Oxides of nitrogen are heavier than air and tend to accumulate in poorly ventilated areas of silos. Monitoring oxygen concentrations in agricultural structures (D) would not provide adequate protection, inasmuch as concentrations of oxides of nitrogen as small as 50 to 500 parts per million can be toxic, even in the presence of adequate oxygen. Screening of workers with chest X-rays and pulmonary function tests (E) are not cost effective and not a reasonable solution, especially if the patient is asymptomatic.

54. **(E)** When bronchiolitis obliterans develops after acute silo filler's disease, patients will have fever, cough, and dyspnea after a period of apparent recovery. This complication can occur one to six weeks after exposure and is primarily an airway disease. The incidence of this complication has decreased in recent decades subsequent to

treatment with steroids. Lymphocytic interstitial pneumonitis (A) is usually seen in association with lymphoproliferative disorders and is very unlikely in our patient. Chronic, massive exposure to the nitrogen oxide gases can result in pulmonary fibrosis (B). But this patient was exposed only once, acutely. Autoimmune disease (C) is not a known complication of silo filler's disease. Recurrence of acute silo filler's disease (D) can be prevented by avoiding exposure to the fresh silage within 48 hours after it has been filled.

55. **(D)** A family history would not be expected to be particularly helpful.

56. **(E)** An upper GI series would not be obtained acutely in the evaluation of this patient.

57. **(C)** This is a common scenario for gastroesophageal reflux.

58. **(A)** Esophageal strictures can result from chronic acid reflux and could contribute to some of this patient's symptoms.

59. **(B)** In a code situation, where there is asystole, transcutaneous pacing is an alternative to attempt to initiate electrical activity.

60. **(C)** Third-degree atrioventricular block is an absolute indication for a permanent pacemaker. However, the patient is hemodynamically stable, and so an emergent transvenous (A) transcutaneous (B) pacer does not need to be used.

61. **(E)** The patient has a hemodynamically stable narrow complex tachycardia. Adenosine should be given to attempt to identify the atrial rhythm and possibly to medicate the patient back to sinus rhythm. In a wide complex tachycardia that is hemodynamically stable, lidocaine should be given first.

62. **(D)** This patient is having a hemodynamically unstable, symptomatic atrial fibrillation, both of which are reasons for immediate electrical cardioversion.

63. **(C)** If patients quit smoking at a young age, within a few years, their epithelium and lung parenchyma will return to normal. All of the other negative things about smoking are true.

64. (C), 65. (A), 66. (B), 67. (D) Although gout is most common in the big toe, it may affect any joint. It is usually monoarticular and joint fluid microscopy reveals needle-shaped crystals which are negatively birefringent (A). Osteoarthritis is a common condition which generally affects weight-bearing or heavily used joints. Heberden's nodes are found on the distal interphalangeal joints, and Bouchard's nodes are seen on the proximal interphalangeal joints. Classic radiographic findings include joint space narrowing, osteophytes, and cysts (B). Rheumatoid arthritis generally occurs in a symmetrical distribution involving large and small joints. Constitutional symptoms, such as fever, are common in severe cases (C). In pseudogout, microscopy of joint fluid aspirate reveals positively birefringent crystals which are rhomboid-shaped. These are calcium pyrophosphate dihydrate crystals (D). Infective arthritis can be caused by numerous organisms, most commonly staphylococcus aureus. Joint fluid aspiration is useful to make the diagnosis based on cell count and culture (E).

68. (D) At this point, no further heroic efforts will save him. His brain and other tissues have been hypoxic for too long for him to recover function.

69. (D) This patient has acute pancreatitis, which is inflammation of the pancreas secondary to a toxin or trauma, which releases pancreatic digestive enzymes and causes necrosis and inflammation of the pancreas. The amylase and lipase levels are elevated, which make the diagnosis of pancreatitis presumptively. Pancreatic cancer (A) would not present with acute abdominal pain. Jaundice, depression, and weight loss would be present initially. The lipase level is also not usually elevated. Chronic pancreatitis (B) can also present this way, but the beta cells in the pancreas would be destroyed and, thus, hypoglycemia or hyperglycemia would be present. This patient has a normal glucose level. In acute cholecystitis (C), there is inflammation of the gallbladder, most likely secondary to gallstones or alcohol. This patient does not have cholecystitis because there is no evidence of jaundice or right upper quadrant pain. The serum alkaline phosphatase level would be elevated in cholecystitis instead of the serum lipase and amylase. This patient had no evidence of trauma or hemorrhage, and therefore bowel perforation (E) is not the correct answer.

70. (B) A CT of the abdomen would show peripancreatic inflammation and edema suggestive of pancreatitis. Laparoscopy (A) is an invasive surgical procedure, which is not useful in making the diagnosis of pancreatitis. It is useful to treat and make the diagnosis of appendicitis and abdominal obstruction secondary to adhesions. An ultrasound of the abdomen (C) is a good test, but it is not very useful in obese patients who have a lot of subcutaneous tissue because a deep, retroperitoneal organ, such as the pancreas, cannot be visualized. X-rays of the abdomen (D) are useful only to make the diagnosis of chronic pancreatitis because of visualization of calcification within the fibrosed pancreas. Abdominal X-rays are not useful in making the diagnosis of acute pancreatitis. Appendicitis, cholecystitis, and abdominal obstruction can all mimic the signs of pancreatitis on the clinical exam (E). A periumbical hematoma called Cullen's sign is, however, suggestive of acute pancreatitis.

71. (C) The most common cause of acute, recurrent pancreatitis is alcohol use. This patient is an alcoholic and, thus, it is the most likely cause of this disorder. Biliary sludge (A) occurs in five percent of the cases of pancreatitis, and nobody really knows the exact reason why sludge occurs and causes pancreatic inflammation. Medications such as Lasix, AZT, DDI, and allopurinol can all cause acute pancreatitis (B). This patient is on no medications. Cholelithiasis is the number two cause of acute pancreatitis in the elderly population. Gallstones (D) cause obstruction of the common bile duct, which in turn causes a backup of bile in the pancreatic duct and subsequent inflammation. A bite of a certain species of spiders can cause pancreatitis, but this is rare. Cytomegalovirus can also on rare occasions cause pancreatitis and cholangitis. It is unusual for bacterial and fungal pathogens to affect the pancreas (E).

72. (E) This patient has acute pancreatitis, for which the treatment of choice is supportive management such as intravenous fluids and nasogastric tube insertion if the patient is vomiting. This can prevent aspiration. Intravenous antibiotics (A) are indicated in sepsis, which this patient does not have. Oxygenation alone (B) is not helpful unless the patient is hypoxemic and other treatment modalities are also used. Morphine sulfate (C) can cause spasm of the sphincter of Oddi, which in turn can exacerbate pancreatitis. Thus, Demerol is often used for pain management in acute pancreatitis. Peritoneal lavage (D) has not been shown to change the outcome in pancreatitis according to multiple clinical studies in the literature.

73. **(E)** Thyroid storm is a severe exacerbation of hyperthyroidism brought on by the stresses of illness or surgical operation. Preoperative evaluation of thyroid function helps to determine the right intraoperative dose of an antithyroid agent to prevent the crisis from happening. Measurements of total serum T4 and T3 (A), TSH (D), radioactive iodine uptake (C), and thyroid resin uptake (B) are all indicated tests in the evaluation of hyperthyroid patients preparing for a surgical procedure.

74. **(C)** Attempts to culture *Borrelia burgdorferi* have not been uniformly successful, and culture results are also not available in a timely fashion. A lumbar puncture (A) is indicated for patients with suspected Lyme disease and neurologic symptoms such as a headache. Cerebral spinal fluid is sent for Lyme titers and polymerase chain reaction. Once Lyme disease is suspected clinically, such as with erythema migrans rash and myalgias and a tick bite, therapy with 21 days of doxycycline (B) should be instituted immediately to prevent late sequela. Most patients will seroconvert within the first four weeks after exposure. If the ELISA serologic test (D) is negative and the suspicion for Lyme disease is high, a Western blot assay should be performed. If part of the tick remains in the skin, then a full body search, even with a magnifying glass, should be carried out (E). The tick should then be carefully removed by the physician.

75. **(B)** A positive correlation between diabetes mellitus (DM) and obesity is a well-established fact. Obesity is believed to suppress insulin secretion and desensitize receptors to insulin actions. Therefore, reducing body weight should be considered as a primary goal in the health maintenance of this diabetic patient. Altering HDL/LDL ratio (A) in favor of LDL would produce an opposite and untoward effect in the primary prevention of diabetes. Treatment of hypertension (C) is an important therapy for this patient, but is unlikely to improve blood glucose irregularities. However, in the presence of obesity, it is not a first priority. Changing sedentary lifestyle (D) and quitting smoking (E) would be good, but they are not mentioned as risk factors in this passage.

76. **(D)** This patient has temporal arteritis, which is a vasculitis of the medium and large arteries. This is most common in the elderly and can masquerade as a routine tension or migraine headache. The immediate treatment of choice is high-dose prednisone to prevent blindness. This can occur because of involvement of the ophthalmic branch of the carotid artery. Temporal artery biopsy (A) is the diagnostic gold standard to make the definitive diagnosis, but this procedure would not be performed right away and, thus, blindness may ensue. Nonsteroidal anti-inflammatory agents (B) are used for migraines and tension headaches, which are usually bilateral. This patient's headache is unilateral and associated with a fever. Antibiotics (C) are needed if this patient has meningitis, which would present with neck stiffness and mental status changes. A lumbar puncture would be needed to make the diagnosis of meningitis. A CT of the brain (E) would be necessary if one suspects an acute stroke or hemorrhage in the brain. This patient has no neurologic findings suggestive of a bleed or stroke.

77. **(A)** Glomerular disease is a renal reason for oliguria or anuria. Volume depletion (B), renal artery compromise (C), shock (D), and heart failure (E) are all prerenal reasons. Some of the postrenal reasons are prostatic obstruction and bilateral ureteral obstruction.

78. **(B)** You are not obliged to obtain a test because a patient wants it, but it is best to explain your reasons to the patient.

79. **(C)** *Strongyloides stercoralis* may be asymptomatic in healthy persons. However, in immunocompromised persons, the larvae may become invasive and disseminate widely, producing a hyperinfection (A), which may be fatal (B). In disseminated disease, filariform larvae invade the gastrointestinal tract, lungs, central nervous system, peritoneum, liver, and kidney (D). Pulmonary symptoms/signs include dyspnea, productive cough, and hemoptysis. Bacteremia probably develops as a result of enteric flora entering through disrupted mucosal barriers (E).

80. **(C)** In the emergency room, one must triage the patients so that the one seen first is not the one who has waited the longest, but the one who is in the most dire need. Of the answers listed, the patient with an acute asthma attack

should be seen first. The other four patients all have conditions necessitating an emergency room visit, but are more stable than the one with an asthma attack.

81. **(D)** This is a primary acute respiratory acidosis without any significant compensatory metabolic alkalosis. The acute opioid overdose will result in hypoventilation, cyanosis, respiratory distress, and, occasionally, pulmonary edema. Treatment is effective and initiated with naloxone intravenously. This is usually quick, however, it may induce a withdrawal reaction. An acute anxiety reaction (A) is typically one of hyperventilation, thus, a primary respiratory alkalosis, and patients will not be hypoxic. Vomiting (B) leads to a loss of acid, thus, a metabolic alkalosis is the primary acid-base disturbance. ARDS (C) is a primary respiratory alkalosis with loss of functional alveoli, resulting in severe hypoxia due to intrapulmonary shunting of blood.

82. **(B)** Morphine can cause spasm of the sphincter of Oddi and worsen the patient's pain. It should be avoided. There are some who would not use aspirin (C) or ibuprofen (E) because of the increased bleeding tendencies, yet there is more of a problem with the pain associated with morphine. Demerol (A) and Tylenol (D) can be used safely.

83. **(A)** The patient should be kept NPO with a nasogastric tube to allow the GI tract to rest and decrease the amount of secretions. Keeping the patient NPO alone will not suffice (B), and by no means should any diet be given [(C), (D), and (E)]. It is also highly unlikely that this patient will have an appetite.

84. **(B)** An ileus results from a slow-down of the GI tract with resultant distension. It can arise as a result of surgery or from any insult to the GI tract. A perforation (A), infection (C), dead bowel (D), or bleeding (E) are possibilities, but the patient would show some peritoneal signs and be much sicker. With a dead bowel that progresses, his life could be at risk.

85. **(B)** A perforated viscous will cause air from the GI tract to enter the abdomen. On an upright film, this air will rise and settle under the diaphragm. A bleeding ulcer (A) would cause blood in the GI tract and lead to melena or hema-

tochezia. An infection (C) would lead to high temperatures and a septic picture. Recurrent cholecystitis (D) would lead to a similar picture as this presentation. Jaundice (E) would present with icterus and elevated bilirubin or elevated liver enzymes.

86. **(D)** A perforated viscous is a surgical emergency and an exploratory laparotomy is warranted in the operating room as soon as possible. Close observation is not sufficient (A). A nasogastric tube (B) or an enema (C) will not solve the problem. A CAT scan (E) may help you diagnose the problem, but you will still need to go to the operating room for an exploration.

87. **(D)** Any patient with an abdominal operation including an incision through the fascia will need six full weeks to heal the incision and make the fascia strong. Lifting anything greater than ten pounds earlier than six weeks may lead to a tear and a hernia. All other activity should be light. Laparoscopic surgery has lessened this requirement.

88. **(D)** Wound infections are unfortunate complications of any surgery. When it occurs, it is best to clean and debride the edges and allow healing. Systemic antibiotics are usually prescribed as a prophylactic measure. Hyperbaric oxygen (B) and topical antibiotics (C) are ineffective. Taking the patient back to the operating room to explore the wound would be unnecessary since the wound breakdown tends to be superficial and not deep (A). Closing the wound (E) is doomed to failure, as it will likely get infected and break down again.

89. **(C)** A male physician should always have a female assistant present when doing gynecologic exams, both for the patient's comfort and to protect himself from false and frivolous allegations of sexual harassment.

90. **(B)** The history and physical findings are consistent with gonococcal arthritis. Disseminated infection is most frequent in females, particularly during the menstrual period. Pharyngeal and urogenital symptoms are typically lacking in this setting. Gonococci are Gram-negative diplococci. If located intracellularly, the diagnosis is highly suspect (B). If the gonococci are located extracellularly or the diplococci are atypical, the

diagnosis is equivocal. The organism is rarely recovered if there are less than 20,000 WBC/cc. However, they are commonly isolated if there are more than 80,000 WBC/cc. The leukocytosis is predominantly neutrophilic. Arthritis caused by other organisms in this particular situation is less likely [(A), (C), (D), and (E)].

91.   **(D)**   Paraplegic patients can sit up and so develop pressure sores while they are in a wheelchair. During this period, the ischial areas support the weight and are prone to the development of the sores. Sacral sores (A) develop in quadriplegic patients who are lying down in bed all the time. Trochanteric pressure sores (B) occur in patients who lie on their sides. Occipital sores (C) also occur on people who lie on their backs and heads and can't even move their heads. Heel sores (E) occur on the feet of those who can't move them, as well.

92.   **(A)**   Since the patient is at risk of harming himself, involuntary admission to a psychiatric facility for 72 hours is appropriate.

93.   **(D)**   This patient has a nonatheromatous inflammatory reaction of the peripheral small arteries and veins leading to superficial thrombophlebitis. In a young male smoker, this disease is called Buerger's disease, or thromboangiitis obliterans, and the main treatment of choice in this vaso-occlusive disease is to discontinue smoking immediately. Venography (A) is an invasive, painful procedure used to verify the presence of deep venous thrombosis when it is suspected. Steroids (B) can be useful if this was a vasculitis such as polyarteritis nodosa or Takayasu's disease. But this disease is associated with a normal ESR and peripheral artery vaso-occlusive disease. Antibiotics (C) could be useful if this was a cellulitis or lymphangitis with a fever and elevated ESR and white count. Conservative therapy with aspirin, local heat (E), and leg elevation is helpful only if cigarette smoking is stopped first.

94.   **(D)**   You must suspect melanoma in this patient, making rectosigmoid examination unnecessary. You are obligated to look at the local lesion as well as regional and metastatic disease. You should therefore examine the skin for other lesions (A), the inguinal lymph nodes (B), the abdomen (C), and the eyes (E).

95.   **(E)**   The vascularity of the lesion is not prognostically significant. However, the A-B-C-D's of melanoma are important:

A   Asymmetry
B   Border
C   Color
D   Depth

Therefore, the size of the lesion (A), the border of the lesion (B), the color of the lesion (C), and the depth of the lesion (D) are all important.

96.   **(D)**   Lentigo maligna melanoma usually occurs on the face of elderly patients. Superficial spreading melanoma (A) is the most common melanoma and occurs on the legs in women and torso in men. Nodular melanoma (B) occurs anywhere on the body and is seen in patients between the third and seventh decades. Acral lentiginous melanoma (C) occurs under the fingernails and toenails. Mucocutaneous melanoma (E) occurs on the mucous membranes.

97.   **(C)**   Melanoma from the ankle may spread to the inguinal region. This worsens the prognosis and will lower the survival rate. Lymphoma (A), Hodgkin's disease (B), venereal disease (D), and regional infection (E) may also involve the inguinal region, but this would be unrelated to the regional spread from melanoma and would not affect the survival rate.

98.   **(B)**   Whereas surgery (C) is still the mainstay for treatment of melanoma, a tissue diagnosis must be made first with a biopsy. There are a lot of lesions that may mimic melanoma, and the clinician must be sure of the diagnosis before treatment begins. Close observation (A) would be inappropriate because melanoma may spread in the interim. Radiation therapy (D) and chemotherapy (E) are adjunctive modalities to surgery and are usually not indicated first.

99.   **(A)**   During the first year after diagnosis and treatment, the patient should be seen every three months. Recurrence may be early. Waiting one (B), two (C), or five (D) years is too long. An oncology patient should always have some form of follow-up (E) because of the chance of recurrent disease.

100.   **(E)**   Exposure to the sun is a major risk factor for melanoma. Smoking (B) and drinking (C)

are high risk factors for cancer of the aerodigestive tract. Lowering cholesterol and eating healthily (D) are important for a long and healthy life, but do not reduce the chance of acquiring melanoma.

101. **(C)** In this patient you would suspect he had resection of his primary lesion as well as some form of lymphadenectomy because of the inguinal involvement. This will very often lead to lymphedema because of the loss of the lymphatics. Congestive heart failure (A), varicose veins (B), and weight gain (E) may lead to a swollen or larger leg, but are less likely in this patient. Recurrent tumor (D) should be considered in every melanoma patient, but would not present like this.

102. **(D)** This is not a case of "duty to warn" because the patient is HIV-negative, is not refusing to practice safe sex, and has two "monogamous" relationships.

103. **(C)** This patient has an acute gouty attack or podagra. It is not necessary to aspirate the joint to look for negatively birefringent crystals because this is a fairly typical case of gout. Alcohol causes an acute elevation of uric acid levels, which drops immediately after eating or when the inflammation occurs. That is why the uric acid level is normal in this case. Only after the acute episode of gouty arthritis subsides does one start allopurinol in hyperexcretors of urinary uric acid. This drug is for chronic use and not used to treat an acute gouty attack. Colchicine (A), given orally or intravenously, works best early in the attack and when the gout is limited to one or two joints only. It should not be given in renal insufficiency. Prednisone (B) is safe and effective if given initially in high doses either orally or intravenously. It can reduce the inflammation of gout significantly. A single intramuscular bolus of corticotropin (D) is an excellent treatment option for gout. This drug works very fast and seems to be more effective than any other treatment options for gout. Indomethacin (E) is given three times a day to alleviate the inflammation of gout. This drug should only be given if the patient has no underlying medical problems such as GI bleed, renal or liver insufficiency, or congestive heart failure.

104. **(D)** Although these symptoms are classic for angina, you need to continue to keep in mind other illnesses in your differential diagnosis. When someone appears very ill, as this patient does, you first need to rule out the potentially fatal illnesses, such as myocardial infarction (A), aortic dissection (B), pulmonary embolism (C), and bowel viscus rupture (E).

105. **(A)** There is no evidence of gastrointestinal bleeding, and the patient is not vomiting profusely; there is no indication for nasogastric tube lavage.

106. **(E)** Gastric ulcer perforation usually presents with severe abdominal pain by history. On physical examination, bowel sounds are diminished significantly or absent, and the patient complains of diffuse abdominal tenderness and notes rebound tenderness consistent with peritonitis.

107. **(A)** Although the electrocardiogram and symptoms are all consistent with an inferior wall myocardial infarction, the widened mediastinum on chest radiograph is very concerning for a concurrent ascending aortic dissection. This needs to be ruled out before thrombolytics are considered.

108. **(D)** Hypotension or shock will merely make thrombolytics less efficacious, but they are not contraindicated. The other answer choices are all absolute contraindications to the use of thrombolytics, as is an aortic dissection.

109. **(C)** All of the other answer choices are appropriate initial management strategies for an acute transmural myocardial infarction. Streptokinase or other thrombolytic agents need to be held until the absolute contraindications are ruled out. All of the other answer choices are appropriate initial management strategies for an acute myocardial infarction.

110. **(C)** The MRI (A), CT (B), and transesophageal echocardiogram (D) all have the same sensitivity and specificity for the diagnosis of an aortic dissection. The choice of which test to order should be based on which can be performed in each clinical situation.

111. **(D)** In an ongoing thoracic aortic dissection, the only treatment option is surgery to repair the dissection. An assessment of the coronary arteries can be done using an intra-operative angiogram. There is no medical treatment for an ongoing thoracic aortic dissection.

112. **(B)** It can cause a disulfiram-type reaction. The other common side effect of metronidazole is that some patients will note a metallic taste in their mouths.

113. **(A)** A deep puncture wound of the foot needs to have the wound thoroughly explored and cleaned (B). An X-ray should be done to look for any foreign body (C). Antibiotics (D) and tetanus administration (E) are routinely given prophylactically. The wound should not be closed since it is dirty and the opening of the wound will allow for the egress of bacteria and inflammatory fluids.

114. **(C)** This geriatric patient has asymptomatic Paget's disease of the bone. Paget's disease is a common bone disorder that involves a "mosaic" pattern in which the cement lines are arranged in a haphazard pattern instead of the normal symmetry of parallel collagen fibers in both cortical and trabecular bone. Most patients are asymptomatic and only have an isolated elevated alkaline phosphatase level coming from the bone. With normal aminotransferase levels, this patient is unlikely to have liver disease and, thus, a liver biopsy (A) and hepatitis profile (B) are not needed. This patient is asymptomatic at this time, and a CT scan of the spine (E) should not be performed to rule out lytic spinal lesions. A bone biopsy (D) is usually never performed in diagnosing Paget's disease. The best management option at this time would be to have another alkaline phosphatase level taken in six months along with another office visit.

115. **(C)** The bone scan (A) is the most sensitive means to detect active lesions of Paget's disease. It would show increased uptake of the radiolabeled scanning agent at the bone site. The earliest manifestation of Paget's disease is a localized osteolytic lesion, most readily detected in the skull. The circumscribed radiolucent area detectable on skull films (B) is termed osteoporosis circumscripta. The urinary hydroxyproline excretion (D) is an index of bone matrix resorption in Paget's disease and it is usually increased. A CT scan of the spine (E) is very useful to assist in the diagnosis of vertebral compression fractures secondary to Paget's disease of the bone. The serum calcitonin level is not useful in making the diagnosis of Paget's disease. An elevated serum calcitonin level (C) is found in medullary thyroid carcinoma. Salmon calcitonin is the treatment of choice for symptomatic Paget's disease of the bone.

116. **(E)** Radiation therapy is used to treat metastatic cancer to the bone and not Paget's disease of the bone. Biphosphonates (A), such as etidronate sodium, are used to treat Paget's disease of the bone by decreasing the osteolytic activity and decreasing the osteoclastic activity in the bone. Biphosphonates are given orally. Calcitonin (C) is a safe and effective therapy for Paget's disease. It is given subcutaneously and is useful for symptoms of high cardiac output, healing of osteolytic lesions, and relief of the bone pain experienced in Paget's disease. Mithramycin (D) is a cytotoxic antibiotic that has been used in patients with marked symptomatology in Paget's disease. It is very potent and has many side effects. Surgery (B), such as occipital craniectomy, may be necessary in patients with basilar decompression. Certain orthopedic procedures, such as tibial osteotomy, total hip replacement, and knee replacement surgery, are required in patients with severe degenerative arthritis secondary to Paget's disease.

117. **(B)** The gallium scan is a radionucleotide scan, which is not used to detect pancreatic carcinoma. The gallium scan is useful to diagnose abscesses, osteomyelitis, and *Pneumocystis carinii* pneumonia. Large, bulky scans (A) are positive in 80% of patients with pancreatic cancer and can be useful to guide percutaneous needle aspiration for obtaining cytology. The endoscopic retrograde cholangiopancreatography (ERCP) (D) is an invasive diagnostic test that is 95% sensitive for pancreatic cancer and provides direct visualization of the pancreatic ducts and peripancreatic tissue. The ERCP also provides for an opportunity to obtain needle-aspiration and a biopsy. The serological marker CA19-9 (E) is 75% sensitive for pancreatic tumor, but it has limited specificity. DU-PAN-2 and peanut lectin are also tumor markers for pancreatic cancer.

118. **(B)** Most often, pancreatic carcinoma presents as a widely metastatic disease. Two of the most common paraneoplastic syndromes associated with pancreatic carcinoma are depression and Trousseau's syndrome, which is migratory venous thrombophlebitis. Jaundice is present in 80% of patients with cancer of the head of the pancreas, which is the most common site (A) of pancreatic cancer. The most consistent type of

genetic damage involves mutations in the K-ras gene, which is present in 85% of pancreatic adenocarcinoma cases. The Philadelphia chromosome (9, 22) is associated with chronic myelogenous leukemia (C). The alkaline phosphatase and bilirubin level are elevated 90% of the time in pancreatic carcinoma. The amylase level is elevated only 17% of the time in pancreatic carcinoma (D). The CEA, CA19-9, and other tumor markers for pancreatic cancer are not specific and sensitive enough to be used alone to make the diagnosis (E). An imaging test is also required, along with a biopsy.

119. **(A)** Surgical excision of the pancreatic tumor is the only modality that offers any chance for long-term, disease-free survival in early stages of the cancer. A pancreaticoduodenal resection (Whipple's procedure) is the operation of choice and offers a three-year survival of 13% in most patients with early-stage pancreatic cancer. Radiation therapy (B) has not had a major impact on the treatment of pancreatic carcinoma, as the tumor is relatively radioresistant and its location makes it a poor candidate for safe radiation therapy. Various chemotherapeutic agents (C) have been tested in the treatment of advanced pancreatic carcinoma, but no regimen substantially improves survival or quality of life. Palliation, and not treatment for cure, is performed by placing a biliary stent (D) for biliary drainage to relieve the obstruction and jaundice. Hormone therapy (E) is not used to treat pancreatic carcinoma. It is used in prostate and breast cancers.

120. **(E)** Diabetes will affect several organ systems including the kidneys, vascular system, nervous system, and ophthalmic system. You may, therefore, see such diseases as hypertension (A), coronary artery disease (B), renal disease (C), and visual changes (D) or blindness. Osteosarcoma would be unrelated.

121. **(A)** Acute ITP is the most common cause of thrombocytopenia in children and sometimes follows viral infections. Acute ITP in adults is not usually associated with viral infections (B). It is not usually associated with life-threatening bleeding (C). It is usually self-limited in duration (D). Bone-marrow transplantation (E) is not indicated in its treatment.

122. **(B)** This is consistent with brain death.

123. **(C)** This patient is mentally impaired.

124. **(D)** Emergency procedures may be performed even if parental consent cannot be obtained first.

125. **(A)** The patient's living will and advanced directives must be honored in determining her care.

126. **(C)**, 127. **(D)**, 128. **(A)**, 129. **(B)** Total lung capacity is the volume of gas contained within the lungs after a maximal inspiration (D). The residual volume is that volume of gas remaining within the lungs at the end of a maximal expiration (A). Both of these measurements are commonly used to diagnose respiratory diseases. The vital capacity is that volume of gas that is exhaled from the lungs in going from the total lung capacity to the residual volume (C). The tidal volume is the volume of gas exchanged during normal resting ventilation (B).

130. **(D)** If a procedure is medically necessary and reasonable for the immediate care of the patient, you can perform it without waiting for his, or his family's, consent. If a procedure is elective or not of an immediate nature, it should await permission of the patient, if he becomes capable, or his next-of-kin. As soon as the patient is stabilized, you should direct your staff to notify the police and try to identify the patient.

131. **(C)** A deep vein thrombosis is a clot that occurs in the deep venous system of the lower extremity due to pooling of the blood. The chance of it occurring increases with the length of surgery (A) and the type of surgery (B). The type of anesthesia (general anesthesia vs. local anesthesia) also has an effect, in that it is higher with the general anesthesia. A previous history of DVT raises the chances for a recurrence (E). Whether surgery is emergent or elective doesn't alter the incidence.

132. **(A)** A pulmonary embolus can develop if a deep vein thrombosis breaks off and embolizes to the pulmonary vasculature. It can lead to severe dyspnea, respiratory failure, or even death. While a myocardial infarction (B) is serious, it does not come directly from a DVT. An ischemic lower extremity (C) is a result of arterial insufficiency. Malignant hyperthermia (D) is an anesthetic complication resulting in very high temperatures and

even death. A deep artery thrombosis (E) is not related to a deep venous thrombosis.

133. **(E)** Coumadin is used to treat a DVT, not prevent it. Coumadin takes two to three days to reach its effect and, thus, can't be used prophylactically. Sequential compression devices (A) and compression stockings (B) work by increasing venous return. This will prevent the pooling of the blood and the resultant thrombosis. Heparin (C) and low molecular weight heparin (D) have quicker onset of action and are used in prevention.

134. **(E)** A deep vein thrombosis may be diagnosed through clinical examination by observing a swollen tender calf (A), ultrasound (B), venogram (C), or plethysmography (D). A radiograph (E) will not reveal a soft tissue clot.

135. **(D)** Physical therapy cannot treat a deep vein thrombosis. Heparin (A), antithrombotic therapy (B), and Coumadin (E) all work to dissolve the clot. Surgical interruption of the vena cava (C) does not treat the DVT per se, but does prevent its migration into the pulmonary vasculature to hopefully prevent a pulmonary embolus.

136. **(C)** The recommended treatment for a deep vein thrombosis after the acute stage is for six months, and it is done with Coumadin as the anticoagulant, after initially using heparin.

137. **(A)** All of the studies have shown that a decreased ejection fraction is associated with a significantly increased long-term mortality.

138. **(D)** This woman has influenza A. The primary mode of transmission of this viral infection is via sneezing, coughing, or talking.

139. **(B)** Amantadine is an effective prophylactic agent in preventing influenza A, but not influenza B. It also is an alternative agent of treatment in patients in whom influenza vaccine is contraindicated.

140. **(D)** The computed tomographic scan of the pelvis shows thickening of the sigmoid colon and gas in the diverticula. The barium enema performed on the same day reveals moderate narrowing of the distal sigmoid colon, with associated mucosal thickening and spasm, consistent with the CT findings. Multiple diverticula are present in the sigmoid colon. These findings, along with the clinical picture, are suggestive of diverticulitis. Early treatment (D) includes bowel rest, surgical consultation, intravenous fluids, and broad spectrum antibiotics combined with anaerobic coverage [(E) and (B)]. There is no evidence of a malignant process on either of these studies [(A) and (C)].

141. **(D)** This computed tomographic scan of the abdomen shows multiple abscesses of the spleen. *Pneumocystis carinii*, other pyogenic organisms, or parasites may produce this picture (D). Autosomal-dominant polycystic renal disease typically presents with multiple renal cysts. Cystic lesions may also occur in other organs, including the ovaries, testes, arachnoid, and pineal. Splenic cysts are extremely rare. The absence of renal cysts on this tomographic cut make this choice less likely (A). There is no evidence of a perforated peptic ulcer (B). The texture of the liver is grainy, but homogenous. Hepatocellular carcinomas can be difficult to diagnose due to the frequent underlying cirrhosis of the liver. There is no evidence of either cirrhosis or a tumor on this section of the liver. In addition, the clinical picture is extremely atypical for this diagnosis (C). The spine does not show any evidence of osteomyelitis. The clinical picture is also atypical (E).

142. **(A)** This specimen demonstrates abundant acid-fast, small, rod-shaped organisms. The acid-fast stain is used to differentiate organisms that are capable of retaining carbol fuchsin dye after disruption by an acid/organic solvent, such as *Mycobacteria* (A). Either the acid-fast (Ziehl-Neelsen) stain or a modification of it may also be used to demonstrate oocysts in cryptosporidial infections (C). *Staphylococci* appear as clumps of Gram-positive cocci on Gram stain (B). Both Gomori's methenamine silver and toluidine blue O, which stain the cyst wall, have been used to identify *Pneumocystis* (D). Morphologic identification of trophozoites in the feces is typically used to diagnose *Entamoeba* infections (E).

143. **(C)** The most common cause of adrenal insufficiency worldwide is tuberculosis. Of the laboratory tests listed, tuberculosis should be a strong consideration. Diagnosis is made by an ACTH stimulation test. A stimulated plasma cortisol greater than 20 micrograms/dL is normal (C).

Plasma renin levels have been advocated by some researchers to evaluate hypertension (A). Thyroid-stimulating hormone is helpful in assessing thyroid dysfunction (B). The hypoglycemia may be due to adrenal insufficiency (D) Consideration must be given to causes of hyponatremia. However, diagnostic evaluation does not include measurement of vasopressin (E).

144. **(B)** Depending on the dose of heroin injected intravenously, traces of morphine (its metabolite) may be detected in the urine for up to 48 hours [(B) and (A)]. Quinine, a common adulterant of street drugs, may persist for a longer period (C). However, quinine is present in many frequently consumed substances, such as tonic water (D). Cannabis may be detected for up to one week following smoking. If may be present for as long as three weeks following chronic, heavy smoking (E).

145. **(B)** With no radiographic evidence of a fracture, either the ankle is broken, but the fracture is so small it can't be seen, or there is a bad sprain. In any event, to treat conservatively is the most appropriate means of treatment. There is no need for surgery (A). Repeating the X-ray is likely to show the same thing unless the first X-ray was technically wrong (D). The patient should not "walk it off," as it may make things worse (E) and convert a stable condition to an unstable one.

146. **(D)** As the name implies, an intentional tort has as a primary component, either the intent to cause harm or, at least, a reasonable certainty that harm will ensue from a given action.

147. **(E)** If the parents or legal guardians of the child bring no action on his or her behalf, then the child may bring action on his or her behalf when the legal age is reached. Under a legal concept, called the "discovery rule," the statute begins at the time the patient discovers the negligence.

148. **(A)** Under vicarious liability, or the doctrine of respondeat superior, the employer is liable for the negligence of the employee. Thus, the hospital is held liable if any health care provider commits a negligent act that leads to damages.

149. **(E)** A physician does not have to accept a patient unless he or she chooses to, or has a contractual obligation to do so, or the emergency nature of the case is self-evident.

150. **(B)** Transient ischemic attacks are focal neurologic defects that last less than 24 hours and resolve spontaneously.

151. **(D)** Palmar erythema is classically found in liver cirrhosis. Stigmata of hyperlipidemia, such as cholesterol plaques (A) and xanthelomas (E), can be found in these patients, as well as signs of carotid artery disease, such as diminished upstrokes (C) and carotid bruits (B).

152. **(A)** The medical treatment for symptomatic carotid artery disease is either aspirin or ticlopidine. Surgery must also be considered.

153. **(C)** Symptomatic patients with a carotid stenosis of greater than 70% should be treated with surgery. Asymptomatic patients should not be treated with surgery.

154. **(B)** A urinary tract infection is an infection anywhere along the urinary tract from the kidneys to the urethra. RBCs and WBCs are often present in addition to leukocyte esterase and nitrites, because bacteria convert nitrates to nitrites. A vaginal yeast infection (A) will have yeast around the vagina with associated itching and occasional reddened skin. Kidney stones (C) will produce RBCs in the urine, but generally not WBCs. Also, there won't always be dysuria. There is often excruciating pain with nephrolithiasis or kidney stones. A bladder tumor (D) may have dysplastic cells in the urine, but there usually are no RBCs or WBCs. A coagulopathy (E) may have RBCs because of the bleeding, but no WBCs or dysuria.

155. **(B)** An antibiotic, such as TMP-SMZ (trimethoprim-sulfamethoxazole) is appropriate for urinary tract infections. An antifungal (A) would be used for a yeast infection. An intravenous pyelogram (C) would be used for the workup of a kidney stone or a tumor. A CAT scan (D) would be used to look for anemia.

156. **(D)** Biopsy of the temporal artery is recommended for anyone suspected of temporal arteritis (giant cell arteritis). In those cases in which the artery appears normal on examination, sections from multiple levels are often necessary. This requires that several centimeters of the artery be resected in order to confirm the diagnosis. This biopsy of the temporal artery demonstrates changes consistent with temporal arteritis, including

interruption of the elastic membrane and granulomatous infiltration (panel A) and a giant cell (panel B). Initial treatment is with high-dose prednisone to prevent visual complications (D). A closely related disorder, polymyalgia rheumatica, responds to prednisone, 10-20 mg/day (C). Wegener's granulomatosis, by contrast, responds to cyclophosphamide, 1-2 mg/kg per day [(A) and (B)]. Interferon alpha-2b, 3 million units three times per week, is used for selected cases of hepatitis (E).

157. **(B)** The Perthes' test is for obstruction of the deep veins, testing for competency and patency. The competence of the saphenofemoral complex (A) is done with the Brodie-Trendelenberg test. Deep vein thrombophlebitis (C) can be detected with calf tenderness and swelling or a Homan's sign. A-V fistulas (D) can be detected by the presence of a thrill over the communication. Muscle atrophy (E) can be determined by inspection and comparison with the contralateral leg.

158. **(E)** According to the U.S. Preventive Services Task Force, lifestyle choices such as smoking, diet, and exercise contribute considerably to mortality and disability of the population. The physician's role as educator and counselor is stressed regarding these choices. The Task Force gives patients more responsibility for their own health. Since many patients visit health care facilities only for acute problems, the Task Force finds it wise and feasible to include preventive measures during those visits.

159. **(B)** This elderly patient has symptoms of benign prostatic hypertrophy, which causes urinary obstruction by compression of the male urethra as it passes through the prostate gland. The obstruction also alters urethral sphincter function and may cause detrusor muscle hypertrophy. The evaluation of benign prostatic hypertrophy begins with a digital rectal examination (E) to palpate nodules in the prostate gland. A transrectal biopsy is not done as an initial assessment unless a nodule or mass lesion is detected by transrectal sonogram (C). A voiding cystourethrogram can also measure voiding pressure and confirm urinary obstruction (A). The prostatic specific antigen (D) is usually mildly elevated in some cases of benign prostatic hypertrophy, and this test should be taken. A transrectal sonogram confirms

prostatic hypertrophy and can be diagnostic for prostate nodules.

160. **(D)** This patient has classic signs and symptoms of urinary tract obstruction secondary to prostatic hypertrophy. The treatment of choice would be to perform a transurethral resection of the prostate (TURP), which has an 85% success rate in alleviating the symptoms of obstruction. A Foley catheter is only a temporary measure in relieving the obstruction. Insertion of a suprapubic catheter (B) is not the treatment of choice. This mode of therapy only alleviates the symptoms, but it does not provide the cure. Nephrostomy tubes (C) should only be placed if there is complete urinary tract obstruction that is not amenable to the definitive cure, which is a transurethral resection of the prostate gland to reduce the urethral obstruction. This patient has no contraindications to the prostate surgery, which will cure his symptoms without subjecting him to permanent catheters and tubes in his body. Alpha-antagonists, such as terazosin and prazosin, may relieve symptoms of bladder outlet obstruction, but this drug takes weeks to work and this patient needs treatment right away (A). Finasteride (E) blocks the conversion of testosterone to dihydrotestosterone and causes regression of the prostate gland. It takes about six months to work and is only effective in about 50% of the patients in reducing the prostate volume.

161. **(C)** The prostate specific antigen is mildly elevated to 6.0 ng/ml and is suggestive of benign prostatic hypertrophy, not carcinoma. Even though carcinoma in-situ was discovered on a transrectal biopsy of the prostate gland (stage A1), studies have not proven that immediate radical prostatectomy (D) or radiation therapy (B) will increase survival—especially when the PSA level is not above 10 ng/ml. The most prudent step to take here would be to repeat the prostate specific antigen level again in six months to see if there is a significant increase suggestive of prostate carcinoma that is spreading. A total orchiectomy (A) is sometimes performed in disseminated stage IV prostate cancer to reduce the level of androgen in the body. Radiation therapy (B) is given to patients with stage B prostate cancer that has spread beyond the capsule. Luteinizing hormone-releasing hormone agonists are also given to patients with disseminated prostate cancer. This patient has no evidence of disseminated prostate cancer (no

bone pain and a normal alkaline phosphatase level).

162. **(D)** Syphilis is the likeliest diagnosis for a 74-year-old male with ataxia and forgetfulness.

163. **(A)** Gonococcal infection is the likeliest diagnosis for a sexually active 20-year-old male with acute arthritis of the knee and erythematous papules.

164. **(E)** Chlamydial infection is the likeliest diagnosis for a 34-year-old woman with infertility.

165. **(C)** Papillomavirus is the likeliest diagnosis for a 40-year-old woman with cervical cancer.

166. **(C)** In contrast to a mentally competent adult refusing a specific therapy, parents cannot legally deny appropriate care to their child because of their own religious beliefs. A court order can rapidly be obtained to at least temporarily take away custody from the parents.

167. **(B)** Tic douloureux is trigeminal neuralgia with an unknown etiology. There is pain along the course of the fifth cranial nerve.

168. **(B)** Acute pancreatitis is a medical emergency. It results in inflammation of the pancreas, usually due to biliary tract disease, surgery, or alcoholism. The patient needs to be admitted (A), kept NPO (C), have an NG tube passed (D), and have amylase levels watched (E). You must rest the pancreas. It is not wise to send the patient home.

169. **(A)** The child has evidence of multiple trauma, and child abuse must be considered the most likely diagnosis at this point.

170. **(D)** A radiograph is likely to show a fracture of the ulna and/or radius, which would be consistent with child abuse. You might subsequently want to obtain other imaging tests, such as an abdominal CT (C) or MRI of the brain (E) if you suspect significant trauma in those sites, but at this point that is not necessary.

171. **(C)** The victim of child abuse rarely receives routine pediatric visits. His malnutrition suggests that no one has been monitoring his ongoing care.

172. **(B)** In this setting, it is best to remove the child from the suspect environment while evaluating both his medical and social condition. Confronting the mother (A) at this point is ill-advised and potentially dangerous for the child if he goes home from the emergency room. The rest of the interventions, including a social work consult, can all be performed in the hospital.

173. **(D)** Men over 40 who present evidence of an increased risk for developing MI should be candidates for low-dose aspirin prophylaxis. The nature of this patient's employment and newly developing symptoms he describes lay reasonable grounds for your decision.

174. **(E)**, 175. **(B)**, 176. **(A)**, 177. **(A)**, 178. **(D)**, 179. **(D)**, and 180. **(B)** The clinical picture of acute laryngotracheobronchitis (croup) consists of brassy cough, inspiratory stridor, and respiratory distress that follow an upper respiratory tract infection. Associated rhinitis and conjunctivitis are highly possible. Symptoms are worse at night.

Parainfluenza viruses are a cause of this condition. Often, viruses of upper airway infections play an allergenic role in the development of bronchial asthma. This boy's URT infection probably is contracted from his younger sister and set the ground work for an asthma attack.

Testing pulmonary function parameters before and after bronchodilator therapy shows an increased MEF and FEV1. Total lung capacity (TLC) and forced vital capacity (FVC) remain unchanged with the administration of a bronchodilator.

According to the current recommendation, administration once or twice a day of inhaled corticosteroids are the agents of first choice. Bronchial asthma is the most common cause of diffuse wheezing over the pulmonary fields. Wheezing can be heard in conditions other than bronchial asthma. Bronchiolitis is the second most common cause of wheezing . Upper airway obstruction by a foreign body is the most common condition associated with localized wheezing.

Approximately 30% of children with asthma experience cough variant asthma with no wheezing.

Although the association between the bronchial asthma and bronchiolitis is uncertain, there is some evidence to suggest that an attack of acute bronchiolitis may set the ground work for asthma.

USMLE Step 3 – Practice Test 3
Day Two – Morning Session

1. **(E)** Pancreatitis would be suspected in a 42-year-old alcoholic male with abdominal pain.

2. **(A)** Pyelonephritis would be suspected in a 33-year-old woman with fever, chills, low-back pain, and vaginal burning.

3. **(B)** Ankylosing spondylitis would be suspected in a 35-year-old male with low-back pain that hurts most in the morning.

4. **(C)** Mechanical back syndrome would be suspected in a 35-year-old male with low-back pain that is worse after being active all day.

5. **(A)** Her symptoms of weakness and high output cardiac state (ejection murmur, hyperdynamic precordium) are consistent with anemia. The normal white count makes leukemia (C) unlikely. Sickle cell disease (D) is all but absent in the non-African-American population. The decreased MCV is consistent with iron deficiency anemia. The ferritin level should be decreased.

6. **(B)** All patients with burns have tremendous bodily fluid shifts. They lose large amounts of fluids and must be resuscitated urgently. The most appropriate first step is intravenous hydration. Placement of a Foley catheter to help monitor fluid replacement is advisable. Antibiotics (A) and tetanus toxoid administration (D) are needed, as well. Chilling a patient (C) and steroids (E) are not indicated.

7. **(C)** Patients with cutaneous burns will also have inhalation injury. It is very uncommon to see an increased carboxyhemoglobin level in burn patients as a result of the inhalation. Urine output will be decreased, not increased. The treatment for this is 100% O_2, which can be delivered in a hyperbaric oxygen chamber.

8. **(B)** An elevated carboxyhemoglobin will normalize on its own even with the patient breathing in room air, but it would take awhile. If, however, you increase the inspired FIO_2 and raise the atmospheric pressure in which it is delivered, then you can effectively lower the carboxyhemoglobin levels back to normal a lot faster. The process by which this is delivered is known as hyperbaric oxygen. To intubate someone (C) would control the amount of inspired O_2, but would not allow you to control the pressure. A chest tube (D) would not change the oxygenation or ventilation, nor would a Foley catheter (E), which is placed in the urethra to measure urinary output.

9. **(D)** Prisoners can rarely participate in clinical trials.

10. **(E)** A sedentary lifestyle or physical inactivity alone can be as significant a risk factor for predisposing for cardiovascular disease as several others combined. For each one percent reduction in serum cholesterol, there is a two percent reduction in the risk of heart disease death (A). Cigarette smoking is associated with 40% of deaths from cardiovascular diseases in persons under the age of 65 (B). Serum cholesterol levels are not increasing, but decreasing, in the United States (C). The percentage of hypertensive patients whose blood pressure is under control is estimated to be 25% (D).

11. **(B)** In emergency situations, you can perform procedures if the guardians are unavailable to provide consent.

12. **(D)** In a non-emergent situation, you must obtain the guardian's permission before performing a procedure.

13. **(A)** The patient has advised you via his advanced directives that he does not want to be resuscitated.

14. **(A)** The patient is competent and has the right to refuse treatment counter to her religious practices.

15. **(E)** This patient has Heerfordt's syndrome, which is sarcoidosis involving the parotid gland,

facial nerve, and uveitis. The gold standard for making the diagnosis of sarcoidosis is by tissue diagnosis, which will reveal noncaseating granulomas. This biopsy is best obtained by transbronchial biopsy or mediastinoscopy of the hilar lymph nodes. Prednisone is the treatment of choice to alleviate the symptoms of uveoparotid fever. A CT scan of the chest alone (A) would only reveal the hilar adenopathy and possible granulomas in the lung parenchyma, but a CT scan-guided lung biopsy would yield a better result. Elevated serum ACE levels (B) occur in sarcoidosis secondary to an increase of this protein in the epitheloid cells of the granuloma. This is an excellent screening test, but false positives do occur, such as in lymphomas. The Kveim test (C) is positive in only 50-60% of patients with sarcoid. It has a low sensitivity. This test is not used anymore in making the diagnosis of sarcoidosis. Gallium scanning (D) of the parotid gland, ocular lesions, and hilar lesions can light up and become positive in active sarcoidosis. But gallium scanning can also be positive in mumps, lymphoma, and infection. Thus, this imaging test is not very specific. A tissue biopsy is required to make a definitive diagnosis of sarcoid.

16. **(E)** Polycythemia vera is not a cause of generalized lymphadenopathy. HIV disease (A) is a common cause of generalized lymphadenopathy, especially in young patients with risk factors. Syphilis (B) may also present with lymphadenopathy. Lymphoma (C), especially non-Hodgkin's lymphoma, may involve several nodal sites. Infectious mononucleosis (D) and CMV infection may cause lymphadenopathy.

17. **(E)** This patient has classic Parkinson's disease, which is diagnosed by history and physical exam. Eventually, sinemet, amantadine, and bromocriptine can be added to the drug regimen to alleviate some of the symptoms of tremors and bradykinesia. A CT of the head, EEG, and MRI of the brain are usually normal. This disease process is severely debilitating and can eventually result in bed sores, incontinence, and wasting. A brain biopsy (A) would be too invasive and not diagnostic for this disease. A lumbar puncture (B) would be normal in Parkinson's disease patients. A lumbar puncture would yield diagnostic results in multiple sclerosis, meningitis, and pseudotumor cerebri. This patient does not have hypothyroidism, and thyroid function tests (C) would not give

us the diagnosis of Parkinson's disease. A spinal cord imaging study such as MRI or CT scan (D) would be normal in a Parkinson's disease patient. It would not be a good test to perform unless one suspects a spinal cord lesion. This patient does not exhibit any specific sign of spinal cord damage.

18. **(E)** This patient has hypertrophic cardiomyopathy, which is an autosomal dominant disorder and is associated with sudden death in young patients. It is characterized by a hypertrophied but nondilated left ventricle in the absence of systemic disease and a functional left-sided obstruction. The ventricle is stiff, with reduced compliance and relaxation of the left ventricle. Diuretics and digoxin are absolutely contraindicated in this disorder because they would lower the left ventricular outflow tract pressure gradient and thus decrease the cardiac output, causing syncope or near-syncope. A family history (A) is very important, since about 25% of those who die suddenly of this disorder have first-degree relatives younger than 50 who experienced sudden nontraumatic death. Thus, since this is an autosomal dominant disease, a cardiovascular screening workup should be initiated on family members. Participation in both dynamic or static strenuous sports activity should be prohibited (B) since this could lead to a decrease in cardiac output and possibly sudden death. Calcium-channel blockers such as diltiazem or verapamil (C), as well as beta-blockers, should be the medical treatment of choice. These drugs would reduce the left ventricular wall stiffness, reduce the elevated diastolic pressures, and also increase exercise tolerance. Surgical myectomy (D) would decrease the septal thickness and hypertrophy and alleviate the functional obstruction from the outflow tract of the left ventricle. This procedure can reduce the symptoms in 75% of patients.

19. **(E)** The presence of *Ascaris lumbricoides* on upper gastrointestinal endoscopy is very unusual because the worm normally resides in the lower intestine (A). Intestinal infection is diagnosed by finding mammillated, oval thick-shelled ascaris eggs in a thick fecal smear (B). Larval migration occurs approximately nine to twelve days following egg ingestion. This is accompanied by eosinophilia, which gradually resolves over several weeks (C). Chest X-rays may reveal evidence of eosinophilic pneumonitis, which is transient (D).

Pulmonary ascariasis cannot be diagnosed by identifying ova in the feces because adult worms have not yet matured and reached the intestinal tract (E).

20. **(C)** These X-rays illustrate osteonecrosis, or skeletal infarction. Shown here are medullary infarcts of the distal femurs and proximal tibias. The most common cause is vascular compromise from fracture or dislocation of the femoral neck. In adults, ethanol abuse or therapy with corticosteroid are the most common causes (C). Osteopetrosis, also known as marble bone disease, is characterized by generalized symmetric osteosclerosis. In severe disease, an "Erlenmeyer flask" deformity is present (B). In osteomyelitis due to hematogenous infection, the earliest X-ray changes are osteopenic or lytic lesions, which may not appear for two to four weeks. Progression of the disease may produce periosteal elevation, thickening, and new bone formation (D). Today, due to earlier detection, hyperparathyroidism rarely produces subperiosteal bone resorption and even more rarely produces osteitis fibrosa cystica (E). Sclerodactyly, which is sclerosis of the skin, is usually accompanied by resorption of the bone of the fingertips (A).

21. **(C)** Articular crepitus is a grating sound whose vibrations may also be palpated. Cracking (A) results from loss of cartilage, allowing bone to rub against bone. Emphysema (B) is subcutaneous air. Popping (D) and creaking (E) are terms not used often in medical literature.

22. **(C)** Thiazide diuretics will increase serum uric acid, rather than decrease uric acid, due to altered renal tubule handling of uric acid. Allopurinol (A) reduces serum uric acid by decreasing production through inhibition of xanthine oxidase. Probenecid (B) and sulfinpyrazone (E) increase uric acid excretion in the urine. Large doses of salicylate (D) reduce serum uric acid, while low doses, (less than 2 grams per day) actually increase uric acid levels.

23. **(B)** For a dog bite, thorough irrigation and debridement is of the utmost importance. The wound should be closed loosely, not tightly (A). There is no need for amputation (C), nor treatment of family members (D), nor observation in the intensive care unit (E).

24. **(D)** This patient has preeclampsia, which is characterized by the triad of hypertension, edema, and proteinuria developing after the 20th week of pregnancy. It occurs more commonly in women who are relatively young or old for pregnancy, diabetics, and women with a family history of preeclampsia. The uric acid is usually elevated in preeclampsia and the peripheral resistance markedly increased. Recent studies have shown that low-dose aspirin (A) can be used to prevent progression of preeclampsia. Patients should be kept on bed rest (B) and methyldopa (C) should be given to lower the high blood pressure. Methyldopa has been shown not to have teratogenic effects on the fetus. Electively delivering the baby by C-section is an option after the 30th week of gestation (E) when there is progression of preeclampsia and the organs are all fully developed and viable in the baby. ACE-inhibitors (D) are contraindicated in pregnancy because they have been shown to cause teratogenic side effects in the fetus and an increase in perinatal mortality and morbidity.

25. **(C)** This patient has now progressed to full-blown eclampsia with seizures and accelerated blood pressure. The treatment of choice is intravenous magnesium sulfate. The patient's urine output, patellar reflex, and respirations need to be monitored while giving magnesium sulfate. Only after the patient has been stabilized would one attempt to deliver the baby; otherwise, the patient is at a high risk of mortality during the delivery (A). Phenytoin (B) is not used to treat seizures and accompanying eclampsia in pregnancy. Calcium gluconate is the treatment of choice for magnesium toxicity. It is not given for eclampsia. Sodium nitroprusside (E) should not be given to lower the elevated blood pressure during eclampsia because the cyanide in nitroprusside can poison the baby.

26. **(D)** Since the patient has no history of any medical illnesses, it is possible that he may have a reversible condition. It is proper for you to try to find such a condition before you decide to do nothing.

27. **(B)** You must treat any correctable cause of coma in this patient.

28. **(D)** Now you work him up as you would any newly diagnosed diabetic.

29. **(A)** This patient should be able to manage his own care at home.

30. **(B)** At the present time, mass screening tools for cancers do not exist. The overall death rate from all cancers has increased in the United States by seven percent over the past two decades (A). Smoking and exposure to increased environmental pollutants made lung cancer the most common cause of cancer death among both men and women (C). Despite all the research, clinical science still is unable to give a clear-cut association between increased mortality rates of cancer and its cause (D). Certain lifestyle choices, such as smoking, alcohol consumption, dietary fat, and excess sun exposure, may be contributing factors in the etiology and pathogenesis (E) of certain forms of cancer. Therefore, avoidance of these risk factors remains the best strategy in preventive measures of cancer.

31. **(E)** This patient has systemic lupus erythematosus, which is a multisystemic disease of unknown origin associated with tissues and organs damaged by deposition of pathogenic antibodies and immune complexes. Virtually any organ can be affected by inflammation. The antinuclear ribonucleoprotein antibody serologic test is usually positive and elevated in patients with mixed connective tissue disease, not lupus. The ANA are elevated in 95% of patients with lupus, but it is not very specific. Anti-double stranded DNA antibody titers (B) are extremely useful in determining if the patient has lupus-induced glomerulonephritis. It is a sensitive and specific assay. A false-positive VDRL level (C) is usually seen in SLE patients because of the autoimmune mechanisms involved. A true-positive VDRL test is suggestive of syphilis infection. The anti-sm antibody test (D) is also positive in lupus patients as well as the presence of the LE cell on the peripheral smear, which is virtually diagnostic for SLE.

32. **(A)** An elevated blood pressure may be secondary to anxiety or nervousness. The "white coat syndrome," where a doctor's or nurse's lab coat causes anxiety, is a reality. You must check it again after the patient has had a chance to relax to be sure it is accurate. To increase the medication (B) or admit to the hospital for further tests (C) or telemetry (D) or ICU (E) may be premature and unnecessary.

33. **(A)** Pallor and maceration of the mucosa of the mouth are typical of angular stomatitis. Macrocheilia (B) is enlargement of the lips. Xerostomia (C) is dryness of the mouth. Gingivitis (D) is inflammation of the gums or gingiva. Periodontitis (E) is an inflammatory disease of the periodontium, or supporting structures of the teeth, which can lead to tooth loss.

34. **(A)** This disease is caused by a deficiency in riboflavin. Niacin (B), pyridoxine (C), cobalamin (D), and folic acid (E) deficiencies will lead to other clinical findings, but do not lead to angular chilitis or stomatitis.

35. **(E)** Riboflavin deficiency may result from liver disease (A), chronic alcoholism (B), chronic diarrhea (C), and a poor diet (D). It generally will not result from lack of vitamin C (E). Lack of vitamin C will result in scurvy.

36. **(B)** Treatment for riboflavin deficiency consists of vitamin supplementation in both oral and IM forms. Surgery (A), total parenteral nutrition (C), and NG tube feeding (D) are not required. Intestinal bypassing (E) will not cure this problem.

37. **(C)** It is permissible to enroll a subject with an IQ of 60 into a clinical trial if the local IRB has approved, in advance, the use of such individuals, provided that consent is obtained from the person responsible for him.

38. **(A)** The innominate artery will present as a pulsatile mass in the suprasternal notch.

39. **(D)** A dewlap is a fatty tumor that is located in the suprasternal notch.

40. **(C)** Tuberculous abscesses present as nonpulsatile, non-fluctuant masses in the suprasternal notch.

41. **(B)** A dermoid cyst will present as a nonpulsatile, fluctuant mass in the suprasternal notch.

42. **(D)** This patient has multiple myeloma, which is a malignant lymphoproliferative disease associated with Bence-Jones protein in the urine, hypercalcemia, and infiltration of plasma cells in the bone marrow. Beta2-microglobulin, an HLA

class I antigen, is a cell-surface component of most nucleated cells. It is secreted in excessive amounts in multiple myeloma and, when elevated, it is associated with a poor prognosis.

43. **(C)** This patient with chronic active hepatitis B is at an increased risk of having a hepatoma. Alpha-fetoprotein is a tumor marker that is associated with liver cancer. This patient has a mass in the liver and weight loss—both suggestive of a hepatoma. Alpha-fetoprotein is used as a screening tool for liver malignancy.

44. **(E)** This patient has signs and symptoms of non-Hodgkin's lymphoma. An elevated lactic dehydrogenase level is associated with a poor prognosis and reflects the growth rate and tumor burden of the lymphoma. A recent multi-institutional study has shown that age, clinical stage, and the pretreatment LDH level can effectively separate patients with a good prognosis using current therapy from those who are unlikely to be cured.

45. **(B)** Prostatic specific antigen is secreted by prostate cells, reaching especially high levels in prostate cancer. Studies with large cohorts of asymptomatic men show that screening with PSA consistently detects approximately one-third more cancers than digital rectal examination. Early detection by prostatic specific antigen has shown little or no effect on disease mortality. The PSA level normally increases with age.

46. **(D)** In hyperthyroidism, the thyroid is overworking and the metabolic rate is speeded up. You would expect to see tachycardia (A), a goiter (B), moist skin (C), and a widened pulse pressure (E). You would not see dry skin.

47. **(A)** The eye signs associated with hyperthyroidism are lid retraction due to the exophthalmos secondary to the increased periorbital fat. Entropion (B), or infolding of the eyelids, does not occur. Ectropion (C), or outfolding of the lids, also does not occur. Blepharitis (D) or conjunctivitis (E), both of which are infections, also do not occur.

48. **(C)** With hyperthyroidism, the serum T3 and T4 are both increased because of increased secretion and conversion.

49. **(E)** Treatment of hyperthyroidism may include surgery (A), iodine (B), propylthiouracil (C),

and methimazole (D). L-thyroxine is used to treat hypothyroidism, not hyperthyroidism.

50. **(B)** Research studies show that there is an increased risk for deep venous thrombosis and pulmonary embolism secondary to the use of estrogen-containing oral contraceptive. Currently, there is no evidence to make any kind of connection between breast (C) or cervical (D) cancer and exogenous estrogens. Benign hepatoma (A) is a recognized complication of oral contraceptives and levels do regress with discontinuation of the pills.

51. **(C)** *Staphylococcus* is the most common organism of the skin. Most of these finger infections start from the skin. The other organisms may be present on the skin but usually will not cause an overt infection. They will usually present themselves differently. *Bacteroides* (A) and *Streptococcus* (B) usually are intraoral. *Clostridium* (D) may be present on the skin but is not as common as *Staphylococcus*. *Herpes* (E) is a viral infection that can occur on the skin following exposure, as occurs with herpetic whitlow.

52. **(B)** First-generation cephalosporins are effective against Gram-positive cocci such as *Staphylococcus*. Second-generation (C) and third-generation (D) cephalosporins are more effective against Gram-negative cocci. Penicillin (A) is more effective against *Streptococcus*. Erythromycin (E) is also more effective against *Streptococcus* than *Staphylococcus*.

53. **(B)** This patient probably has a sexually transmitted disease such as gonorrhea or chlamydia trachomatis. A penile swab and culture is the most practical and cost-effective test to make the diagnosis and subsequently treat the patient with the correct antibiotics. CT scan of the pelvis (A) can be used to diagnose a penile abscess. This patient is not febrile and, thus, an abscess is unlikely. This patient does not have dysuria and burning or urgency on voiding and, thus, a urinary tract infection is unlikely. Urinary tract infections in men are unusual, but if one suspects it, then a urine culture (C) would be useful. A prostate exam (D) is a requirement in any male over the age of 40. This prostate exam would include a stool guaiac exam and an evaluation the prostate for nodules, but it will not make the correct diagnosis unless prostatitis is suspected. A serum VDRL (E) or RPR

is used to make a diagnosis of latent or suspected syphilis exposure. This patient does not have condyloma lata or venereal warts to suspect syphilis.

54. **(C)** A pneumothorax results from air in the pleural cavity. A patient will complain of a spontaneous, sharp pain that radiates to the cervical area. Dyspnea and cyanosis may result. Angina (A) is cardiac chest pain from myocardial ischemia. Myocardial infarction (B) is damage to the heart muscle from ischemia. A fractured rib (D) may cause pain and a pneumothorax, but is unlikely to occur spontaneously—it will often follow trauma. Bronchitis (E) is an infectious disease that will not usually lead to a pneumothorax.

55. **(C)**, 56. **(A)**, 57. **(E)**, 58. **(B)** Small-cell carcinoma commonly secretes hormonal substances such as ACTH and is also associated with neurologic syndromes such as Eaton-Lambert syndrome, a condition that presents with muscle weakness, which improves with repetition. Adenocarcinoma is the most common lung tumor in nonsmokers but can also occur in smokers. Histology is characterized by glandular formation with mucin-producing cells. Squamous cell carcinoma is the most common lung tumor to cause hypercalcemia, which may be mediated through bone metastasis, PTH-like action, prostaglandins, or osteoclast activating factor. Large cell carcinoma is less common and may represent a poorly differentiated adenocarcinoma. Carcinoid tumors of the lung may occasionally present with carcinoid syndrome although much less commonly than small bowel carcinoids. Symptoms include flushing and diarrhea.

59. **(B)** At this time, there is no evidence to suggest that the number of postoperative complications is reduced in outpatient surgical care.

60. **(A)** Adult-onset diabetes mellitus (NIDDM) patients who receive oral hypoglycemic agents are at high risk for postoperative complications, as are patients with juvenile-onset diabetes (IDDM) and, thus, they must be carefully monitored in the perioperative period.

61. **(A)** For patients to be considered candidates for outpatient ambulatory surgical operation, they should be in a relatively stable medical condition. As a general rule, less invasive intervention is performed on patients who may be less healthy, and more invasive intervention is considered for patients who are in good health. In-and-out surgery is best suited for the pediatric population. Pediatric patients are free of severe, concomitant systemic illnesses, and surgical procedures commonly performed on children are shorter, less extensive, and less invasive. Immunocompromised patients, such as those with HIV seropositivity and post-transplant status and cancer patients on chemo- and radiotherapy, are also good candidates for this type of surgical care. Unless suffering from a concomitant serious medical condition, many geriatric patients, too, can be immunocompromised. Therefore, they may acquire nosocomial infections in a hospital setting.

62. **(D)** Criteria that must be met before the patient may leave the ambulatory surgery facility include stabilized vital signs (A), pain adequately controlled, absence of surgical bleeding, tolerable nausea (E), and ability to void (C). Guidelines for safe discharge also include capability to tolerate oral intake of fluids and presence of an escort.

63. **(E)** The escort in ambulatory surgery should be able to receive and comprehend postoperative instructions (C), be available to call for medical assistance if needed (B), accompany the patient home (A), and serve as a companion during the first 24 hours postoperatively.

64. **(E)** The incidence rate of unscheduled hospitalization of patients from ambulatory surgery facilities is one to four percent. Reasons for this can be surgical, medical, and anesthesia-related. Surgical causes include intraoperative surgical or medical complications. Medical reasons include requirements for IV antibiotic therapy or poorly controlled concomitant cardiac or pulmonary disorders, hypertension, and diabetes mellitus. Anesthesia-related causes include uncontrollable nausea, vomiting, or pain, and aspiration pneumonia.

65. **(E)** Following some surgical procedures, patients may experience significant postoperative pain that is manageable in a recovery care facility, called an aftercare center. If it is unavailable, appropriate use of home care services may still allow a patient to avoid inpatient postoperative care.

66. **(D)** Follow-up telephone calls should be made to all patients on the first postoperative day to ensure quality as well as patient satisfaction. Postage-paid postcards may be sent to patients requesting information on their overall experience.

67. **(C)** This patient has post-splenectomy reactivation malarial syndrome. The malaria was latent and dormant in the liver and, subsequent to splenectomy, reactivation occurred. Encapsulated bacteria such as *Streptococcus* and *Haemophilus influenzae* are the most common organisms associated with post-splenectomy sepsis. This patient had negative blood cultures and no toxic granulations in the blood smear to suggest an abscess (A). A splenic hematoma (B) would show up on a CT scan of the abdomen, but it is an unlikely case in this situation because of the normal HCT. Hemolytic anemia (D) can also present with fever and joint pains, but the LDH would be elevated and the HCT would be decreased. This is not the case in this scenario. In lymphoma (E), the LDH would be elevated and it would not generally present right after a splenectomy. Chemotherapy is the correct treatment in lymphoma.

68. **(E)** There are no scientific data supporting the linkage of smoking and colonic carcinoma. The other malignancies are linked to cigarette smoking. Other carcinomas, such as of the mouth, stomach, bladder, and uterine cervix, also occur in increased incidence in smokers.

69. **(C)** Cardiac output is the product of heart rate and stroke volume. Vagal (A) and beta-adrenergic (B) stimulation both affect heart rate. Contractility (D) and ventricular end-diastolic volume (E) both affect stroke volume. Systemic vascular resistance is an independent entity from cardiac output.

70. **(B)** At this point, it is wise to discuss your options with someone with more experience.

71. **(D)** Directly confronting the patient with threats is unwise and not likely to be useful.

72. **(D)** Your obligation here includes warning the potential victim. Notifying the police and hospital security is also useful, as is continuing your effort to dissuade the patient from his plans.

73. **(C)** This case is an example of the "duty to warn" obligation of a physician informed of a potentially harmful situation.

74. **(A)** The risk to a person's safety takes priority over doctor-patient confidentiality privileges.

75. **(B)** A person cannot be committed for threatening like this.

76. **(B)** He cannot be arrested because he has not committed a crime, unless he does not have a permit for the gun. He cannot be put on probation unless he has committed a crime.

77. **(A)** This would make it a crime for the patient to come within a given distance of his wife.

78. **(A)** Cretinism, or infantile hypothyroidism, results from an enzymatic defect or iodine deficiency. Tall stature (A) is not a sign. Short stature is, as well as thick lips (B), obesity (C), short hands (D), and thick fingers (E).

79. **(B)** If the patient is unconscious, but not brain dead, a decision may be made by the court to discontinue life support. There must be documented evidence or testimony that this was the patient's last wish prior to the loss of consciousness. If there is no indication concerning the patient's wishes, life support may not be withdrawn unless the Harvard criteria of brain death have been established.

80. **(D)** Urethral symptoms in a sexually active male without other localizing renal complaints are most consistent with chlamydial urethritis.

81. **(E)** Behçet's syndrome can affect the joints and eyes but rarely causes significant diarrhea and is not seen much in people of Scandinavian ancestry. On the other hand, *Yersinia enterocolitica* (A) is a relatively common cause of a clinical picture such as this in people from Scandinavia. Reiter's syndrome (B), which can be related to yersinial infection, chlamydial infection (C), and inflammatory bowel disease (D) also can be associated with a presentation like this.

82. **(B)** Patients with severe diabetic peripheral neuropathy can have severe trauma to their extremities, especially the feet, and not feel the injury or the resulting infection.

83. **(D)** This clinical picture of menometrorrhagia is most consistent with uterine fibroids.

84. **(D)** Aspirin (A), beta-blockers (B), nitroglycerin (C), and cholesterol-lowering agents (E) have all been shown to decrease mortality in patients with coronary artery disease. Calcium channel blockers have failed to show this benefit, and, in fact, the shorter-acting ones have been shown to cause a slightly increased incidence of death in patients with coronary artery disease.

85. **(B)** In patients who are known to be non-compliant, clonidine can be dangerous. If clonidine is taken and then stopped suddenly, a rebound hypertension can occur. Other antihypertensives that don't have bad effects in patients who are non-compliant would be more appropriate.

86. **(C)** In patients who have difficult-to-control diabetes mellitus, the symptoms associated with hypoglycemia, such as sweating, tachycardia, anxiety, can be blocked by beta-blocker therapy. If they don't know that they're hypoglycemic, they can continue with hypoglycemia without knowing and without wanting to eat or drink; this can be potentially very dangerous.

87. **(A)** In patients with decreased renal perfusion, such as renal artery stenosis or severe congestive heart failure, ACE inhibitor usage can be associated with hyperkalemia and renal failure.

88. **(A)** In patients who are on chronic NSAIDs, ACE inhibitors can be very dangerous. Together, the two medications can precipitate acute renal failure.

89. **(A)** This elderly patient has temporal or giant cell arteritis, which is a vasculitic syndrome associated with intermittent jaw claudication, visual symptoms, and an elevated ESR. This disease affects the geriatric population usually in the large and medium-sized arteries supplying the neck, and extracranial structures of the head and arms are involved. The treatment of choice is steroids. Headache is the most common presenting symptom in this disorder.

90. **(C)** This young female has Takayasu's arteritis. This syndrome is more common in females. It is an inflammatory vasculitis involving the aortic arch and branches. It is also called "pulseless disease" because of the absent pulses in the upper extremities from occlusion of the major vessels. Transient ischemic attacks, syncope, and claudication of the upper extremities are common presenting symptoms in this disorder. Treatment is with steroids.

91. **(B)** This Turkish male has Behçet's disease. This mucocutaneous disease is more commonly found in patients of Mediterranean areas such as Turkey and the Middle East. Constitutional signs such as fever and weight loss are present in 63% of patients with this disorder. Twenty-five percent of patients with this disorder have phlebitis or arteritis. Oral ulcers are the most common finding and they are painful. Genital ulcers, uveitis, joint pain, and aseptic meningitis are also other typical findings associated with Behçet's disease. Colchicine, cyclosporine, and steroids have all been tried as therapy for this disorder.

92. **(E)** This male patient has allergic angiitis, or granulomatous vasculitis (Churg-Strauss disease). This disorder involves the small and medium arteries of the lung parenchyma and is associated with eosinophilia. Wheezing and interstitial lung disease are common. In the skin, dermal small and larger muscular arteries in the subcutaneous tissues are involved. Males are more commonly affected, as well as people with allergies.

93. **(C)** Urine screening is not recommended in asymptomatic persons even with childhood urine abnormalities. All individuals with DM [(A) and (B)] should be screened. Pregnancy [(B) and (D)] is another indication for periodic urine testing. A family history of lupus nephritis (E) is always an indication for screening by urine testing.

94. **(E)** An ectopic pregnancy occurs anywhere outside the endometrium. It occurs 1:100 to 1:200 diagnosed pregnancies. The treatment is surgical. A spontaneous abortion (A) is loss of the normal products of conception up until 20 weeks of gestation. It is also known as a miscarriage. Threatened abortion (B) is any bleeding or cramping occurring in the first 20 weeks of pregnancy. Hyperemesis gravidarum (C) is malignant excess vomiting due to the pregnancy. It is malignant in that it leads to dehydration and acidosis. Hospitalization and hydration are required. Preeclampsia (D) is the development of hypertension, edema and albuminuria after the 20th week of pregnancy

that may lead to full-blown eclampsia and sei-zures.

95.   **(D)**   Negatively birefringent crystals are classic for gout. The joint aspirate is consistent with an inflammatory disease; a septic joint [(A) and (B)] would commonly have greater than 100,000 nucleated cells.

96. **(C)**, 97. **(D)**, 98. **(B)**, 99. **(A)** Leukemia is a condition in which the bone marrow is replaced with a clone of malignant lymphocytic or granulocytic cells. There are particular clinical, histopathological, and cytogenetic methods to help to distinguish different forms of leukemia. CML is usually a disease of adults and often presents with leukocytosis and thrombocytosis. There is a cytogenetic abnormality present in approximately 90% of patients with CML, known as the Philadelphia chromosome (reciprocal translocation of part of the long arm of chromosome 22 to chromosome 9). CLL usually afflicts older patients and is characterized by the presence of a positive Coombs' test in 30% of patients. Hypogammaglobulinemia is also often present with a subsequent increase in susceptibility to bacterial infection. ALL is primarily a disease of children and can be distinguished from AML histochemically by a lack of staining for myeloperoxidase and lack of staining for Auer rods (coalescence of cytoplasmic granules which stain pink with Wright's stain). Acute monocytic leukemia is a subtype of AML, which is characterized by leukemic infiltrates in the gums and skin with subsequent bleeding. Histochemical staining commonly reveals Auer rods and myeloperoxidase-positive cells.

100.   **(A)**   It is ethical and correct for you to identify yourself and do what you can. If you cannot do a procedure, either under the conditions of the airplane or under the best of conditions, you should not do it. If indicated, you can ask the pilot to land.

101.   **(A)**   Hyperthyroidism, not hypothyroidism, commonly predisposes toward the development of atrial fibrillation. Both pulmonary embolus (B) and pericarditis (C) can lead to the development of acute atrial fibrillation. Heavy ethanol binging (D) can lead to atrial fibrillation, termed "holiday heart." Hypertension (E), through left atrial enlargement, can lead to chronic atrial fibrillation.

102.   **(E)**   Bretylium is indicated in patients with life-threatening ventricular tachycardiacs that do not respond to other agents, such as lidocaine. Digitalis (B) and propranolol (C) are both useful in controlling ventricular rate in patients with atrial fibrillation. Amiodarone (A) at low doses and quinidine (D) can be effective in terminating atrial tachyrhythmias.

103.   **(A)**   Irregular P-P interval is characteristic of multifocal atrial tachycardia (MAT). There is variation of P-wave morphology, not QRS morphology (B). Atrial rates in MAT tend to range between 100-130, not 200 (C). Retrograde P-waves (D) are associated with junctional rhythms. A reduced P-R interval (E) is observed in Wolff-Parkinson-White syndrome.

104.   **(A)**   MAT is associated with pulmonary diseases and is best treated by improving the underlying pulmonary condition. Zollinger-Ellison syndrome (B) results in hypergastrinemia and ulcers and has no cardiac manifestations. Pericarditis (C) predisposes toward atrial fibrillation and flutter, but not MAT. Atrial myxoma (D) is a rare atrial tumor unassociated with MAT.

105.   **(C)**   Left supraclavicular adenopathy would provide the best clue. In patients with gastric carcinoma, a hard lymph node there is very specific for cancer and is called Virchow's node.

106.   **(C)**   A peptic ulcer presents classically with epigastric pain (A), one to four hours postprandially (B), is relieved by H2 blockers (D) and is rhythmic and periodic (E) in pain character. A peptic ulcer is also classically relieved with food, not increased with food (C).

107.   **(B)**   The patient has a primary acute respiratory acidosis. Patients with chronic obstructive pulmonary disease often are baseline slightly hypoxemic and require that to drive their respirations. If you over-oxygenate them, they lose their drive to breathe and begin to underventilate, causing an acute respiratory acidosis which can cause neurologic deterioration.

108.   **(C)**   The median age for fibrocystic breast disease is 30. Menarche is usually at age 13 (A). Fibroadenoma has a median age of 20 (B). Intraductal papilloma has a median age of 40 (D). Carcinoma has a median age of 54 (E).

109. **(A)** The patient described appears to have pneumonia. Auscultation often reveals rales in the affected lung field. Bilateral wheezing is a more common finding in patients with asthma or congestive heart failure ("cardiac asthma") (B). Subcutaneous emphysema may present with crepitus over the anterior clavicle and is not a common finding in pneumonia (C). The ausculatory findings of pneumothorax include absent breath sounds and hyperresonance in the area of the collapsed lung (D). Although there may be normal breath sounds in patients with pneumonia, rales in the affected area are more common (E).

110. **(A)** The most common organism causing community-acquired pneumonia is the *Pneumococcus*. Gram stain reveals Gram-positive diplococci and chains. *S. aureus* is commonly seen as Gram-positive cocci in clusters. This organism is not as common a cause of community-acquired pneumonia as the pneumococcus (B). Diptheroids are not common causes of pneumonia (C). Gram-negative organisms are more common in nosocomial pneumonia rather than community-acquired pneumonia (D). Acid-fast bacilli suggest tuberculous infection, a less common cause of community-acquired pneumonia (E).

111. **(A)** The patient should be treated with in-hospital intravenous antibiotics due to his age, fever, and tachypnea. Oxacillin is an active agent against most *S. aureus* organisms and should be used in this situation. There is a significant resistance of *S. aureus* to penicillin due to the ability of this organism to produce beta-lactamase (B). Intravenous vancomycin should be limited to cases of oxacillin-resistant *S. aureus* due to the increasing development of vancomycin-resistant organisms with injudicious use of this agent (C). Oral vancomycin is not well absorbed and is not effective for pneumonia (D). First-generation cephalosporins are active against *S. aureus*, however, intravenous antibiotics are indicated in the patient described (E).

112. **(E)** Pulmonary examination and X-ray findings lag behind clinical improvement and may take weeks to months before resolving. Therefore, management should be based on clinical improvement rather than improvement on X-ray. Malignancy is not yet a consideration based on a five-day interval chest X-ray (A). If there is clinical improvement, broadening of antibiotic cover-age is not indicated (B). Daily chest X-rays are not indicated for management of community-acquired pneumonia (C). Open lung biopsy is not indicated based on these X-ray findings (D).

113. **(C)** *Legionella pneumonia* usually presents in older smokers. In patients under 60 years old and with community-acquired pneumonia, the most common organisms are *Streptococcus pneumonia* (A), *Mycoplasma pneumoniae* (B), and *Chlamydia pneumoniae* (E). *Haemophilus influenzae* (D) can be found as well, especially in smokers.

114. **(A)** Smoking increases the incidence of *Haemophilus influenzae* as the causative organism. Ethanol intake (B) can increase the chance of aspiration pneumonia, making anaerobic organisms more likely. Cystic fibrosis patients (C) are most commonly infected with *Pseudomonas aeruginosa*.

115. **(C)** The macrolide derivatives have good effect against pneumococcus, as well as some of the atypicals, such as *Mycoplasma* and *Chlamydia*. Fluroquinolones, such as cipronoxacin (A), should not be used in community-acquired pneumonia because of a poor effect against *Pneumococcus*. One dose of a third-generation cephalosporin (D) is probably not enough duration of treatment. Vancomycin (E) should only be considered in nosocomial pneumonias where penicillin-resistant organisms are a concern. Penicillin (B) is ineffective against many of the *Pneumococcus* species and has poor coverage against atypicals.

116. **(C)** Abnormalities can take up to six weeks to resolve. Effective treatment can be judged by clinical status.

117. **(E)** Stridor, a crowing sound, is generally caused by obstruction of the airway between the nose and larger bronchi. All of the other choices: foreign body aspiration (A), croup (B), epiglottitis (C), and lyngomalacia (D) affect the upper airway. Asthma usually causes wheezing. The site of airway obstruction is in the large and small bronchioles.

118. **(D)** Acute epiglottis, not viral croup, is an emergency. The patient should be kept in a quiet area free from agitation until the airway can be visualized and secured to prevent acute obstruction.

In addition to parainfluenza Type I and II and RSV, croup can also be caused by influenza virus (A). In spasmodic croup, one usually observes the sudden onset of hoarseness and barking cough at night, which resolves with humidified air (B). A frontal radiographic view of the neck shows a classic "steeple" sign (C) of the gubglottic area where the airway narrows, appearing like a point of a pencil or steeple. Racemic epinephrine (E) is often used to manage croup.

119. **(D)** Although the overall death rate from all malignancies has increased by approximately seven percent in the U.S. over the past decades, lung cancer is now the number one cause of cancer death among men and women. This overall increase is associated with an aging population. Breast cancer mortality (C) is relatively unchanged over the period. However, colon (A) and prostate (E) cancer mortalities have slightly increased.

120. **(D)** Adrenalcortical hypofunction leads to diastolic hypotension. Pheochromocytoma (A), acromegaly (B), adrenalcortical hyperfunction (C), and carcinoid (E) all lead to diastolic hypertension, in which the heightened diastolic pressure represents the minimal continuous load to which the peripheral circulation is subjected.

121. **(B)** Patients may present with "pseudo-thrombocytopenia." This benign condition results when a routine blood sample is anticoagulated with EDTA. When the blood sample is anticoagulated with heparin (B), which prevents in vitro clumping, the platelet count normalizes [(A) and (C)]. In this condition, as illustrated, platelets agglutinate or adhere to leukocytes (D). When platelets are counted by an electronic counting machine, the platelet clumps are misidentified (E).

122. **(B)** An abdominal ultrasound would help delineate the amount of ascites and identify masses.

123. **(A)** A pelvic examination is a critical part of any woman's routine physical, even after menopause.

124. **(E)** Cytologic studies are essential in this patient.

125. **(D)** An EEG would not contribute much to the evaluation of this patient.

126. **(C)** Meigs' syndrome is metastatic ovarian cancer with malignant ascites.

127. **(B)** While this is an incurable disease, there are drug combinations that can ameliorate the symptoms and slow the progress in some people. Many of these are in experimental stages of development, however.

128. **(B)** A genetic counselor can best discuss the risks of disease in her family members.

129. **(C)** Just because your patient has terminal cancer does not mean you do not need to follow her. She may live for a long time and need your help. Furthermore, a routine follow-up appointment is one small way to give her some hope for the future.

130. **(C)** Again, you must have the patient's written permission before you release information about his health to anyone.

131. **(A)** In a hemodynamically stable narrow-complex tachycardia, the first intervention should be intravenous adenosine. In this healthy patient, the most likely etiology is paroxysmal supraventricular tachycardia, which can often be broken by intravenous adenosine.

132. **(A)** MMR contains live attenuated viruses; the others do not. DTP (D) contains toxoids and inactivated bacteria. IPV (B) contains inactivated viruses. Hepatitis B vaccine (C) contains inactivated viral antigen. Hib (E) contains polysaccharide-protein conjugate.

133. **(C)** A pneumoperitoneum is air in the peritoneal cavity resulting from perforation of a hollow viscus. On physical exam, there is a tympanitic abdomen and no bowel sounds. A radiograph would reveal air between the viscera.

134. **(E)** Melena results from the breakdown of blood anywhere along the GI tract. It is not normal and should be worked-up. A stool hemoccult (A) will confirm the presence of blood rather than just black tarry stools that may have resulted from food or medications. A rectal exam (B) may note the presence of masses or strictures or any other cause of bleeding. Sigmoidoscopy (C) will allow you to visualize directly the distal colon. A barium enema (D) will allow you to radiographically

examine the colon. There is no immediate need for a CAT scan of the abdomen. Depending on what the workup reveals, it may be ordered later.

135. **(E)** Aortic rupture is not one of the known complications of a spinal tap (E). However, infection (A), headache (B), nerve injury (C), and herniation (D) are all potential complications of performing a spinal tap to study the cerebrospinal fluid and should be explained while obtaining informed consent.

136. **(D)** The likeliest cause for a positive hemoccult test in this patient is a rectal lesion, so a sigmoidoscopy is the most useful first test to perform.

137. **(A)** People who take chronic nonsteroidals are at risk for peptic ulcerations.

138. **(D)** This patient and his brother both have herpes whitlow, caused by infection with herpes simplex virus. The lesion is usually painful and associated with swelling and local adenopathy. Primary cutaneous inoculation with herpes simplex virus often occurs secondary to transmission via saliva and mucocutaneous membranes. Treatment is with acyclovir, which is an antiviral agent. Steroids (A) are contraindicated in this infection and would make the infection worse and cause dissemination as well. Antibiotics (B) are used for bacterial infections, which this patient does not have. Antibiotics can be used if a bacterial infection is superimposed on a viral infection. In that case, the patient would have an associated fever. Topical antifungal creams (C) are used for athlete's foot and "jock itch." This patient has a viral infection and not a fungal infection. If this wound was secondary to a human bite or animal bite, then debridement and irrigation with saline (E) would be adequate. This lesion is not secondary to a bite, but to a viral infection.

139. **(B)** The sputum with congestive heart failure is classically pink and frothy.

140. **(A)** The most common cause of congestive heart failure is myocardial infarction. Calcium channel blockers (E) can sometimes exacerbate congestive heart failure, but usually are not a primary cause.

141. **(B)** A systolic flow murmur is either benign or a sign of slightly increased cardiac output. All of the other signs are consistent with heart failure.

142. **(C)** All of the other answers are reasonable tests to order initially. A cardiac catheterization may be considered if the stress test is grossly positive.

143. **(C)** Beta-blockers (A) have been shown to decrease mortality after a myocardial infarction. The ACE inhibitors (B), nitrates (D), and hydralazine (E) have all been shown to decrease mortality in patients with congestive heart failure.

144. **(E)** Side effects include cough, renal failure, and hyperkalemia. However, studies have shown all of the other effects of ACE inhibitors to be true.

145. **(D)** ACE inhibitors have been shown to cause all of these side effects and complications, except pruritus.

146. **(A)** In a patient with known coronary artery disease, it's reasonable to try a beta-blocker, as numerous studies have shown a decreased mortality in post-myocardial infarction patients who are placed on a beta-blocker.

147. **(A)** The PAS-stained material obtained from the periorbital lesion, shown in Panel A, demonstrates typical irregularly shaped broad hyphae with right-angle branching. In Panel B, stained with lactophenol blue, characteristic sporangia and rhizoids of the pathogen, rhizopus, are evident. Rhizopus and mucor are the most common pathogens that produce mucormycosis. In poorly controlled diabetics, the nose and paranasal sinuses are most commonly involved. Treatment is with amphotericin B (A), the only drug with proven clinical efficacy. In addition, surgical debridement and management of the underlying medical problems are essential.

148. **(C)** Temporal arteritis is one of the necrotizing vasculitides named for the principal cranial artery involved. It is often associated with polymyalgia rheumatica. It is unilateral or bilateral and can last from three months to three years. Jaw claudication is frequent.

149. **(D)** The overlying skin is not normal, but is red and swollen. The involved artery feels hard and nodular (A). The artery is tender (B) and pulsatile (C). There is associated weakness, malaise, and prostration (E).

150. **(E)** With temporal arteritis, vision is often impaired (A), and there is ophthalmoplegia (B), retinal changes (C), and unilateral or bilateral eye involvement (D).

151. **(E)** The headache from a brain tumor is not due to a vascular cause, but rather to mass effect-displacement. Fever headaches (A), hypertensive headaches (B), cluster headaches (C), and atypical migraines (D) are all vascular headaches.

152. **(D)** The physician can decide what to do in a medical emergency in a minor patient when the guardian is not immediately available.

153. **(C)** The legal guardian must be contacted for permission for non-emergency procedures in a minor.

154. **(A)** A competent patient can give permission for postmortem use of his/her organs.

155. **(A)** A competent patient has the right to refuse treatment.

156. **(B)** This patient has classic enteric fever or *Salmonella typhi* infection. He acquired the infection from the fecal-oral route from an endemic part of India. The rash is called "rose spots" and is highly suggestive of *Salmonella typhi*, along with the leukopenia and relative bradycardia. The gold standard for diagnosis is a few sets of blood cultures which would grow the organism. The treatment is intravenous ceftriaxone or oral ciprofloxacin. Stool cultures for *Salmonella* (A) usually grow the organism in two to three weeks after the fever has started, so this would not aid in the acute infectious process. Stool for ova and parasites would not yield anything. A bone marrow aspirate (C) can also grow *Salmonella*, but this does not have a better diagnostic sensitivity than blood cultures. Looking under the microscope at the peripheral smear would be diagnostic for malaria, not *Salmonella*. A chest X-ray (E) would be negative in *Salmonella* infection because this is an enteric disease. A vaccine is now available to protect against *Salmonella typhi* when travelling to endemic areas. It is given in three doses, and it is a live oral avirulent Ty21a vaccine. Protection lasts for several years. Protection in food handling is important in chronic carriers of the infection, as well as environmental sanitation measures.

157. **(D)** Postexposure immunization measures against salmonellosis do not exist. All other infectious conditions would have less severe presentation with early immunizations after the exposure.

158. **(C)** This patient has hairy cell leukemia, which is a rare disorder and more common in males. Patients have symptoms due to anemia, fatigue, fever, weight loss, and abdominal fullness and early satiety secondary to splenomegaly. Clinical lymphadenopathy is rare and the white count is usually low. In addition to the cytopenias, the peripheral blood film usually demonstrates absolute lymphocytosis with cells having cytoplasmic projections—hairy cells. Hairy cells exhibit a reaction that is positive for tartaric acid. The prognosis for this disorder is poor and the treatment of choice is interferon.

159. **(A)** This patient has clinical signs and symptoms of chronic myelogenous leukemia. Chronic myelogenous leukemia is a disease characterized by overproduction of cells of the granulocytic, monocytic series A characteristic cytogenetic abnormality (the Philadelphia chromosome) and is present in the bone marrow cells in more than 95% of cases. Splenomegaly is usually present and all untreated patients with CML have an elevated white blood cell count. CML is a myeloproliferative disorder. Blast crises in CML is associated with a poor prognosis. The leukocyte alkaline phosphatase level is decreased in patients with chronic myelogenous leukemia.

160. **(E)** This unfortunate man has an acute thrombotic stroke with hemiparesis secondary to thrombosis from an increase in blood viscosity. He has polycythemia vera, which is a myeloproliferative disorder characterized by splenomegaly, increased red blood cell mass, hyperviscosity, and occasionally an increase in blood pressure. Generalized pruritus and headaches are common symptoms in polycythemia vera. Patients also may have an increase in platelet counts, leukocyte counts, and vitamin B12 levels. Thrombohemorrhagic complications are also common. Frequent phlebotomy and interferon-alpha are the

recommended treatments of choice for polycythemia vera. This disorder runs in families.

161. **(B)** This patient has essential thrombocythemia, which is associated with an increase in platelet counts over 600,000/uL and absence of conditions associated with reactive thrombocytosis. Usually, there is a normal red blood cell count and normal spleen size. There are megakaryocyte clusters associated with essential thrombocythemia in the bone marrow. Iron stores are usually diminished and patients are usually asymptomatic, although acute strokes and transient ischemic attacks can occur secondary to thrombosis.

162. **(D)** Amyloidosis is a disturbance of endogenous protein metabolism leading to organ dysfunction. Signs include macroglossia, hypertension, hepatosplenomegaly, edema, muscle and joint pain, and nephrotic syndrome.

163. **(D)** Testing for visual acuity in the elderly requires sufficient grounds for doing so (e.g., persistent headaches or the presence of symptoms of DM). School-age children (B), preferably at age three (A), and DM in any age group are indications for screening [(C) and (E)].

164. **(C)** Rales and hyperresonant percussion are seen with pulmonary emphysema. In a closed pneumothorax (A), there is resonant percussion and no rales. In an open pneumothorax (B), there is hyperresonant percussion and no rales. In a hydropneumothorax (D), there is flat or hyperresonant percussion and no rales.

165. **(C)** In a patient with known history of timely boosters of tetanus toxoid, the emergency care of clean wounds does not mandate another injection at the time of injury. It is administered in pediatric patients in DTP combination (A) at ten-year intervals (B). Since a small proportion of vaccines does not maintain an effective level or lasting immunity against tetanus for ten years, dirty or lacerated wounds always require a booster dose (D). No records of immunization is another indication for toxoid administration (E).

166. **(C)** Flumazenil is appropriate treatment for benzodiazepine overdose. Appropriate treatment for ethylene glycol ingestion include gastric lavage (A), intravenous ethanol (B), and thiamin (D). Hemodialysis (E) is sometimes very effective.

167. **(C)** The most common cause of small-bowel obstruction in patients who have had previous abdominal surgery is adhesions. The other common etiologies include cancer (B) and incarcerated hernias (A).

168. **(C)** The chest X-ray demonstrates a left hilar mass, for which, in this clinical setting, the most likely diagnosis is lung carcinoma (C). In primary pulmonary hypertension, the chest X-ray shows enlarged central pulmonary arteries (A). In grade 1 sarcoidosis, there is bilateral hilar lymph node enlargement; in grade 2A, lymph node enlargement is associated with parenchymal changes; in grade 3, parenchymal changes are present in the absence of adenopathy (B). In lung abscess, X-rays typically show a parenchymal infiltrate with a cavity containing an air-fluid level (D). There is no evidence of metastatic breast cancer on this X-ray (E).

169. **(A)** Small-cell carcinoma pulmonary malignancy is not associated with rheumatoid arthritis. Pulmonary nodules are associated with rheumatoid arthritis (B). In Caplan's syndrome, patients with rheumatoid arthritis who are exposed to industrial agents develop pulmonary nodules. Obliterative bronchiolitis and fibrosing alveolitis may develop in rheumatoid arthritis in a manner similar to lupus or scleroderma [(C) and (E)]. Pleural effusions are common in rheumatoid arthritis and other connective tissue diseases (D).

170. **(E)** There are numerous extra-articular manifestations of rheumatoid arthritis. However, urethral discharge is not associated with rheumatoid arthritis; rather it is a manifestation of the rheumatoid factor negative arthropathy, Reiter's syndrome. Episcleritis occurs in approximately one percent of patients with rheumatoid arthritis (B). Felty's syndrome is a condition consisting of rheumatoid arthritis, splenomegaly, leukopenia, and thrombocytopenia (C). Pericarditis is often seen in patients with rheumatoid arthritis, although it is usually asymptomatic (D).

171. **(A)** This patient has Raynaud's phenomenon, which is a vasospastic disorder of the

digital arteries after exposure to cold. This results in ischemia of the digits and subsequent pain. This disorder can be associated with scleroderma and the CREST syndrome. Women are most commonly affected. The initial treatment of choice would be conservative. This would include keeping the hands warm and discontinuing cigarette smoking, which would increase the vasospasm. Vasodilating drugs, such as calcium-channel blockers (nifedipine) and reserpine are occasionally helpful, but the side effects, such as orthostatic hypotension, may preclude their use (B). Steroids (C) are not useful in this isolated disorder. If scleroderma is also involved, then steroids are used to treat the vasculitis. Treatment of Raynaud's phenomenon is available, so choice (D) is incorrect. Sympathectomy (E) provides only transient benefit in most patients, but should be considered when a patient has progressive ulceration or gangrene of the digits that fails to improve after a conservative regimen.

172. **(E)** Because this patient is experiencing an early phase of the infection, she would benefit from vaccinations. It will protect her from the further development of hepatitis.

173. **(B)** Surgery with resection of the bowel has not been shown to improve survival in metastatic colon cancer, especially when the cancer has spread to the liver. 5-fluorouracil (A) is a chemotherapeutic agent that has been used to treat metastatic colon carcinoma for over 30 years. It can be given by the intravenous route, arterial infusion, intraperitoneally, or orally. Its side effects include leukopenia, diarrhea, stomatitis, and intractable vomiting. Levamisole (C) is an immune system stimulator and when it is given in combination with 5-fluorouracil, there is a significant reduction in recurrence rate and death rate. Leucovorin (folinic acid) in combination with 5-fluorouracil (D) has been shown to produce a small but significant three-year survival benefit. Because hepatic metastases obtain most of their blood supply from the hepatic artery rather than the ptoral vein, arterial rather than systemic infusion of adjuvant agents allows higher drug levels to reach the tumor site with lower systemic toxicity and less possibility of the development of drug resistance (E). Studies have shown that the com-

bination of floxuridine and dexamethasone sodium phosphate increases the two-year survival to 60%.

174. **(D)** All of the answers except red cell casts are found in bacterial cystitis; red cell casts are found in glomerular diseases, such as glomerulonephritis.

175. **(D)** Risk factors for esophageal cancer include chronic alcoholism (A), smoking (B), and damage to the esophageal epithelium with substances such as lye (E). Chronic gastroesophageal reflux (C) disease can lead to a transformation of the epithelium to Barrett's esophagus, which is a pre-malignant state.

176. **(A)** The incidence of male breast carcinoma is one percent of that in women. It must always be included in the differential for males with an unknown breast mass that is suspicious.

177. **(C)** This patient probably has missed her menstrual cycles because of stress. If her endometrium is primed and ready for menstruation, then administering oral progesterone (10 mg) will result in withdrawal bleeding. If withdrawal bleeding does not occur, then further work-up is necessary. An endometrial biopsy (A) is needed only if administering oral progesterone does not result in withdrawal bleeding. Colposcopy (B) is an invasive procedure that involves taking a biopsy and scraping from the cervix. This procedure is done only after a Pap smear comes back with abnormal cells on cytopathology. Oral estrogen administration (D) alone will not result in withdrawal bleeding and, thus, will not aid in the management of this patient. An elevated serum prolactin level can also result in oligomenorrhea (E), but this patient has no signs of lactation or cranial adenomas. Obtaining a serum prolactin level would be useful only if the progesterone withdrawal test did not happen.

178. **(C)** This patient's presentation is highly suggestive of the anti-phospholipid antibody syndrome, which sometimes has features similar to systemic lupus and which can cause thrombotic phenomena and fetal wastage. Choice (A) is not correct since this is not the picture of an Rh

incompatibility. (B) is not correct because anti-smooth muscle antibodies are not associated with such a syndrome. Similarly, (D) is incorrect. (E) is incorrect since rheumatoid factor-positive conditions are not associated with a syndrome such as this.

179. **(A)** Cor pulmonale, or pulmonary hypertension, results from such diseases as hypertension, mitral stenosis, pulmonary emphysema, left-to-right cardiac shunts, pulmonary fibrosis, and scleroderma. It is not associated with mitral regurgitation (B), pulmonary hypotension (C), or cardiac hypotension (D).

180. **(D)** Although aspirin can block platelet action, it does not cause thrombocytopenia as can heparin (A), famotidine (B), gold salts (C), and quinidine (E).

USMLE Step 3 – Practice Test 3
Day Two – Afternoon Session

1. **(E)** Her symptoms are consistent with nephrolithiasis, which patients will often state is the worst pain in their lives (sometimes worse than childbirth). Typically, urinalysis will show hematuria. The gold standard test is the intravenous pyelogram. Treatment includes pain control and hydration, after which the stone commonly passes spontaneously. If it doesn't, lithotripsy or surgical treatment can be done.

2. **(B)** Chest pain at rest is known as unstable angina and is very serious. It is more dangerous than stable angina, which occurs on exertion (A). A myocardial infarction (C) or heart attack (D) implies damage to the heart muscle from the ischemia, whereas, with angina, the ischemia leads to no heart damage.

3. **(C)** This patient most likely has had a myocardial infraction. She needs to be admitted to a coronary intensive care unit. Here she will be closely observed, monitored, and protected against further progression of her infarction. To discharge home (A) or admit to a floor bed (B) is not sufficient. To schedule the patient with a cardiologist (D) or simply start the patient on aspirin and nitroglycerin (E) also are insufficient and do not treat the patient.

4. **(B)** If there were an infarction, then there is probably myocardial damage. The heart will not pump as well and you would expect to see decreased wall motion on the echocardiogram. It is unlikely that it will be normal (A) or increased (C). To have no wall motion at all (D), would imply a non-beating heart and clinical death.

5. **(C)** Prior to coronary artery bypass grafting, the surgeon must know where the blockages of the coronary vessels are. The only way to know this for sure is with a cardiac catheterization. It will delineate the vessels of the heart and show the occlusions. A CT (A) or MRI (B) of the chest will not adequately reveal the vessels. A chest X-ray (D) similarly will not reveal the vessels. Left ventricular end diastolic pressure (E) may be an important measurement, but will not help the surgeon with the bypass.

6. **(C)** Most surgeons will agree that the results of bypass grafting will last between five and ten years. After that time, the vessels may reocclude and surgery may be indicated again.

7. **(E)** After successful bypass grafting, the patient must be reeducated. The reeducation includes an exercise regimen (A), an improved diet (B) that is low in cholesterol and fat, smoking cessation (C), and stress and lifestyle modification (D). In an ambulatory patient, there is no need to teach the patient about the avoidance of pressure sores.

8. **(B)** In this age group, an otitis media is a very common source of an infection and subsequent temperature. The other otitides [(A) and (C)] may occur, but are more common in other age groups. Sinusitis (D) and meningitis (E) also occur, but not as frequently. Also, with these diseases, there usually isn't tugging on the ears.

9. **(D)** The return of the bulbocavernosus reflex signifies the end of spinal shock. During spinal shock, the reflex will be absent (C) and the patient may appear to have a complete spinal cord lesion. Only after spinal shock, which usually resolves in 24 hours, can the level of the lesion be adequately assessed. The return of the reflex offers no information regarding prognosis or recovery of other levels presented in choices (A), (B), or (E).

10. **(D)**, 11. **(B)**, 12. **(A)**, and 13. **(E)** Alcoholic liver disease (A) covers a spectrum of liver dysfunction, ranging from fatty liver to alcoholic hepatitis to alcoholic cirrhosis. Liver function tests commonly show an SGOT which is more that twice that of the SGPT. Total bilirubin is often elevated when alcoholic liver disease has progressed to alcoholic hepatitis or alcoholic cirrhosis. Other findings in

alcoholic cirrhosis include spider angiomata (tiny blanching cutaneous vessels) and muscle wasting. Viral hepatitis (B), due to hepatitis B and C, is often due to bloodborne transmission such as intravenous drug use. Constitutional symptoms are often associated with viral hepatitis and liver function tests usually show an SGPT which is greater than the SGOT. Cholangiocarcinoma (C) is a tumor of the bile ducts. It commonly presents as progressive jaundice, and weight loss in elderly patients or patients with a history of primary sclerosing cholangitis. Liver function tests show an elevated total bilirubin and alkaline phosphatase. Acute cholangitis (D) is an infection of the biliary tree, most commonly secondary to an impacted stone in the common bile duct. Patients present with pain, jaundice, and fever. Liver function tests show an elevated alkaline phosphatase and total bilirubin count, although transaminases are usually also elevated during the early period. Acute cholecystitis (E) usually occurs secondary to a stone impacted in the neck of the gall bladder. Liver function tests are often normal, as there is no obstruction of bile from the liver.

14.　**(A)**　This patient has necrotizing fascitis, which is usually caused by the infectious organism *Streptococcus pyogenes*. It occurs suddenly and in young, healthy individuals. The immediate treatment is fasciotomy by the surgical team because death is otherwise imminent. The affected arm is subsequently debrided and irrigated. Clindamycin alone (B) is an inappropriate choice. Antibiotic combinations, such as ampicillin/sulbactam plus clindamycin, are given only after surgery is performed. Hyperbaric oxygen chamber usage (C) is good for patients with anaerobic infections. This patient has infection with a Grampositive aerobic toxin-producing bacteria. This patient has weakness and decreased sensation of the left upper extremity secondary to an infectious process and not to a stroke. Thus, a CT of the head (D) is useless and would only delay the necessary surgical intervention. Thrombolytic therapy (E) is also contraindicated because this patient does not have a thromboembolic stroke causing the weakness, but a severe infection affecting the subcutaneous tissue and muscles of the left upper limb.

15.　**(D)**　In patients who have had an aortic graft placed and who present with gastrointestinal bleeding, the diagnosis of aorto-enteric fistula should be assumed until ruled out. These patients can exsanguinate within minutes and need to be taken to laparotomy immediately to rule out fistula.

16.　**(B)**　This patient has acute ethylene glycol intoxication by ingestion of antifreeze. This causes renal failure secondary to oxalate build-up in the renal tubules, and the key to survival is to save the kidneys. Immediate dialysis is necessary in this patient to prevent uremia and permanent kidney failure. Hemoperfusion (A) may be indicated for chloramphenicol and hypnotic sedative overdoses. Activated charcoal (C) is given orally or by nasogastric tube to prevent absorption of the toxic substance. In this case, giving charcoal is futile because the antifreeze was already absorbed and the kidneys already damaged, as reflected by the elevated BUN and creatinine. Gastric lavage (D) is used to prevent absorption of toxic substances recently ingested such as aspirin, Tylenol, and tricyclic antidepressants. This patient has already absorbed the ethylene glycol. Forced alkaline diuresis (E) enhances the elimination of chlorphenoxyacetic acid herbicides, phenobarbital, and salicylates. If this patient can urinate, then regular hydration can flush out the oxalate crystals in the urine. Intravenous ethanol is also used to treat ethylene glycol intoxication by inhibiting alcohol dehydrogenase.

17.　**(B)**　Cataplexy is a symptom associated with narcolepsy, not OSA. Although narcolepsy is another cause of excessive daytime sleepiness, this disorder also consists of symptoms of hypnagogic hallucinations and sleep paralysis, symptoms not seen in OSA. The other symptoms are all commonly seen in patients with OSA, although the symptoms are commonly identified by a patient's family member rather than the patient.

18.　**(A)**　Nocturnal myoclonus, or periodic limb movement disorder, is another condition associated with excessive daytime sleepiness and insomnia. Schizophrenic patients (B) usually sleep well. Somnambulism (C), or sleep-walking, does not result in daytime sleepiness. Sleep terrors (D), also called parvis nocturnes, occurs primarily in young children, but patients do not recall the events the next day and do not have daytime sleepiness.

19.　**(A)**　Increased upper airway muscle activity is not a pathophysiological mechanism related to the development of OSA, rather a decreased upper airway muscle activity that is characteristic of patients with OSA. Structural compromise of airway patency (B) can often be demonstrated clinically as "pharyngeal crowding" and is related to the development of OSA. High airway compliance (C) results in an airway more prone to collapse and obstruction. High nasal resistance (D) contributes to collapse of the upper airway through increased subatmospheric pressure generated in the pharynx during inspiration (E).

20.   **(C)**   Polysomnography, commonly known as a sleep study, is the definitive test for the diagnosis of OSA and allows for the determination of the various sleep stages, ventilatory variables, oxygen saturation, and heart rate during sleep. Holter monitoring (A) and electroencephalography (B) may reveal abnormalities in patients with OSA, but are not definitive diagnostic tests. Pharyngeal nerve conduction studies (D) are not clinically useful for this diagnosis.

21.   **(B)**   Falls in oxygen saturation during apneic episodes are characteristic of OSA. Episodes of airflow cessation during sleep are also common but are associated with respiratory effort (A). A lack of respiratory effort is more suggestive of central sleep apnea. Direct wake-to-REM sleep transitions (C) are common in patients with narcolepsy. Seizure activity during non-REM sleep (D) is not characteristic of OSA.

22.   **(D)**   Tracheostomy is not indicated as a first-line therapy in patients with OSA, and is only used when all other treatment options have failed. Weight reduction (A) increases upper airway lumen size. Avoidance of alcohol (B) improves upper airway muscle tone. Nasal CPAP (C) is one of the most successful approaches to treatment by maintaining pharyngeal patency with positive pressure. Uvulopalatopharyngoplasty (E) is useful in patients with redundant pharyngeal tissue.

23.   **(E)**   Anemia is unlikely to be related to OSA, as this condition usually results in polycythemia due to chronic hypoxemia. OSA is likely to have contributed to this patient's systemic hypertension (A). Right-sided heart failure (B) may result from chronic hypoxemia (D) and pulmonary hypertension. Dysrhythmias (C) are thought to be the result of apneic episodes.

24.   **(E)**   The most likely mechanism of nocturnal sudden death in patients with OSA is from tachy- and bradyrhythmias. OSA by itself does not cause coronary artery disease or myocardial infarction (A), pulmonary embolus (B), stroke (C), or pneumothorax (D).

25.   **(B)**   Dysentery occurs secondary to mucosal invasion of the pathogenic organism. Common causes include *Shigella* and enteroinvasive *E. coli*. Ulcerative erosions into arterial vessels are a mechanism of GI bleeding from peptic ulcer disease (A). Dysentery is not generally associated with a systemic coagulopathy unless sepsis and disseminated intravascular coagulation develop (C). Thrombosis of submucosal capillaries does not occur in dysentery (D). Bowel necrosis is a cause of bleeding in ischemic bowel disease, but is not common in infectious dysentery (E).

26.   **(C)**   Sodium fluoride improves bone-mineral density by stimulating osteoblasts. High doses of plain sodium fluoride have been shown to decrease spine fractures, but increase the incidence of new hip fractures by increasing bone fragility. Recently, slow-release sodium fluoride has been associated with an increased formation of normal bone. Alendronate (A) is a biphosphonate, which has been shown to decrease bone turnover and inhibit osteoclast activity. This drug is now available and approved by the FDA for treatment of postmenopausal osteoporosis. It is extremely important that there is adequate lighting (B) and fall-proof carpets and furniture, along with adequate bathroom fixtures that can prevent future falls and fractures in this elderly female. Estrogen replacement (D) can protect postmenopausal women against osteoporosis and decrease the incidence of hip and spine fractures by 50% in some studies. Adding progesterone to estrogen decreases the incidence of endometrial carcinoma. Nasal salmon calcitonin (E) in a dose of 200 IU per day has been shown to increase bone-mineral density and reduce the rate of new fractures. Nausea and nasal dryness are some of the side effects of this new drug.

27.   **(B)**   Plummer-Vinson syndrome is a postcricoid esophageal web associated in patients with iron deficiency. Dysphagia is present due to the webbing.

28. **(A)** This synovial fluid analysis is most consistent with septic arthritis. Rheumatoid arthritis (B) and factor negative spondyloarthropathies (C) usually present with a lower number of WBC in the fluid and only about 50% PMN. Glucose in these conditions is also generally lower than serum levels. Traumatic injury to the knee (D) results in a much smaller number of WBC and a glucose level similar to that of blood.

29. **(D)** There are no medical indications for travelers to take blood with them. If urgent resuscitation is needed, use of plasma expanders can be recommended. The limited storage period of blood does not make this option feasible in cases of international travel. Traveler's diarrhea (A) is common. It usually presents with watery diarrhea associated with cramping and is secondary to an *E. coli* toxin. Treatment options include doxycycline, trimethoprim, bismuth subsalicylate, Ciprofloxin, and antimotility agents such as loperamide. These medications can provide fast, effective relief from this common overseas problem. All raw food (B) can become contaminated with bacteria such as *Salmonella* and, thus, avoidance of raw meats, vegetables, and unpasteurized milk and dairy products is prudent. The patient can reduce the risk of mosquito bites by avoiding outdoor activity in the evening and twilight hours and wearing clothing that covers exposed skin when possible (C). This can prevent malaria. When chlorinated water is unavailable, or where hygiene and sanitation are poor, beverages and ice should be made from boiling water. Whenever feasible, canned or bottled carbonated water or soda should be ingested (E).

30. **(B)** Culture-proven gonorrhea is a condition that must be reported to the local Board of Health.

31. **(E)** Questions important in this evaluation include any pain associated with swallowing (A), intentional weight loss (B), smoking and drinking history (C), and types of food giving difficulty (D). These will help guide your diagnosis as to suspect cancer or a non-neoplastic cause as well as localizing the pain. Tasting foods (E) may be important with some diseases of the oral cavity, but with a dysphagia workup, there are more pertinent questions to be asked.

32. **(B)** Dysphagia is difficulty in swallowing. Odynophagia (A) is painful swallowing. Regurgitation (C) is refluxing food. Obstruction (D) is the blockage of food along the GI tract. Emesis (E) is vomiting.

33. **(B)** Pain from the oropharynx, not the nasopharynx (A), localizes in the neck. Esophageal pain (C) localizes in the chest. Swallowing does not occur in the stomach (D) or duodenum (E) per se.

34. **(D)** Painful dysphagia from intrinsic lesions, which can be detected from inspection of the oropharynx include: tonsillitis (A), angioneurotic edema (B), carcinoma (C), and pharyngitis (E). Esophagitis (D) cannot be detected in this way.

35. **(D)** One of the diagnoses you should be considering high on your list is HIV/AIDS. At this point, the patient's family history is not likely to be contributory to his present illness.

36. **(A)** This patient has a spondyloarthropathy called ankylosing spondylitis, which is characterized by chronic low back pain for over three months, age below 40, improved lower back pain with increasing activity, and a positive HLA-B27. The diagnostic test of choice is plain X-rays of the sacroiliac joint, which would reveal sacroiliitis. Serum rheumatoid factor (B) would be positive in rheumatoid arthritis, which is an inflammatory arthritis usually in the metatarsophalangeal joint (wrist joint). Arthrocentesis of the first metatarsophalangeal joint (C) is diagnostic for gouty arthritis. This patient has no pain in that area. Plain films of the spine (D) would give information to diagnose degenerative joint disease, which is usually present in older patients and patients with osteoarthritis. The lumbar films would show sclerosis and joint space narrowing. The straight-leg testing examination (E) is nonspecific. It reveals sciatic pain or nerve entrapment which would cause the lower back pain.

37. **(C)** Traveler's diarrhea is endemic in areas where hygiene is poor. Therefore, individuals planning on trips to those areas should be advised to strictly follow rules on personal hygiene. Prophylaxis against traveler's diarrhea is not

recommended (A). Quinoline derivatives (e.g., Ciprofloxin), as well as bismuth subsalicylate or trimethoprim-sulfamethoxazole, should be given as soon as symptoms of diarrhea begin to develop and are diagnosed by a physician as traveler's diarrhea (D). Trying to stop the patient from making a trip (B) generally is beyond the scope of the medical profession. Waiting for the patient's next visit to treat him for his diarrhea, instead of counseling on precautions, is not a professional approach (E).

38. **(B)** The so-called Somogyi phenomenon is a condition in which a patient develops rebound hyperglycemia because his dose of insulin is sufficiently high to give him some degree of hypoglycemia. It is evidence of some residual pancreatic function.

39. **(C)** SLE may flare or present for the first time right after delivery. In patients with known SLE, this is a period during which they need to be closely watched for signs of exacerbation. Hormonal alterations are thought to contribute to this timing.

40. **(D)** Allergic reactions to antibiotics often manifest as truncal rashes.

41. **(A)** Sepsis should be considered a likely cause of spiking fevers and confusion in an elderly patient with a known site of infection.

42. **(C)** An IVP is not indicated at this point and might well worsen the patient's condition by its osmotic load.

43. **(E)** This is a typical abdominal crisis in a patient with sickle cell anemia.

44. **(A)** Hypomagnesemia is not associated with sickle crises. The other conditions are. An elevated BUN (E) might be seen because of dehydration.

45. **(B)** Neither the time nor site of a patient's crisis can be predicted.

46. **(B)** Iron deficiency, as well as zinc and calcium deficiency, is associated with increased absorption of ingested lead. Anorexia nervosa (A) does not alter lead absorption. Hypercalcemia (C)

is not associated with increased absorption of lead. No association between increased lead absorption and the measles (D) or ulcerative colitis (E) is known.

47. **(D)** The prothrombin time remains the best way to monitor adequacy of Coumadin dosage.

48. **(B)** Oral contraceptives have been associated with pulmonary emboli.

49. **(C)** Cellulitis of the lower extremities is fairly common in diabetics, mainly due to increased atherosclerosis and decreased circulation.

50. **(D)** Acute bronchitis often occurs in smokers with COPD.

51. **(A)** A patient with SLE can become pregnant, just like other young women, and this is the likeliest cause of amenorrhea.

52. **(D)** The patient has none of the characteristic signs of Wernicke-Korsakoff psychosis, including confabulation.

53. **(B)** Sedation is necessary to continue the patient's evaluation.

54. **(A)** It is appropriate to admit such a patient. Attempts at counseling him regarding the dangers of alcoholism should await his recovery.

55. **(C)** The patient has delirium tremens, which can be fatal, but usually is not, if appropriately treated.

56. **(E)** An individual receiving chronic steroid treatment is very likely to develop cataracts, which can impair vision.

57. **(B)** In the postoperative setting, with this constellation of symptoms and findings, pneumonia is the most likely diagnosis and should be treated.

58. **(E)** A chest radiograph is the first test that should be done when a patient has a positive PPD and it is not known if he/she had a positive test in the past.

59. **(B)** Most nursing homes require three negative serial sputum cultures for tuberculosis in this setting before they will accept a patient such as this for transfer.

60. **(D)** The delay in transfer should be explained to the family.

61. **(D)** A recent outdoor camping trip in the upper Midwest should cause concern regarding the possibility of an insect bite that could cause a syndrome such as this. None of the other conditions would be expected in this setting.

62. **(D)** The date of her most recent PPD is not relevant at this point, while the answers to all of the questions are.

63. **(E)** The specific rash is called erythema chronicum migrans.

64. **(A)** The drug of choice for the initial treatment of Lyme disease is tetracycline. Sometimes, if patients are allergic to this or do not respond to an initial course, other agents, such as ampicillin, need to be used.

65. **(C)** The patient should be told that something is wrong and needs to be examined further.

66. **(D)** The patient does not need to be admitted to the ICU at this time, but all of the other steps are necessary.

67. **(A)** Obtaining tissue diagnosis is critical at this juncture, since different tissue types will require different therapeutic and/or palliative measures and will have different prognoses.

68. **(C)** The patient's 90-pack-year history of cigarette smoking is most likely to be associated with the tumor type.

69. **(E)** This is an untreatable tumor, but judicious use of radiotherapy can reduce the size of the tumor, the degree of obstruction, and the patient's symptoms for a while. She will probably eventually need morphine (D) and possibly oxygen (C). At present, no chemotherapy regimens (A) are known to be useful and, thus, bone marrow transplantation (B) is not indicated.

70. **(D)** It is not appropriate to give someone a definite period of time [(A) and (C)] in this situation because it is unpredictable. It is also unfair to offer them the false hope of a new treatment when none is even being discussed in the oncologic community (B). It is also not considered generally acceptable medical practice to recommend unconventional treatments like high-dose vitamins for cancer (E). Such agents can have adverse side effects that can make patients feel even worse.

71. **(C)** Unless the patient chooses to return to her family physician, it is unreasonable for you to stop seeing her because she is "terminal." This will only increase her already likely sense of hopelessness.

72. **(B)** You must rule out the possibility of a brain tumor causing increased intracranial pressure. This condition could explain the patient's personality changes and symptoms. You would not send him out without evaluation (A). You would not perform an LP in the absence of a fever with a suspicion of increased intracranial pressure (C). Referral to a psychiatrist is inappropriate at this point (D). It is unlikely that a surgical abdomen would result in these symptoms (E).

73. **(B)** Asthma most commonly presents with wheezing and cough in this age group and can cause some hypoxia. Pneumonia (A) would likely cause a febrile illness and usually would not be recurrent. Bronchitis (C) and obliterative alveolitis (D) are unusual in young children. Tuberculosis (E) usually does not cause wheezing.

74. **(D)** Beta-blockers worsen bronchoconstriction.

75. **(C)** A lung scan is not helpful in evaluating this condition.

76. **(B)** Many children with asthma developing at an early age "outgrow" it as they get older.

77. **(C)** A patient on steroids may be PPD-negative, or anergic, despite active infection. A chest radiograph would show a lesion. Skin tests for common antigens, such as *Candida,* should be placed since their positivity would prove the patient was not anergic. A repeat PPD (B) would not be useful.

78. **(B)** The likeliest cause of this patient's discomfort is a Colles' fracture of the forearm, which will be easily detectable by radiography.

79. **(C)** Esophageal varices most commonly cause acute hematemesis. Peptic ulcers (B) occasionally can, but this is much less common.

80. **(D)** A Mallory-Weiss tear of the esophagus commonly follows a period of prolonged retching and is manifested by hematemesis.

81. **(A)** Hemorrhoidal bleeding most commonly presents as blood streaking on toilet paper.

82. **(B)** Peptic ulcers are often associated with melena due to degradation of the blood by the gastric acid and then passage through the colon.

83. **(B)** A miscarriage is the most common cause of cramping and vaginal bleeding at this stage of pregnancy.

84. **(D)** Controlling the patient's heart rate at this point is most important. His condition is sufficiently stable to permit medical treatment while evaluation of the underlying pathology is begun.

85. **(A)** This patient's clinical features on morning rounds are most consistent with alcohol withdrawal.

86. **(D)** Fibrin split products are not abnormal in alcohol withdrawal. In this patient, one would expect the amylase (A) and lipase (C) to be elevated because the patient presented with symptoms consistent with pancreatitis. The stool hemoccult (B) would be positive because the patient has had some GI bleeding. The albumin (E) is likely to be low because of some degree of liver disease due to alcohol consumption.

87. **(C)** It would be inappropriate to send this individual home [(A) and (D)]. Surgery is not indicated (B). He does not need to be in an ICU (E).

88. **(D)** Delirium tremens and other forms of alcohol withdrawal are not benign.

89. **(E)** Erythema nodosum is not usually associated with otitis media, while all of the other conditions can be.

90. **(E)** Blood transfusions are not part of the treatment of lupus-related hemolytic anemia. The anemia and thrombocytopenia usually respond to high-dose corticosteroids (A). IV gammaglobulin (B) and immunosuppressive drugs (C) may be used in severe cases. Splenectomy (D) may be indicated in patients that fail to respond to the other measures.

91. **(D)** Insulin is only necessary if there is excessive hyperglycemia. Volume replacement (A), narcotics (B) for pain control, and nasogastric suctioning (C) to place the pancreas at rest are the principal treatment options for pancreatitis. In patients that develop hypocalcemia, calcium supplementation (E) is necessary.

92. **(D)** This patient's signs and symptoms are consistent with trichomonal infection. The treatment consists of a single dose of metronidazole for both patient and partner. Tetracycline [(A), (B), and (E)] is used to treat *Chlamydia* infection, while miconazole (E) is used to treat *Candidiasis*.

93. **(B)** Recurrent dislocations of the shoulder are usually anterior.

94. **(A)** The single most important correlate with newborn mortality is birth weight. The lower the birth weight, the higher the incidence of neonatal mortality. Extremes of birth weight, both low and high are associated with greater neonatal morbidity and possible birth trauma.

95. **(E)** Paget's disease is a bone disorder that may be associated with paramyxovirus infections. Bone destruction is severe in Paget's disease, yet calcium levels remain normal. A diagnostic feature of Paget's disease is an increase in serum osteocalcin levels with increases in alkaline phosphatase levels, as well.

96. **(C)** The anion gap is defined as Na+ = (HCO3- + Cl-), which is 135- (15 + 100) = 20 mEq/ L in this case. The other choices do not reflect the true anion gap. A value of greater than 12-15 mEq/ L is generally considered abnormal. Causes of a high anion gap include salicylates, lactate, uremia, methanol, paraldehyde, ethanol, and diabetic ketoacidosis (mnemonic is "SLUMPED").

97. **(C)** Iodine deficiency is not associated with hyperthyroidism. Struma ovarii (ovarian tumors that contain mainly thyroid tissue) and all of the other conditions presented can produce hyperthyroidism.

98. **(E)** Humans are the only natural reservoir for *Corynebacterium diphtheriae* (A). Spread occurs in close-contact settings via respiratory droplets from persons with clinical disease (B). However, most individuals with nasopharyngeal infection do not develop clinical disease. These asymptomatic carriers are also important in transmission of the organism (D). The organism survives for weeks on environmental surfaces including dust (C). Diphtheria immunization prevents clinical disease but does not prevent the carrier state (E).

99. **(D)** Interval CPK screening is not useful in detection of susceptible persons (D). Malignant hyperthermia consists of a group of inherited disorders characterized by a rapid temperature elevation in response to inhalational anesthetics or muscle relaxants. Triggering anesthetics release calcium from the membrane of the muscle cell's sarcoplasmic reticulum, which is defective in storing this ion (E). This results in a sudden increase in myoplasmic calcium, which activates myosin ATPase. Ultimately, sudden massive muscle contraction occurs, leading to a rapid rise in body temperature (A). A linkage to mutations in the skeletal muscle ryanodine receptor (RYR1) has been observed in some families with the autosomal dominant disorder (B). In individuals with one form of autosomally dominant inherited disease, biopsied muscle contracts on exposure to caffeine or halothane at concentrations that do not alter normal muscle contraction (C).

100. **(B)** This is a typical presentation of diarrhea due to overgrowth of *Clostridium difficile* following antibiotic therapy.

101. **(A)** An urticarial rash is often a manifestation of an allergic reaction to a drug, commonly an antibiotic such as penicillin or sulfa.

102. **(B)** This condition is frequently associated with recurrent urinary infections.

103. **(E)** Renal calculi are associated with recurrent UTIs and can occur in a familial pattern.

104. **(D)** All of the other tests are useful at this point, but a 24-hour urine for protein quantitation is not indicated now.

105. **(B)** You are most concerned that this patient has renal calculi, which should be seen emergently if an attack occurs. Not only can the patient's symptoms be treated, but a diagnosis is most easily made during an attack.

106. **(B)** No P waves are seen in atrial fibrillation.

107. **(C)** Hyperthyroidism can be an etiology of atrial fibrillation as well as chest pain and shortness of breath. The only way to make this diagnosis in a patient such as this is via thyroid function tests.

108. **(D)** None of the other tests would likely be helpful at this time.

109. **(B)** The other conditions are common etiologies of atrial fibrillation.

110. **(C)** One of the etiologies of atrial fibrillation is a pulmonary embolus, and the V/P scan is a relatively quick and simple screening test.

111. **(A)** The elevated T4 indicates oversecretion of the hormone by the thyroid, and the low TSH shows that the pituitary is appropriately suppressed by the high levels of hormone. Medullary thyroid cancer does not usually produce significant, if any, hyperthyroidism.

112. **(D)** Management of the patient's hyperthyroidism will best alleviate her symptoms and signs.

113. **(A)** It may be necessary to control the patient's atrial fibrillation acutely by cardioversion before the definitive therapy can act.

114. **(A)** A child with multiple fractures of different ages should be assumed to be the victim of abuse until proven otherwise.

115. **(A)** A simple fall in an elderly person, especially a woman, can cause a fracture that would not occur in a younger individual and that might not be particularly symptomatic.

116. **(B)** This development is consistent with alcohol withdrawal if the patient is a heavy drinker.

117. **(D)** The patient likely has either placenta previa or abruptio placentae, both of which require close observation and often emergency intervention.

118. **(B)** Hyaline membrane disease is responsible for approximately 30% of neonatal deaths in this country.

119. **(A)** Hyaline membrane disease is associated with a deficiency of surfactant in the lungs. This condition is most common in prematurity, but is not specifically associated with any of the other conditions listed here.

120. **(D)** All of the other conditions have been associated with this condition.

121. **(D)** All of the other modalities can be beneficial.

122. **(D)** Seizures can be a delayed sequelae of blunt head trauma that may have resulted in a focal bleed.

123. **(A)** Some urinary tract infections can present with hemorrhagic cystitis. The absence of colicky pain or cramping makes nephrolithiasis (C) very unlikely.

124. **(B)** This woman should be considered to be experiencing unstable angina, which is a medical emergency, and should be transported to the hospital under observation immediately.

125. **(C)** Hemarthrosis is most likely in this setting of an apparently non-inflammatory effusion that developed after minimal exertion to the joint.

126. **(C)** These are likely to be nocturnal hot flashes.

127. **(D)** Marfan's is associated with tallness, family history, ectopia lentis, and cardiac involvement, among other features.

128. **(E)** One should first inquire when a patient's last dose of medication was before deciding that the medicine no longer works.

129. **(D)** The renal stone may have been obstructing the urinary outflow, and, hence, was responsible for development of the infection. Impending passage of the stone could cause the pain and bleeding.

130. **(B)** In this setting, infection is not particularly likely (E). The headaches are significant enough, and are increasing in severity, to require a workup rather than mere follow-up (A).

131. **(B)** Children with JRA are often seronegative and have a pauciarticular (fewer than five joints involved) arthritis.

132. **(D)** Trimethoprim-sulfamethoxazole is commonly used for prophylaxis of *Pneumocystis carinii* pneumonia in patients with AIDS and is associated with a high incidence of rash in these individuals.

133. **(B)** This patient has "peau d'orange," which usually indicates a fairly longstanding tumor. Her prognosis is not good.

134. **(B)** Unstable angina is the term for a sharp chest pain at rest.

135. **(A)** Pleurisy is the term for a sharp chest pain with breathing.

136. **(D)** Cervical disk disease is the term for neck pain radiating to the left arm.

137. **(C)** Acute myocardial infarction is the condition associated with acute severe substernal chest pain.

138. **(C)** A lumbar puncture is indicated because of the high likelihood of meningitis in this setting. Bacterial meningitis is potentially a life-threatening condition, which should be identified and treated as soon as possible.

139. **(C)** The patient's symptoms and travel should at least raise the possibility of Lyme disease.

140. **(C)** The patient's symptoms are most consistent with the vegetative features of depression.

141. **(D)** The most likely diagnosis in this setting is pulmonary embolus. Fat emboli are not uncommon after major fractures, such as femoral.

142. **(A)** This is likely to represent a traumatic fracture, which is best diagnosed via radiography.

143. **(A)** Diabetes mellitus can cause hyperosmolarity as a result of the increased glucose and ketones in circulation.

144. **(C)** This is associated with acute renal failure because of failure of the kidneys to properly control magnesium balance.

145. **(B)** Most diuretics, except the spironolactones, are associated with potassium-wasting by the kidneys.

146. **(A)** Hypoglycemia can occur as an early manifestation of diabetes mellitus or as a result of excess dosage of insulin.

147. **(D)** Evaluation of the anemia should begin with the size, shape, and staining of the red cells. The patient's anemia is most likely due to her chronic disease of rheumatoid arthritis, and thus will be normocytic and normochromic. Treatment and bone marrow biopsy are not indicated at this point.

148. **(B)** As long as her vital signs and condition are stable, a good evaluation is the best first step.

149. **(B)** ST segment elevation is most likely to be associated with this patient's condition.

150. **(B)** This condition is associated with a normal CPK.

151. **(C)** A flu-like illness can precede this condition.

152. **(A)** This is an inflammatory treatment and can often be adequately treated with nonsteroidal anti-inflammatory agents or with steroids.

153. **(E)** A pleural rub is likely to be heard.

154. **(D)** The chest radiograph is usually normal in this condition.

155. **(C)** This patient has pleurisy, which is probably viral in origin, and most often resolves without residua.

156. **(B)** An ambulance should be called and you should see the patient.

157. **(E)** Drug-induced lupus presents clinically and immunologically differently compared with the spontaneous form of the disease (E). A genetic predisposition for systemic lupus erythematosis (SLE) is suggested by the increased concordance in monozygotic as compared with dizygotic twins, a ten percent frequency of patients with more than one affected family member, and correlations of MHC class II and III genes with the disease (A). The increased prevalence of the disease in women of childbearing age (B), as well as abnormalities of estrogens and androgens in affected persons, suggests a hormonal influence in the development of the disease. The more genes susceptibility a person has, the greater the relative risk for developing SLE. It has been calculated that at least three or four genes are necessary for the disease to develop (C). Ultraviolet light, especially UV-B, causes the disease to flare in more than half the cases (D).

158. **(B)** People with bipolar disorders classically spend large quantities of money, which they often do not have, when they are in a manic phase.

159. **(D)** This patient is suicidal and depressed, but is apparently reacting to a specific situation.

160. **(A)** This is an example of the typical confabulation associated with Wernicke-Korsakoff syndrome.

161. **(C)** This patient is exhibiting the delusional paranoia typical of a paranoid schizophrenic.

162. **(D)** A chest radiograph is not indicated at this point.

163. **(B)** The barium enema result is consistent with inflammatory bowel disease, specifically ulcerative colitis, but a colonoscopic examination with biopsy is the definitive way to make the diagnosis.

164. **(A)** This pattern is not consistent with any of the other conditions. Peptic ulcer disease (C) does not occur in the colon. The other conditions do not cause such histology or pathology.

165. **(D)** The principal diagnosis that must be eliminated in this setting is Crohn's disease, which can involve the colon like this, but also usually affects the upper bowel.

166. **(A)** The initial treatment of choice is medical management, especially with steroids.

167. **(D)** Annual colonoscopy is recommended for early identification of some of the more serious complications of this condition.

168. **(C)** Ulcerative colitis increases the risk of colon cancer, early detection of which can be provided by annual colonoscopy.

169. **(B)** Removal of the colon prevents colitis. However, if necessary, it is usually a late intervention for this condition.

170. **(C)** At this point, dilatation and curettage is not necessary. After the rest of the workup, it may be.

171. **(B)** This patient's age and findings are most consistent with impending menopause.

172. **(D)** Noncompliance must be carefully evaluated before a new drug is added to the regimen.

173. **(D)** This patient has no evidence of having been pregnant. Pseudocyesis is a psychiatric condition in which the patient's body attempts to mimic pregnancy, and the patient is convinced that she is pregnant although she is not.

174. **(D)** Induction of emesis in a patient with possible acid or base ingestion is contraindicated because of repeated injury to the esophagus if the toxin is made to pass through it again.

175. **(B)** A barium swallow is not indicated because there is no evidence at this point of abnormal esophageal motility.

176. **(E)** In the setting of excessive alcohol ingestion, abdominal pain, elevated amylase, leukocytosis, and focal ileus on radiograph, acute pancreatitis is the most likely diagnosis. The other conditions would not cause this array of signs and symptoms.

177. **(B)** This patient should not receive anything by mouth at this point.

178. **(D)** Pancreatic pseudocyst is a complication of pancreatitis.

179. **(C)** This patient's history and presentation is quite suggestive of HIV/AIDS. The results of an HIV test, which requires the patient's consent, would be very helpful in her treatment.

180. **(B)** Acute cessation of allopurinol in a patient undergoing surgery can cause a gouty attack postoperatively.

USMLE STEP 3

Answer Sheets

USMLE STEP 3
PRACTICE TEST 1

Day One – Morning Session

ANSWER SHEET

1. Ⓐ Ⓑ Ⓒ Ⓓ Ⓔ	31. Ⓐ Ⓑ Ⓒ Ⓓ Ⓔ	61. Ⓐ Ⓑ Ⓒ Ⓓ Ⓔ
2. Ⓐ Ⓑ Ⓒ Ⓓ Ⓔ	32. Ⓐ Ⓑ Ⓒ Ⓓ Ⓔ	62. Ⓐ Ⓑ Ⓒ Ⓓ Ⓔ
3. Ⓐ Ⓑ Ⓒ Ⓓ Ⓔ	33. Ⓐ Ⓑ Ⓒ Ⓓ Ⓔ	63. Ⓐ Ⓑ Ⓒ Ⓓ Ⓔ
4. Ⓐ Ⓑ Ⓒ Ⓓ Ⓔ	34. Ⓐ Ⓑ Ⓒ Ⓓ Ⓔ	64. Ⓐ Ⓑ Ⓒ Ⓓ Ⓔ
5. Ⓐ Ⓑ Ⓒ Ⓓ Ⓔ	35. Ⓐ Ⓑ Ⓒ Ⓓ Ⓔ	65. Ⓐ Ⓑ Ⓒ Ⓓ Ⓔ
6. Ⓐ Ⓑ Ⓒ Ⓓ Ⓔ	36. Ⓐ Ⓑ Ⓒ Ⓓ Ⓔ	66. Ⓐ Ⓑ Ⓒ Ⓓ Ⓔ
7. Ⓐ Ⓑ Ⓒ Ⓓ Ⓔ	37. Ⓐ Ⓑ Ⓒ Ⓓ Ⓔ	67. Ⓐ Ⓑ Ⓒ Ⓓ Ⓔ
8. Ⓐ Ⓑ Ⓒ Ⓓ Ⓔ	38. Ⓐ Ⓑ Ⓒ Ⓓ Ⓔ	68. Ⓐ Ⓑ Ⓒ Ⓓ Ⓔ
9. Ⓐ Ⓑ Ⓒ Ⓓ Ⓔ	39. Ⓐ Ⓑ Ⓒ Ⓓ Ⓔ	69. Ⓐ Ⓑ Ⓒ Ⓓ Ⓔ
10. Ⓐ Ⓑ Ⓒ Ⓓ Ⓔ	40. Ⓐ Ⓑ Ⓒ Ⓓ Ⓔ	70. Ⓐ Ⓑ Ⓒ Ⓓ Ⓔ
11. Ⓐ Ⓑ Ⓒ Ⓓ Ⓔ	41. Ⓐ Ⓑ Ⓒ Ⓓ Ⓔ	71. Ⓐ Ⓑ Ⓒ Ⓓ Ⓔ
12. Ⓐ Ⓑ Ⓒ Ⓓ Ⓔ	42. Ⓐ Ⓑ Ⓒ Ⓓ Ⓔ	72. Ⓐ Ⓑ Ⓒ Ⓓ Ⓔ
13. Ⓐ Ⓑ Ⓒ Ⓓ Ⓔ	43. Ⓐ Ⓑ Ⓒ Ⓓ Ⓔ	73. Ⓐ Ⓑ Ⓒ Ⓓ Ⓔ
14. Ⓐ Ⓑ Ⓒ Ⓓ Ⓔ	44. Ⓐ Ⓑ Ⓒ Ⓓ Ⓔ	74. Ⓐ Ⓑ Ⓒ Ⓓ Ⓔ
15. Ⓐ Ⓑ Ⓒ Ⓓ Ⓔ	45. Ⓐ Ⓑ Ⓒ Ⓓ Ⓔ	75. Ⓐ Ⓑ Ⓒ Ⓓ Ⓔ
16. Ⓐ Ⓑ Ⓒ Ⓓ Ⓔ	46. Ⓐ Ⓑ Ⓒ Ⓓ Ⓔ	76. Ⓐ Ⓑ Ⓒ Ⓓ Ⓔ
17. Ⓐ Ⓑ Ⓒ Ⓓ Ⓔ	47. Ⓐ Ⓑ Ⓒ Ⓓ Ⓔ	77. Ⓐ Ⓑ Ⓒ Ⓓ Ⓔ
18. Ⓐ Ⓑ Ⓒ Ⓓ Ⓔ	48. Ⓐ Ⓑ Ⓒ Ⓓ Ⓔ	78. Ⓐ Ⓑ Ⓒ Ⓓ Ⓔ
19. Ⓐ Ⓑ Ⓒ Ⓓ Ⓔ	49. Ⓐ Ⓑ Ⓒ Ⓓ Ⓔ	79. Ⓐ Ⓑ Ⓒ Ⓓ Ⓔ
20. Ⓐ Ⓑ Ⓒ Ⓓ Ⓔ	50. Ⓐ Ⓑ Ⓒ Ⓓ Ⓔ	80. Ⓐ Ⓑ Ⓒ Ⓓ Ⓔ
21. Ⓐ Ⓑ Ⓒ Ⓓ Ⓔ	51. Ⓐ Ⓑ Ⓒ Ⓓ Ⓔ	81. Ⓐ Ⓑ Ⓒ Ⓓ Ⓔ
22. Ⓐ Ⓑ Ⓒ Ⓓ Ⓔ	52. Ⓐ Ⓑ Ⓒ Ⓓ Ⓔ	82. Ⓐ Ⓑ Ⓒ Ⓓ Ⓔ
23. Ⓐ Ⓑ Ⓒ Ⓓ Ⓔ	53. Ⓐ Ⓑ Ⓒ Ⓓ Ⓔ	83. Ⓐ Ⓑ Ⓒ Ⓓ Ⓔ
24. Ⓐ Ⓑ Ⓒ Ⓓ Ⓔ	54. Ⓐ Ⓑ Ⓒ Ⓓ Ⓔ	84. Ⓐ Ⓑ Ⓒ Ⓓ Ⓔ
25. Ⓐ Ⓑ Ⓒ Ⓓ Ⓔ	55. Ⓐ Ⓑ Ⓒ Ⓓ Ⓔ	85. Ⓐ Ⓑ Ⓒ Ⓓ Ⓔ
26. Ⓐ Ⓑ Ⓒ Ⓓ Ⓔ	56. Ⓐ Ⓑ Ⓒ Ⓓ Ⓔ	86. Ⓐ Ⓑ Ⓒ Ⓓ Ⓔ
27. Ⓐ Ⓑ Ⓒ Ⓓ Ⓔ	57. Ⓐ Ⓑ Ⓒ Ⓓ Ⓔ	87. Ⓐ Ⓑ Ⓒ Ⓓ Ⓔ
28. Ⓐ Ⓑ Ⓒ Ⓓ Ⓔ	58. Ⓐ Ⓑ Ⓒ Ⓓ Ⓔ	88. Ⓐ Ⓑ Ⓒ Ⓓ Ⓔ
29. Ⓐ Ⓑ Ⓒ Ⓓ Ⓔ	59. Ⓐ Ⓑ Ⓒ Ⓓ Ⓔ	89. Ⓐ Ⓑ Ⓒ Ⓓ Ⓔ
30. Ⓐ Ⓑ Ⓒ Ⓓ Ⓔ	60. Ⓐ Ⓑ Ⓒ Ⓓ Ⓔ	90. Ⓐ Ⓑ Ⓒ Ⓓ Ⓔ

91. Ⓐ Ⓑ Ⓒ Ⓓ Ⓔ
92. Ⓐ Ⓑ Ⓒ Ⓓ Ⓔ
93. Ⓐ Ⓑ Ⓒ Ⓓ Ⓔ
94. Ⓐ Ⓑ Ⓒ Ⓓ Ⓔ
95. Ⓐ Ⓑ Ⓒ Ⓓ Ⓔ
96. Ⓐ Ⓑ Ⓒ Ⓓ Ⓔ
97. Ⓐ Ⓑ Ⓒ Ⓓ Ⓔ
98. Ⓐ Ⓑ Ⓒ Ⓓ Ⓔ
99. Ⓐ Ⓑ Ⓒ Ⓓ Ⓔ
100. Ⓐ Ⓑ Ⓒ Ⓓ Ⓔ
101. Ⓐ Ⓑ Ⓒ Ⓓ Ⓔ
102. Ⓐ Ⓑ Ⓒ Ⓓ Ⓔ
103. Ⓐ Ⓑ Ⓒ Ⓓ Ⓔ
104. Ⓐ Ⓑ Ⓒ Ⓓ Ⓔ
105. Ⓐ Ⓑ Ⓒ Ⓓ Ⓔ
106. Ⓐ Ⓑ Ⓒ Ⓓ Ⓔ
107. Ⓐ Ⓑ Ⓒ Ⓓ Ⓔ
108. Ⓐ Ⓑ Ⓒ Ⓓ Ⓔ
109. Ⓐ Ⓑ Ⓒ Ⓓ Ⓔ
110. Ⓐ Ⓑ Ⓒ Ⓓ Ⓔ
111. Ⓐ Ⓑ Ⓒ Ⓓ Ⓔ
112. Ⓐ Ⓑ Ⓒ Ⓓ Ⓔ
113. Ⓐ Ⓑ Ⓒ Ⓓ Ⓔ
114. Ⓐ Ⓑ Ⓒ Ⓓ Ⓔ
115. Ⓐ Ⓑ Ⓒ Ⓓ Ⓔ
116. Ⓐ Ⓑ Ⓒ Ⓓ Ⓔ
117. Ⓐ Ⓑ Ⓒ Ⓓ Ⓔ
118. Ⓐ Ⓑ Ⓒ Ⓓ Ⓔ
119. Ⓐ Ⓑ Ⓒ Ⓓ Ⓔ
120. Ⓐ Ⓑ Ⓒ Ⓓ Ⓔ

121. Ⓐ Ⓑ Ⓒ Ⓓ Ⓔ
122. Ⓐ Ⓑ Ⓒ Ⓓ Ⓔ
123. Ⓐ Ⓑ Ⓒ Ⓓ Ⓔ
124. Ⓐ Ⓑ Ⓒ Ⓓ Ⓔ
125. Ⓐ Ⓑ Ⓒ Ⓓ Ⓔ
126. Ⓐ Ⓑ Ⓒ Ⓓ Ⓔ
127. Ⓐ Ⓑ Ⓒ Ⓓ Ⓔ
128. Ⓐ Ⓑ Ⓒ Ⓓ Ⓔ
129. Ⓐ Ⓑ Ⓒ Ⓓ Ⓔ
130. Ⓐ Ⓑ Ⓒ Ⓓ Ⓔ
131. Ⓐ Ⓑ Ⓒ Ⓓ Ⓔ
132. Ⓐ Ⓑ Ⓒ Ⓓ Ⓔ
133. Ⓐ Ⓑ Ⓒ Ⓓ Ⓔ
134. Ⓐ Ⓑ Ⓒ Ⓓ Ⓔ
135. Ⓐ Ⓑ Ⓒ Ⓓ Ⓔ
136. Ⓐ Ⓑ Ⓒ Ⓓ Ⓔ
137. Ⓐ Ⓑ Ⓒ Ⓓ Ⓔ
138. Ⓐ Ⓑ Ⓒ Ⓓ Ⓔ
139. Ⓐ Ⓑ Ⓒ Ⓓ Ⓔ
140. Ⓐ Ⓑ Ⓒ Ⓓ Ⓔ
141. Ⓐ Ⓑ Ⓒ Ⓓ Ⓔ
142. Ⓐ Ⓑ Ⓒ Ⓓ Ⓔ
143. Ⓐ Ⓑ Ⓒ Ⓓ Ⓔ
144. Ⓐ Ⓑ Ⓒ Ⓓ Ⓔ
145. Ⓐ Ⓑ Ⓒ Ⓓ Ⓔ
146. Ⓐ Ⓑ Ⓒ Ⓓ Ⓔ
147. Ⓐ Ⓑ Ⓒ Ⓓ Ⓔ
148. Ⓐ Ⓑ Ⓒ Ⓓ Ⓔ
149. Ⓐ Ⓑ Ⓒ Ⓓ Ⓔ
150. Ⓐ Ⓑ Ⓒ Ⓓ Ⓔ

151. Ⓐ Ⓑ Ⓒ Ⓓ Ⓔ
152. Ⓐ Ⓑ Ⓒ Ⓓ Ⓔ
153. Ⓐ Ⓑ Ⓒ Ⓓ Ⓔ
154. Ⓐ Ⓑ Ⓒ Ⓓ Ⓔ
155. Ⓐ Ⓑ Ⓒ Ⓓ Ⓔ
156. Ⓐ Ⓑ Ⓒ Ⓓ Ⓔ
157. Ⓐ Ⓑ Ⓒ Ⓓ Ⓔ
158. Ⓐ Ⓑ Ⓒ Ⓓ Ⓔ
159. Ⓐ Ⓑ Ⓒ Ⓓ Ⓔ
160. Ⓐ Ⓑ Ⓒ Ⓓ Ⓔ
161. Ⓐ Ⓑ Ⓒ Ⓓ Ⓔ
162. Ⓐ Ⓑ Ⓒ Ⓓ Ⓔ
163. Ⓐ Ⓑ Ⓒ Ⓓ Ⓔ
164. Ⓐ Ⓑ Ⓒ Ⓓ Ⓔ
165. Ⓐ Ⓑ Ⓒ Ⓓ Ⓔ
166. Ⓐ Ⓑ Ⓒ Ⓓ Ⓔ
167. Ⓐ Ⓑ Ⓒ Ⓓ Ⓔ
168. Ⓐ Ⓑ Ⓒ Ⓓ Ⓔ
169. Ⓐ Ⓑ Ⓒ Ⓓ Ⓔ
170. Ⓐ Ⓑ Ⓒ Ⓓ Ⓔ
171. Ⓐ Ⓑ Ⓒ Ⓓ Ⓔ
172. Ⓐ Ⓑ Ⓒ Ⓓ Ⓔ
173. Ⓐ Ⓑ Ⓒ Ⓓ Ⓔ
174. Ⓐ Ⓑ Ⓒ Ⓓ Ⓔ
175. Ⓐ Ⓑ Ⓒ Ⓓ Ⓔ
176. Ⓐ Ⓑ Ⓒ Ⓓ Ⓔ
177. Ⓐ Ⓑ Ⓒ Ⓓ Ⓔ
178. Ⓐ Ⓑ Ⓒ Ⓓ Ⓔ
179. Ⓐ Ⓑ Ⓒ Ⓓ Ⓔ
180. Ⓐ Ⓑ Ⓒ Ⓓ Ⓔ

USMLE STEP 3
PRACTICE TEST 1

Day One – Afternoon Session

ANSWER SHEET

1. Ⓐ Ⓑ Ⓒ Ⓓ Ⓔ
2. Ⓐ Ⓑ Ⓒ Ⓓ Ⓔ
3. Ⓐ Ⓑ Ⓒ Ⓓ Ⓔ
4. Ⓐ Ⓑ Ⓒ Ⓓ Ⓔ
5. Ⓐ Ⓑ Ⓒ Ⓓ Ⓔ
6. Ⓐ Ⓑ Ⓒ Ⓓ Ⓔ
7. Ⓐ Ⓑ Ⓒ Ⓓ Ⓔ
8. Ⓐ Ⓑ Ⓒ Ⓓ Ⓔ
9. Ⓐ Ⓑ Ⓒ Ⓓ Ⓔ
10. Ⓐ Ⓑ Ⓒ Ⓓ Ⓔ
11. Ⓐ Ⓑ Ⓒ Ⓓ Ⓔ
12. Ⓐ Ⓑ Ⓒ Ⓓ Ⓔ
13. Ⓐ Ⓑ Ⓒ Ⓓ Ⓔ
14. Ⓐ Ⓑ Ⓒ Ⓓ Ⓔ
15. Ⓐ Ⓑ Ⓒ Ⓓ Ⓔ
16. Ⓐ Ⓑ Ⓒ Ⓓ Ⓔ
17. Ⓐ Ⓑ Ⓒ Ⓓ Ⓔ
18. Ⓐ Ⓑ Ⓒ Ⓓ Ⓔ
19. Ⓐ Ⓑ Ⓒ Ⓓ Ⓔ
20. Ⓐ Ⓑ Ⓒ Ⓓ Ⓔ
21. Ⓐ Ⓑ Ⓒ Ⓓ Ⓔ
22. Ⓐ Ⓑ Ⓒ Ⓓ Ⓔ
23. Ⓐ Ⓑ Ⓒ Ⓓ Ⓔ
24. Ⓐ Ⓑ Ⓒ Ⓓ Ⓔ
25. Ⓐ Ⓑ Ⓒ Ⓓ Ⓔ
26. Ⓐ Ⓑ Ⓒ Ⓓ Ⓔ
27. Ⓐ Ⓑ Ⓒ Ⓓ Ⓔ
28. Ⓐ Ⓑ Ⓒ Ⓓ Ⓔ
29. Ⓐ Ⓑ Ⓒ Ⓓ Ⓔ
30. Ⓐ Ⓑ Ⓒ Ⓓ Ⓔ

31. Ⓐ Ⓑ Ⓒ Ⓓ Ⓔ
32. Ⓐ Ⓑ Ⓒ Ⓓ Ⓔ
33. Ⓐ Ⓑ Ⓒ Ⓓ Ⓔ
34. Ⓐ Ⓑ Ⓒ Ⓓ Ⓔ
35. Ⓐ Ⓑ Ⓒ Ⓓ Ⓔ
36. Ⓐ Ⓑ Ⓒ Ⓓ Ⓔ
37. Ⓐ Ⓑ Ⓒ Ⓓ Ⓔ
38. Ⓐ Ⓑ Ⓒ Ⓓ Ⓔ
39. Ⓐ Ⓑ Ⓒ Ⓓ Ⓔ
40. Ⓐ Ⓑ Ⓒ Ⓓ Ⓔ
41. Ⓐ Ⓑ Ⓒ Ⓓ Ⓔ
42. Ⓐ Ⓑ Ⓒ Ⓓ Ⓔ
43. Ⓐ Ⓑ Ⓒ Ⓓ Ⓔ
44. Ⓐ Ⓑ Ⓒ Ⓓ Ⓔ
45. Ⓐ Ⓑ Ⓒ Ⓓ Ⓔ
46. Ⓐ Ⓑ Ⓒ Ⓓ Ⓔ
47. Ⓐ Ⓑ Ⓒ Ⓓ Ⓔ
48. Ⓐ Ⓑ Ⓒ Ⓓ Ⓔ
49. Ⓐ Ⓑ Ⓒ Ⓓ Ⓔ
50. Ⓐ Ⓑ Ⓒ Ⓓ Ⓔ
51. Ⓐ Ⓑ Ⓒ Ⓓ Ⓔ
52. Ⓐ Ⓑ Ⓒ Ⓓ Ⓔ
53. Ⓐ Ⓑ Ⓒ Ⓓ Ⓔ
54. Ⓐ Ⓑ Ⓒ Ⓓ Ⓔ
55. Ⓐ Ⓑ Ⓒ Ⓓ Ⓔ
56. Ⓐ Ⓑ Ⓒ Ⓓ Ⓔ
57. Ⓐ Ⓑ Ⓒ Ⓓ Ⓔ
58. Ⓐ Ⓑ Ⓒ Ⓓ Ⓔ
59. Ⓐ Ⓑ Ⓒ Ⓓ Ⓔ
60. Ⓐ Ⓑ Ⓒ Ⓓ Ⓔ

61. Ⓐ Ⓑ Ⓒ Ⓓ Ⓔ
62. Ⓐ Ⓑ Ⓒ Ⓓ Ⓔ
63. Ⓐ Ⓑ Ⓒ Ⓓ Ⓔ
64. Ⓐ Ⓑ Ⓒ Ⓓ Ⓔ
65. Ⓐ Ⓑ Ⓒ Ⓓ Ⓔ
66. Ⓐ Ⓑ Ⓒ Ⓓ Ⓔ
67. Ⓐ Ⓑ Ⓒ Ⓓ Ⓔ
68. Ⓐ Ⓑ Ⓒ Ⓓ Ⓔ
69. Ⓐ Ⓑ Ⓒ Ⓓ Ⓔ
70. Ⓐ Ⓑ Ⓒ Ⓓ Ⓔ
71. Ⓐ Ⓑ Ⓒ Ⓓ Ⓔ
72. Ⓐ Ⓑ Ⓒ Ⓓ Ⓔ
73. Ⓐ Ⓑ Ⓒ Ⓓ Ⓔ
74. Ⓐ Ⓑ Ⓒ Ⓓ Ⓔ
75. Ⓐ Ⓑ Ⓒ Ⓓ Ⓔ
76. Ⓐ Ⓑ Ⓒ Ⓓ Ⓔ
77. Ⓐ Ⓑ Ⓒ Ⓓ Ⓔ
78. Ⓐ Ⓑ Ⓒ Ⓓ Ⓔ
79. Ⓐ Ⓑ Ⓒ Ⓓ Ⓔ
80. Ⓐ Ⓑ Ⓒ Ⓓ Ⓔ
81. Ⓐ Ⓑ Ⓒ Ⓓ Ⓔ
82. Ⓐ Ⓑ Ⓒ Ⓓ Ⓔ
83. Ⓐ Ⓑ Ⓒ Ⓓ Ⓔ
84. Ⓐ Ⓑ Ⓒ Ⓓ Ⓔ
85. Ⓐ Ⓑ Ⓒ Ⓓ Ⓔ
86. Ⓐ Ⓑ Ⓒ Ⓓ Ⓔ
87. Ⓐ Ⓑ Ⓒ Ⓓ Ⓔ
88. Ⓐ Ⓑ Ⓒ Ⓓ Ⓔ
89. Ⓐ Ⓑ Ⓒ Ⓓ Ⓔ
90. Ⓐ Ⓑ Ⓒ Ⓓ Ⓔ

91. Ⓐ Ⓑ Ⓒ Ⓓ Ⓔ
92. Ⓐ Ⓑ Ⓒ Ⓓ Ⓔ
93. Ⓐ Ⓑ Ⓒ Ⓓ Ⓔ
94. Ⓐ Ⓑ Ⓒ Ⓓ Ⓔ
95. Ⓐ Ⓑ Ⓒ Ⓓ Ⓔ
96. Ⓐ Ⓑ Ⓒ Ⓓ Ⓔ
97. Ⓐ Ⓑ Ⓒ Ⓓ Ⓔ
98. Ⓐ Ⓑ Ⓒ Ⓓ Ⓔ
99. Ⓐ Ⓑ Ⓒ Ⓓ Ⓔ
100. Ⓐ Ⓑ Ⓒ Ⓓ Ⓔ
101. Ⓐ Ⓑ Ⓒ Ⓓ Ⓔ
102. Ⓐ Ⓑ Ⓒ Ⓓ Ⓔ
103. Ⓐ Ⓑ Ⓒ Ⓓ Ⓔ
104. Ⓐ Ⓑ Ⓒ Ⓓ Ⓔ
105. Ⓐ Ⓑ Ⓒ Ⓓ Ⓔ
106. Ⓐ Ⓑ Ⓒ Ⓓ Ⓔ
107. Ⓐ Ⓑ Ⓒ Ⓓ Ⓔ
108. Ⓐ Ⓑ Ⓒ Ⓓ Ⓔ
109. Ⓐ Ⓑ Ⓒ Ⓓ Ⓔ
110. Ⓐ Ⓑ Ⓒ Ⓓ Ⓔ
111. Ⓐ Ⓑ Ⓒ Ⓓ Ⓔ
112. Ⓐ Ⓑ Ⓒ Ⓓ Ⓔ
113. Ⓐ Ⓑ Ⓒ Ⓓ Ⓔ
114. Ⓐ Ⓑ Ⓒ Ⓓ Ⓔ
115. Ⓐ Ⓑ Ⓒ Ⓓ Ⓔ
116. Ⓐ Ⓑ Ⓒ Ⓓ Ⓔ
117. Ⓐ Ⓑ Ⓒ Ⓓ Ⓔ
118. Ⓐ Ⓑ Ⓒ Ⓓ Ⓔ
119. Ⓐ Ⓑ Ⓒ Ⓓ Ⓔ
120. Ⓐ Ⓑ Ⓒ Ⓓ Ⓔ

121. Ⓐ Ⓑ Ⓒ Ⓓ Ⓔ
122. Ⓐ Ⓑ Ⓒ Ⓓ Ⓔ
123. Ⓐ Ⓑ Ⓒ Ⓓ Ⓔ
124. Ⓐ Ⓑ Ⓒ Ⓓ Ⓔ
125. Ⓐ Ⓑ Ⓒ Ⓓ Ⓔ
126. Ⓐ Ⓑ Ⓒ Ⓓ Ⓔ
127. Ⓐ Ⓑ Ⓒ Ⓓ Ⓔ
128. Ⓐ Ⓑ Ⓒ Ⓓ Ⓔ
129. Ⓐ Ⓑ Ⓒ Ⓓ Ⓔ
130. Ⓐ Ⓑ Ⓒ Ⓓ Ⓔ
131. Ⓐ Ⓑ Ⓒ Ⓓ Ⓔ
132. Ⓐ Ⓑ Ⓒ Ⓓ Ⓔ
133. Ⓐ Ⓑ Ⓒ Ⓓ Ⓔ
134. Ⓐ Ⓑ Ⓒ Ⓓ Ⓔ
135. Ⓐ Ⓑ Ⓒ Ⓓ Ⓔ
136. Ⓐ Ⓑ Ⓒ Ⓓ Ⓔ
137. Ⓐ Ⓑ Ⓒ Ⓓ Ⓔ
138. Ⓐ Ⓑ Ⓒ Ⓓ Ⓔ
139. Ⓐ Ⓑ Ⓒ Ⓓ Ⓔ
140. Ⓐ Ⓑ Ⓒ Ⓓ Ⓔ
141. Ⓐ Ⓑ Ⓒ Ⓓ Ⓔ
142. Ⓐ Ⓑ Ⓒ Ⓓ Ⓔ
143. Ⓐ Ⓑ Ⓒ Ⓓ Ⓔ
144. Ⓐ Ⓑ Ⓒ Ⓓ Ⓔ
145. Ⓐ Ⓑ Ⓒ Ⓓ Ⓔ
146. Ⓐ Ⓑ Ⓒ Ⓓ Ⓔ
147. Ⓐ Ⓑ Ⓒ Ⓓ Ⓔ
148. Ⓐ Ⓑ Ⓒ Ⓓ Ⓔ
149. Ⓐ Ⓑ Ⓒ Ⓓ Ⓔ
150. Ⓐ Ⓑ Ⓒ Ⓓ Ⓔ

151. Ⓐ Ⓑ Ⓒ Ⓓ Ⓔ
152. Ⓐ Ⓑ Ⓒ Ⓓ Ⓔ
153. Ⓐ Ⓑ Ⓒ Ⓓ Ⓔ
154. Ⓐ Ⓑ Ⓒ Ⓓ Ⓔ
155. Ⓐ Ⓑ Ⓒ Ⓓ Ⓔ
156. Ⓐ Ⓑ Ⓒ Ⓓ Ⓔ
157. Ⓐ Ⓑ Ⓒ Ⓓ Ⓔ
158. Ⓐ Ⓑ Ⓒ Ⓓ Ⓔ
159. Ⓐ Ⓑ Ⓒ Ⓓ Ⓔ
160. Ⓐ Ⓑ Ⓒ Ⓓ Ⓔ
161. Ⓐ Ⓑ Ⓒ Ⓓ Ⓔ
162. Ⓐ Ⓑ Ⓒ Ⓓ Ⓔ
163. Ⓐ Ⓑ Ⓒ Ⓓ Ⓔ
164. Ⓐ Ⓑ Ⓒ Ⓓ Ⓔ
165. Ⓐ Ⓑ Ⓒ Ⓓ Ⓔ
166. Ⓐ Ⓑ Ⓒ Ⓓ Ⓔ
167. Ⓐ Ⓑ Ⓒ Ⓓ Ⓔ
168. Ⓐ Ⓑ Ⓒ Ⓓ Ⓔ
169. Ⓐ Ⓑ Ⓒ Ⓓ Ⓔ
170. Ⓐ Ⓑ Ⓒ Ⓓ Ⓔ
171. Ⓐ Ⓑ Ⓒ Ⓓ Ⓔ
172. Ⓐ Ⓑ Ⓒ Ⓓ Ⓔ
173. Ⓐ Ⓑ Ⓒ Ⓓ Ⓔ
174. Ⓐ Ⓑ Ⓒ Ⓓ Ⓔ
175. Ⓐ Ⓑ Ⓒ Ⓓ Ⓔ
176. Ⓐ Ⓑ Ⓒ Ⓓ Ⓔ
177. Ⓐ Ⓑ Ⓒ Ⓓ Ⓔ
178. Ⓐ Ⓑ Ⓒ Ⓓ Ⓔ
179. Ⓐ Ⓑ Ⓒ Ⓓ Ⓔ
180. Ⓐ Ⓑ Ⓒ Ⓓ Ⓔ

USMLE STEP 3
PRACTICE TEST 1

Day Two – Morning Session

ANSWER SHEET

1. Ⓐ Ⓑ Ⓒ Ⓓ Ⓔ
2. Ⓐ Ⓑ Ⓒ Ⓓ Ⓔ
3. Ⓐ Ⓑ Ⓒ Ⓓ Ⓔ
4. Ⓐ Ⓑ Ⓒ Ⓓ Ⓔ
5. Ⓐ Ⓑ Ⓒ Ⓓ Ⓔ
6. Ⓐ Ⓑ Ⓒ Ⓓ Ⓔ
7. Ⓐ Ⓑ Ⓒ Ⓓ Ⓔ
8. Ⓐ Ⓑ Ⓒ Ⓓ Ⓔ
9. Ⓐ Ⓑ Ⓒ Ⓓ Ⓔ
10. Ⓐ Ⓑ Ⓒ Ⓓ Ⓔ
11. Ⓐ Ⓑ Ⓒ Ⓓ Ⓔ
12. Ⓐ Ⓑ Ⓒ Ⓓ Ⓔ
13. Ⓐ Ⓑ Ⓒ Ⓓ Ⓔ
14. Ⓐ Ⓑ Ⓒ Ⓓ Ⓔ
15. Ⓐ Ⓑ Ⓒ Ⓓ Ⓔ
16. Ⓐ Ⓑ Ⓒ Ⓓ Ⓔ
17. Ⓐ Ⓑ Ⓒ Ⓓ Ⓔ
18. Ⓐ Ⓑ Ⓒ Ⓓ Ⓔ
19. Ⓐ Ⓑ Ⓒ Ⓓ Ⓔ
20. Ⓐ Ⓑ Ⓒ Ⓓ Ⓔ
21. Ⓐ Ⓑ Ⓒ Ⓓ Ⓔ
22. Ⓐ Ⓑ Ⓒ Ⓓ Ⓔ
23. Ⓐ Ⓑ Ⓒ Ⓓ Ⓔ
24. Ⓐ Ⓑ Ⓒ Ⓓ Ⓔ
25. Ⓐ Ⓑ Ⓒ Ⓓ Ⓔ
26. Ⓐ Ⓑ Ⓒ Ⓓ Ⓔ
27. Ⓐ Ⓑ Ⓒ Ⓓ Ⓔ
28. Ⓐ Ⓑ Ⓒ Ⓓ Ⓔ
29. Ⓐ Ⓑ Ⓒ Ⓓ Ⓔ
30. Ⓐ Ⓑ Ⓒ Ⓓ Ⓔ

31. Ⓐ Ⓑ Ⓒ Ⓓ Ⓔ
32. Ⓐ Ⓑ Ⓒ Ⓓ Ⓔ
33. Ⓐ Ⓑ Ⓒ Ⓓ Ⓔ
34. Ⓐ Ⓑ Ⓒ Ⓓ Ⓔ
35. Ⓐ Ⓑ Ⓒ Ⓓ Ⓔ
36. Ⓐ Ⓑ Ⓒ Ⓓ Ⓔ
37. Ⓐ Ⓑ Ⓒ Ⓓ Ⓔ
38. Ⓐ Ⓑ Ⓒ Ⓓ Ⓔ
39. Ⓐ Ⓑ Ⓒ Ⓓ Ⓔ
40. Ⓐ Ⓑ Ⓒ Ⓓ Ⓔ
41. Ⓐ Ⓑ Ⓒ Ⓓ Ⓔ
42. Ⓐ Ⓑ Ⓒ Ⓓ Ⓔ
43. Ⓐ Ⓑ Ⓒ Ⓓ Ⓔ
44. Ⓐ Ⓑ Ⓒ Ⓓ Ⓔ
45. Ⓐ Ⓑ Ⓒ Ⓓ Ⓔ
46. Ⓐ Ⓑ Ⓒ Ⓓ Ⓔ
47. Ⓐ Ⓑ Ⓒ Ⓓ Ⓔ
48. Ⓐ Ⓑ Ⓒ Ⓓ Ⓔ
49. Ⓐ Ⓑ Ⓒ Ⓓ Ⓔ
50. Ⓐ Ⓑ Ⓒ Ⓓ Ⓔ
51. Ⓐ Ⓑ Ⓒ Ⓓ Ⓔ
52. Ⓐ Ⓑ Ⓒ Ⓓ Ⓔ
53. Ⓐ Ⓑ Ⓒ Ⓓ Ⓔ
54. Ⓐ Ⓑ Ⓒ Ⓓ Ⓔ
55. Ⓐ Ⓑ Ⓒ Ⓓ Ⓔ
56. Ⓐ Ⓑ Ⓒ Ⓓ Ⓔ
57. Ⓐ Ⓑ Ⓒ Ⓓ Ⓔ
58. Ⓐ Ⓑ Ⓒ Ⓓ Ⓔ
59. Ⓐ Ⓑ Ⓒ Ⓓ Ⓔ
60. Ⓐ Ⓑ Ⓒ Ⓓ Ⓔ

61. Ⓐ Ⓑ Ⓒ Ⓓ Ⓔ
62. Ⓐ Ⓑ Ⓒ Ⓓ Ⓔ
63. Ⓐ Ⓑ Ⓒ Ⓓ Ⓔ
64. Ⓐ Ⓑ Ⓒ Ⓓ Ⓔ
65. Ⓐ Ⓑ Ⓒ Ⓓ Ⓔ
66. Ⓐ Ⓑ Ⓒ Ⓓ Ⓔ
67. Ⓐ Ⓑ Ⓒ Ⓓ Ⓔ
68. Ⓐ Ⓑ Ⓒ Ⓓ Ⓔ
69. Ⓐ Ⓑ Ⓒ Ⓓ Ⓔ
70. Ⓐ Ⓑ Ⓒ Ⓓ Ⓔ
71. Ⓐ Ⓑ Ⓒ Ⓓ Ⓔ
72. Ⓐ Ⓑ Ⓒ Ⓓ Ⓔ
73. Ⓐ Ⓑ Ⓒ Ⓓ Ⓔ
74. Ⓐ Ⓑ Ⓒ Ⓓ Ⓔ
75. Ⓐ Ⓑ Ⓒ Ⓓ Ⓔ
76. Ⓐ Ⓑ Ⓒ Ⓓ Ⓔ
77. Ⓐ Ⓑ Ⓒ Ⓓ Ⓔ
78. Ⓐ Ⓑ Ⓒ Ⓓ Ⓔ
79. Ⓐ Ⓑ Ⓒ Ⓓ Ⓔ
80. Ⓐ Ⓑ Ⓒ Ⓓ Ⓔ
81. Ⓐ Ⓑ Ⓒ Ⓓ Ⓔ
82. Ⓐ Ⓑ Ⓒ Ⓓ Ⓔ
83. Ⓐ Ⓑ Ⓒ Ⓓ Ⓔ
84. Ⓐ Ⓑ Ⓒ Ⓓ Ⓔ
85. Ⓐ Ⓑ Ⓒ Ⓓ Ⓔ
86. Ⓐ Ⓑ Ⓒ Ⓓ Ⓔ
87. Ⓐ Ⓑ Ⓒ Ⓓ Ⓔ
88. Ⓐ Ⓑ Ⓒ Ⓓ Ⓔ
89. Ⓐ Ⓑ Ⓒ Ⓓ Ⓔ
90. Ⓐ Ⓑ Ⓒ Ⓓ Ⓔ

91. Ⓐ Ⓑ Ⓒ Ⓓ Ⓔ
92. Ⓐ Ⓑ Ⓒ Ⓓ Ⓔ
93. Ⓐ Ⓑ Ⓒ Ⓓ Ⓔ
94. Ⓐ Ⓑ Ⓒ Ⓓ Ⓔ
95. Ⓐ Ⓑ Ⓒ Ⓓ Ⓔ
96. Ⓐ Ⓑ Ⓒ Ⓓ Ⓔ
97. Ⓐ Ⓑ Ⓒ Ⓓ Ⓔ
98. Ⓐ Ⓑ Ⓒ Ⓓ Ⓔ
99. Ⓐ Ⓑ Ⓒ Ⓓ Ⓔ
100. Ⓐ Ⓑ Ⓒ Ⓓ Ⓔ
101. Ⓐ Ⓑ Ⓒ Ⓓ Ⓔ
102. Ⓐ Ⓑ Ⓒ Ⓓ Ⓔ
103. Ⓐ Ⓑ Ⓒ Ⓓ Ⓔ
104. Ⓐ Ⓑ Ⓒ Ⓓ Ⓔ
105. Ⓐ Ⓑ Ⓒ Ⓓ Ⓔ
106. Ⓐ Ⓑ Ⓒ Ⓓ Ⓔ
107. Ⓐ Ⓑ Ⓒ Ⓓ Ⓔ
108. Ⓐ Ⓑ Ⓒ Ⓓ Ⓔ
109. Ⓐ Ⓑ Ⓒ Ⓓ Ⓔ
110. Ⓐ Ⓑ Ⓒ Ⓓ Ⓔ
111. Ⓐ Ⓑ Ⓒ Ⓓ Ⓔ
112. Ⓐ Ⓑ Ⓒ Ⓓ Ⓔ
113. Ⓐ Ⓑ Ⓒ Ⓓ Ⓔ
114. Ⓐ Ⓑ Ⓒ Ⓓ Ⓔ
115. Ⓐ Ⓑ Ⓒ Ⓓ Ⓔ
116. Ⓐ Ⓑ Ⓒ Ⓓ Ⓔ
117. Ⓐ Ⓑ Ⓒ Ⓓ Ⓔ
118. Ⓐ Ⓑ Ⓒ Ⓓ Ⓔ
119. Ⓐ Ⓑ Ⓒ Ⓓ Ⓔ
120. Ⓐ Ⓑ Ⓒ Ⓓ Ⓔ

121. Ⓐ Ⓑ Ⓒ Ⓓ Ⓔ
122. Ⓐ Ⓑ Ⓒ Ⓓ Ⓔ
123. Ⓐ Ⓑ Ⓒ Ⓓ Ⓔ
124. Ⓐ Ⓑ Ⓒ Ⓓ Ⓔ
125. Ⓐ Ⓑ Ⓒ Ⓓ Ⓔ
126. Ⓐ Ⓑ Ⓒ Ⓓ Ⓔ
127. Ⓐ Ⓑ Ⓒ Ⓓ Ⓔ
128. Ⓐ Ⓑ Ⓒ Ⓓ Ⓔ
129. Ⓐ Ⓑ Ⓒ Ⓓ Ⓔ
130. Ⓐ Ⓑ Ⓒ Ⓓ Ⓔ
131. Ⓐ Ⓑ Ⓒ Ⓓ Ⓔ
132. Ⓐ Ⓑ Ⓒ Ⓓ Ⓔ
133. Ⓐ Ⓑ Ⓒ Ⓓ Ⓔ
134. Ⓐ Ⓑ Ⓒ Ⓓ Ⓔ
135. Ⓐ Ⓑ Ⓒ Ⓓ Ⓔ
136. Ⓐ Ⓑ Ⓒ Ⓓ Ⓔ
137. Ⓐ Ⓑ Ⓒ Ⓓ Ⓔ
138. Ⓐ Ⓑ Ⓒ Ⓓ Ⓔ
139. Ⓐ Ⓑ Ⓒ Ⓓ Ⓔ
140. Ⓐ Ⓑ Ⓒ Ⓓ Ⓔ
141. Ⓐ Ⓑ Ⓒ Ⓓ Ⓔ
142. Ⓐ Ⓑ Ⓒ Ⓓ Ⓔ
143. Ⓐ Ⓑ Ⓒ Ⓓ Ⓔ
144. Ⓐ Ⓑ Ⓒ Ⓓ Ⓔ
145. Ⓐ Ⓑ Ⓒ Ⓓ Ⓔ
146. Ⓐ Ⓑ Ⓒ Ⓓ Ⓔ
147. Ⓐ Ⓑ Ⓒ Ⓓ Ⓔ
148. Ⓐ Ⓑ Ⓒ Ⓓ Ⓔ
149. Ⓐ Ⓑ Ⓒ Ⓓ Ⓔ
150. Ⓐ Ⓑ Ⓒ Ⓓ Ⓔ

151. Ⓐ Ⓑ Ⓒ Ⓓ Ⓔ
152. Ⓐ Ⓑ Ⓒ Ⓓ Ⓔ
153. Ⓐ Ⓑ Ⓒ Ⓓ Ⓔ
154. Ⓐ Ⓑ Ⓒ Ⓓ Ⓔ
155. Ⓐ Ⓑ Ⓒ Ⓓ Ⓔ
156. Ⓐ Ⓑ Ⓒ Ⓓ Ⓔ
157. Ⓐ Ⓑ Ⓒ Ⓓ Ⓔ
158. Ⓐ Ⓑ Ⓒ Ⓓ Ⓔ
159. Ⓐ Ⓑ Ⓒ Ⓓ Ⓔ
160. Ⓐ Ⓑ Ⓒ Ⓓ Ⓔ
161. Ⓐ Ⓑ Ⓒ Ⓓ Ⓔ
162. Ⓐ Ⓑ Ⓒ Ⓓ Ⓔ
163. Ⓐ Ⓑ Ⓒ Ⓓ Ⓔ
164. Ⓐ Ⓑ Ⓒ Ⓓ Ⓔ
165. Ⓐ Ⓑ Ⓒ Ⓓ Ⓔ
166. Ⓐ Ⓑ Ⓒ Ⓓ Ⓔ
167. Ⓐ Ⓑ Ⓒ Ⓓ Ⓔ
168. Ⓐ Ⓑ Ⓒ Ⓓ Ⓔ
169. Ⓐ Ⓑ Ⓒ Ⓓ Ⓔ
170. Ⓐ Ⓑ Ⓒ Ⓓ Ⓔ
171. Ⓐ Ⓑ Ⓒ Ⓓ Ⓔ
172. Ⓐ Ⓑ Ⓒ Ⓓ Ⓔ
173. Ⓐ Ⓑ Ⓒ Ⓓ Ⓔ
174. Ⓐ Ⓑ Ⓒ Ⓓ Ⓔ
175. Ⓐ Ⓑ Ⓒ Ⓓ Ⓔ
176. Ⓐ Ⓑ Ⓒ Ⓓ Ⓔ
177. Ⓐ Ⓑ Ⓒ Ⓓ Ⓔ
178. Ⓐ Ⓑ Ⓒ Ⓓ Ⓔ
179. Ⓐ Ⓑ Ⓒ Ⓓ Ⓔ
180. Ⓐ Ⓑ Ⓒ Ⓓ Ⓔ

USMLE STEP 3
PRACTICE TEST 1

Day Two – Afternoon Session

ANSWER SHEET

1. Ⓐ Ⓑ Ⓒ Ⓓ Ⓔ	31. Ⓐ Ⓑ Ⓒ Ⓓ Ⓔ	61. Ⓐ Ⓑ Ⓒ Ⓓ Ⓔ
2. Ⓐ Ⓑ Ⓒ Ⓓ Ⓔ	32. Ⓐ Ⓑ Ⓒ Ⓓ Ⓔ	62. Ⓐ Ⓑ Ⓒ Ⓓ Ⓔ
3. Ⓐ Ⓑ Ⓒ Ⓓ Ⓔ	33. Ⓐ Ⓑ Ⓒ Ⓓ Ⓔ	63. Ⓐ Ⓑ Ⓒ Ⓓ Ⓔ
4. Ⓐ Ⓑ Ⓒ Ⓓ Ⓔ	34. Ⓐ Ⓑ Ⓒ Ⓓ Ⓔ	64. Ⓐ Ⓑ Ⓒ Ⓓ Ⓔ
5. Ⓐ Ⓑ Ⓒ Ⓓ Ⓔ	35. Ⓐ Ⓑ Ⓒ Ⓓ Ⓔ	65. Ⓐ Ⓑ Ⓒ Ⓓ Ⓔ
6. Ⓐ Ⓑ Ⓒ Ⓓ Ⓔ	36. Ⓐ Ⓑ Ⓒ Ⓓ Ⓔ	66. Ⓐ Ⓑ Ⓒ Ⓓ Ⓔ
7. Ⓐ Ⓑ Ⓒ Ⓓ Ⓔ	37. Ⓐ Ⓑ Ⓒ Ⓓ Ⓔ	67. Ⓐ Ⓑ Ⓒ Ⓓ Ⓔ
8. Ⓐ Ⓑ Ⓒ Ⓓ Ⓔ	38. Ⓐ Ⓑ Ⓒ Ⓓ Ⓔ	68. Ⓐ Ⓑ Ⓒ Ⓓ Ⓔ
9. Ⓐ Ⓑ Ⓒ Ⓓ Ⓔ	39. Ⓐ Ⓑ Ⓒ Ⓓ Ⓔ	69. Ⓐ Ⓑ Ⓒ Ⓓ Ⓔ
10. Ⓐ Ⓑ Ⓒ Ⓓ Ⓔ	40. Ⓐ Ⓑ Ⓒ Ⓓ Ⓔ	70. Ⓐ Ⓑ Ⓒ Ⓓ Ⓔ
11. Ⓐ Ⓑ Ⓒ Ⓓ Ⓔ	41. Ⓐ Ⓑ Ⓒ Ⓓ Ⓔ	71. Ⓐ Ⓑ Ⓒ Ⓓ Ⓔ
12. Ⓐ Ⓑ Ⓒ Ⓓ Ⓔ	42. Ⓐ Ⓑ Ⓒ Ⓓ Ⓔ	72. Ⓐ Ⓑ Ⓒ Ⓓ Ⓔ
13. Ⓐ Ⓑ Ⓒ Ⓓ Ⓔ	43. Ⓐ Ⓑ Ⓒ Ⓓ Ⓔ	73. Ⓐ Ⓑ Ⓒ Ⓓ Ⓔ
14. Ⓐ Ⓑ Ⓒ Ⓓ Ⓔ	44. Ⓐ Ⓑ Ⓒ Ⓓ Ⓔ	74. Ⓐ Ⓑ Ⓒ Ⓓ Ⓔ
15. Ⓐ Ⓑ Ⓒ Ⓓ Ⓔ	45. Ⓐ Ⓑ Ⓒ Ⓓ Ⓔ	75. Ⓐ Ⓑ Ⓒ Ⓓ Ⓔ
16. Ⓐ Ⓑ Ⓒ Ⓓ Ⓔ	46. Ⓐ Ⓑ Ⓒ Ⓓ Ⓔ	76. Ⓐ Ⓑ Ⓒ Ⓓ Ⓔ
17. Ⓐ Ⓑ Ⓒ Ⓓ Ⓔ	47. Ⓐ Ⓑ Ⓒ Ⓓ Ⓔ	77. Ⓐ Ⓑ Ⓒ Ⓓ Ⓔ
18. Ⓐ Ⓑ Ⓒ Ⓓ Ⓔ	48. Ⓐ Ⓑ Ⓒ Ⓓ Ⓔ	78. Ⓐ Ⓑ Ⓒ Ⓓ Ⓔ
19. Ⓐ Ⓑ Ⓒ Ⓓ Ⓔ	49. Ⓐ Ⓑ Ⓒ Ⓓ Ⓔ	79. Ⓐ Ⓑ Ⓒ Ⓓ Ⓔ
20. Ⓐ Ⓑ Ⓒ Ⓓ Ⓔ	50. Ⓐ Ⓑ Ⓒ Ⓓ Ⓔ	80. Ⓐ Ⓑ Ⓒ Ⓓ Ⓔ
21. Ⓐ Ⓑ Ⓒ Ⓓ Ⓔ	51. Ⓐ Ⓑ Ⓒ Ⓓ Ⓔ	81. Ⓐ Ⓑ Ⓒ Ⓓ Ⓔ
22. Ⓐ Ⓑ Ⓒ Ⓓ Ⓔ	52. Ⓐ Ⓑ Ⓒ Ⓓ Ⓔ	82. Ⓐ Ⓑ Ⓒ Ⓓ Ⓔ
23. Ⓐ Ⓑ Ⓒ Ⓓ Ⓔ	53. Ⓐ Ⓑ Ⓒ Ⓓ Ⓔ	83. Ⓐ Ⓑ Ⓒ Ⓓ Ⓔ
24. Ⓐ Ⓑ Ⓒ Ⓓ Ⓔ	54. Ⓐ Ⓑ Ⓒ Ⓓ Ⓔ	84. Ⓐ Ⓑ Ⓒ Ⓓ Ⓔ
25. Ⓐ Ⓑ Ⓒ Ⓓ Ⓔ	55. Ⓐ Ⓑ Ⓒ Ⓓ Ⓔ	85. Ⓐ Ⓑ Ⓒ Ⓓ Ⓔ
26. Ⓐ Ⓑ Ⓒ Ⓓ Ⓔ	56. Ⓐ Ⓑ Ⓒ Ⓓ Ⓔ	86. Ⓐ Ⓑ Ⓒ Ⓓ Ⓔ
27. Ⓐ Ⓑ Ⓒ Ⓓ Ⓔ	57. Ⓐ Ⓑ Ⓒ Ⓓ Ⓔ	87. Ⓐ Ⓑ Ⓒ Ⓓ Ⓔ
28. Ⓐ Ⓑ Ⓒ Ⓓ Ⓔ	58. Ⓐ Ⓑ Ⓒ Ⓓ Ⓔ	88. Ⓐ Ⓑ Ⓒ Ⓓ Ⓔ
29. Ⓐ Ⓑ Ⓒ Ⓓ Ⓔ	59. Ⓐ Ⓑ Ⓒ Ⓓ Ⓔ	89. Ⓐ Ⓑ Ⓒ Ⓓ Ⓔ
30. Ⓐ Ⓑ Ⓒ Ⓓ Ⓔ	60. Ⓐ Ⓑ Ⓒ Ⓓ Ⓔ	90. Ⓐ Ⓑ Ⓒ Ⓓ Ⓔ

91. Ⓐ Ⓑ Ⓒ Ⓓ Ⓔ	121. Ⓐ Ⓑ Ⓒ Ⓓ Ⓔ	151. Ⓐ Ⓑ Ⓒ Ⓓ Ⓔ
92. Ⓐ Ⓑ Ⓒ Ⓓ Ⓔ	122. Ⓐ Ⓑ Ⓒ Ⓓ Ⓔ	152. Ⓐ Ⓑ Ⓒ Ⓓ Ⓔ
93. Ⓐ Ⓑ Ⓒ Ⓓ Ⓔ	123. Ⓐ Ⓑ Ⓒ Ⓓ Ⓔ	153. Ⓐ Ⓑ Ⓒ Ⓓ Ⓔ
94. Ⓐ Ⓑ Ⓒ Ⓓ Ⓔ	124. Ⓐ Ⓑ Ⓒ Ⓓ Ⓔ	154. Ⓐ Ⓑ Ⓒ Ⓓ Ⓔ
95. Ⓐ Ⓑ Ⓒ Ⓓ Ⓔ	125. Ⓐ Ⓑ Ⓒ Ⓓ Ⓔ	155. Ⓐ Ⓑ Ⓒ Ⓓ Ⓔ
96. Ⓐ Ⓑ Ⓒ Ⓓ Ⓔ	126. Ⓐ Ⓑ Ⓒ Ⓓ Ⓔ	156. Ⓐ Ⓑ Ⓒ Ⓓ Ⓔ
97. Ⓐ Ⓑ Ⓒ Ⓓ Ⓔ	127. Ⓐ Ⓑ Ⓒ Ⓓ Ⓔ	157. Ⓐ Ⓑ Ⓒ Ⓓ Ⓔ
98. Ⓐ Ⓑ Ⓒ Ⓓ Ⓔ	128. Ⓐ Ⓑ Ⓒ Ⓓ Ⓔ	158. Ⓐ Ⓑ Ⓒ Ⓓ Ⓔ
99. Ⓐ Ⓑ Ⓒ Ⓓ Ⓔ	129. Ⓐ Ⓑ Ⓒ Ⓓ Ⓔ	159. Ⓐ Ⓑ Ⓒ Ⓓ Ⓔ
100. Ⓐ Ⓑ Ⓒ Ⓓ Ⓔ	130. Ⓐ Ⓑ Ⓒ Ⓓ Ⓔ	160. Ⓐ Ⓑ Ⓒ Ⓓ Ⓔ
101. Ⓐ Ⓑ Ⓒ Ⓓ Ⓔ	131. Ⓐ Ⓑ Ⓒ Ⓓ Ⓔ	161. Ⓐ Ⓑ Ⓒ Ⓓ Ⓔ
102. Ⓐ Ⓑ Ⓒ Ⓓ Ⓔ	132. Ⓐ Ⓑ Ⓒ Ⓓ Ⓔ	162. Ⓐ Ⓑ Ⓒ Ⓓ Ⓔ
103. Ⓐ Ⓑ Ⓒ Ⓓ Ⓔ	133. Ⓐ Ⓑ Ⓒ Ⓓ Ⓔ	163. Ⓐ Ⓑ Ⓒ Ⓓ Ⓔ
104. Ⓐ Ⓑ Ⓒ Ⓓ Ⓔ	134. Ⓐ Ⓑ Ⓒ Ⓓ Ⓔ	164. Ⓐ Ⓑ Ⓒ Ⓓ Ⓔ
105. Ⓐ Ⓑ Ⓒ Ⓓ Ⓔ	135. Ⓐ Ⓑ Ⓒ Ⓓ Ⓔ	165. Ⓐ Ⓑ Ⓒ Ⓓ Ⓔ
106. Ⓐ Ⓑ Ⓒ Ⓓ Ⓔ	136. Ⓐ Ⓑ Ⓒ Ⓓ Ⓔ	166. Ⓐ Ⓑ Ⓒ Ⓓ Ⓔ
107. Ⓐ Ⓑ Ⓒ Ⓓ Ⓔ	137. Ⓐ Ⓑ Ⓒ Ⓓ Ⓔ	167. Ⓐ Ⓑ Ⓒ Ⓓ Ⓔ
108. Ⓐ Ⓑ Ⓒ Ⓓ Ⓔ	138. Ⓐ Ⓑ Ⓒ Ⓓ Ⓔ	168. Ⓐ Ⓑ Ⓒ Ⓓ Ⓔ
109. Ⓐ Ⓑ Ⓒ Ⓓ Ⓔ	139. Ⓐ Ⓑ Ⓒ Ⓓ Ⓔ	169. Ⓐ Ⓑ Ⓒ Ⓓ Ⓔ
110. Ⓐ Ⓑ Ⓒ Ⓓ Ⓔ	140. Ⓐ Ⓑ Ⓒ Ⓓ Ⓔ	170. Ⓐ Ⓑ Ⓒ Ⓓ Ⓔ
111. Ⓐ Ⓑ Ⓒ Ⓓ Ⓔ	141. Ⓐ Ⓑ Ⓒ Ⓓ Ⓔ	171. Ⓐ Ⓑ Ⓒ Ⓓ Ⓔ
112. Ⓐ Ⓑ Ⓒ Ⓓ Ⓔ	142. Ⓐ Ⓑ Ⓒ Ⓓ Ⓔ	172. Ⓐ Ⓑ Ⓒ Ⓓ Ⓔ
113. Ⓐ Ⓑ Ⓒ Ⓓ Ⓔ	143. Ⓐ Ⓑ Ⓒ Ⓓ Ⓔ	173. Ⓐ Ⓑ Ⓒ Ⓓ Ⓔ
114. Ⓐ Ⓑ Ⓒ Ⓓ Ⓔ	144. Ⓐ Ⓑ Ⓒ Ⓓ Ⓔ	174. Ⓐ Ⓑ Ⓒ Ⓓ Ⓔ
115. Ⓐ Ⓑ Ⓒ Ⓓ Ⓔ	145. Ⓐ Ⓑ Ⓒ Ⓓ Ⓔ	175. Ⓐ Ⓑ Ⓒ Ⓓ Ⓔ
116. Ⓐ Ⓑ Ⓒ Ⓓ Ⓔ	146. Ⓐ Ⓑ Ⓒ Ⓓ Ⓔ	176. Ⓐ Ⓑ Ⓒ Ⓓ Ⓔ
117. Ⓐ Ⓑ Ⓒ Ⓓ Ⓔ	147. Ⓐ Ⓑ Ⓒ Ⓓ Ⓔ	177. Ⓐ Ⓑ Ⓒ Ⓓ Ⓔ
118. Ⓐ Ⓑ Ⓒ Ⓓ Ⓔ	148. Ⓐ Ⓑ Ⓒ Ⓓ Ⓔ	178. Ⓐ Ⓑ Ⓒ Ⓓ Ⓔ
119. Ⓐ Ⓑ Ⓒ Ⓓ Ⓔ	149. Ⓐ Ⓑ Ⓒ Ⓓ Ⓔ	179. Ⓐ Ⓑ Ⓒ Ⓓ Ⓔ
120. Ⓐ Ⓑ Ⓒ Ⓓ Ⓔ	150. Ⓐ Ⓑ Ⓒ Ⓓ Ⓔ	180. Ⓐ Ⓑ Ⓒ Ⓓ Ⓔ

USMLE STEP 3
PRACTICE TEST 2

Day One – Morning Session

ANSWER SHEET

1. Ⓐ Ⓑ Ⓒ Ⓓ Ⓔ
2. Ⓐ Ⓑ Ⓒ Ⓓ Ⓔ
3. Ⓐ Ⓑ Ⓒ Ⓓ Ⓔ
4. Ⓐ Ⓑ Ⓒ Ⓓ Ⓔ
5. Ⓐ Ⓑ Ⓒ Ⓓ Ⓔ
6. Ⓐ Ⓑ Ⓒ Ⓓ Ⓔ
7. Ⓐ Ⓑ Ⓒ Ⓓ Ⓔ
8. Ⓐ Ⓑ Ⓒ Ⓓ Ⓔ
9. Ⓐ Ⓑ Ⓒ Ⓓ Ⓔ
10. Ⓐ Ⓑ Ⓒ Ⓓ Ⓔ
11. Ⓐ Ⓑ Ⓒ Ⓓ Ⓔ
12. Ⓐ Ⓑ Ⓒ Ⓓ Ⓔ
13. Ⓐ Ⓑ Ⓒ Ⓓ Ⓔ
14. Ⓐ Ⓑ Ⓒ Ⓓ Ⓔ
15. Ⓐ Ⓑ Ⓒ Ⓓ Ⓔ
16. Ⓐ Ⓑ Ⓒ Ⓓ Ⓔ
17. Ⓐ Ⓑ Ⓒ Ⓓ Ⓔ
18. Ⓐ Ⓑ Ⓒ Ⓓ Ⓔ
19. Ⓐ Ⓑ Ⓒ Ⓓ Ⓔ
20. Ⓐ Ⓑ Ⓒ Ⓓ Ⓔ
21. Ⓐ Ⓑ Ⓒ Ⓓ Ⓔ
22. Ⓐ Ⓑ Ⓒ Ⓓ Ⓔ
23. Ⓐ Ⓑ Ⓒ Ⓓ Ⓔ
24. Ⓐ Ⓑ Ⓒ Ⓓ Ⓔ
25. Ⓐ Ⓑ Ⓒ Ⓓ Ⓔ
26. Ⓐ Ⓑ Ⓒ Ⓓ Ⓔ
27. Ⓐ Ⓑ Ⓒ Ⓓ Ⓔ
28. Ⓐ Ⓑ Ⓒ Ⓓ Ⓔ
29. Ⓐ Ⓑ Ⓒ Ⓓ Ⓔ
30. Ⓐ Ⓑ Ⓒ Ⓓ Ⓔ

31. Ⓐ Ⓑ Ⓒ Ⓓ Ⓔ
32. Ⓐ Ⓑ Ⓒ Ⓓ Ⓔ
33. Ⓐ Ⓑ Ⓒ Ⓓ Ⓔ
34. Ⓐ Ⓑ Ⓒ Ⓓ Ⓔ
35. Ⓐ Ⓑ Ⓒ Ⓓ Ⓔ
36. Ⓐ Ⓑ Ⓒ Ⓓ Ⓔ
37. Ⓐ Ⓑ Ⓒ Ⓓ Ⓔ
38. Ⓐ Ⓑ Ⓒ Ⓓ Ⓔ
39. Ⓐ Ⓑ Ⓒ Ⓓ Ⓔ
40. Ⓐ Ⓑ Ⓒ Ⓓ Ⓔ
41. Ⓐ Ⓑ Ⓒ Ⓓ Ⓔ
42. Ⓐ Ⓑ Ⓒ Ⓓ Ⓔ
43. Ⓐ Ⓑ Ⓒ Ⓓ Ⓔ
44. Ⓐ Ⓑ Ⓒ Ⓓ Ⓔ
45. Ⓐ Ⓑ Ⓒ Ⓓ Ⓔ
46. Ⓐ Ⓑ Ⓒ Ⓓ Ⓔ
47. Ⓐ Ⓑ Ⓒ Ⓓ Ⓔ
48. Ⓐ Ⓑ Ⓒ Ⓓ Ⓔ
49. Ⓐ Ⓑ Ⓒ Ⓓ Ⓔ
50. Ⓐ Ⓑ Ⓒ Ⓓ Ⓔ
51. Ⓐ Ⓑ Ⓒ Ⓓ Ⓔ
52. Ⓐ Ⓑ Ⓒ Ⓓ Ⓔ
53. Ⓐ Ⓑ Ⓒ Ⓓ Ⓔ
54. Ⓐ Ⓑ Ⓒ Ⓓ Ⓔ
55. Ⓐ Ⓑ Ⓒ Ⓓ Ⓔ
56. Ⓐ Ⓑ Ⓒ Ⓓ Ⓔ
57. Ⓐ Ⓑ Ⓒ Ⓓ Ⓔ
58. Ⓐ Ⓑ Ⓒ Ⓓ Ⓔ
59. Ⓐ Ⓑ Ⓒ Ⓓ Ⓔ
60. Ⓐ Ⓑ Ⓒ Ⓓ Ⓔ

61. Ⓐ Ⓑ Ⓒ Ⓓ Ⓔ
62. Ⓐ Ⓑ Ⓒ Ⓓ Ⓔ
63. Ⓐ Ⓑ Ⓒ Ⓓ Ⓔ
64. Ⓐ Ⓑ Ⓒ Ⓓ Ⓔ
65. Ⓐ Ⓑ Ⓒ Ⓓ Ⓔ
66. Ⓐ Ⓑ Ⓒ Ⓓ Ⓔ
67. Ⓐ Ⓑ Ⓒ Ⓓ Ⓔ
68. Ⓐ Ⓑ Ⓒ Ⓓ Ⓔ
69. Ⓐ Ⓑ Ⓒ Ⓓ Ⓔ
70. Ⓐ Ⓑ Ⓒ Ⓓ Ⓔ
71. Ⓐ Ⓑ Ⓒ Ⓓ Ⓔ
72. Ⓐ Ⓑ Ⓒ Ⓓ Ⓔ
73. Ⓐ Ⓑ Ⓒ Ⓓ Ⓔ
74. Ⓐ Ⓑ Ⓒ Ⓓ Ⓔ
75. Ⓐ Ⓑ Ⓒ Ⓓ Ⓔ
76. Ⓐ Ⓑ Ⓒ Ⓓ Ⓔ
77. Ⓐ Ⓑ Ⓒ Ⓓ Ⓔ
78. Ⓐ Ⓑ Ⓒ Ⓓ Ⓔ
79. Ⓐ Ⓑ Ⓒ Ⓓ Ⓔ
80. Ⓐ Ⓑ Ⓒ Ⓓ Ⓔ
81. Ⓐ Ⓑ Ⓒ Ⓓ Ⓔ
82. Ⓐ Ⓑ Ⓒ Ⓓ Ⓔ
83. Ⓐ Ⓑ Ⓒ Ⓓ Ⓔ
84. Ⓐ Ⓑ Ⓒ Ⓓ Ⓔ
85. Ⓐ Ⓑ Ⓒ Ⓓ Ⓔ
86. Ⓐ Ⓑ Ⓒ Ⓓ Ⓔ
87. Ⓐ Ⓑ Ⓒ Ⓓ Ⓔ
88. Ⓐ Ⓑ Ⓒ Ⓓ Ⓔ
89. Ⓐ Ⓑ Ⓒ Ⓓ Ⓔ
90. Ⓐ Ⓑ Ⓒ Ⓓ Ⓔ

91. Ⓐ Ⓑ Ⓒ Ⓓ Ⓔ
92. Ⓐ Ⓑ Ⓒ Ⓓ Ⓔ
93. Ⓐ Ⓑ Ⓒ Ⓓ Ⓔ
94. Ⓐ Ⓑ Ⓒ Ⓓ Ⓔ
95. Ⓐ Ⓑ Ⓒ Ⓓ Ⓔ
96. Ⓐ Ⓑ Ⓒ Ⓓ Ⓔ
97. Ⓐ Ⓑ Ⓒ Ⓓ Ⓔ
98. Ⓐ Ⓑ Ⓒ Ⓓ Ⓔ
99. Ⓐ Ⓑ Ⓒ Ⓓ Ⓔ
100. Ⓐ Ⓑ Ⓒ Ⓓ Ⓔ
101. Ⓐ Ⓑ Ⓒ Ⓓ Ⓔ
102. Ⓐ Ⓑ Ⓒ Ⓓ Ⓔ
103. Ⓐ Ⓑ Ⓒ Ⓓ Ⓔ
104. Ⓐ Ⓑ Ⓒ Ⓓ Ⓔ
105. Ⓐ Ⓑ Ⓒ Ⓓ Ⓔ
106. Ⓐ Ⓑ Ⓒ Ⓓ Ⓔ
107. Ⓐ Ⓑ Ⓒ Ⓓ Ⓔ
108. Ⓐ Ⓑ Ⓒ Ⓓ Ⓔ
109. Ⓐ Ⓑ Ⓒ Ⓓ Ⓔ
110. Ⓐ Ⓑ Ⓒ Ⓓ Ⓔ
111. Ⓐ Ⓑ Ⓒ Ⓓ Ⓔ
112. Ⓐ Ⓑ Ⓒ Ⓓ Ⓔ
113. Ⓐ Ⓑ Ⓒ Ⓓ Ⓔ
114. Ⓐ Ⓑ Ⓒ Ⓓ Ⓔ
115. Ⓐ Ⓑ Ⓒ Ⓓ Ⓔ
116. Ⓐ Ⓑ Ⓒ Ⓓ Ⓔ
117. Ⓐ Ⓑ Ⓒ Ⓓ Ⓔ
118. Ⓐ Ⓑ Ⓒ Ⓓ Ⓔ
119. Ⓐ Ⓑ Ⓒ Ⓓ Ⓔ
120. Ⓐ Ⓑ Ⓒ Ⓓ Ⓔ

121. Ⓐ Ⓑ Ⓒ Ⓓ Ⓔ
122. Ⓐ Ⓑ Ⓒ Ⓓ Ⓔ
123. Ⓐ Ⓑ Ⓒ Ⓓ Ⓔ
124. Ⓐ Ⓑ Ⓒ Ⓓ Ⓔ
125. Ⓐ Ⓑ Ⓒ Ⓓ Ⓔ
126. Ⓐ Ⓑ Ⓒ Ⓓ Ⓔ
127. Ⓐ Ⓑ Ⓒ Ⓓ Ⓔ
128. Ⓐ Ⓑ Ⓒ Ⓓ Ⓔ
129. Ⓐ Ⓑ Ⓒ Ⓓ Ⓔ
130. Ⓐ Ⓑ Ⓒ Ⓓ Ⓔ
131. Ⓐ Ⓑ Ⓒ Ⓓ Ⓔ
132. Ⓐ Ⓑ Ⓒ Ⓓ Ⓔ
133. Ⓐ Ⓑ Ⓒ Ⓓ Ⓔ
134. Ⓐ Ⓑ Ⓒ Ⓓ Ⓔ
135. Ⓐ Ⓑ Ⓒ Ⓓ Ⓔ
136. Ⓐ Ⓑ Ⓒ Ⓓ Ⓔ
137. Ⓐ Ⓑ Ⓒ Ⓓ Ⓔ
138. Ⓐ Ⓑ Ⓒ Ⓓ Ⓔ
139. Ⓐ Ⓑ Ⓒ Ⓓ Ⓔ
140. Ⓐ Ⓑ Ⓒ Ⓓ Ⓔ
141. Ⓐ Ⓑ Ⓒ Ⓓ Ⓔ
142. Ⓐ Ⓑ Ⓒ Ⓓ Ⓔ
143. Ⓐ Ⓑ Ⓒ Ⓓ Ⓔ
144. Ⓐ Ⓑ Ⓒ Ⓓ Ⓔ
145. Ⓐ Ⓑ Ⓒ Ⓓ Ⓔ
146. Ⓐ Ⓑ Ⓒ Ⓓ Ⓔ
147. Ⓐ Ⓑ Ⓒ Ⓓ Ⓔ
148. Ⓐ Ⓑ Ⓒ Ⓓ Ⓔ
149. Ⓐ Ⓑ Ⓒ Ⓓ Ⓔ
150. Ⓐ Ⓑ Ⓒ Ⓓ Ⓔ

151. Ⓐ Ⓑ Ⓒ Ⓓ Ⓔ
152. Ⓐ Ⓑ Ⓒ Ⓓ Ⓔ
153. Ⓐ Ⓑ Ⓒ Ⓓ Ⓔ
154. Ⓐ Ⓑ Ⓒ Ⓓ Ⓔ
155. Ⓐ Ⓑ Ⓒ Ⓓ Ⓔ
156. Ⓐ Ⓑ Ⓒ Ⓓ Ⓔ
157. Ⓐ Ⓑ Ⓒ Ⓓ Ⓔ
158. Ⓐ Ⓑ Ⓒ Ⓓ Ⓔ
159. Ⓐ Ⓑ Ⓒ Ⓓ Ⓔ
160. Ⓐ Ⓑ Ⓒ Ⓓ Ⓔ
161. Ⓐ Ⓑ Ⓒ Ⓓ Ⓔ
162. Ⓐ Ⓑ Ⓒ Ⓓ Ⓔ
163. Ⓐ Ⓑ Ⓒ Ⓓ Ⓔ
164. Ⓐ Ⓑ Ⓒ Ⓓ Ⓔ
165. Ⓐ Ⓑ Ⓒ Ⓓ Ⓔ
166. Ⓐ Ⓑ Ⓒ Ⓓ Ⓔ
167. Ⓐ Ⓑ Ⓒ Ⓓ Ⓔ
168. Ⓐ Ⓑ Ⓒ Ⓓ Ⓔ
169. Ⓐ Ⓑ Ⓒ Ⓓ Ⓔ
170. Ⓐ Ⓑ Ⓒ Ⓓ Ⓔ
171. Ⓐ Ⓑ Ⓒ Ⓓ Ⓔ
172. Ⓐ Ⓑ Ⓒ Ⓓ Ⓔ
173. Ⓐ Ⓑ Ⓒ Ⓓ Ⓔ
174. Ⓐ Ⓑ Ⓒ Ⓓ Ⓔ
175. Ⓐ Ⓑ Ⓒ Ⓓ Ⓔ
176. Ⓐ Ⓑ Ⓒ Ⓓ Ⓔ
177. Ⓐ Ⓑ Ⓒ Ⓓ Ⓔ
178. Ⓐ Ⓑ Ⓒ Ⓓ Ⓔ
179. Ⓐ Ⓑ Ⓒ Ⓓ Ⓔ
180. Ⓐ Ⓑ Ⓒ Ⓓ Ⓔ

USMLE STEP 3
PRACTICE TEST 2

Day One – Afternoon Session

ANSWER SHEET

1. Ⓐ Ⓑ Ⓒ Ⓓ Ⓔ	31. Ⓐ Ⓑ Ⓒ Ⓓ Ⓔ	61. Ⓐ Ⓑ Ⓒ Ⓓ Ⓔ
2. Ⓐ Ⓑ Ⓒ Ⓓ Ⓔ	32. Ⓐ Ⓑ Ⓒ Ⓓ Ⓔ	62. Ⓐ Ⓑ Ⓒ Ⓓ Ⓔ
3. Ⓐ Ⓑ Ⓒ Ⓓ Ⓔ	33. Ⓐ Ⓑ Ⓒ Ⓓ Ⓔ	63. Ⓐ Ⓑ Ⓒ Ⓓ Ⓔ
4. Ⓐ Ⓑ Ⓒ Ⓓ Ⓔ	34. Ⓐ Ⓑ Ⓒ Ⓓ Ⓔ	64. Ⓐ Ⓑ Ⓒ Ⓓ Ⓔ
5. Ⓐ Ⓑ Ⓒ Ⓓ Ⓔ	35. Ⓐ Ⓑ Ⓒ Ⓓ Ⓔ	65. Ⓐ Ⓑ Ⓒ Ⓓ Ⓔ
6. Ⓐ Ⓑ Ⓒ Ⓓ Ⓔ	36. Ⓐ Ⓑ Ⓒ Ⓓ Ⓔ	66. Ⓐ Ⓑ Ⓒ Ⓓ Ⓔ
7. Ⓐ Ⓑ Ⓒ Ⓓ Ⓔ	37. Ⓐ Ⓑ Ⓒ Ⓓ Ⓔ	67. Ⓐ Ⓑ Ⓒ Ⓓ Ⓔ
8. Ⓐ Ⓑ Ⓒ Ⓓ Ⓔ	38. Ⓐ Ⓑ Ⓒ Ⓓ Ⓔ	68. Ⓐ Ⓑ Ⓒ Ⓓ Ⓔ
9. Ⓐ Ⓑ Ⓒ Ⓓ Ⓔ	39. Ⓐ Ⓑ Ⓒ Ⓓ Ⓔ	69. Ⓐ Ⓑ Ⓒ Ⓓ Ⓔ
10. Ⓐ Ⓑ Ⓒ Ⓓ Ⓔ	40. Ⓐ Ⓑ Ⓒ Ⓓ Ⓔ	70. Ⓐ Ⓑ Ⓒ Ⓓ Ⓔ
11. Ⓐ Ⓑ Ⓒ Ⓓ Ⓔ	41. Ⓐ Ⓑ Ⓒ Ⓓ Ⓔ	71. Ⓐ Ⓑ Ⓒ Ⓓ Ⓔ
12. Ⓐ Ⓑ Ⓒ Ⓓ Ⓔ	42. Ⓐ Ⓑ Ⓒ Ⓓ Ⓔ	72. Ⓐ Ⓑ Ⓒ Ⓓ Ⓔ
13. Ⓐ Ⓑ Ⓒ Ⓓ Ⓔ	43. Ⓐ Ⓑ Ⓒ Ⓓ Ⓔ	73. Ⓐ Ⓑ Ⓒ Ⓓ Ⓔ
14. Ⓐ Ⓑ Ⓒ Ⓓ Ⓔ	44. Ⓐ Ⓑ Ⓒ Ⓓ Ⓔ	74. Ⓐ Ⓑ Ⓒ Ⓓ Ⓔ
15. Ⓐ Ⓑ Ⓒ Ⓓ Ⓔ	45. Ⓐ Ⓑ Ⓒ Ⓓ Ⓔ	75. Ⓐ Ⓑ Ⓒ Ⓓ Ⓔ
16. Ⓐ Ⓑ Ⓒ Ⓓ Ⓔ	46. Ⓐ Ⓑ Ⓒ Ⓓ Ⓔ	76. Ⓐ Ⓑ Ⓒ Ⓓ Ⓔ
17. Ⓐ Ⓑ Ⓒ Ⓓ Ⓔ	47. Ⓐ Ⓑ Ⓒ Ⓓ Ⓔ	77. Ⓐ Ⓑ Ⓒ Ⓓ Ⓔ
18. Ⓐ Ⓑ Ⓒ Ⓓ Ⓔ	48. Ⓐ Ⓑ Ⓒ Ⓓ Ⓔ	78. Ⓐ Ⓑ Ⓒ Ⓓ Ⓔ
19. Ⓐ Ⓑ Ⓒ Ⓓ Ⓔ	49. Ⓐ Ⓑ Ⓒ Ⓓ Ⓔ	79. Ⓐ Ⓑ Ⓒ Ⓓ Ⓔ
20. Ⓐ Ⓑ Ⓒ Ⓓ Ⓔ	50. Ⓐ Ⓑ Ⓒ Ⓓ Ⓔ	80. Ⓐ Ⓑ Ⓒ Ⓓ Ⓔ
21. Ⓐ Ⓑ Ⓒ Ⓓ Ⓔ	51. Ⓐ Ⓑ Ⓒ Ⓓ Ⓔ	81. Ⓐ Ⓑ Ⓒ Ⓓ Ⓔ
22. Ⓐ Ⓑ Ⓒ Ⓓ Ⓔ	52. Ⓐ Ⓑ Ⓒ Ⓓ Ⓔ	82. Ⓐ Ⓑ Ⓒ Ⓓ Ⓔ
23. Ⓐ Ⓑ Ⓒ Ⓓ Ⓔ	53. Ⓐ Ⓑ Ⓒ Ⓓ Ⓔ	83. Ⓐ Ⓑ Ⓒ Ⓓ Ⓔ
24. Ⓐ Ⓑ Ⓒ Ⓓ Ⓔ	54. Ⓐ Ⓑ Ⓒ Ⓓ Ⓔ	84. Ⓐ Ⓑ Ⓒ Ⓓ Ⓔ
25. Ⓐ Ⓑ Ⓒ Ⓓ Ⓔ	55. Ⓐ Ⓑ Ⓒ Ⓓ Ⓔ	85. Ⓐ Ⓑ Ⓒ Ⓓ Ⓔ
26. Ⓐ Ⓑ Ⓒ Ⓓ Ⓔ	56. Ⓐ Ⓑ Ⓒ Ⓓ Ⓔ	86. Ⓐ Ⓑ Ⓒ Ⓓ Ⓔ
27. Ⓐ Ⓑ Ⓒ Ⓓ Ⓔ	57. Ⓐ Ⓑ Ⓒ Ⓓ Ⓔ	87. Ⓐ Ⓑ Ⓒ Ⓓ Ⓔ
28. Ⓐ Ⓑ Ⓒ Ⓓ Ⓔ	58. Ⓐ Ⓑ Ⓒ Ⓓ Ⓔ	88. Ⓐ Ⓑ Ⓒ Ⓓ Ⓔ
29. Ⓐ Ⓑ Ⓒ Ⓓ Ⓔ	59. Ⓐ Ⓑ Ⓒ Ⓓ Ⓔ	89. Ⓐ Ⓑ Ⓒ Ⓓ Ⓔ
30. Ⓐ Ⓑ Ⓒ Ⓓ Ⓔ	60. Ⓐ Ⓑ Ⓒ Ⓓ Ⓔ	90. Ⓐ Ⓑ Ⓒ Ⓓ Ⓔ

91. Ⓐ Ⓑ Ⓒ Ⓓ Ⓔ	121. Ⓐ Ⓑ Ⓒ Ⓓ Ⓔ	151. Ⓐ Ⓑ Ⓒ Ⓓ Ⓔ
92. Ⓐ Ⓑ Ⓒ Ⓓ Ⓔ	122. Ⓐ Ⓑ Ⓒ Ⓓ Ⓔ	152. Ⓐ Ⓑ Ⓒ Ⓓ Ⓔ
93. Ⓐ Ⓑ Ⓒ Ⓓ Ⓔ	123. Ⓐ Ⓑ Ⓒ Ⓓ Ⓔ	153. Ⓐ Ⓑ Ⓒ Ⓓ Ⓔ
94. Ⓐ Ⓑ Ⓒ Ⓓ Ⓔ	124. Ⓐ Ⓑ Ⓒ Ⓓ Ⓔ	154. Ⓐ Ⓑ Ⓒ Ⓓ Ⓔ
95. Ⓐ Ⓑ Ⓒ Ⓓ Ⓔ	125. Ⓐ Ⓑ Ⓒ Ⓓ Ⓔ	155. Ⓐ Ⓑ Ⓒ Ⓓ Ⓔ
96. Ⓐ Ⓑ Ⓒ Ⓓ Ⓔ	126. Ⓐ Ⓑ Ⓒ Ⓓ Ⓔ	156. Ⓐ Ⓑ Ⓒ Ⓓ Ⓔ
97. Ⓐ Ⓑ Ⓒ Ⓓ Ⓔ	127. Ⓐ Ⓑ Ⓒ Ⓓ Ⓔ	157. Ⓐ Ⓑ Ⓒ Ⓓ Ⓔ
98. Ⓐ Ⓑ Ⓒ Ⓓ Ⓔ	128. Ⓐ Ⓑ Ⓒ Ⓓ Ⓔ	158. Ⓐ Ⓑ Ⓒ Ⓓ Ⓔ
99. Ⓐ Ⓑ Ⓒ Ⓓ Ⓔ	129. Ⓐ Ⓑ Ⓒ Ⓓ Ⓔ	159. Ⓐ Ⓑ Ⓒ Ⓓ Ⓔ
100. Ⓐ Ⓑ Ⓒ Ⓓ Ⓔ	130. Ⓐ Ⓑ Ⓒ Ⓓ Ⓔ	160. Ⓐ Ⓑ Ⓒ Ⓓ Ⓔ
101. Ⓐ Ⓑ Ⓒ Ⓓ Ⓔ	131. Ⓐ Ⓑ Ⓒ Ⓓ Ⓔ	161. Ⓐ Ⓑ Ⓒ Ⓓ Ⓔ
102. Ⓐ Ⓑ Ⓒ Ⓓ Ⓔ	132. Ⓐ Ⓑ Ⓒ Ⓓ Ⓔ	162. Ⓐ Ⓑ Ⓒ Ⓓ Ⓔ
103. Ⓐ Ⓑ Ⓒ Ⓓ Ⓔ	133. Ⓐ Ⓑ Ⓒ Ⓓ Ⓔ	163. Ⓐ Ⓑ Ⓒ Ⓓ Ⓔ
104. Ⓐ Ⓑ Ⓒ Ⓓ Ⓔ	134. Ⓐ Ⓑ Ⓒ Ⓓ Ⓔ	164. Ⓐ Ⓑ Ⓒ Ⓓ Ⓔ
105. Ⓐ Ⓑ Ⓒ Ⓓ Ⓔ	135. Ⓐ Ⓑ Ⓒ Ⓓ Ⓔ	165. Ⓐ Ⓑ Ⓒ Ⓓ Ⓔ
106. Ⓐ Ⓑ Ⓒ Ⓓ Ⓔ	136. Ⓐ Ⓑ Ⓒ Ⓓ Ⓔ	166. Ⓐ Ⓑ Ⓒ Ⓓ Ⓔ
107. Ⓐ Ⓑ Ⓒ Ⓓ Ⓔ	137. Ⓐ Ⓑ Ⓒ Ⓓ Ⓔ	167. Ⓐ Ⓑ Ⓒ Ⓓ Ⓔ
108. Ⓐ Ⓑ Ⓒ Ⓓ Ⓔ	138. Ⓐ Ⓑ Ⓒ Ⓓ Ⓔ	168. Ⓐ Ⓑ Ⓒ Ⓓ Ⓔ
109. Ⓐ Ⓑ Ⓒ Ⓓ Ⓔ	139. Ⓐ Ⓑ Ⓒ Ⓓ Ⓔ	169. Ⓐ Ⓑ Ⓒ Ⓓ Ⓔ
110. Ⓐ Ⓑ Ⓒ Ⓓ Ⓔ	140. Ⓐ Ⓑ Ⓒ Ⓓ Ⓔ	170. Ⓐ Ⓑ Ⓒ Ⓓ Ⓔ
111. Ⓐ Ⓑ Ⓒ Ⓓ Ⓔ	141. Ⓐ Ⓑ Ⓒ Ⓓ Ⓔ	171. Ⓐ Ⓑ Ⓒ Ⓓ Ⓔ
112. Ⓐ Ⓑ Ⓒ Ⓓ Ⓔ	142. Ⓐ Ⓑ Ⓒ Ⓓ Ⓔ	172. Ⓐ Ⓑ Ⓒ Ⓓ Ⓔ
113. Ⓐ Ⓑ Ⓒ Ⓓ Ⓔ	143. Ⓐ Ⓑ Ⓒ Ⓓ Ⓔ	173. Ⓐ Ⓑ Ⓒ Ⓓ Ⓔ
114. Ⓐ Ⓑ Ⓒ Ⓓ Ⓔ	144. Ⓐ Ⓑ Ⓒ Ⓓ Ⓔ	174. Ⓐ Ⓑ Ⓒ Ⓓ Ⓔ
115. Ⓐ Ⓑ Ⓒ Ⓓ Ⓔ	145. Ⓐ Ⓑ Ⓒ Ⓓ Ⓔ	175. Ⓐ Ⓑ Ⓒ Ⓓ Ⓔ
116. Ⓐ Ⓑ Ⓒ Ⓓ Ⓔ	146. Ⓐ Ⓑ Ⓒ Ⓓ Ⓔ	176. Ⓐ Ⓑ Ⓒ Ⓓ Ⓔ
117. Ⓐ Ⓑ Ⓒ Ⓓ Ⓔ	147. Ⓐ Ⓑ Ⓒ Ⓓ Ⓔ	177. Ⓐ Ⓑ Ⓒ Ⓓ Ⓔ
118. Ⓐ Ⓑ Ⓒ Ⓓ Ⓔ	148. Ⓐ Ⓑ Ⓒ Ⓓ Ⓔ	178. Ⓐ Ⓑ Ⓒ Ⓓ Ⓔ
119. Ⓐ Ⓑ Ⓒ Ⓓ Ⓔ	149. Ⓐ Ⓑ Ⓒ Ⓓ Ⓔ	179. Ⓐ Ⓑ Ⓒ Ⓓ Ⓔ
120. Ⓐ Ⓑ Ⓒ Ⓓ Ⓔ	150. Ⓐ Ⓑ Ⓒ Ⓓ Ⓔ	180. Ⓐ Ⓑ Ⓒ Ⓓ Ⓔ

USMLE STEP 3
PRACTICE TEST 2

Day Two – Morning Session

ANSWER SHEET

1. Ⓐ Ⓑ Ⓒ Ⓓ Ⓔ
2. Ⓐ Ⓑ Ⓒ Ⓓ Ⓔ
3. Ⓐ Ⓑ Ⓒ Ⓓ Ⓔ
4. Ⓐ Ⓑ Ⓒ Ⓓ Ⓔ
5. Ⓐ Ⓑ Ⓒ Ⓓ Ⓔ
6. Ⓐ Ⓑ Ⓒ Ⓓ Ⓔ
7. Ⓐ Ⓑ Ⓒ Ⓓ Ⓔ
8. Ⓐ Ⓑ Ⓒ Ⓓ Ⓔ
9. Ⓐ Ⓑ Ⓒ Ⓓ Ⓔ
10. Ⓐ Ⓑ Ⓒ Ⓓ Ⓔ
11. Ⓐ Ⓑ Ⓒ Ⓓ Ⓔ
12. Ⓐ Ⓑ Ⓒ Ⓓ Ⓔ
13. Ⓐ Ⓑ Ⓒ Ⓓ Ⓔ
14. Ⓐ Ⓑ Ⓒ Ⓓ Ⓔ
15. Ⓐ Ⓑ Ⓒ Ⓓ Ⓔ
16. Ⓐ Ⓑ Ⓒ Ⓓ Ⓔ
17. Ⓐ Ⓑ Ⓒ Ⓓ Ⓔ
18. Ⓐ Ⓑ Ⓒ Ⓓ Ⓔ
19. Ⓐ Ⓑ Ⓒ Ⓓ Ⓔ
20. Ⓐ Ⓑ Ⓒ Ⓓ Ⓔ
21. Ⓐ Ⓑ Ⓒ Ⓓ Ⓔ
22. Ⓐ Ⓑ Ⓒ Ⓓ Ⓔ
23. Ⓐ Ⓑ Ⓒ Ⓓ Ⓔ
24. Ⓐ Ⓑ Ⓒ Ⓓ Ⓔ
25. Ⓐ Ⓑ Ⓒ Ⓓ Ⓔ
26. Ⓐ Ⓑ Ⓒ Ⓓ Ⓔ
27. Ⓐ Ⓑ Ⓒ Ⓓ Ⓔ
28. Ⓐ Ⓑ Ⓒ Ⓓ Ⓔ
29. Ⓐ Ⓑ Ⓒ Ⓓ Ⓔ
30. Ⓐ Ⓑ Ⓒ Ⓓ Ⓔ

31. Ⓐ Ⓑ Ⓒ Ⓓ Ⓔ
32. Ⓐ Ⓑ Ⓒ Ⓓ Ⓔ
33. Ⓐ Ⓑ Ⓒ Ⓓ Ⓔ
34. Ⓐ Ⓑ Ⓒ Ⓓ Ⓔ
35. Ⓐ Ⓑ Ⓒ Ⓓ Ⓔ
36. Ⓐ Ⓑ Ⓒ Ⓓ Ⓔ
37. Ⓐ Ⓑ Ⓒ Ⓓ Ⓔ
38. Ⓐ Ⓑ Ⓒ Ⓓ Ⓔ
39. Ⓐ Ⓑ Ⓒ Ⓓ Ⓔ
40. Ⓐ Ⓑ Ⓒ Ⓓ Ⓔ
41. Ⓐ Ⓑ Ⓒ Ⓓ Ⓔ
42. Ⓐ Ⓑ Ⓒ Ⓓ Ⓔ
43. Ⓐ Ⓑ Ⓒ Ⓓ Ⓔ
44. Ⓐ Ⓑ Ⓒ Ⓓ Ⓔ
45. Ⓐ Ⓑ Ⓒ Ⓓ Ⓔ
46. Ⓐ Ⓑ Ⓒ Ⓓ Ⓔ
47. Ⓐ Ⓑ Ⓒ Ⓓ Ⓔ
48. Ⓐ Ⓑ Ⓒ Ⓓ Ⓔ
49. Ⓐ Ⓑ Ⓒ Ⓓ Ⓔ
50. Ⓐ Ⓑ Ⓒ Ⓓ Ⓔ
51. Ⓐ Ⓑ Ⓒ Ⓓ Ⓔ
52. Ⓐ Ⓑ Ⓒ Ⓓ Ⓔ
53. Ⓐ Ⓑ Ⓒ Ⓓ Ⓔ
54. Ⓐ Ⓑ Ⓒ Ⓓ Ⓔ
55. Ⓐ Ⓑ Ⓒ Ⓓ Ⓔ
56. Ⓐ Ⓑ Ⓒ Ⓓ Ⓔ
57. Ⓐ Ⓑ Ⓒ Ⓓ Ⓔ
58. Ⓐ Ⓑ Ⓒ Ⓓ Ⓔ
59. Ⓐ Ⓑ Ⓒ Ⓓ Ⓔ
60. Ⓐ Ⓑ Ⓒ Ⓓ Ⓔ

61. Ⓐ Ⓑ Ⓒ Ⓓ Ⓔ
62. Ⓐ Ⓑ Ⓒ Ⓓ Ⓔ
63. Ⓐ Ⓑ Ⓒ Ⓓ Ⓔ
64. Ⓐ Ⓑ Ⓒ Ⓓ Ⓔ
65. Ⓐ Ⓑ Ⓒ Ⓓ Ⓔ
66. Ⓐ Ⓑ Ⓒ Ⓓ Ⓔ
67. Ⓐ Ⓑ Ⓒ Ⓓ Ⓔ
68. Ⓐ Ⓑ Ⓒ Ⓓ Ⓔ
69. Ⓐ Ⓑ Ⓒ Ⓓ Ⓔ
70. Ⓐ Ⓑ Ⓒ Ⓓ Ⓔ
71. Ⓐ Ⓑ Ⓒ Ⓓ Ⓔ
72. Ⓐ Ⓑ Ⓒ Ⓓ Ⓔ
73. Ⓐ Ⓑ Ⓒ Ⓓ Ⓔ
74. Ⓐ Ⓑ Ⓒ Ⓓ Ⓔ
75. Ⓐ Ⓑ Ⓒ Ⓓ Ⓔ
76. Ⓐ Ⓑ Ⓒ Ⓓ Ⓔ
77. Ⓐ Ⓑ Ⓒ Ⓓ Ⓔ
78. Ⓐ Ⓑ Ⓒ Ⓓ Ⓔ
79. Ⓐ Ⓑ Ⓒ Ⓓ Ⓔ
80. Ⓐ Ⓑ Ⓒ Ⓓ Ⓔ
81. Ⓐ Ⓑ Ⓒ Ⓓ Ⓔ
82. Ⓐ Ⓑ Ⓒ Ⓓ Ⓔ
83. Ⓐ Ⓑ Ⓒ Ⓓ Ⓔ
84. Ⓐ Ⓑ Ⓒ Ⓓ Ⓔ
85. Ⓐ Ⓑ Ⓒ Ⓓ Ⓔ
86. Ⓐ Ⓑ Ⓒ Ⓓ Ⓔ
87. Ⓐ Ⓑ Ⓒ Ⓓ Ⓔ
88. Ⓐ Ⓑ Ⓒ Ⓓ Ⓔ
89. Ⓐ Ⓑ Ⓒ Ⓓ Ⓔ
90. Ⓐ Ⓑ Ⓒ Ⓓ Ⓔ

91. Ⓐ Ⓑ Ⓒ Ⓓ Ⓔ
92. Ⓐ Ⓑ Ⓒ Ⓓ Ⓔ
93. Ⓐ Ⓑ Ⓒ Ⓓ Ⓔ
94. Ⓐ Ⓑ Ⓒ Ⓓ Ⓔ
95. Ⓐ Ⓑ Ⓒ Ⓓ Ⓔ
96. Ⓐ Ⓑ Ⓒ Ⓓ Ⓔ
97. Ⓐ Ⓑ Ⓒ Ⓓ Ⓔ
98. Ⓐ Ⓑ Ⓒ Ⓓ Ⓔ
99. Ⓐ Ⓑ Ⓒ Ⓓ Ⓔ
100. Ⓐ Ⓑ Ⓒ Ⓓ Ⓔ
101. Ⓐ Ⓑ Ⓒ Ⓓ Ⓔ
102. Ⓐ Ⓑ Ⓒ Ⓓ Ⓔ
103. Ⓐ Ⓑ Ⓒ Ⓓ Ⓔ
104. Ⓐ Ⓑ Ⓒ Ⓓ Ⓔ
105. Ⓐ Ⓑ Ⓒ Ⓓ Ⓔ
106. Ⓐ Ⓑ Ⓒ Ⓓ Ⓔ
107. Ⓐ Ⓑ Ⓒ Ⓓ Ⓔ
108. Ⓐ Ⓑ Ⓒ Ⓓ Ⓔ
109. Ⓐ Ⓑ Ⓒ Ⓓ Ⓔ
110. Ⓐ Ⓑ Ⓒ Ⓓ Ⓔ
111. Ⓐ Ⓑ Ⓒ Ⓓ Ⓔ
112. Ⓐ Ⓑ Ⓒ Ⓓ Ⓔ
113. Ⓐ Ⓑ Ⓒ Ⓓ Ⓔ
114. Ⓐ Ⓑ Ⓒ Ⓓ Ⓔ
115. Ⓐ Ⓑ Ⓒ Ⓓ Ⓔ
116. Ⓐ Ⓑ Ⓒ Ⓓ Ⓔ
117. Ⓐ Ⓑ Ⓒ Ⓓ Ⓔ
118. Ⓐ Ⓑ Ⓒ Ⓓ Ⓔ
119. Ⓐ Ⓑ Ⓒ Ⓓ Ⓔ
120. Ⓐ Ⓑ Ⓒ Ⓓ Ⓔ

121. Ⓐ Ⓑ Ⓒ Ⓓ Ⓔ
122. Ⓐ Ⓑ Ⓒ Ⓓ Ⓔ
123. Ⓐ Ⓑ Ⓒ Ⓓ Ⓔ
124. Ⓐ Ⓑ Ⓒ Ⓓ Ⓔ
125. Ⓐ Ⓑ Ⓒ Ⓓ Ⓔ
126. Ⓐ Ⓑ Ⓒ Ⓓ Ⓔ
127. Ⓐ Ⓑ Ⓒ Ⓓ Ⓔ
128. Ⓐ Ⓑ Ⓒ Ⓓ Ⓔ
129. Ⓐ Ⓑ Ⓒ Ⓓ Ⓔ
130. Ⓐ Ⓑ Ⓒ Ⓓ Ⓔ
131. Ⓐ Ⓑ Ⓒ Ⓓ Ⓔ
132. Ⓐ Ⓑ Ⓒ Ⓓ Ⓔ
133. Ⓐ Ⓑ Ⓒ Ⓓ Ⓔ
134. Ⓐ Ⓑ Ⓒ Ⓓ Ⓔ
135. Ⓐ Ⓑ Ⓒ Ⓓ Ⓔ
136. Ⓐ Ⓑ Ⓒ Ⓓ Ⓔ
137. Ⓐ Ⓑ Ⓒ Ⓓ Ⓔ
138. Ⓐ Ⓑ Ⓒ Ⓓ Ⓔ
139. Ⓐ Ⓑ Ⓒ Ⓓ Ⓔ
140. Ⓐ Ⓑ Ⓒ Ⓓ Ⓔ
141. Ⓐ Ⓑ Ⓒ Ⓓ Ⓔ
142. Ⓐ Ⓑ Ⓒ Ⓓ Ⓔ
143. Ⓐ Ⓑ Ⓒ Ⓓ Ⓔ
144. Ⓐ Ⓑ Ⓒ Ⓓ Ⓔ
145. Ⓐ Ⓑ Ⓒ Ⓓ Ⓔ
146. Ⓐ Ⓑ Ⓒ Ⓓ Ⓔ
147. Ⓐ Ⓑ Ⓒ Ⓓ Ⓔ
148. Ⓐ Ⓑ Ⓒ Ⓓ Ⓔ
149. Ⓐ Ⓑ Ⓒ Ⓓ Ⓔ
150. Ⓐ Ⓑ Ⓒ Ⓓ Ⓔ

151. Ⓐ Ⓑ Ⓒ Ⓓ Ⓔ
152. Ⓐ Ⓑ Ⓒ Ⓓ Ⓔ
153. Ⓐ Ⓑ Ⓒ Ⓓ Ⓔ
154. Ⓐ Ⓑ Ⓒ Ⓓ Ⓔ
155. Ⓐ Ⓑ Ⓒ Ⓓ Ⓔ
156. Ⓐ Ⓑ Ⓒ Ⓓ Ⓔ
157. Ⓐ Ⓑ Ⓒ Ⓓ Ⓔ
158. Ⓐ Ⓑ Ⓒ Ⓓ Ⓔ
159. Ⓐ Ⓑ Ⓒ Ⓓ Ⓔ
160. Ⓐ Ⓑ Ⓒ Ⓓ Ⓔ
161. Ⓐ Ⓑ Ⓒ Ⓓ Ⓔ
162. Ⓐ Ⓑ Ⓒ Ⓓ Ⓔ
163. Ⓐ Ⓑ Ⓒ Ⓓ Ⓔ
164. Ⓐ Ⓑ Ⓒ Ⓓ Ⓔ
165. Ⓐ Ⓑ Ⓒ Ⓓ Ⓔ
166. Ⓐ Ⓑ Ⓒ Ⓓ Ⓔ
167. Ⓐ Ⓑ Ⓒ Ⓓ Ⓔ
168. Ⓐ Ⓑ Ⓒ Ⓓ Ⓔ
169. Ⓐ Ⓑ Ⓒ Ⓓ Ⓔ
170. Ⓐ Ⓑ Ⓒ Ⓓ Ⓔ
171. Ⓐ Ⓑ Ⓒ Ⓓ Ⓔ
172. Ⓐ Ⓑ Ⓒ Ⓓ Ⓔ
173. Ⓐ Ⓑ Ⓒ Ⓓ Ⓔ
174. Ⓐ Ⓑ Ⓒ Ⓓ Ⓔ
175. Ⓐ Ⓑ Ⓒ Ⓓ Ⓔ
176. Ⓐ Ⓑ Ⓒ Ⓓ Ⓔ
177. Ⓐ Ⓑ Ⓒ Ⓓ Ⓔ
178. Ⓐ Ⓑ Ⓒ Ⓓ Ⓔ
179. Ⓐ Ⓑ Ⓒ Ⓓ Ⓔ
180. Ⓐ Ⓑ Ⓒ Ⓓ Ⓔ

USMLE STEP 3
PRACTICE TEST 2

Day Two – Afternoon Session

ANSWER SHEET

1. Ⓐ Ⓑ Ⓒ Ⓓ Ⓔ
2. Ⓐ Ⓑ Ⓒ Ⓓ Ⓔ
3. Ⓐ Ⓑ Ⓒ Ⓓ Ⓔ
4. Ⓐ Ⓑ Ⓒ Ⓓ Ⓔ
5. Ⓐ Ⓑ Ⓒ Ⓓ Ⓔ
6. Ⓐ Ⓑ Ⓒ Ⓓ Ⓔ
7. Ⓐ Ⓑ Ⓒ Ⓓ Ⓔ
8. Ⓐ Ⓑ Ⓒ Ⓓ Ⓔ
9. Ⓐ Ⓑ Ⓒ Ⓓ Ⓔ
10. Ⓐ Ⓑ Ⓒ Ⓓ Ⓔ
11. Ⓐ Ⓑ Ⓒ Ⓓ Ⓔ
12. Ⓐ Ⓑ Ⓒ Ⓓ Ⓔ
13. Ⓐ Ⓑ Ⓒ Ⓓ Ⓔ
14. Ⓐ Ⓑ Ⓒ Ⓓ Ⓔ
15. Ⓐ Ⓑ Ⓒ Ⓓ Ⓔ
16. Ⓐ Ⓑ Ⓒ Ⓓ Ⓔ
17. Ⓐ Ⓑ Ⓒ Ⓓ Ⓔ
18. Ⓐ Ⓑ Ⓒ Ⓓ Ⓔ
19. Ⓐ Ⓑ Ⓒ Ⓓ Ⓔ
20. Ⓐ Ⓑ Ⓒ Ⓓ Ⓔ
21. Ⓐ Ⓑ Ⓒ Ⓓ Ⓔ
22. Ⓐ Ⓑ Ⓒ Ⓓ Ⓔ
23. Ⓐ Ⓑ Ⓒ Ⓓ Ⓔ
24. Ⓐ Ⓑ Ⓒ Ⓓ Ⓔ
25. Ⓐ Ⓑ Ⓒ Ⓓ Ⓔ
26. Ⓐ Ⓑ Ⓒ Ⓓ Ⓔ
27. Ⓐ Ⓑ Ⓒ Ⓓ Ⓔ
28. Ⓐ Ⓑ Ⓒ Ⓓ Ⓔ
29. Ⓐ Ⓑ Ⓒ Ⓓ Ⓔ
30. Ⓐ Ⓑ Ⓒ Ⓓ Ⓔ
31. Ⓐ Ⓑ Ⓒ Ⓓ Ⓔ
32. Ⓐ Ⓑ Ⓒ Ⓓ Ⓔ
33. Ⓐ Ⓑ Ⓒ Ⓓ Ⓔ
34. Ⓐ Ⓑ Ⓒ Ⓓ Ⓔ
35. Ⓐ Ⓑ Ⓒ Ⓓ Ⓔ
36. Ⓐ Ⓑ Ⓒ Ⓓ Ⓔ
37. Ⓐ Ⓑ Ⓒ Ⓓ Ⓔ
38. Ⓐ Ⓑ Ⓒ Ⓓ Ⓔ
39. Ⓐ Ⓑ Ⓒ Ⓓ Ⓔ
40. Ⓐ Ⓑ Ⓒ Ⓓ Ⓔ
41. Ⓐ Ⓑ Ⓒ Ⓓ Ⓔ
42. Ⓐ Ⓑ Ⓒ Ⓓ Ⓔ
43. Ⓐ Ⓑ Ⓒ Ⓓ Ⓔ
44. Ⓐ Ⓑ Ⓒ Ⓓ Ⓔ
45. Ⓐ Ⓑ Ⓒ Ⓓ Ⓔ
46. Ⓐ Ⓑ Ⓒ Ⓓ Ⓔ
47. Ⓐ Ⓑ Ⓒ Ⓓ Ⓔ
48. Ⓐ Ⓑ Ⓒ Ⓓ Ⓔ
49. Ⓐ Ⓑ Ⓒ Ⓓ Ⓔ
50. Ⓐ Ⓑ Ⓒ Ⓓ Ⓔ
51. Ⓐ Ⓑ Ⓒ Ⓓ Ⓔ
52. Ⓐ Ⓑ Ⓒ Ⓓ Ⓔ
53. Ⓐ Ⓑ Ⓒ Ⓓ Ⓔ
54. Ⓐ Ⓑ Ⓒ Ⓓ Ⓔ
55. Ⓐ Ⓑ Ⓒ Ⓓ Ⓔ
56. Ⓐ Ⓑ Ⓒ Ⓓ Ⓔ
57. Ⓐ Ⓑ Ⓒ Ⓓ Ⓔ
58. Ⓐ Ⓑ Ⓒ Ⓓ Ⓔ
59. Ⓐ Ⓑ Ⓒ Ⓓ Ⓔ
60. Ⓐ Ⓑ Ⓒ Ⓓ Ⓔ
61. Ⓐ Ⓑ Ⓒ Ⓓ Ⓔ
62. Ⓐ Ⓑ Ⓒ Ⓓ Ⓔ
63. Ⓐ Ⓑ Ⓒ Ⓓ Ⓔ
64. Ⓐ Ⓑ Ⓒ Ⓓ Ⓔ
65. Ⓐ Ⓑ Ⓒ Ⓓ Ⓔ
66. Ⓐ Ⓑ Ⓒ Ⓓ Ⓔ
67. Ⓐ Ⓑ Ⓒ Ⓓ Ⓔ
68. Ⓐ Ⓑ Ⓒ Ⓓ Ⓔ
69. Ⓐ Ⓑ Ⓒ Ⓓ Ⓔ
70. Ⓐ Ⓑ Ⓒ Ⓓ Ⓔ
71. Ⓐ Ⓑ Ⓒ Ⓓ Ⓔ
72. Ⓐ Ⓑ Ⓒ Ⓓ Ⓔ
73. Ⓐ Ⓑ Ⓒ Ⓓ Ⓔ
74. Ⓐ Ⓑ Ⓒ Ⓓ Ⓔ
75. Ⓐ Ⓑ Ⓒ Ⓓ Ⓔ
76. Ⓐ Ⓑ Ⓒ Ⓓ Ⓔ
77. Ⓐ Ⓑ Ⓒ Ⓓ Ⓔ
78. Ⓐ Ⓑ Ⓒ Ⓓ Ⓔ
79. Ⓐ Ⓑ Ⓒ Ⓓ Ⓔ
80. Ⓐ Ⓑ Ⓒ Ⓓ Ⓔ
81. Ⓐ Ⓑ Ⓒ Ⓓ Ⓔ
82. Ⓐ Ⓑ Ⓒ Ⓓ Ⓔ
83. Ⓐ Ⓑ Ⓒ Ⓓ Ⓔ
84. Ⓐ Ⓑ Ⓒ Ⓓ Ⓔ
85. Ⓐ Ⓑ Ⓒ Ⓓ Ⓔ
86. Ⓐ Ⓑ Ⓒ Ⓓ Ⓔ
87. Ⓐ Ⓑ Ⓒ Ⓓ Ⓔ
88. Ⓐ Ⓑ Ⓒ Ⓓ Ⓔ
89. Ⓐ Ⓑ Ⓒ Ⓓ Ⓔ
90. Ⓐ Ⓑ Ⓒ Ⓓ Ⓔ

91. Ⓐ Ⓑ Ⓒ Ⓓ Ⓔ	121. Ⓐ Ⓑ Ⓒ Ⓓ Ⓔ	151. Ⓐ Ⓑ Ⓒ Ⓓ Ⓔ
92. Ⓐ Ⓑ Ⓒ Ⓓ Ⓔ	122. Ⓐ Ⓑ Ⓒ Ⓓ Ⓔ	152. Ⓐ Ⓑ Ⓒ Ⓓ Ⓔ
93. Ⓐ Ⓑ Ⓒ Ⓓ Ⓔ	123. Ⓐ Ⓑ Ⓒ Ⓓ Ⓔ	153. Ⓐ Ⓑ Ⓒ Ⓓ Ⓔ
94. Ⓐ Ⓑ Ⓒ Ⓓ Ⓔ	124. Ⓐ Ⓑ Ⓒ Ⓓ Ⓔ	154. Ⓐ Ⓑ Ⓒ Ⓓ Ⓔ
95. Ⓐ Ⓑ Ⓒ Ⓓ Ⓔ	125. Ⓐ Ⓑ Ⓒ Ⓓ Ⓔ	155. Ⓐ Ⓑ Ⓒ Ⓓ Ⓔ
96. Ⓐ Ⓑ Ⓒ Ⓓ Ⓔ	126. Ⓐ Ⓑ Ⓒ Ⓓ Ⓔ	156. Ⓐ Ⓑ Ⓒ Ⓓ Ⓔ
97. Ⓐ Ⓑ Ⓒ Ⓓ Ⓔ	127. Ⓐ Ⓑ Ⓒ Ⓓ Ⓔ	157. Ⓐ Ⓑ Ⓒ Ⓓ Ⓔ
98. Ⓐ Ⓑ Ⓒ Ⓓ Ⓔ	128. Ⓐ Ⓑ Ⓒ Ⓓ Ⓔ	158. Ⓐ Ⓑ Ⓒ Ⓓ Ⓔ
99. Ⓐ Ⓑ Ⓒ Ⓓ Ⓔ	129. Ⓐ Ⓑ Ⓒ Ⓓ Ⓔ	159. Ⓐ Ⓑ Ⓒ Ⓓ Ⓔ
100. Ⓐ Ⓑ Ⓒ Ⓓ Ⓔ	130. Ⓐ Ⓑ Ⓒ Ⓓ Ⓔ	160. Ⓐ Ⓑ Ⓒ Ⓓ Ⓔ
101. Ⓐ Ⓑ Ⓒ Ⓓ Ⓔ	131. Ⓐ Ⓑ Ⓒ Ⓓ Ⓔ	161. Ⓐ Ⓑ Ⓒ Ⓓ Ⓔ
102. Ⓐ Ⓑ Ⓒ Ⓓ Ⓔ	132. Ⓐ Ⓑ Ⓒ Ⓓ Ⓔ	162. Ⓐ Ⓑ Ⓒ Ⓓ Ⓔ
103. Ⓐ Ⓑ Ⓒ Ⓓ Ⓔ	133. Ⓐ Ⓑ Ⓒ Ⓓ Ⓔ	163. Ⓐ Ⓑ Ⓒ Ⓓ Ⓔ
104. Ⓐ Ⓑ Ⓒ Ⓓ Ⓔ	134. Ⓐ Ⓑ Ⓒ Ⓓ Ⓔ	164. Ⓐ Ⓑ Ⓒ Ⓓ Ⓔ
105. Ⓐ Ⓑ Ⓒ Ⓓ Ⓔ	135. Ⓐ Ⓑ Ⓒ Ⓓ Ⓔ	165. Ⓐ Ⓑ Ⓒ Ⓓ Ⓔ
106. Ⓐ Ⓑ Ⓒ Ⓓ Ⓔ	136. Ⓐ Ⓑ Ⓒ Ⓓ Ⓔ	166. Ⓐ Ⓑ Ⓒ Ⓓ Ⓔ
107. Ⓐ Ⓑ Ⓒ Ⓓ Ⓔ	137. Ⓐ Ⓑ Ⓒ Ⓓ Ⓔ	167. Ⓐ Ⓑ Ⓒ Ⓓ Ⓔ
108. Ⓐ Ⓑ Ⓒ Ⓓ Ⓔ	138. Ⓐ Ⓑ Ⓒ Ⓓ Ⓔ	168. Ⓐ Ⓑ Ⓒ Ⓓ Ⓔ
109. Ⓐ Ⓑ Ⓒ Ⓓ Ⓔ	139. Ⓐ Ⓑ Ⓒ Ⓓ Ⓔ	169. Ⓐ Ⓑ Ⓒ Ⓓ Ⓔ
110. Ⓐ Ⓑ Ⓒ Ⓓ Ⓔ	140. Ⓐ Ⓑ Ⓒ Ⓓ Ⓔ	170. Ⓐ Ⓑ Ⓒ Ⓓ Ⓔ
111. Ⓐ Ⓑ Ⓒ Ⓓ Ⓔ	141. Ⓐ Ⓑ Ⓒ Ⓓ Ⓔ	171. Ⓐ Ⓑ Ⓒ Ⓓ Ⓔ
112. Ⓐ Ⓑ Ⓒ Ⓓ Ⓔ	142. Ⓐ Ⓑ Ⓒ Ⓓ Ⓔ	172. Ⓐ Ⓑ Ⓒ Ⓓ Ⓔ
113. Ⓐ Ⓑ Ⓒ Ⓓ Ⓔ	143. Ⓐ Ⓑ Ⓒ Ⓓ Ⓔ	173. Ⓐ Ⓑ Ⓒ Ⓓ Ⓔ
114. Ⓐ Ⓑ Ⓒ Ⓓ Ⓔ	144. Ⓐ Ⓑ Ⓒ Ⓓ Ⓔ	174. Ⓐ Ⓑ Ⓒ Ⓓ Ⓔ
115. Ⓐ Ⓑ Ⓒ Ⓓ Ⓔ	145. Ⓐ Ⓑ Ⓒ Ⓓ Ⓔ	175. Ⓐ Ⓑ Ⓒ Ⓓ Ⓔ
116. Ⓐ Ⓑ Ⓒ Ⓓ Ⓔ	146. Ⓐ Ⓑ Ⓒ Ⓓ Ⓔ	176. Ⓐ Ⓑ Ⓒ Ⓓ Ⓔ
117. Ⓐ Ⓑ Ⓒ Ⓓ Ⓔ	147. Ⓐ Ⓑ Ⓒ Ⓓ Ⓔ	177. Ⓐ Ⓑ Ⓒ Ⓓ Ⓔ
118. Ⓐ Ⓑ Ⓒ Ⓓ Ⓔ	148. Ⓐ Ⓑ Ⓒ Ⓓ Ⓔ	178. Ⓐ Ⓑ Ⓒ Ⓓ Ⓔ
119. Ⓐ Ⓑ Ⓒ Ⓓ Ⓔ	149. Ⓐ Ⓑ Ⓒ Ⓓ Ⓔ	179. Ⓐ Ⓑ Ⓒ Ⓓ Ⓔ
120. Ⓐ Ⓑ Ⓒ Ⓓ Ⓔ	150. Ⓐ Ⓑ Ⓒ Ⓓ Ⓔ	180. Ⓐ Ⓑ Ⓒ Ⓓ Ⓔ

USMLE STEP 3
PRACTICE TEST 3

Day One – Morning Session

ANSWER SHEET

1. Ⓐ Ⓑ Ⓒ Ⓓ Ⓔ	31. Ⓐ Ⓑ Ⓒ Ⓓ Ⓔ	61. Ⓐ Ⓑ Ⓒ Ⓓ Ⓔ
2. Ⓐ Ⓑ Ⓒ Ⓓ Ⓔ	32. Ⓐ Ⓑ Ⓒ Ⓓ Ⓔ	62. Ⓐ Ⓑ Ⓒ Ⓓ Ⓔ
3. Ⓐ Ⓑ Ⓒ Ⓓ Ⓔ	33. Ⓐ Ⓑ Ⓒ Ⓓ Ⓔ	63. Ⓐ Ⓑ Ⓒ Ⓓ Ⓔ
4. Ⓐ Ⓑ Ⓒ Ⓓ Ⓔ	34. Ⓐ Ⓑ Ⓒ Ⓓ Ⓔ	64. Ⓐ Ⓑ Ⓒ Ⓓ Ⓔ
5. Ⓐ Ⓑ Ⓒ Ⓓ Ⓔ	35. Ⓐ Ⓑ Ⓒ Ⓓ Ⓔ	65. Ⓐ Ⓑ Ⓒ Ⓓ Ⓔ
6. Ⓐ Ⓑ Ⓒ Ⓓ Ⓔ	36. Ⓐ Ⓑ Ⓒ Ⓓ Ⓔ	66. Ⓐ Ⓑ Ⓒ Ⓓ Ⓔ
7. Ⓐ Ⓑ Ⓒ Ⓓ Ⓔ	37. Ⓐ Ⓑ Ⓒ Ⓓ Ⓔ	67. Ⓐ Ⓑ Ⓒ Ⓓ Ⓔ
8. Ⓐ Ⓑ Ⓒ Ⓓ Ⓔ	38. Ⓐ Ⓑ Ⓒ Ⓓ Ⓔ	68. Ⓐ Ⓑ Ⓒ Ⓓ Ⓔ
9. Ⓐ Ⓑ Ⓒ Ⓓ Ⓔ	39. Ⓐ Ⓑ Ⓒ Ⓓ Ⓔ	69. Ⓐ Ⓑ Ⓒ Ⓓ Ⓔ
10. Ⓐ Ⓑ Ⓒ Ⓓ Ⓔ	40. Ⓐ Ⓑ Ⓒ Ⓓ Ⓔ	70. Ⓐ Ⓑ Ⓒ Ⓓ Ⓔ
11. Ⓐ Ⓑ Ⓒ Ⓓ Ⓔ	41. Ⓐ Ⓑ Ⓒ Ⓓ Ⓔ	71. Ⓐ Ⓑ Ⓒ Ⓓ Ⓔ
12. Ⓐ Ⓑ Ⓒ Ⓓ Ⓔ	42. Ⓐ Ⓑ Ⓒ Ⓓ Ⓔ	72. Ⓐ Ⓑ Ⓒ Ⓓ Ⓔ
13. Ⓐ Ⓑ Ⓒ Ⓓ Ⓔ	43. Ⓐ Ⓑ Ⓒ Ⓓ Ⓔ	73. Ⓐ Ⓑ Ⓒ Ⓓ Ⓔ
14. Ⓐ Ⓑ Ⓒ Ⓓ Ⓔ	44. Ⓐ Ⓑ Ⓒ Ⓓ Ⓔ	74. Ⓐ Ⓑ Ⓒ Ⓓ Ⓔ
15. Ⓐ Ⓑ Ⓒ Ⓓ Ⓔ	45. Ⓐ Ⓑ Ⓒ Ⓓ Ⓔ	75. Ⓐ Ⓑ Ⓒ Ⓓ Ⓔ
16. Ⓐ Ⓑ Ⓒ Ⓓ Ⓔ	46. Ⓐ Ⓑ Ⓒ Ⓓ Ⓔ	76. Ⓐ Ⓑ Ⓒ Ⓓ Ⓔ
17. Ⓐ Ⓑ Ⓒ Ⓓ Ⓔ	47. Ⓐ Ⓑ Ⓒ Ⓓ Ⓔ	77. Ⓐ Ⓑ Ⓒ Ⓓ Ⓔ
18. Ⓐ Ⓑ Ⓒ Ⓓ Ⓔ	48. Ⓐ Ⓑ Ⓒ Ⓓ Ⓔ	78. Ⓐ Ⓑ Ⓒ Ⓓ Ⓔ
19. Ⓐ Ⓑ Ⓒ Ⓓ Ⓔ	49. Ⓐ Ⓑ Ⓒ Ⓓ Ⓔ	79. Ⓐ Ⓑ Ⓒ Ⓓ Ⓔ
20. Ⓐ Ⓑ Ⓒ Ⓓ Ⓔ	50. Ⓐ Ⓑ Ⓒ Ⓓ Ⓔ	80. Ⓐ Ⓑ Ⓒ Ⓓ Ⓔ
21. Ⓐ Ⓑ Ⓒ Ⓓ Ⓔ	51. Ⓐ Ⓑ Ⓒ Ⓓ Ⓔ	81. Ⓐ Ⓑ Ⓒ Ⓓ Ⓔ
22. Ⓐ Ⓑ Ⓒ Ⓓ Ⓔ	52. Ⓐ Ⓑ Ⓒ Ⓓ Ⓔ	82. Ⓐ Ⓑ Ⓒ Ⓓ Ⓔ
23. Ⓐ Ⓑ Ⓒ Ⓓ Ⓔ	53. Ⓐ Ⓑ Ⓒ Ⓓ Ⓔ	83. Ⓐ Ⓑ Ⓒ Ⓓ Ⓔ
24. Ⓐ Ⓑ Ⓒ Ⓓ Ⓔ	54. Ⓐ Ⓑ Ⓒ Ⓓ Ⓔ	84. Ⓐ Ⓑ Ⓒ Ⓓ Ⓔ
25. Ⓐ Ⓑ Ⓒ Ⓓ Ⓔ	55. Ⓐ Ⓑ Ⓒ Ⓓ Ⓔ	85. Ⓐ Ⓑ Ⓒ Ⓓ Ⓔ
26. Ⓐ Ⓑ Ⓒ Ⓓ Ⓔ	56. Ⓐ Ⓑ Ⓒ Ⓓ Ⓔ	86. Ⓐ Ⓑ Ⓒ Ⓓ Ⓔ
27. Ⓐ Ⓑ Ⓒ Ⓓ Ⓔ	57. Ⓐ Ⓑ Ⓒ Ⓓ Ⓔ	87. Ⓐ Ⓑ Ⓒ Ⓓ Ⓔ
28. Ⓐ Ⓑ Ⓒ Ⓓ Ⓔ	58. Ⓐ Ⓑ Ⓒ Ⓓ Ⓔ	88. Ⓐ Ⓑ Ⓒ Ⓓ Ⓔ
29. Ⓐ Ⓑ Ⓒ Ⓓ Ⓔ	59. Ⓐ Ⓑ Ⓒ Ⓓ Ⓔ	89. Ⓐ Ⓑ Ⓒ Ⓓ Ⓔ
30. Ⓐ Ⓑ Ⓒ Ⓓ Ⓔ	60. Ⓐ Ⓑ Ⓒ Ⓓ Ⓔ	90. Ⓐ Ⓑ Ⓒ Ⓓ Ⓔ

91. Ⓐ Ⓑ Ⓒ Ⓓ Ⓔ
92. Ⓐ Ⓑ Ⓒ Ⓓ Ⓔ
93. Ⓐ Ⓑ Ⓒ Ⓓ Ⓔ
94. Ⓐ Ⓑ Ⓒ Ⓓ Ⓔ
95. Ⓐ Ⓑ Ⓒ Ⓓ Ⓔ
96. Ⓐ Ⓑ Ⓒ Ⓓ Ⓔ
97. Ⓐ Ⓑ Ⓒ Ⓓ Ⓔ
98. Ⓐ Ⓑ Ⓒ Ⓓ Ⓔ
99. Ⓐ Ⓑ Ⓒ Ⓓ Ⓔ
100. Ⓐ Ⓑ Ⓒ Ⓓ Ⓔ
101. Ⓐ Ⓑ Ⓒ Ⓓ Ⓔ
102. Ⓐ Ⓑ Ⓒ Ⓓ Ⓔ
103. Ⓐ Ⓑ Ⓒ Ⓓ Ⓔ
104. Ⓐ Ⓑ Ⓒ Ⓓ Ⓔ
105. Ⓐ Ⓑ Ⓒ Ⓓ Ⓔ
106. Ⓐ Ⓑ Ⓒ Ⓓ Ⓔ
107. Ⓐ Ⓑ Ⓒ Ⓓ Ⓔ
108. Ⓐ Ⓑ Ⓒ Ⓓ Ⓔ
109. Ⓐ Ⓑ Ⓒ Ⓓ Ⓔ
110. Ⓐ Ⓑ Ⓒ Ⓓ Ⓔ
111. Ⓐ Ⓑ Ⓒ Ⓓ Ⓔ
112. Ⓐ Ⓑ Ⓒ Ⓓ Ⓔ
113. Ⓐ Ⓑ Ⓒ Ⓓ Ⓔ
114. Ⓐ Ⓑ Ⓒ Ⓓ Ⓔ
115. Ⓐ Ⓑ Ⓒ Ⓓ Ⓔ
116. Ⓐ Ⓑ Ⓒ Ⓓ Ⓔ
117. Ⓐ Ⓑ Ⓒ Ⓓ Ⓔ
118. Ⓐ Ⓑ Ⓒ Ⓓ Ⓔ
119. Ⓐ Ⓑ Ⓒ Ⓓ Ⓔ
120. Ⓐ Ⓑ Ⓒ Ⓓ Ⓔ

121. Ⓐ Ⓑ Ⓒ Ⓓ Ⓔ
122. Ⓐ Ⓑ Ⓒ Ⓓ Ⓔ
123. Ⓐ Ⓑ Ⓒ Ⓓ Ⓔ
124. Ⓐ Ⓑ Ⓒ Ⓓ Ⓔ
125. Ⓐ Ⓑ Ⓒ Ⓓ Ⓔ
126. Ⓐ Ⓑ Ⓒ Ⓓ Ⓔ
127. Ⓐ Ⓑ Ⓒ Ⓓ Ⓔ
128. Ⓐ Ⓑ Ⓒ Ⓓ Ⓔ
129. Ⓐ Ⓑ Ⓒ Ⓓ Ⓔ
130. Ⓐ Ⓑ Ⓒ Ⓓ Ⓔ
131. Ⓐ Ⓑ Ⓒ Ⓓ Ⓔ
132. Ⓐ Ⓑ Ⓒ Ⓓ Ⓔ
133. Ⓐ Ⓑ Ⓒ Ⓓ Ⓔ
134. Ⓐ Ⓑ Ⓒ Ⓓ Ⓔ
135. Ⓐ Ⓑ Ⓒ Ⓓ Ⓔ
136. Ⓐ Ⓑ Ⓒ Ⓓ Ⓔ
137. Ⓐ Ⓑ Ⓒ Ⓓ Ⓔ
138. Ⓐ Ⓑ Ⓒ Ⓓ Ⓔ
139. Ⓐ Ⓑ Ⓒ Ⓓ Ⓔ
140. Ⓐ Ⓑ Ⓒ Ⓓ Ⓔ
141. Ⓐ Ⓑ Ⓒ Ⓓ Ⓔ
142. Ⓐ Ⓑ Ⓒ Ⓓ Ⓔ
143. Ⓐ Ⓑ Ⓒ Ⓓ Ⓔ
144. Ⓐ Ⓑ Ⓒ Ⓓ Ⓔ
145. Ⓐ Ⓑ Ⓒ Ⓓ Ⓔ
146. Ⓐ Ⓑ Ⓒ Ⓓ Ⓔ
147. Ⓐ Ⓑ Ⓒ Ⓓ Ⓔ
148. Ⓐ Ⓑ Ⓒ Ⓓ Ⓔ
149. Ⓐ Ⓑ Ⓒ Ⓓ Ⓔ
150. Ⓐ Ⓑ Ⓒ Ⓓ Ⓔ

151. Ⓐ Ⓑ Ⓒ Ⓓ Ⓔ
152. Ⓐ Ⓑ Ⓒ Ⓓ Ⓔ
153. Ⓐ Ⓑ Ⓒ Ⓓ Ⓔ
154. Ⓐ Ⓑ Ⓒ Ⓓ Ⓔ
155. Ⓐ Ⓑ Ⓒ Ⓓ Ⓔ
156. Ⓐ Ⓑ Ⓒ Ⓓ Ⓔ
157. Ⓐ Ⓑ Ⓒ Ⓓ Ⓔ
158. Ⓐ Ⓑ Ⓒ Ⓓ Ⓔ
159. Ⓐ Ⓑ Ⓒ Ⓓ Ⓔ
160. Ⓐ Ⓑ Ⓒ Ⓓ Ⓔ
161. Ⓐ Ⓑ Ⓒ Ⓓ Ⓔ
162. Ⓐ Ⓑ Ⓒ Ⓓ Ⓔ
163. Ⓐ Ⓑ Ⓒ Ⓓ Ⓔ
164. Ⓐ Ⓑ Ⓒ Ⓓ Ⓔ
165. Ⓐ Ⓑ Ⓒ Ⓓ Ⓔ
166. Ⓐ Ⓑ Ⓒ Ⓓ Ⓔ
167. Ⓐ Ⓑ Ⓒ Ⓓ Ⓔ
168. Ⓐ Ⓑ Ⓒ Ⓓ Ⓔ
169. Ⓐ Ⓑ Ⓒ Ⓓ Ⓔ
170. Ⓐ Ⓑ Ⓒ Ⓓ Ⓔ
171. Ⓐ Ⓑ Ⓒ Ⓓ Ⓔ
172. Ⓐ Ⓑ Ⓒ Ⓓ Ⓔ
173. Ⓐ Ⓑ Ⓒ Ⓓ Ⓔ
174. Ⓐ Ⓑ Ⓒ Ⓓ Ⓔ
175. Ⓐ Ⓑ Ⓒ Ⓓ Ⓔ
176. Ⓐ Ⓑ Ⓒ Ⓓ Ⓔ
177. Ⓐ Ⓑ Ⓒ Ⓓ Ⓔ
178. Ⓐ Ⓑ Ⓒ Ⓓ Ⓔ
179. Ⓐ Ⓑ Ⓒ Ⓓ Ⓔ
180. Ⓐ Ⓑ Ⓒ Ⓓ Ⓔ

USMLE STEP 3
PRACTICE TEST 3

Day One – Afternoon Session

ANSWER SHEET

1. Ⓐ Ⓑ Ⓒ Ⓓ Ⓔ	31. Ⓐ Ⓑ Ⓒ Ⓓ Ⓔ	61. Ⓐ Ⓑ Ⓒ Ⓓ Ⓔ
2. Ⓐ Ⓑ Ⓒ Ⓓ Ⓔ	32. Ⓐ Ⓑ Ⓒ Ⓓ Ⓔ	62. Ⓐ Ⓑ Ⓒ Ⓓ Ⓔ
3. Ⓐ Ⓑ Ⓒ Ⓓ Ⓔ	33. Ⓐ Ⓑ Ⓒ Ⓓ Ⓔ	63. Ⓐ Ⓑ Ⓒ Ⓓ Ⓔ
4. Ⓐ Ⓑ Ⓒ Ⓓ Ⓔ	34. Ⓐ Ⓑ Ⓒ Ⓓ Ⓔ	64. Ⓐ Ⓑ Ⓒ Ⓓ Ⓔ
5. Ⓐ Ⓑ Ⓒ Ⓓ Ⓔ	35. Ⓐ Ⓑ Ⓒ Ⓓ Ⓔ	65. Ⓐ Ⓑ Ⓒ Ⓓ Ⓔ
6. Ⓐ Ⓑ Ⓒ Ⓓ Ⓔ	36. Ⓐ Ⓑ Ⓒ Ⓓ Ⓔ	66. Ⓐ Ⓑ Ⓒ Ⓓ Ⓔ
7. Ⓐ Ⓑ Ⓒ Ⓓ Ⓔ	37. Ⓐ Ⓑ Ⓒ Ⓓ Ⓔ	67. Ⓐ Ⓑ Ⓒ Ⓓ Ⓔ
8. Ⓐ Ⓑ Ⓒ Ⓓ Ⓔ	38. Ⓐ Ⓑ Ⓒ Ⓓ Ⓔ	68. Ⓐ Ⓑ Ⓒ Ⓓ Ⓔ
9. Ⓐ Ⓑ Ⓒ Ⓓ Ⓔ	39. Ⓐ Ⓑ Ⓒ Ⓓ Ⓔ	69. Ⓐ Ⓑ Ⓒ Ⓓ Ⓔ
10. Ⓐ Ⓑ Ⓒ Ⓓ Ⓔ	40. Ⓐ Ⓑ Ⓒ Ⓓ Ⓔ	70. Ⓐ Ⓑ Ⓒ Ⓓ Ⓔ
11. Ⓐ Ⓑ Ⓒ Ⓓ Ⓔ	41. Ⓐ Ⓑ Ⓒ Ⓓ Ⓔ	71. Ⓐ Ⓑ Ⓒ Ⓓ Ⓔ
12. Ⓐ Ⓑ Ⓒ Ⓓ Ⓔ	42. Ⓐ Ⓑ Ⓒ Ⓓ Ⓔ	72. Ⓐ Ⓑ Ⓒ Ⓓ Ⓔ
13. Ⓐ Ⓑ Ⓒ Ⓓ Ⓔ	43. Ⓐ Ⓑ Ⓒ Ⓓ Ⓔ	73. Ⓐ Ⓑ Ⓒ Ⓓ Ⓔ
14. Ⓐ Ⓑ Ⓒ Ⓓ Ⓔ	44. Ⓐ Ⓑ Ⓒ Ⓓ Ⓔ	74. Ⓐ Ⓑ Ⓒ Ⓓ Ⓔ
15. Ⓐ Ⓑ Ⓒ Ⓓ Ⓔ	45. Ⓐ Ⓑ Ⓒ Ⓓ Ⓔ	75. Ⓐ Ⓑ Ⓒ Ⓓ Ⓔ
16. Ⓐ Ⓑ Ⓒ Ⓓ Ⓔ	46. Ⓐ Ⓑ Ⓒ Ⓓ Ⓔ	76. Ⓐ Ⓑ Ⓒ Ⓓ Ⓔ
17. Ⓐ Ⓑ Ⓒ Ⓓ Ⓔ	47. Ⓐ Ⓑ Ⓒ Ⓓ Ⓔ	77. Ⓐ Ⓑ Ⓒ Ⓓ Ⓔ
18. Ⓐ Ⓑ Ⓒ Ⓓ Ⓔ	48. Ⓐ Ⓑ Ⓒ Ⓓ Ⓔ	78. Ⓐ Ⓑ Ⓒ Ⓓ Ⓔ
19. Ⓐ Ⓑ Ⓒ Ⓓ Ⓔ	49. Ⓐ Ⓑ Ⓒ Ⓓ Ⓔ	79. Ⓐ Ⓑ Ⓒ Ⓓ Ⓔ
20. Ⓐ Ⓑ Ⓒ Ⓓ Ⓔ	50. Ⓐ Ⓑ Ⓒ Ⓓ Ⓔ	80. Ⓐ Ⓑ Ⓒ Ⓓ Ⓔ
21. Ⓐ Ⓑ Ⓒ Ⓓ Ⓔ	51. Ⓐ Ⓑ Ⓒ Ⓓ Ⓔ	81. Ⓐ Ⓑ Ⓒ Ⓓ Ⓔ
22. Ⓐ Ⓑ Ⓒ Ⓓ Ⓔ	52. Ⓐ Ⓑ Ⓒ Ⓓ Ⓔ	82. Ⓐ Ⓑ Ⓒ Ⓓ Ⓔ
23. Ⓐ Ⓑ Ⓒ Ⓓ Ⓔ	53. Ⓐ Ⓑ Ⓒ Ⓓ Ⓔ	83. Ⓐ Ⓑ Ⓒ Ⓓ Ⓔ
24. Ⓐ Ⓑ Ⓒ Ⓓ Ⓔ	54. Ⓐ Ⓑ Ⓒ Ⓓ Ⓔ	84. Ⓐ Ⓑ Ⓒ Ⓓ Ⓔ
25. Ⓐ Ⓑ Ⓒ Ⓓ Ⓔ	55. Ⓐ Ⓑ Ⓒ Ⓓ Ⓔ	85. Ⓐ Ⓑ Ⓒ Ⓓ Ⓔ
26. Ⓐ Ⓑ Ⓒ Ⓓ Ⓔ	56. Ⓐ Ⓑ Ⓒ Ⓓ Ⓔ	86. Ⓐ Ⓑ Ⓒ Ⓓ Ⓔ
27. Ⓐ Ⓑ Ⓒ Ⓓ Ⓔ	57. Ⓐ Ⓑ Ⓒ Ⓓ Ⓔ	87. Ⓐ Ⓑ Ⓒ Ⓓ Ⓔ
28. Ⓐ Ⓑ Ⓒ Ⓓ Ⓔ	58. Ⓐ Ⓑ Ⓒ Ⓓ Ⓔ	88. Ⓐ Ⓑ Ⓒ Ⓓ Ⓔ
29. Ⓐ Ⓑ Ⓒ Ⓓ Ⓔ	59. Ⓐ Ⓑ Ⓒ Ⓓ Ⓔ	89. Ⓐ Ⓑ Ⓒ Ⓓ Ⓔ
30. Ⓐ Ⓑ Ⓒ Ⓓ Ⓔ	60. Ⓐ Ⓑ Ⓒ Ⓓ Ⓔ	90. Ⓐ Ⓑ Ⓒ Ⓓ Ⓔ

91. Ⓐ Ⓑ Ⓒ Ⓓ Ⓔ
92. Ⓐ Ⓑ Ⓒ Ⓓ Ⓔ
93. Ⓐ Ⓑ Ⓒ Ⓓ Ⓔ
94. Ⓐ Ⓑ Ⓒ Ⓓ Ⓔ
95. Ⓐ Ⓑ Ⓒ Ⓓ Ⓔ
96. Ⓐ Ⓑ Ⓒ Ⓓ Ⓔ
97. Ⓐ Ⓑ Ⓒ Ⓓ Ⓔ
98. Ⓐ Ⓑ Ⓒ Ⓓ Ⓔ
99. Ⓐ Ⓑ Ⓒ Ⓓ Ⓔ
100. Ⓐ Ⓑ Ⓒ Ⓓ Ⓔ
101. Ⓐ Ⓑ Ⓒ Ⓓ Ⓔ
102. Ⓐ Ⓑ Ⓒ Ⓓ Ⓔ
103. Ⓐ Ⓑ Ⓒ Ⓓ Ⓔ
104. Ⓐ Ⓑ Ⓒ Ⓓ Ⓔ
105. Ⓐ Ⓑ Ⓒ Ⓓ Ⓔ
106. Ⓐ Ⓑ Ⓒ Ⓓ Ⓔ
107. Ⓐ Ⓑ Ⓒ Ⓓ Ⓔ
108. Ⓐ Ⓑ Ⓒ Ⓓ Ⓔ
109. Ⓐ Ⓑ Ⓒ Ⓓ Ⓔ
110. Ⓐ Ⓑ Ⓒ Ⓓ Ⓔ
111. Ⓐ Ⓑ Ⓒ Ⓓ Ⓔ
112. Ⓐ Ⓑ Ⓒ Ⓓ Ⓔ
113. Ⓐ Ⓑ Ⓒ Ⓓ Ⓔ
114. Ⓐ Ⓑ Ⓒ Ⓓ Ⓔ
115. Ⓐ Ⓑ Ⓒ Ⓓ Ⓔ
116. Ⓐ Ⓑ Ⓒ Ⓓ Ⓔ
117. Ⓐ Ⓑ Ⓒ Ⓓ Ⓔ
118. Ⓐ Ⓑ Ⓒ Ⓓ Ⓔ
119. Ⓐ Ⓑ Ⓒ Ⓓ Ⓔ
120. Ⓐ Ⓑ Ⓒ Ⓓ Ⓔ

121. Ⓐ Ⓑ Ⓒ Ⓓ Ⓔ
122. Ⓐ Ⓑ Ⓒ Ⓓ Ⓔ
123. Ⓐ Ⓑ Ⓒ Ⓓ Ⓔ
124. Ⓐ Ⓑ Ⓒ Ⓓ Ⓔ
125. Ⓐ Ⓑ Ⓒ Ⓓ Ⓔ
126. Ⓐ Ⓑ Ⓒ Ⓓ Ⓔ
127. Ⓐ Ⓑ Ⓒ Ⓓ Ⓔ
128. Ⓐ Ⓑ Ⓒ Ⓓ Ⓔ
129. Ⓐ Ⓑ Ⓒ Ⓓ Ⓔ
130. Ⓐ Ⓑ Ⓒ Ⓓ Ⓔ
131. Ⓐ Ⓑ Ⓒ Ⓓ Ⓔ
132. Ⓐ Ⓑ Ⓒ Ⓓ Ⓔ
133. Ⓐ Ⓑ Ⓒ Ⓓ Ⓔ
134. Ⓐ Ⓑ Ⓒ Ⓓ Ⓔ
135. Ⓐ Ⓑ Ⓒ Ⓓ Ⓔ
136. Ⓐ Ⓑ Ⓒ Ⓓ Ⓔ
137. Ⓐ Ⓑ Ⓒ Ⓓ Ⓔ
138. Ⓐ Ⓑ Ⓒ Ⓓ Ⓔ
139. Ⓐ Ⓑ Ⓒ Ⓓ Ⓔ
140. Ⓐ Ⓑ Ⓒ Ⓓ Ⓔ
141. Ⓐ Ⓑ Ⓒ Ⓓ Ⓔ
142. Ⓐ Ⓑ Ⓒ Ⓓ Ⓔ
143. Ⓐ Ⓑ Ⓒ Ⓓ Ⓔ
144. Ⓐ Ⓑ Ⓒ Ⓓ Ⓔ
145. Ⓐ Ⓑ Ⓒ Ⓓ Ⓔ
146. Ⓐ Ⓑ Ⓒ Ⓓ Ⓔ
147. Ⓐ Ⓑ Ⓒ Ⓓ Ⓔ
148. Ⓐ Ⓑ Ⓒ Ⓓ Ⓔ
149. Ⓐ Ⓑ Ⓒ Ⓓ Ⓔ
150. Ⓐ Ⓑ Ⓒ Ⓓ Ⓔ

151. Ⓐ Ⓑ Ⓒ Ⓓ Ⓔ
152. Ⓐ Ⓑ Ⓒ Ⓓ Ⓔ
153. Ⓐ Ⓑ Ⓒ Ⓓ Ⓔ
154. Ⓐ Ⓑ Ⓒ Ⓓ Ⓔ
155. Ⓐ Ⓑ Ⓒ Ⓓ Ⓔ
156. Ⓐ Ⓑ Ⓒ Ⓓ Ⓔ
157. Ⓐ Ⓑ Ⓒ Ⓓ Ⓔ
158. Ⓐ Ⓑ Ⓒ Ⓓ Ⓔ
159. Ⓐ Ⓑ Ⓒ Ⓓ Ⓔ
160. Ⓐ Ⓑ Ⓒ Ⓓ Ⓔ
161. Ⓐ Ⓑ Ⓒ Ⓓ Ⓔ
162. Ⓐ Ⓑ Ⓒ Ⓓ Ⓔ
163. Ⓐ Ⓑ Ⓒ Ⓓ Ⓔ
164. Ⓐ Ⓑ Ⓒ Ⓓ Ⓔ
165. Ⓐ Ⓑ Ⓒ Ⓓ Ⓔ
166. Ⓐ Ⓑ Ⓒ Ⓓ Ⓔ
167. Ⓐ Ⓑ Ⓒ Ⓓ Ⓔ
168. Ⓐ Ⓑ Ⓒ Ⓓ Ⓔ
169. Ⓐ Ⓑ Ⓒ Ⓓ Ⓔ
170. Ⓐ Ⓑ Ⓒ Ⓓ Ⓔ
171. Ⓐ Ⓑ Ⓒ Ⓓ Ⓔ
172. Ⓐ Ⓑ Ⓒ Ⓓ Ⓔ
173. Ⓐ Ⓑ Ⓒ Ⓓ Ⓔ
174. Ⓐ Ⓑ Ⓒ Ⓓ Ⓔ
175. Ⓐ Ⓑ Ⓒ Ⓓ Ⓔ
176. Ⓐ Ⓑ Ⓒ Ⓓ Ⓔ
177. Ⓐ Ⓑ Ⓒ Ⓓ Ⓔ
178. Ⓐ Ⓑ Ⓒ Ⓓ Ⓔ
179. Ⓐ Ⓑ Ⓒ Ⓓ Ⓔ
180. Ⓐ Ⓑ Ⓒ Ⓓ Ⓔ

USMLE STEP 3
PRACTICE TEST 3

Day Two – Morning Session

ANSWER SHEET

1. Ⓐ Ⓑ Ⓒ Ⓓ Ⓔ
2. Ⓐ Ⓑ Ⓒ Ⓓ Ⓔ
3. Ⓐ Ⓑ Ⓒ Ⓓ Ⓔ
4. Ⓐ Ⓑ Ⓒ Ⓓ Ⓔ
5. Ⓐ Ⓑ Ⓒ Ⓓ Ⓔ
6. Ⓐ Ⓑ Ⓒ Ⓓ Ⓔ
7. Ⓐ Ⓑ Ⓒ Ⓓ Ⓔ
8. Ⓐ Ⓑ Ⓒ Ⓓ Ⓔ
9. Ⓐ Ⓑ Ⓒ Ⓓ Ⓔ
10. Ⓐ Ⓑ Ⓒ Ⓓ Ⓔ
11. Ⓐ Ⓑ Ⓒ Ⓓ Ⓔ
12. Ⓐ Ⓑ Ⓒ Ⓓ Ⓔ
13. Ⓐ Ⓑ Ⓒ Ⓓ Ⓔ
14. Ⓐ Ⓑ Ⓒ Ⓓ Ⓔ
15. Ⓐ Ⓑ Ⓒ Ⓓ Ⓔ
16. Ⓐ Ⓑ Ⓒ Ⓓ Ⓔ
17. Ⓐ Ⓑ Ⓒ Ⓓ Ⓔ
18. Ⓐ Ⓑ Ⓒ Ⓓ Ⓔ
19. Ⓐ Ⓑ Ⓒ Ⓓ Ⓔ
20. Ⓐ Ⓑ Ⓒ Ⓓ Ⓔ
21. Ⓐ Ⓑ Ⓒ Ⓓ Ⓔ
22. Ⓐ Ⓑ Ⓒ Ⓓ Ⓔ
23. Ⓐ Ⓑ Ⓒ Ⓓ Ⓔ
24. Ⓐ Ⓑ Ⓒ Ⓓ Ⓔ
25. Ⓐ Ⓑ Ⓒ Ⓓ Ⓔ
26. Ⓐ Ⓑ Ⓒ Ⓓ Ⓔ
27. Ⓐ Ⓑ Ⓒ Ⓓ Ⓔ
28. Ⓐ Ⓑ Ⓒ Ⓓ Ⓔ
29. Ⓐ Ⓑ Ⓒ Ⓓ Ⓔ
30. Ⓐ Ⓑ Ⓒ Ⓓ Ⓔ

31. Ⓐ Ⓑ Ⓒ Ⓓ Ⓔ
32. Ⓐ Ⓑ Ⓒ Ⓓ Ⓔ
33. Ⓐ Ⓑ Ⓒ Ⓓ Ⓔ
34. Ⓐ Ⓑ Ⓒ Ⓓ Ⓔ
35. Ⓐ Ⓑ Ⓒ Ⓓ Ⓔ
36. Ⓐ Ⓑ Ⓒ Ⓓ Ⓔ
37. Ⓐ Ⓑ Ⓒ Ⓓ Ⓔ
38. Ⓐ Ⓑ Ⓒ Ⓓ Ⓔ
39. Ⓐ Ⓑ Ⓒ Ⓓ Ⓔ
40. Ⓐ Ⓑ Ⓒ Ⓓ Ⓔ
41. Ⓐ Ⓑ Ⓒ Ⓓ Ⓔ
42. Ⓐ Ⓑ Ⓒ Ⓓ Ⓔ
43. Ⓐ Ⓑ Ⓒ Ⓓ Ⓔ
44. Ⓐ Ⓑ Ⓒ Ⓓ Ⓔ
45. Ⓐ Ⓑ Ⓒ Ⓓ Ⓔ
46. Ⓐ Ⓑ Ⓒ Ⓓ Ⓔ
47. Ⓐ Ⓑ Ⓒ Ⓓ Ⓔ
48. Ⓐ Ⓑ Ⓒ Ⓓ Ⓔ
49. Ⓐ Ⓑ Ⓒ Ⓓ Ⓔ
50. Ⓐ Ⓑ Ⓒ Ⓓ Ⓔ
51. Ⓐ Ⓑ Ⓒ Ⓓ Ⓔ
52. Ⓐ Ⓑ Ⓒ Ⓓ Ⓔ
53. Ⓐ Ⓑ Ⓒ Ⓓ Ⓔ
54. Ⓐ Ⓑ Ⓒ Ⓓ Ⓔ
55. Ⓐ Ⓑ Ⓒ Ⓓ Ⓔ
56. Ⓐ Ⓑ Ⓒ Ⓓ Ⓔ
57. Ⓐ Ⓑ Ⓒ Ⓓ Ⓔ
58. Ⓐ Ⓑ Ⓒ Ⓓ Ⓔ
59. Ⓐ Ⓑ Ⓒ Ⓓ Ⓔ
60. Ⓐ Ⓑ Ⓒ Ⓓ Ⓔ

61. Ⓐ Ⓑ Ⓒ Ⓓ Ⓔ
62. Ⓐ Ⓑ Ⓒ Ⓓ Ⓔ
63. Ⓐ Ⓑ Ⓒ Ⓓ Ⓔ
64. Ⓐ Ⓑ Ⓒ Ⓓ Ⓔ
65. Ⓐ Ⓑ Ⓒ Ⓓ Ⓔ
66. Ⓐ Ⓑ Ⓒ Ⓓ Ⓔ
67. Ⓐ Ⓑ Ⓒ Ⓓ Ⓔ
68. Ⓐ Ⓑ Ⓒ Ⓓ Ⓔ
69. Ⓐ Ⓑ Ⓒ Ⓓ Ⓔ
70. Ⓐ Ⓑ Ⓒ Ⓓ Ⓔ
71. Ⓐ Ⓑ Ⓒ Ⓓ Ⓔ
72. Ⓐ Ⓑ Ⓒ Ⓓ Ⓔ
73. Ⓐ Ⓑ Ⓒ Ⓓ Ⓔ
74. Ⓐ Ⓑ Ⓒ Ⓓ Ⓔ
75. Ⓐ Ⓑ Ⓒ Ⓓ Ⓔ
76. Ⓐ Ⓑ Ⓒ Ⓓ Ⓔ
77. Ⓐ Ⓑ Ⓒ Ⓓ Ⓔ
78. Ⓐ Ⓑ Ⓒ Ⓓ Ⓔ
79. Ⓐ Ⓑ Ⓒ Ⓓ Ⓔ
80. Ⓐ Ⓑ Ⓒ Ⓓ Ⓔ
81. Ⓐ Ⓑ Ⓒ Ⓓ Ⓔ
82. Ⓐ Ⓑ Ⓒ Ⓓ Ⓔ
83. Ⓐ Ⓑ Ⓒ Ⓓ Ⓔ
84. Ⓐ Ⓑ Ⓒ Ⓓ Ⓔ
85. Ⓐ Ⓑ Ⓒ Ⓓ Ⓔ
86. Ⓐ Ⓑ Ⓒ Ⓓ Ⓔ
87. Ⓐ Ⓑ Ⓒ Ⓓ Ⓔ
88. Ⓐ Ⓑ Ⓒ Ⓓ Ⓔ
89. Ⓐ Ⓑ Ⓒ Ⓓ Ⓔ
90. Ⓐ Ⓑ Ⓒ Ⓓ Ⓔ

91. Ⓐ Ⓑ Ⓒ Ⓓ Ⓔ	121. Ⓐ Ⓑ Ⓒ Ⓓ Ⓔ	151. Ⓐ Ⓑ Ⓒ Ⓓ Ⓔ
92. Ⓐ Ⓑ Ⓒ Ⓓ Ⓔ	122. Ⓐ Ⓑ Ⓒ Ⓓ Ⓔ	152. Ⓐ Ⓑ Ⓒ Ⓓ Ⓔ
93. Ⓐ Ⓑ Ⓒ Ⓓ Ⓔ	123. Ⓐ Ⓑ Ⓒ Ⓓ Ⓔ	153. Ⓐ Ⓑ Ⓒ Ⓓ Ⓔ
94. Ⓐ Ⓑ Ⓒ Ⓓ Ⓔ	124. Ⓐ Ⓑ Ⓒ Ⓓ Ⓔ	154. Ⓐ Ⓑ Ⓒ Ⓓ Ⓔ
95. Ⓐ Ⓑ Ⓒ Ⓓ Ⓔ	125. Ⓐ Ⓑ Ⓒ Ⓓ Ⓔ	155. Ⓐ Ⓑ Ⓒ Ⓓ Ⓔ
96. Ⓐ Ⓑ Ⓒ Ⓓ Ⓔ	126. Ⓐ Ⓑ Ⓒ Ⓓ Ⓔ	156. Ⓐ Ⓑ Ⓒ Ⓓ Ⓔ
97. Ⓐ Ⓑ Ⓒ Ⓓ Ⓔ	127. Ⓐ Ⓑ Ⓒ Ⓓ Ⓔ	157. Ⓐ Ⓑ Ⓒ Ⓓ Ⓔ
98. Ⓐ Ⓑ Ⓒ Ⓓ Ⓔ	128. Ⓐ Ⓑ Ⓒ Ⓓ Ⓔ	158. Ⓐ Ⓑ Ⓒ Ⓓ Ⓔ
99. Ⓐ Ⓑ Ⓒ Ⓓ Ⓔ	129. Ⓐ Ⓑ Ⓒ Ⓓ Ⓔ	159. Ⓐ Ⓑ Ⓒ Ⓓ Ⓔ
100. Ⓐ Ⓑ Ⓒ Ⓓ Ⓔ	130. Ⓐ Ⓑ Ⓒ Ⓓ Ⓔ	160. Ⓐ Ⓑ Ⓒ Ⓓ Ⓔ
101. Ⓐ Ⓑ Ⓒ Ⓓ Ⓔ	131. Ⓐ Ⓑ Ⓒ Ⓓ Ⓔ	161. Ⓐ Ⓑ Ⓒ Ⓓ Ⓔ
102. Ⓐ Ⓑ Ⓒ Ⓓ Ⓔ	132. Ⓐ Ⓑ Ⓒ Ⓓ Ⓔ	162. Ⓐ Ⓑ Ⓒ Ⓓ Ⓔ
103. Ⓐ Ⓑ Ⓒ Ⓓ Ⓔ	133. Ⓐ Ⓑ Ⓒ Ⓓ Ⓔ	163. Ⓐ Ⓑ Ⓒ Ⓓ Ⓔ
104. Ⓐ Ⓑ Ⓒ Ⓓ Ⓔ	134. Ⓐ Ⓑ Ⓒ Ⓓ Ⓔ	164. Ⓐ Ⓑ Ⓒ Ⓓ Ⓔ
105. Ⓐ Ⓑ Ⓒ Ⓓ Ⓔ	135. Ⓐ Ⓑ Ⓒ Ⓓ Ⓔ	165. Ⓐ Ⓑ Ⓒ Ⓓ Ⓔ
106. Ⓐ Ⓑ Ⓒ Ⓓ Ⓔ	136. Ⓐ Ⓑ Ⓒ Ⓓ Ⓔ	166. Ⓐ Ⓑ Ⓒ Ⓓ Ⓔ
107. Ⓐ Ⓑ Ⓒ Ⓓ Ⓔ	137. Ⓐ Ⓑ Ⓒ Ⓓ Ⓔ	167. Ⓐ Ⓑ Ⓒ Ⓓ Ⓔ
108. Ⓐ Ⓑ Ⓒ Ⓓ Ⓔ	138. Ⓐ Ⓑ Ⓒ Ⓓ Ⓔ	168. Ⓐ Ⓑ Ⓒ Ⓓ Ⓔ
109. Ⓐ Ⓑ Ⓒ Ⓓ Ⓔ	139. Ⓐ Ⓑ Ⓒ Ⓓ Ⓔ	169. Ⓐ Ⓑ Ⓒ Ⓓ Ⓔ
110. Ⓐ Ⓑ Ⓒ Ⓓ Ⓔ	140. Ⓐ Ⓑ Ⓒ Ⓓ Ⓔ	170. Ⓐ Ⓑ Ⓒ Ⓓ Ⓔ
111. Ⓐ Ⓑ Ⓒ Ⓓ Ⓔ	141. Ⓐ Ⓑ Ⓒ Ⓓ Ⓔ	171. Ⓐ Ⓑ Ⓒ Ⓓ Ⓔ
112. Ⓐ Ⓑ Ⓒ Ⓓ Ⓔ	142. Ⓐ Ⓑ Ⓒ Ⓓ Ⓔ	172. Ⓐ Ⓑ Ⓒ Ⓓ Ⓔ
113. Ⓐ Ⓑ Ⓒ Ⓓ Ⓔ	143. Ⓐ Ⓑ Ⓒ Ⓓ Ⓔ	173. Ⓐ Ⓑ Ⓒ Ⓓ Ⓔ
114. Ⓐ Ⓑ Ⓒ Ⓓ Ⓔ	144. Ⓐ Ⓑ Ⓒ Ⓓ Ⓔ	174. Ⓐ Ⓑ Ⓒ Ⓓ Ⓔ
115. Ⓐ Ⓑ Ⓒ Ⓓ Ⓔ	145. Ⓐ Ⓑ Ⓒ Ⓓ Ⓔ	175. Ⓐ Ⓑ Ⓒ Ⓓ Ⓔ
116. Ⓐ Ⓑ Ⓒ Ⓓ Ⓔ	146. Ⓐ Ⓑ Ⓒ Ⓓ Ⓔ	176. Ⓐ Ⓑ Ⓒ Ⓓ Ⓔ
117. Ⓐ Ⓑ Ⓒ Ⓓ Ⓔ	147. Ⓐ Ⓑ Ⓒ Ⓓ Ⓔ	177. Ⓐ Ⓑ Ⓒ Ⓓ Ⓔ
118. Ⓐ Ⓑ Ⓒ Ⓓ Ⓔ	148. Ⓐ Ⓑ Ⓒ Ⓓ Ⓔ	178. Ⓐ Ⓑ Ⓒ Ⓓ Ⓔ
119. Ⓐ Ⓑ Ⓒ Ⓓ Ⓔ	149. Ⓐ Ⓑ Ⓒ Ⓓ Ⓔ	179. Ⓐ Ⓑ Ⓒ Ⓓ Ⓔ
120. Ⓐ Ⓑ Ⓒ Ⓓ Ⓔ	150. Ⓐ Ⓑ Ⓒ Ⓓ Ⓔ	180. Ⓐ Ⓑ Ⓒ Ⓓ Ⓔ

USMLE STEP 3
PRACTICE TEST 3

Day Two – Afternoon Session

ANSWER SHEET

1. Ⓐ Ⓑ Ⓒ Ⓓ Ⓔ	31. Ⓐ Ⓑ Ⓒ Ⓓ Ⓔ	61. Ⓐ Ⓑ Ⓒ Ⓓ Ⓔ
2. Ⓐ Ⓑ Ⓒ Ⓓ Ⓔ	32. Ⓐ Ⓑ Ⓒ Ⓓ Ⓔ	62. Ⓐ Ⓑ Ⓒ Ⓓ Ⓔ
3. Ⓐ Ⓑ Ⓒ Ⓓ Ⓔ	33. Ⓐ Ⓑ Ⓒ Ⓓ Ⓔ	63. Ⓐ Ⓑ Ⓒ Ⓓ Ⓔ
4. Ⓐ Ⓑ Ⓒ Ⓓ Ⓔ	34. Ⓐ Ⓑ Ⓒ Ⓓ Ⓔ	64. Ⓐ Ⓑ Ⓒ Ⓓ Ⓔ
5. Ⓐ Ⓑ Ⓒ Ⓓ Ⓔ	35. Ⓐ Ⓑ Ⓒ Ⓓ Ⓔ	65. Ⓐ Ⓑ Ⓒ Ⓓ Ⓔ
6. Ⓐ Ⓑ Ⓒ Ⓓ Ⓔ	36. Ⓐ Ⓑ Ⓒ Ⓓ Ⓔ	66. Ⓐ Ⓑ Ⓒ Ⓓ Ⓔ
7. Ⓐ Ⓑ Ⓒ Ⓓ Ⓔ	37. Ⓐ Ⓑ Ⓒ Ⓓ Ⓔ	67. Ⓐ Ⓑ Ⓒ Ⓓ Ⓔ
8. Ⓐ Ⓑ Ⓒ Ⓓ Ⓔ	38. Ⓐ Ⓑ Ⓒ Ⓓ Ⓔ	68. Ⓐ Ⓑ Ⓒ Ⓓ Ⓔ
9. Ⓐ Ⓑ Ⓒ Ⓓ Ⓔ	39. Ⓐ Ⓑ Ⓒ Ⓓ Ⓔ	69. Ⓐ Ⓑ Ⓒ Ⓓ Ⓔ
10. Ⓐ Ⓑ Ⓒ Ⓓ Ⓔ	40. Ⓐ Ⓑ Ⓒ Ⓓ Ⓔ	70. Ⓐ Ⓑ Ⓒ Ⓓ Ⓔ
11. Ⓐ Ⓑ Ⓒ Ⓓ Ⓔ	41. Ⓐ Ⓑ Ⓒ Ⓓ Ⓔ	71. Ⓐ Ⓑ Ⓒ Ⓓ Ⓔ
12. Ⓐ Ⓑ Ⓒ Ⓓ Ⓔ	42. Ⓐ Ⓑ Ⓒ Ⓓ Ⓔ	72. Ⓐ Ⓑ Ⓒ Ⓓ Ⓔ
13. Ⓐ Ⓑ Ⓒ Ⓓ Ⓔ	43. Ⓐ Ⓑ Ⓒ Ⓓ Ⓔ	73. Ⓐ Ⓑ Ⓒ Ⓓ Ⓔ
14. Ⓐ Ⓑ Ⓒ Ⓓ Ⓔ	44. Ⓐ Ⓑ Ⓒ Ⓓ Ⓔ	74. Ⓐ Ⓑ Ⓒ Ⓓ Ⓔ
15. Ⓐ Ⓑ Ⓒ Ⓓ Ⓔ	45. Ⓐ Ⓑ Ⓒ Ⓓ Ⓔ	75. Ⓐ Ⓑ Ⓒ Ⓓ Ⓔ
16. Ⓐ Ⓑ Ⓒ Ⓓ Ⓔ	46. Ⓐ Ⓑ Ⓒ Ⓓ Ⓔ	76. Ⓐ Ⓑ Ⓒ Ⓓ Ⓔ
17. Ⓐ Ⓑ Ⓒ Ⓓ Ⓔ	47. Ⓐ Ⓑ Ⓒ Ⓓ Ⓔ	77. Ⓐ Ⓑ Ⓒ Ⓓ Ⓔ
18. Ⓐ Ⓑ Ⓒ Ⓓ Ⓔ	48. Ⓐ Ⓑ Ⓒ Ⓓ Ⓔ	78. Ⓐ Ⓑ Ⓒ Ⓓ Ⓔ
19. Ⓐ Ⓑ Ⓒ Ⓓ Ⓔ	49. Ⓐ Ⓑ Ⓒ Ⓓ Ⓔ	79. Ⓐ Ⓑ Ⓒ Ⓓ Ⓔ
20. Ⓐ Ⓑ Ⓒ Ⓓ Ⓔ	50. Ⓐ Ⓑ Ⓒ Ⓓ Ⓔ	80. Ⓐ Ⓑ Ⓒ Ⓓ Ⓔ
21. Ⓐ Ⓑ Ⓒ Ⓓ Ⓔ	51. Ⓐ Ⓑ Ⓒ Ⓓ Ⓔ	81. Ⓐ Ⓑ Ⓒ Ⓓ Ⓔ
22. Ⓐ Ⓑ Ⓒ Ⓓ Ⓔ	52. Ⓐ Ⓑ Ⓒ Ⓓ Ⓔ	82. Ⓐ Ⓑ Ⓒ Ⓓ Ⓔ
23. Ⓐ Ⓑ Ⓒ Ⓓ Ⓔ	53. Ⓐ Ⓑ Ⓒ Ⓓ Ⓔ	83. Ⓐ Ⓑ Ⓒ Ⓓ Ⓔ
24. Ⓐ Ⓑ Ⓒ Ⓓ Ⓔ	54. Ⓐ Ⓑ Ⓒ Ⓓ Ⓔ	84. Ⓐ Ⓑ Ⓒ Ⓓ Ⓔ
25. Ⓐ Ⓑ Ⓒ Ⓓ Ⓔ	55. Ⓐ Ⓑ Ⓒ Ⓓ Ⓔ	85. Ⓐ Ⓑ Ⓒ Ⓓ Ⓔ
26. Ⓐ Ⓑ Ⓒ Ⓓ Ⓔ	56. Ⓐ Ⓑ Ⓒ Ⓓ Ⓔ	86. Ⓐ Ⓑ Ⓒ Ⓓ Ⓔ
27. Ⓐ Ⓑ Ⓒ Ⓓ Ⓔ	57. Ⓐ Ⓑ Ⓒ Ⓓ Ⓔ	87. Ⓐ Ⓑ Ⓒ Ⓓ Ⓔ
28. Ⓐ Ⓑ Ⓒ Ⓓ Ⓔ	58. Ⓐ Ⓑ Ⓒ Ⓓ Ⓔ	88. Ⓐ Ⓑ Ⓒ Ⓓ Ⓔ
29. Ⓐ Ⓑ Ⓒ Ⓓ Ⓔ	59. Ⓐ Ⓑ Ⓒ Ⓓ Ⓔ	89. Ⓐ Ⓑ Ⓒ Ⓓ Ⓔ
30. Ⓐ Ⓑ Ⓒ Ⓓ Ⓔ	60. Ⓐ Ⓑ Ⓒ Ⓓ Ⓔ	90. Ⓐ Ⓑ Ⓒ Ⓓ Ⓔ

91. Ⓐ Ⓑ Ⓒ Ⓓ Ⓔ	121. Ⓐ Ⓑ Ⓒ Ⓓ Ⓔ	151. Ⓐ Ⓑ Ⓒ Ⓓ Ⓔ
92. Ⓐ Ⓑ Ⓒ Ⓓ Ⓔ	122. Ⓐ Ⓑ Ⓒ Ⓓ Ⓔ	152. Ⓐ Ⓑ Ⓒ Ⓓ Ⓔ
93. Ⓐ Ⓑ Ⓒ Ⓓ Ⓔ	123. Ⓐ Ⓑ Ⓒ Ⓓ Ⓔ	153. Ⓐ Ⓑ Ⓒ Ⓓ Ⓔ
94. Ⓐ Ⓑ Ⓒ Ⓓ Ⓔ	124. Ⓐ Ⓑ Ⓒ Ⓓ Ⓔ	154. Ⓐ Ⓑ Ⓒ Ⓓ Ⓔ
95. Ⓐ Ⓑ Ⓒ Ⓓ Ⓔ	125. Ⓐ Ⓑ Ⓒ Ⓓ Ⓔ	155. Ⓐ Ⓑ Ⓒ Ⓓ Ⓔ
96. Ⓐ Ⓑ Ⓒ Ⓓ Ⓔ	126. Ⓐ Ⓑ Ⓒ Ⓓ Ⓔ	156. Ⓐ Ⓑ Ⓒ Ⓓ Ⓔ
97. Ⓐ Ⓑ Ⓒ Ⓓ Ⓔ	127. Ⓐ Ⓑ Ⓒ Ⓓ Ⓔ	157. Ⓐ Ⓑ Ⓒ Ⓓ Ⓔ
98. Ⓐ Ⓑ Ⓒ Ⓓ Ⓔ	128. Ⓐ Ⓑ Ⓒ Ⓓ Ⓔ	158. Ⓐ Ⓑ Ⓒ Ⓓ Ⓔ
99. Ⓐ Ⓑ Ⓒ Ⓓ Ⓔ	129. Ⓐ Ⓑ Ⓒ Ⓓ Ⓔ	159. Ⓐ Ⓑ Ⓒ Ⓓ Ⓔ
100. Ⓐ Ⓑ Ⓒ Ⓓ Ⓔ	130. Ⓐ Ⓑ Ⓒ Ⓓ Ⓔ	160. Ⓐ Ⓑ Ⓒ Ⓓ Ⓔ
101. Ⓐ Ⓑ Ⓒ Ⓓ Ⓔ	131. Ⓐ Ⓑ Ⓒ Ⓓ Ⓔ	161. Ⓐ Ⓑ Ⓒ Ⓓ Ⓔ
102. Ⓐ Ⓑ Ⓒ Ⓓ Ⓔ	132. Ⓐ Ⓑ Ⓒ Ⓓ Ⓔ	162. Ⓐ Ⓑ Ⓒ Ⓓ Ⓔ
103. Ⓐ Ⓑ Ⓒ Ⓓ Ⓔ	133. Ⓐ Ⓑ Ⓒ Ⓓ Ⓔ	163. Ⓐ Ⓑ Ⓒ Ⓓ Ⓔ
104. Ⓐ Ⓑ Ⓒ Ⓓ Ⓔ	134. Ⓐ Ⓑ Ⓒ Ⓓ Ⓔ	164. Ⓐ Ⓑ Ⓒ Ⓓ Ⓔ
105. Ⓐ Ⓑ Ⓒ Ⓓ Ⓔ	135. Ⓐ Ⓑ Ⓒ Ⓓ Ⓔ	165. Ⓐ Ⓑ Ⓒ Ⓓ Ⓔ
106. Ⓐ Ⓑ Ⓒ Ⓓ Ⓔ	136. Ⓐ Ⓑ Ⓒ Ⓓ Ⓔ	166. Ⓐ Ⓑ Ⓒ Ⓓ Ⓔ
107. Ⓐ Ⓑ Ⓒ Ⓓ Ⓔ	137. Ⓐ Ⓑ Ⓒ Ⓓ Ⓔ	167. Ⓐ Ⓑ Ⓒ Ⓓ Ⓔ
108. Ⓐ Ⓑ Ⓒ Ⓓ Ⓔ	138. Ⓐ Ⓑ Ⓒ Ⓓ Ⓔ	168. Ⓐ Ⓑ Ⓒ Ⓓ Ⓔ
109. Ⓐ Ⓑ Ⓒ Ⓓ Ⓔ	139. Ⓐ Ⓑ Ⓒ Ⓓ Ⓔ	169. Ⓐ Ⓑ Ⓒ Ⓓ Ⓔ
110. Ⓐ Ⓑ Ⓒ Ⓓ Ⓔ	140. Ⓐ Ⓑ Ⓒ Ⓓ Ⓔ	170. Ⓐ Ⓑ Ⓒ Ⓓ Ⓔ
111. Ⓐ Ⓑ Ⓒ Ⓓ Ⓔ	141. Ⓐ Ⓑ Ⓒ Ⓓ Ⓔ	171. Ⓐ Ⓑ Ⓒ Ⓓ Ⓔ
112. Ⓐ Ⓑ Ⓒ Ⓓ Ⓔ	142. Ⓐ Ⓑ Ⓒ Ⓓ Ⓔ	172. Ⓐ Ⓑ Ⓒ Ⓓ Ⓔ
113. Ⓐ Ⓑ Ⓒ Ⓓ Ⓔ	143. Ⓐ Ⓑ Ⓒ Ⓓ Ⓔ	173. Ⓐ Ⓑ Ⓒ Ⓓ Ⓔ
114. Ⓐ Ⓑ Ⓒ Ⓓ Ⓔ	144. Ⓐ Ⓑ Ⓒ Ⓓ Ⓔ	174. Ⓐ Ⓑ Ⓒ Ⓓ Ⓔ
115. Ⓐ Ⓑ Ⓒ Ⓓ Ⓔ	145. Ⓐ Ⓑ Ⓒ Ⓓ Ⓔ	175. Ⓐ Ⓑ Ⓒ Ⓓ Ⓔ
116. Ⓐ Ⓑ Ⓒ Ⓓ Ⓔ	146. Ⓐ Ⓑ Ⓒ Ⓓ Ⓔ	176. Ⓐ Ⓑ Ⓒ Ⓓ Ⓔ
117. Ⓐ Ⓑ Ⓒ Ⓓ Ⓔ	147. Ⓐ Ⓑ Ⓒ Ⓓ Ⓔ	177. Ⓐ Ⓑ Ⓒ Ⓓ Ⓔ
118. Ⓐ Ⓑ Ⓒ Ⓓ Ⓔ	148. Ⓐ Ⓑ Ⓒ Ⓓ Ⓔ	178. Ⓐ Ⓑ Ⓒ Ⓓ Ⓔ
119. Ⓐ Ⓑ Ⓒ Ⓓ Ⓔ	149. Ⓐ Ⓑ Ⓒ Ⓓ Ⓔ	179. Ⓐ Ⓑ Ⓒ Ⓓ Ⓔ
120. Ⓐ Ⓑ Ⓒ Ⓓ Ⓔ	150. Ⓐ Ⓑ Ⓒ Ⓓ Ⓔ	180. Ⓐ Ⓑ Ⓒ Ⓓ Ⓔ